Examination Paediatrics

A guide to paediatric training

Third edition

Dedication

To the late Dr Paul Stuart McCarthy,
(15.10.1974 – 2.4.2005)
'Merv',
a true hero

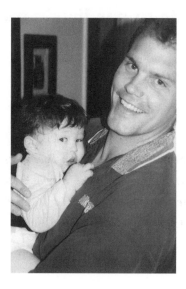

Merv was the finest medical student, resident, colleague, air force squadron leader, volunteer medical officer, adventurer and friend that anyone could wish to encounter. I was honoured to have the privilege to teach him paediatrics as a student, and later to have him work alongside me as a resident whom few, if any, could equal in enthusiasm, dedication, selflessness and caring.

Merv embodied all that is noble in medicine and human endeavour. An exceptional man in every sense of the word, he was a brilliant doctor, and a respected and admired squadron leader in the Royal Australian Air Force.

Merv was a remarkable sportsman, having rowed the Atlantic Ocean (with his closest friend Dr Patrick Weinrauch, 'Moshe') in their two-man boat 'Freedom' in an international race, the Ward Evans Atlantic Rowing Challenge ('Two people, four oars, 3000 miles'). Representing Australia against many other countries' best rowers, Merv and Moshe took 45 days to complete the journey, and came second in the world in the process.

He was an unsurpassed humanitarian, aiding thousands of tsunami victims over many months in Indonesia in 2004. He died tragically in a helicopter accident (the Sea King helicopter tragedy) in April 2005 when returning yet again to aid victims of after-shocks in Indonesia, after a brief return home to Australia.

The fact that there can be people in this world as good and selfless as Paul McCarthy should give everyone hope for the future.

Examination Paediatrics

A guide to paediatric training

Third edition

Wayne Harris

MBBS, MRCP (UK), FRACP

Senior Staff Specialist in Paediatrics,
Sunshine Coast Health Service District
Senior Lecturer, Department of Paediatrics and Child Health,
University of Queensland, Brisbane

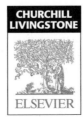

CHURCHILL
LIVINGSTONE

ELSEVIER

Sydney Edinburgh London New York Philadelphia St Louis Toronto

ELSEVIER

Churchill Livingstone
is an imprint of Elsevier

Elsevier Australia
(a division of Reed International Books Australia Pty Ltd)
30–52 Smidmore Street, Marrickville, NSW 2204
ACN 001 002 357

This edition © 2006 Elsevier Australia
Second edition © 2002
First edition © 1992

National Library of Australia Cataloguing-in-Publication Data

---

Harris, Wayne, 1958– .
      Examination paediatrics.

      3rd ed.
      Includes index.
      For medical students.
      ISBN-13: 978-0-7295-3772-8.
      ISBN-10: 0-7295-3772-2.

      1. Pediatrics. 2. Pediatrics – Examinations, questions, etc. I. Title.

      618.92

Publisher: Debbie Lee
Publishing Editor: Sophie Kaliniecki
Developmental Editor: Samantha Bensch
Publishing Services Manager: Helena Klijn
Edited and project managed by Carol Natsis
Proofread by Tim Learner
Indexed by Forsyth Publishing Services
Design by Tania Edwards
Typeset by Midland Typesetters
Printed by Southwood Press

Contents

Contents

Preface

Be excellent to each other.

Rufus, Bill and Ted's Excellent Adventure

The first edition of this book was written in 1992 to assist candidates preparing for the Fellowship of the Royal Australasian College of Physicians (Part 1) Examination in Paediatrics, or for the Membership of the Royal College of Physicians (Part 2) Examination in Paediatrics, inspired by Talley and O'Connor's book *Examination Medicine*. The second edition came out in 2002, and much to our amazement, sold well enough to justify a third edition. The day came when our book was listed on the RACP's website under recommended reading. That made us feel that the book was worth keeping as an ongoing concern.

My previous co-authors Brian Timms and Robin Choong have handed me the reins fully now, and I shall continue to update this book regularly for as long as it is found useful. Knowing the book is used in Ireland, Canada, New Zealand and Southeast Asia inspires me to improve it with each edition.

I shall try to continue in Talley and O'Connor's adult-sized footsteps, and hope this edition is yet more useful than the previous one. I believe there is much of relevance to senior medical students and general practitioners, as well as to paediatric trainees. There are new long cases, new short cases, new expanded sections of previous chapters, new mnemonics and broader background information. There are new sections covering autism, Down syndrome, Turner's syndrome, anorexia nervosa and congenital adrenal hyperplasia. As noted in previous editions, this is not the 'Einstein Encyclopaedia of Paediatrics'; its purpose is to make the hurdle of any paediatric examination easier to clear.

Don't panic! Good luck!

Wayne Harris
April 2006

Preface to the first edition

Don't panic.

Douglas Adams, The Hitchhiker's Guide to the Galaxy

This book has been written to assist candidates preparing for the Fellowship of the Royal Australasian College of Physicians (Part 1) Examination in Paediatrics. It is also intended to assist candidates preparing for the Membership of the Royal College of Physicians (Part 2) Examination in Paediatrics. It was inspired by Talley and O'Connor's book *Examination Medicine,* written to assist in the preparation for the Royal Australasian College of Physicians' Internal Medicine (Part I) Examination.

We have tried to present a structured and comprehensive approach to the clinical examination of the paediatric patient in a way that is particularly relevant for the post-graduate degrees of the FRACP (Part 1) and the MRCP (Part 2). Approaches are presented for most of the common-examination long and short cases.

This book is not designed to be the 'Einstein Encyclopaedia of Paediatrics'. As a supplement to the major texts and journal articles, it aims to demonstrate approaches that the authors have found successful.

Our combined experience of the FRACP examination comprises six written examinations, and six clinical examinations (including two 'extra time' cases), and for the MRCP, one clinical examination. This broad coverage of most conceivable contingencies ensures that many of the approaches have been tested (successfully) in the actual examination settings by the authors, while others have been tested by our peers in their examinations.

We hope that this book will be useful for examination candidates, and also helpful to paediatric residents/house officers, senior medical students and general practitioners who deal with children.

While every effort has been made to ensure the accuracy of the information herein, especially with regard to drug selection and dosage, appropriate information sources should be consulted, particularly for new or uncommon drugs. It is the clinician's responsibility to check the appropriateness of an opinion in relation to acute clinical situations and new developments. Any comments or suggestions will be gratefully and humbly received, so that future editions of this book may prove to be more useful.

Good luck!

Wayne Harris
Brian Timms
Robin Choong
1992

Acknowledgments

Special thanks

To my family for supporting me throughout the months spent producing this edition.

To my friends and colleagues, Dr Brian Timms and Dr Robin Choong, two of my favourite people, for supporting me as co-authors over the first and second editions of this book, and for encouraging me to complete this edition.

To the following wonderful people, for your unwavering support, and encouragement: Dr John Arranga, Dr Tim Bradshaw, Dr Andrew Burke, Dr Jonathan Chahal, Dr Aaron Chambers, Ms Danielle Cohen, Dr Anita Cohn, Dr Steve Cook, Mr Richard Cranbrook, Ms Catherine Downey, Dr Leanne Faithfull, Dr Stephanie Hogarth, Mr Steve Irwin, Mrs Terri Irwin, Dr David Koskuba, Mlle Lydie Le Febvre, Dr Sara Lucas, Dr Charley McNabb, Dr Romayne Moore, Dr Herminia Narvaez, Dr Joseph Pasion, Mr Rob Penfold, Dr Sonia Reichert, Dr Kate Rodwell, Ms Junko Tanaka, Mr Charles Waterstreet, Dr Patrick Weinrauch, and Dr Luke Wheatley.

Reviewers

I would like to thank the following specialists who were kind enough to review different sections of the book. Their comments were invaluable. However, the book does not necessarily reflect the opinions of these specialists.

Associate Professor DB Appleton, FRCP (Edin), FRACP, Paediatric Neurologist, The Royal Children's Hospital, Brisbane.

Dr C Barnes, FRACP, Paediatric Haematologist, The Royal Children's Hospital, Melbourne.

Professor A Carmichael, MD, FRACP, Dean, Faculty of Health Science, University of Tasmania, Hobart.

Associate Professor A Chang, FRACP, Paediatric Respiratory Consultant, The Royal Children's Hospital, Brisbane.

Dr R Choong, FRACP, AIMM, Senior Staff Specialist, Paediatric Intensive Care and Paediatric Emergency Medicine, The Children's Hospital at Westmead.

Professor G Cleghorn, FRACP, FACG, Head, Discipline of Paediatrics and Child Health, University of Queensland; Clinical Director, the Children's Nutrition Research Centre, Royal Children's Hospital, Brisbane.

Dr L Dalla Pozza, FRACP, Paediatric Oncologist, The Children's Hospital at Westmead.

Dr D Dossetor, MA, DCH, FRCP (UK), FRCPsych (UK), FRANZCP, MD, Senior Staff Specialist, Area Director for Mental Health, The Children's Hospital at Westmead; Clinical Senior Lecturer, University of Sydney.

Dr P Francis, FRACP, Paediatric Respiratory Physician, Royal Children's Hospital, Brisbane.

Dr E Hodson, FRACP, Paediatric Nephrologist, The Children's Hospital at Westmead.

Dr J Lawson, FRACP, Paediatric Neurologist, Sydney Children's Hospital.

Associate Professor M McDowell, FRACP, Developmental Paediatrician, Mater Misericordiae Children's Hospital, Brisbane.

Dr J McGill, FRACP, Director, Department of Metabolic Medicine, Royal Children's Hospital, Brisbane.

Dr S Madden, FRANZP, Child and Adolescent Psychiatrist, The Children's Hospital at Westmead.

Dr C Marraffa, FRACP, Consultant Paediatrician, Royal Children's Hospital, Melbourne.

Dr J Munro, FRACP, Paediatric Rheumatologist, Royal Children's Hospital, Melbourne.

Professor K North, MD, FRACP, Douglas Burroughs Professor of Paediatrics, Associate Dean and Head of Discipline, Paediatrics and Child Health, Faculty of Medicine, University of Sydney; Head, Neurogenetics Research Unit, The Children's Hospital at Westmead.

Professor D Roberton, MD, FRACP, FRCPA, McGregor-Reid Professor of Paediatrics, University of Adelaide; Head, Department of Paediatrics, Women's and Children's Hospital, Adelaide.

Dr B Timms, FRACP, Consultant Paediatrician, Consultant Neonatologist, Melbourne.

Dr C Wainwright, FRACP, Paediatric Respiratory Physician, Royal Children's Hospital, Brisbane.

Professor G Warne, FRACP, Paediatric Endocrinologist, Royal Children's Hospital, Melbourne.

Dr C Whight, FRACP, Paediatric Cardiologist, Royal Children's Hospital, Brisbane.

Introduction

This book is designed primarily to assist candidates in passing clinical examinations in paediatrics, particularly at the postgraduate level. The first edition was found helpful in many countries with many different clinical examination scenarios, although it was specifically designed to tackle the clinical section of the FRACP Part 1 Examination in Paediatrics and the MRCP (now the MRCPCH) Part 2 examination. Written examinations, which must be passed in most countries before any clinical examination can be sat, are not covered other than in the brief outline given below.

Basic training requirements

Most potential candidates should be familiar with these. Comprehensive information on training can be obtained and downloaded from the websites of the various learned colleges. For Australia, New Zealand, the United Kingdom and Canada, the relevant addresses are:

- Fellowship in the Royal Australasian College of Physicians (FRACP): <http://www.racp.edu.au/paed/index.htm>.
- Membership of the Royal College of Paediatrics and Child Health (MRCPCH): <http://www.rcpch.ac.uk/rcpch/index.htm>.
- Fellowship of the Royal College of Physicians of Canada (FRCPC): <http://rcpsc.medical.org/english/index> (click on 'Residency Education' for this one).

The written examination

In Australia, the written component of the FRACP examination comprises two papers taken on the same day. Paper 1 contains 70 A-type questions (best single response of five alternatives) testing knowledge of basic sciences and lasts two hours, while paper 2 consists of 100 A-type questions assessing investigational material, clinical paediatrics and therapeutics, and lasts three hours. It is held annually.

In the UK, the MRCPCH Part I examination lasts two and a half hours, and comprises 60 multiple-choice questions (MCQs), 15 of which are common to the MRCPCH and the MRCP(UK). The written component of the MRCPCH Part II examination comprises three short answer papers: the first is the case history paper, containing four or more compulsory questions and lasting 55 minutes; the second is the data interpretation paper, containing 10 compulsory questions and lasting 45 minutes; the third is the photographic material paper containing 20 compulsory questions and lasting 50 minutes.

The best preparation for any written examination involves doing as many past examination questions as possible, and extensive reading of major texts and journals. The most useful textbooks and journals are listed under Suggested Reading at the end of the book. There are no set curricula specified for most paediatric examinations.

The college regularly releases previous examination papers. These are essential reading. There are also a number of papers that are composites of remembered questions that previous candidates have written down after their examination, which have been 'handed down' over the years. The main problem with 'remembered' papers is their inaccuracy. However, most candidates seem to find these helpful.

The RACP produces self-assessment questions for paediatricians, the Australian Self-Assessment Programme (ASAP), which are strongly recommended.

The clinical examination

This book is aimed at assisting in preparing for clinical examinations. Chapter 1 details a general approach. It will be noted that certain cases are emphasised, not because they are more important than others but because they are good examples of the complicated material required for long and short cases.

Achievement psychology: the psychology of passing

Chapter 4 discusses the psychological aspects of the preparation for, and performance in, the examination. This is a very important area that should not be overlooked.

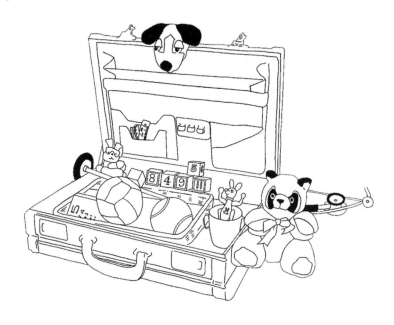

Approach to the examination

Positive mindset

All paediatric clinical examinations test the following aspects:

1. Clinical skills—history taking, physical examination, interpretation of findings, construction of a diagnosis or differential diagnoses, method of investigation, overall management of the patient.
2. Attitudes.
3. Interpersonal relationships.

Candidates invited to postgraduate clinical examinations have usually satisfied their relevant learned college regarding their factual knowledge. Consequently, their factual knowledge should be at a standard appropriate for making management decisions in the case being examined.

Clinical skills are usually taught adequately to most candidates at the hospitals where they were trained. However, little if any attention is paid to developing proper attitudes and interpersonal relationship skills. Advertisers and sales representatives know the importance of personal contact. They realise that appearance, personality and speech are crucial in successful negotiations. The 'viva' is very similar in that candidates have to 'sell' themselves and their knowledge to the examiners. Successful candidates usually possess certain characteristics, namely:

1. A positive, confident response to personal confrontation. People with strong personalities have little trouble but those who are easily embarrassed and shy away from confrontation between equals may do poorly. This response can be changed by methods described in this book.
2. Ability to sort out relevant from irrelevant information. Those who 'think', ask questions, seek explanations and try to understand rather than learn by rote do well.
3. Familiarity with the method of examination.
4. Endurance. Candidates who are 'street-wise' and naturally confident tend to have little difficulty, whereas their less confident colleagues are left to learn the hard way and eventually succeed or fail.

Preparation for the 'viva' requires effective communication skills during physical confrontation. Attitudes, interpersonal skills and projection of a confident, professional consultant image can be learned and developed.

Techniques include:

1. Mental rehearsal, visualisation, affirmations (see Chapter 4).
2. Body language.

3. Eye contact.
4. Breath control.
5. Dress sense.
6. Speech training.
7. Development of equanimity.
8. Ability to summarise.
9. Reasoning skills.
10. Examiner assessment.

Body language

Non-verbal communication in the form of a person's gestures are very accurate indicators of his or her attitudes, emotions, thoughts and desires.

In order to learn body language, set aside a couple of minutes a day to study and read other people's gestures. Examine your own body language. Copy the body language of people you admire and respect, such as a consultant who you feel would have no difficulty passing the clinical examination. The model you choose does not necessarily have to be a real person: he or she may be a composite of ideal body language.

There is an old saying: 'If you would be powerful, pretend to be powerful.' One way to adopt an attitude that helps you achieve any objective is to act 'as if' you were already there. If you change your posture, your breathing patterns, your muscle tension, your tone of voice, you instantly change the way you feel. For example, if you feel depressed, consciously stand up straight, throw your shoulders back, breathe deeply and look upward. See if you can feel depressed in that posture. You'll find yourself feeling alert, vital and confident.

An important component of body language is consistency. If you are giving what you think is a positive message, but your voice is weak, high-pitched and tentative and your gestures reveal poor self-confidence, you will be unconvincing and ineffective. Individuals who consistently succeed are those who can commit all of their resources, mental and physical, towards reaching a goal. One way to develop consistency is to model yourself on individuals who are consistent. Copy the way they stand, sit and move, their key facial expressions and gestures, their tone of voice, their vocabulary, their breathing patterns and so on. You will begin to generate the same attitudes that they experience, and experience the same successful results. Effectiveness comes from delivering one unified message.

When you next attend a place where people meet and interact, study the individuals who have adopted the gestures and postures of the individuals with whom they are talking. This mimicry is how one individual tells another that he or she is in agreement with their thoughts and attitudes. You can use this unconscious mimicry to your advantage. One of the best ways of establishing effective personal communication is through mimicking the breathing patterns, posture, tone of voice, gestures, words and phrases of the person or people with whom you are interacting. Once you establish contact with someone, you create a bond and reach a stage where you begin to initiate change rather than just mimicking the other person, a stage where you have established so much mutual contact that when you change, the other person unconsciously follows you. If, when you try to lead someone, they do not follow, it simply means there is insufficient rapport. Mimic, strengthen the mutual contact and try again.

Eye contact

When answering questions or making a point, look the examiner straight in the eye. Powerful individuals have always been characterised by exceptional eyes. If you have difficulty maintaining eye contact, there are a few techniques you can use to develop a more effective gaze.

Work on not blinking. Practise unblinking eye contact, especially when under pressure. If you are intimidated and unable to look directly into the examiner's eyes, a little trick is to concentrate your gaze on a point midway between the examiner's eyes. Another helpful hint is to imagine a triangle on the examiner's forehead with the apex at the highest point and the base of the triangle formed by an imaginary line between both eyes. Keep your gaze directed at this area. In the mirror, practise narrowing your lids a bit but do not squint. When you move your eyes from one point to another (as from one examiner to another), do it without blinking. When you look from one person to another without blinking, it is unnerving for anyone watching you. To further emphasise this powerful gaze, move your eyes first without blinking and then follow with your head movement just behind the eye movement. Slightly lowering your head forwards while maintaining the gaze also adds power to the eye movement.

Breath control

Often, especially in a viva voce or an important interview, you find yourself struck by a sudden panic attack. Breath control can be particularly useful to regain composure, prevent fear, reduce stress or fatigue, and generate energy. It is a technique developed by the samurai to regain control during life and death struggles. Take a deep breath, then exhale slowly and imperceptibly. As you are exhaling, contract your abdominal muscles so that you feel like you are tightening a corset. Relax the muscles at the end of exhalation. Do not expel all the air. Leave about 20% in the lungs. Then inhale gently. Your lips should be slightly parted, expelling your breath over your lower teeth with your tongue gently touching your hard palate. You may repeat breath control as often as required. Practise breath control until it is second nature and then use it whenever you are under any physical or mental stress.

Dress and grooming

You have to 'sell' yourself and your knowledge. Your appearance is your most important 'equipment' for the clinical examination. It must reflect the public expectations of the professional person. Look around at what is worn by successful individuals in the respected professions (such as your examiners). Ask yourself: 'Do I look like a mature, careful, conservative and respected junior consultant?' Male candidates should avoid colourful suits, jackets and trousers, and unusual ties. Dark suits (greys, navy blue, pin-stripes, noncommittal ties, red ties) are more suitable (this is termed 'power dressing' by image consultants). Female candidates should preferably avoid revealing or tight dresses as well as showy jewellery. Footwear should be clean and appropriate.

Long hair and beards should probably be avoided, but if you cannot bear to shave your beard, at least keep it neat and trimmed. It is safer to be clean shaven and have tidy hair. Visit the hairdresser a couple of days before (and not on the day of) the clinical examination so that it does not appear as though you have had it done just for the examinations.

If you have difficulties with perspiration when under pressure, use an unscented antiperspirant on the day of the examination. Apply the antiperspirant to your forehead, hairline and neck to prevent beads of sweat appearing during the 'viva' (one of the previous co-authors used this method successfully).

Speech training

Poor speech will definitely adversely affect your 'viva' performance and is surprisingly common. By poor speech we mean poor diction, inaudible voice and bad vocabulary. Tape-record yourself speaking or have someone sit about 2 metres from you and listen to you speak. Then note:

1. Whether or not every word was heard clearly.
2. Whether or not what you said was understood.
3. Whether or not you used jargon, slang or abbreviations.

Addressing these three points will help you assess whether or not your speech is a problem. Take note of your pitch and rapidity of speech. If you do speak too quickly, make a conscious effort to slow down by reading aloud at a pace that allows a listener to make a note of the content of your speech. Another useful exercise is to study the speech of newsreaders. Note that they speak clearly, concisely and slowly so that every word is understood. They also use very little jargon, slang or abbreviations. Try mimicking a newsreader's speaking style the next time you present a case.

Other methods of improving your speech are:

1. Enrolment with a professional teacher.
2. Using a video camera to film your efforts and then playing back the result.

Equanimity

Sir William Osler suggested that physicians should possess equanimity: composure under pressure, and when faced with the adversities of life. This is particularly true during the clinical examination, where your long case may be an uncooperative, crying child, for example. Candidates may experience stress as a result of physical confrontation, inadequate knowledge, low self-confidence and poor physical health. Equanimity, although coming more easily to phlegmatic personalities, may be cultivated. Knowledge and experience create confidence, which in turn leads to calmness. The above causes of stress can all be overcome by more study (to improve knowledge base), more practice, mental reprogramming and then actively seeking out stressful situations to increase experience. Adequate exercise, a well-balanced diet and enough sleep should go a long way towards maintaining physical health.

Ability to summarise

The ability to summarise, encapsulate the essence and emphasise the major issues without losing too much detail requires understanding and experience. However, it is a necessary skill for the physician, and therefore needs to be developed through practice. Remember: practice makes the impossible possible. Note that the limit of effective retention of verbal information is usually less than 15 seconds, so the better you can convey the essential details to the examiners in the 'viva', the greater the effect.

Reasoning skills

Reasoning skills involve the ability to analyse a problem rapidly, break it down into manageable parts and then formulate a solution. An adequate knowledge base, experience and rational thinking are needed.

To assist in developing these skills, make a habit of meticulously examining every detail of a child's clinical records. Analyse the data, learn to pick out any vital information that is missing and ignore irrelevant information. Deduce from available data what other information you need to justify your conclusions.

Assessment of examiner

An ancient Chinese general, Sun Tze, once stated, 'Know the enemy and know yourself, and you can fight a hundred battles with no danger of defeat'. Although examiners are not exactly the enemy, you still need to assess:

1. Whether or not the examiner is friendly or unhelpful.
2. The quality of communication between the examiner and yourself.
3. The strength of the examiner's personality compared to yours.

On occasions, it may be worthwhile doing some reconnaissance work and finding out some information about your potential examiners (likes, dislikes, areas of interest).

The clinical examination

Preparation

The road to success in any 'viva' usually entails doing a large number of long and short cases. You need to begin seeing cases at least several months before the clinical examination. Your service commitment should provide you with all the material you require for training and preparation. Treat each patient you see during the course of your daily work as a practice long or short case. Endeavour to do at least one (but preferably two or three) long case(s) per week. Try to expose yourself to as many different examiners as possible.

Preparation for the short case requires much practice, especially when more candidates fail their short cases than their long cases. If possible, visit other hospitals, especially if these have a reputation for teaching. Experience as a 'bulldog' (i.e. observing an actual examination and assisting the candidate) is also invaluable in gaining insight about the conduct of the examination and expectations of the examiners. Taking turns as an examiner during practice sessions with your colleagues is worthwhile because it allows you to experience first-hand the annoying habits of candidates. Mental rehearsal of short cases (and long cases) will accelerate learning (see Chapter 4, Achievement psychology).

Most major teaching hospitals hold trial and mock examinations a few weeks before the actual 'viva'. These simulated examinations provide invaluable feedback about your progress.

Part of your preparation involves obtaining all the relevant information from the appropriate learned college about the requirements for paediatric training; this is invariably available in booklet form or is downloadable from the college's website. Familiarise yourself well with the contents and study the regulations. About 6 months before the examination write to the college for an application form. Fill in your application form a few months before the examination and ensure that the form and your examination fee reach the college before the closing date. Remember to apply for examination leave from your employer.

If possible, in the last few weeks before the 'viva', do some reconnaisance work and locate the examination venue as far as you can. Check it out in relation to where you will be staying, ascertain the suitable modes of transport, public transport timetables and the length of time it will take to travel to the venue at the times scheduled for the examinations. Remember to check your accommodation arrangements in advance.

In the week before the examination, check the clothing you intend to wear (make sure it fits!), check that you have the right equipment and remember the appointment with the hairdresser. In the few days before the examination try to get some mental rest and leave study aside. Avoid any major changes in your daily routine and lifestyle.

A checklist (prepared in advance) of what you need to do on the day may be helpful.

Make sure you arrive at least 30 minutes before the examination is due to start, so that you can recover from the trip, relax, go to the bathroom and so on. The longer the travelling distance, the more provision you need to make to cover for delays during travel (one of the previous co-authors experienced car trouble on the day of the 'viva').

There are certain 'rules' that you need to obey at the 'viva'. Do not enter the examiner's room until asked. Do not sit down until invited. Do not slouch when seated but sit four-square and upright (it creates the impression that you mean what you say). Minimise nervous hand movements. If you tend to fidget, turn your hand movements into gestures. Bags should be placed under the chair (or given to the 'bulldog') and removed when leaving. Do not stare, smile politely and always answer courteously. Remember to speak up and be as brief and factual as possible. Avoid jargon, slang, clichés, abbreviations, brand names (of medications), meaningless expressions, and rising inflections at the end of sentences. Most importantly, do not antagonise or argue with the examiners. You will always lose! Some examples of antagonising behaviour include patronising answers, appearing to show little or no interest in the subject matter and a negative response to criticism.

If you decide to use beta-blockers during the examination, it would be wise to use the drug during at least one practice session, particularly if you have asthma. It would be inconvenient to have an asthma attack at the examination, as happened to a colleague who took what is considered a cardioselective beta-blocker. After at least 12 puffs or so of salbutamol, he passed.

Equipment

Equipment is always available at the examination. However, it would be wise to take the following with you:

1. Pens (more than one and make sure they work), pencils and paper.
2. Your own stethoscope.
3. A hand-held eye chart for testing visual acuity (with a piece of string attached to the chart, the length of which is the recommended distance from eye to chart; this allows you to quickly position the chart at the correct distance from eye).
4. Cottonwool (fine sensation), new blunt pins.
5. Watch, preferably with a sweeping second hand.
6. Pocket tape measure.
7. Torch with new batteries and bulb.
8. A red-topped hat pin for visual field testing in the older child.
9. Toys, red woollen ball on a thread to test visual fields in infants, small container of hundreds and thousands (or equivalent) to test hearing, raisins (pincer grip), coloured cubes for developmental assessment.
10. Other: pocket ophthalmoscope, pocket tendon hammer, spatulas, tuning forks, Denver II developmental chart, percentile charts for height, weight and head circumference.

Most candidates have a small leather briefcase (or equivalent carrying bag) for their equipment. Be absolutely familiar with the equipment you have in your bag. Nothing looks worse than a candidate fumbling through his or her bag or, worse still, his or her pockets at the vital moment.

2

The long case

In the long-case section of a clinical examination, the candidate usually is given 60 minutes with a child and parent(s); then the case is presented and the candidate questioned by the examiners. Usually 20–30 minutes is spent with the examiners; this is what happens in the FRACP and the MRCPCH. In that time the candidate must take a full history, perform a relevant physical examination and synthesise a management plan that is sensible and appropriate for the particular child. Practice is the key to success.

Practising long cases is extremely beneficial for improving your clinical skills, irrespective of the examination looming in the distance. Practice cases should be performed under examination conditions whenever possible. Most consultant paediatricians are quite willing to spare 20–30 minutes to listen to candidates presenting cases. Advanced trainees who have recently passed are also usually prepared to act as examiners for candidates.

Obtaining the history

The aim of the long case is chiefly to assess how you would manage the child, his problems and his family. The examiners want to know whether or not you can competently care for a patient in practice. The history in the majority of cases will provide you with the diagnoses.

You must allocate your time with care. Generally, 20 minutes should be spent on the history, 10–15 minutes on the physical examination and the remainder of the time on recording, reviewing and organising the information for presentation. This time spent on organisation is the most important.

Making notes is vital. Two commonly used methods are:

1. Using a small spiral-bound pad.
2. Using a small card system: numbering the cards, and using headings such as 'examination findings'.

Remember to keep to the essentials and to include the following:

1. Identification of the child's details—age, date of birth, home address.
2. Identification of the clinical problem(s).
3. Specific inquiry of system involvement.
4. Relevant past medical history: include birth history, immunisation history.
5. Present treatment.
6. Growth and development.
7. Social history: always ask about parental relationships, number of children, family income, financial support, other siblings' reactions to the patient's illness, schooling.

Always introduce yourself to the child and parent(s). Always be courteous, diplomatic and tactful, use basic English and never order them about. Explain to the parent(s) that this is a very important examination.

The following questions have been found useful by many candidates.

1. What exactly is wrong with your child?
2. Is your child an inpatient at the moment?
3. What are the names of the doctors taking care of your child?
4. What tests have been done on your child? Have any new tests been done lately? How often do you come for review? How many times has your child been admitted?
5. What treatment is your child on? Have there been any recent changes in your child's treatment?
6. What is worrying you the most?
7. What is worrying the doctors the most?
8. What is worrying the child the most?
9. What complications of treatment are there?
10. What of the future? For the family? For the patient?
11. Is there anything else that someone else has done or asked that I haven't done or asked?

Remember, do not accept the patient's history without questioning.

Make a list of all the important problems and then organise this list so that the most important or current issue is presented first, followed by the other problems in decreasing order of importance.

Physical examination

Remember to keep to essentials and look at the front, back and both sides. Ask the parent(s) what the examiners looked for when they examined the child. A detailed examination should be done of those regions related to the child's main complaint. Following the specific examination, other systems need to be assessed. Remember to assess growth parameters, blood pressure, oral cavity and the skin.

Preparation to meet the examiners

After completing the history and examination, always ask yourself: 'Have I left anything out?' and 'Can this be anything else?'

Study your notes thoughtfully, underline or highlight positive findings and 'box' all relevant negative findings. This is the information you will present to the examiners.

Ask yourself whether the case is mainly a management or a diagnostic problem. If it is a diagnostic problem, remember that 'common things occur commonly'. If more than half of your findings support your first diagnosis, then it is most likely the correct one. For your alternative diagnoses, take the main positive findings and have three possible diagnoses for each. Make a summary of the possible diagnoses that occur three or more times.

Create an introduction that is clear, concise, arouses interest and summarises the main problems. It should last no longer than 30 seconds. Remember: first impressions are important, so spend time mentally rehearsing the delivery of your introduction. (See below for a long-case proforma.)

Mentally rehearse your order of presentation; present the most important issues first. Keep some issues in reserve so that when the examiners ask you about them, you will be able to provide immediate answers, rather than laying all your cards on the table immediately. Your conclusion should re-emphasise the main problems in order of decreasing importance. The entire presentation should last no longer than 7 minutes.

Try to anticipate possible lines of questioning, and think up reasonable answers in advance. Common questions asked by examiners include:

1. 'Tell me about your patient.' You should be able to give a clear, concise presentation lasting less than 7 minutes.
2. 'What is your conclusion about this case?' You should respond by giving a most likely diagnosis and differential diagnoses. Avoid giving an overcomprehensive list of differential diagnoses.
3. 'How would you manage this patient?' You should prepare an outline of management and be able to support it. You are probably going to be asked about relevant investigations. You should have reasons for doing the test and be able to discuss the test in detail. Write down any test results given and comment on their significance.

Assume that the examiners are there to help you. If an examiner continues to ask a question even though you do not immediately know the answer, he or she may be attempting to establish a very basic fact. Try to step back mentally for a moment; the answer is often forthcoming. Do not waffle. If you do not know the answer to a question, do not be afraid to admit it, but do so confidently. It allows the examiner to change the line of questioning and, hopefully, ask you a question which you *can* answer. Always be prepared to justify any statement you make in the 'viva'.

A long-case proforma

Although proformas cannot be taken into the examination, it is very useful to have a standard commencement to a long-case presentation that is second nature to you. It is suggested that you may use proformas in practice cases; the author used the proforma below successfully with each and every long case.

Opening statement

'I have just seen [name of child], a [age in months or years] old boy/girl with a [duration of time] history of [presenting complaint], who is currently in hospital for [reason for being in hospital that day]. [Name of child]'s problems include [list of each diagnosis in order of importance, or in the case of a multisystem disease, each aspect as it arose in chronological order]. I shall discuss the history of each problem in this order.'

Details and history

Next the presenting complaint is set out in detail.

Then, for each problem listed in the opening statement, make four columns, with the headings *Dates (or age of child)*, *Past history*, *Current status*, *Recent changes*. The history is listed in chronological order under each heading. For example, if the problem was nephrotic syndrome it could be listed as in Table 2.1.

Table 2.1			
Dates (or age of child)	**Past history**	**Current status**	**Recent changes**
12 months	Presented with generalised oedema		
16 months	Renal biopsy diagnosed MCGN, started cyclophosphamide		
24 months	Moved interstate and weaned off prednisolone		
2 years 3 months	Changed hospitals and management reintroduced steroids		
4 years	Prednisolone stopped		
4 years 3 months	Admitted with oedema		
Present		On alternate day prednisolone	Reintroduction of steroids after representation with oedema

Remaining history

When you have completed the problem listing sheets, remember to ask the parent supplying the history, 'What did the examiners ask you?' Then the rest of the history can be obtained. The prompts given in Table 2.2 may help.

Examination

For the examination, it is always best to start with a general description of the patient, as if you were describing a photograph over the telephone. Again using the example of nephrotic syndrome, an opening line could be: 'On examination [name] was a 4-year-old Cushingoid boy, with moon face, a swollen abdomen and a swollen scrotum, with an intravenous line in the left forearm.'

Next describe the parameters (head circumference, weight, height) and show the examiners the centile chart (which you have of course plotted at high speed). The vital signs (pulse, respiratory rate, blood pressure, temperature and, if relevant to the presentation, urinalysis) may then be given, and then the findings in the organ system most relevant to the child's current clinical problems. Again, using the nephrotic syndrome example, this would be similar to the following: 'Examination of the renal system was as follows: periorbital oedema, ascites, tense scrotum, no effusions, Cushingoid features (buffalo hump, loss of supraclavicular fossa), but no striae, cataracts, not short, no acne, no bone pain, no bruising.'

During the examination of the child, ask the parent again, 'What did the examiners look at yesterday?' After the relevant system, examine the other systems too: cardiovascular, chest, abdomen, ear, nose and throat, central nervous system, and where appropriate, developmental assessment.

Table 2.2

Birth history

Date of birth.............../ Birth weight.............../ Hospital.........................
Pregnancy: Drugs.................../ Bleeding.............../Illnesses.....................
      Hyper/hypotension......................./ Hospitalisations.....................
      Ultrasounds........................../ Other tests............................
      Polyhydramnios:......................./ Fetal movements:.......................
      Planned?............./ Gestation.................../ Delivery method..............
      Apgar scores...........at 1 minute ....at 5 minutes

Perinatal history

Respiratory distress......................./ Oxygen requirement........................
Feeding: Breast................./ Bottle........................../ Tube........................
Jaundice................./ Weight gain.................../ Other problems..............
Discharge date/age...................../ Discharge weight.............................

Feeding history

Currently.................../ Breast/bottle: until.............../ Solids: since.............
Past feeding history...

Milestones

Good baby?......................./ Hearing..................../ Smiled................
Compared to sibs.............../ Sat.................../ Sleeping behaviour............
Crawled........................./ Feeding self..................../ Walking..............
Toilet trained...................../ Talking: single words...........Sentences.............
School compared to sibs.........................../ Vision.............................
Current developmental abilities/problems:
Vision........................../ Hearing.................../ Gross motor...............
Fine motor.............../ Language..................../ Personal social................

Family history

Mother: Name........................Age...... Job..................... Health............
Father: Name......................Age...... Job.................... Health............
Note any consanguinity.................../ Planning any more children?.............
Relevant family history.................../ Other diseases in family....................
Previous marriages...
Past pregnancies: Terminations......................./ Miscarriages.....................
Children who have died..
Family interactions........................./ Family supports...........................
Family's understanding of disease: Mother / Father / Sibs............................

Social history (can be the most important)

Financial status........................./ Private health insurance......................
Home......................./ Car......................./ Allowances........................
Family supports.........................../ Other supports...........................
Societies........................../ Magazines................................
How long in Australia?..

School history

School attended........................./ Grade.............../ Performance................
Subjects........................./ Sports.........................../ Friends..............
Ambitions...................../ How much school has been missed?......................

Continued

Table 2.2 *(Continued)*

Parents
Change in social life........................./ Parents' friends.....................................
Last holiday?................................./ Respite care? ....

Home
Any structural changes to cope with the illness...

Transport to school/doctor
Need for special transport.............../ Financial burden of transport................

Other past history
Infections.................................../ Fractures.....................................
Operations.................................../ Hospitalisations.............................

Immunisation
Up to date?.............................../ Given on time?...................................
Any missed?........................../ Adverse reactions?................................

Allergies
Presenting symptoms: Rash........./ Angio-oedema........./ Anaphylaxis..............
Requirement for adrenaline?......../ Medicalert bracelet...............................

Most serious problem
Mother's opinion.........................../ Father's opinion................................
Patient's opinion.........................../ Doctor's opinion................................

Parents' understanding of disease
....

Compliance
....

Alternative medicine
....

Systems review
Cardiovascular / Respiratory / Ear, nose, throat / Eyes / Gastrointestinal tract /
Central nervous system / Skin / Joints / Endocrine / Renal / Haematological

Home management

Medications	Side effects	Levels

Note: List the above under headings: many long-case patients are on multiple drugs.

Other management
Physiotherapy.............................../ Occupational therapy............................
Speech therapy ..../ Other therapy...................................
Daily routine..
Clinics attended..
Specialists seen regularly (what do they ask / do / examine?)...........................
Local doctor..
Paediatrician ....

After the examination, present a summary, reiterating the important points. Following this you have the opportunity to discuss the management plan that you, the candidate, would initiate. There are several useful phrases that may help you start this discussion, such as:

- 'As regards management, my main concerns are…', *or*
- 'With respect to [problem], as the paediatrician looking after [patient], I would …', *or*
- 'In the line of investigations, I would …',

Remember to have a list of issues ready to discuss confidently.

3
CHAPTER

The short case

The short-case section of any postgraduate examination covers a number of systems (typically cardiovascular, respiratory, abdomen, neurological), and different countries' learned colleges vary in their approach. In Australia, the individual FRACP short case tends to have a lead-in that is fairly broad, for example 'Examine the gait', and a comprehensive examination is expected, lasting anywhere between 5 and 10 minutes on average. In the UK, the individual MRCPCH short cases tend to have a lead-in that is more directed, so a more focussed examination is in order: the examiner may say 'Listen to the heart', and that is what the candidate must do, not pick up the hands, take the pulse and look for clubbing, but get the stethoscope and listen. The short cases here are deliberately set out in the 'comprehensive' approach; it is easy to adapt the relevant portion of the examination to whichever lead-in the examiner gives. A short case tests the candidate's ability to examine a child with the ease and accuracy of a consultant paediatrician, rather than a paediatric registrar, although the examiners are judging the candidate at his/her expected level of training.

A short-case examination should be sufficiently comprehensive for the lead-in given, but directed. It should be confidently performed, quick enough to be within the confines of examination timing, and above all conducted kindly and with consideration for the patient and the parent.

The emphasis is as much on the method of physical examination as on the interpretation of the signs elicited. Remember that the examiners are judging you as a (future) peer. Thus a high standard is mandatory.

Proficiency in short cases, even more so than in long cases, is dependent upon months of practice, preferably on a daily basis, perfecting a coherent approach to every possible clinical problem likely to be presented. Several examination problems, such as short stature or precocious puberty, require a great deal of clinical material to be covered in under 10 minutes, so a well prepared routine is essential. This book gives an outline of an approach to most of the commonly seen short-case topics.

For several of the short cases outlined, there is an accompanying diagram that visually supplements the content of the text. The author found it easier to remember a diagram than a long list written on a card.

The time allotted to the short-case section varies between countries. Irrespective of the time allocated, it is usual that at least four systems are assessed. Often the examiners will instruct that you may either talk as you proceed, or examine in silence and summarise at the completion of the examination. Most candidates prefer the former method, as it allows the examiners to see, and hear, how you think, and should a questionable finding be noted, the examiners may guide you at that point.

It is crucial to listen carefully to the examiners' 'lead-in'. It usually comprises a brief history followed by a direction for the examination: for example, 'Derek is a 4-year-old boy who has been having increasing difficulty walking; would you please examine his gait'. Several points here need emphasising. Firstly, the introduction used is the same for all candidates who see that patient and has been carefully formulated by the examiners. Secondly, the introduction can contain some very useful hints as to the diagnosis, so do be very aware of this. Thirdly, do what the examiners ask. If the request is to perform an abdominal examination, do not start with the hands, start with the abdomen.

In any short case, it is always worthwhile spending at least 20–30 seconds standing back and getting an overall impression of the patient, otherwise signs such as chest or limb asymmetry, or a recognisable pattern of dysmorphism, may well be overlooked.

It helps to visualise yourself as a consultant before you commence any short case. It may be useful to imagine you are a locum paediatrician, being asked for a second opinion on any child you see. One sign of being stuck in 'registrar mode' is prefacing every potential action with 'I'd like to'. Do not say 'I would now like to look at'…, just do it! You do not see one consultant asking another's permission to proceed during each step of an examination.

However, do not overstep the boundaries of confidence. Do not argue with the examiners under any circumstances. Very rarely you may be right, but you may fail and be thought arrogant. If you become angry with an uncooperative child, you may fail; if you inadvertently hurt a child, such as in a joint examination, you may well fail. If you do not follow the examiners' 'lead-in', you will fail; as one examiner was heard to say (in a mock exam, thankfully): 'Answer the bloody question!'.

At the completion of your examination, you may mention further areas which you would examine next, should time permit, and then present a succinct summary of your findings with the most likely diagnosis, followed by a logically presented differential diagnosis. The differential diagnosis need not be exhaustive. In particular, it should never be a rote-learnt list for a certain type of case, but should be relevant only to the particular child you have just examined. Be careful that the first diseases you mention are not inappropriate suggestions. For example, an infant with jaundice and a Kasai scar on the abdomen should not be given a diagnosis of metabolic liver disease as the most likely possibility. So, beware of 'automatic list' responses.

Should you see a particularly confusing patient, and you are quite unable to work out their signs, do not bluff. It would be appropriate to admit that you find the signs confusing, but approach this methodically and logically. For example, if a child has a large array of heart murmurs, and the underlying diagnosis is completely unclear, it may be sensible to say, 'This child has complex congenital heart disease, but I am uncertain as to the exact anatomical diagnosis. However, taking each murmur individually…', and proceed to give a differential diagnosis for each murmur, mentioning that an electrocardiogram and a chest X-ray may clarify the diagnostic possibilities. You do not have to get the diagnosis absolutely correct to pass. Conversely, getting the diagnosis correct does not equal passing: if a child has an obvious aortic stenosis, missing neck auscultation for murmur radiation, and giving no thought to assessing the severity of the lesion, will not help you to pass.

Many candidates over the years have had acting lessons and training in elocution to improve their presentation. For many, overcoming mumbling is a major hurdle. A successful solution for some candidates has been to record their performance on audio- or videotape and then replay this to see how they would appear to the examiners.

An important point in presentation is correct coinage. Do not use terms such as 'I think there perhaps might be a little bit of asymmetry of the chest'; either there is asymmetry, or there is not. Similarly 'perhaps a tinge cyanosed' is not an appropriate description. You should try to eliminate words of uncertainty from your vocabulary.

As well as avoiding the 'I think perhaps' syndrome, you need to consciously tighten up your description of the patient's signs: for example, 'acyanotic' is far preferable to 'pink', and 'paucity of spontaneous lower limb movement' is preferable to the 'legs aren't moving quite as much as I'd expect them to'. Use the correct medical terminology every time; avoid all colloquialisms.

Do be aware that the examiners themselves have examined the children on the morning of the examination, without the aid of the child's notes and with a similar introduction to the one that the candidates receive. This means that they too have examined the child 'blind', and thus any conflicting or questionable findings can be noted so as to maximise the suitability of the case, and assess whether the lead-in is appropriate.

The most useful form of practice is to be critically assessed by a consultant, and optimally one who is an examiner. Being examined by an advanced trainee who has recently passed is also very beneficial. The most easily accessible form of practice is, of course, with your fellow candidates.

It makes sense to practise at a number of different hospitals and to be exposed to as many different examiners as possible, so as not to become accustomed to one particular pattern of criticism and questioning.

Achievement psychology

Positive mindset

> As a man thinketh in his heart, so is he.
>
> *Proverbs 23:7*

The essence of any successful candidate's mental attitude is positive thinking. If you expect success, you get success; but if you expect failure, you eventually get failure. Negativism is one of life's great cop-outs because it allows you to accept life's little failures without embarrassment. If you expect to fail—and you have communicated this belief to those around you—you will not look that bad when you do fail. But if you expect and communicate success, then fail, you end up looking a fool.

It is risky to expect positive things to happen to you but positive self-expectancy is the only sure way of being successful. 'What can be conceived and believed can be achieved'—but it takes more than saying 'I can' to pass exams or achieve any other goal. One of the presuppositions of neurolinguistic programming is that *if one person can do something, anyone can learn to do it*. Therefore confidence, self-discipline, self-esteem, mental toughness, persuasion, concentration and decisiveness are all qualities and skills you can learn and develop, just as you have learned to tie your shoelaces, drive a car or ride a bicycle. You need to develop an effective strategy by using role models. Find someone who is achieving the success you want. Find out what that individual is doing. Do the same things and you will achieve the same results. The price you pay is to take consistent action and to do it repeatedly until you acquire the winning habits that will allow you to achieve those results. This chapter will provide you with strategies that will empower you to realise your goals.

Self-motivation

> Great souls have wills, feeble ones have only wishes.
>
> *Chinese proverb*

Candidates who do not persist with their desire to succeed do so out of choice! They have chosen not to exercise self-discipline and persistence to work diligently towards their goal. You can choose to be a success or failure: 'Whether you think you can or think you can't, you're right'. Realise that nothing is final until you accept it as such. We all make mistakes, we all fall down and we have all at some time given up under adversity. However, to stay down once you've fallen is a matter of choice.

Commitment

If success has an entry fee, the cost is total commitment.

Denis Waitley

There is no lasting success without absolute commitment. Achievers are willing to *do whatever it takes* to succeed. This commitment to 'paying the price' is the essential quality in the mindset of an achiever. Heed Goethe's advice:

> Until one is committed, there is hesitancy, the chance to draw back, always ineffectiveness. Concerning all acts of initiative (and creation), there is one elementary truth the ignorance of which kills countless ideas and splendid plans: that the moment one definitely commits oneself, then Providence moves too. All sorts of things occur to help one that would never otherwise have occurred...Whatever you can do or dream you can, begin it now. Boldness has genius, power, and magic in it.

Remember the words of the Jedi Master Yoda in *Star Wars*: 'Try not. Do, or do not. There is no try'.

Why do you do the things you do?

If you cannot answer this question, you are just going through the motions, drifting. 'I guess I'm doing what I'm supposed to' becomes the theme of your life. This lack of total commitment may keep you from regressing, but it does not encourage peak performance. Successful candidates always have a *purpose* in mind for their actions. The quality of your life is directly related to your willingness to put your plans into action. Purpose creates motivation. If you want the power of purpose, you need to identify your mission and always act in a way that will further your efforts to reach it.

Create a priority purpose—a *mission* for yourself. Ask yourself:

1. Why do I do the things I do?
2. What is most important to me?
3. What am I willing to invest?
4. How much am I willing to endure?
5. What am I willing to give up?
6. How much responsibility am I willing to take?
7. Am I willing to begin where I am?
8. Am I willing to settle for anything less than my full potential?

Answering these questions will aid you in determining your mission. *Focus* on that mission in your thoughts and actions.

To further your efforts to fulfil your mission, ask yourself:

1. Do I understand the aims and requirements of the examination?
2. Do I have the determination to study seriously? Do I give top priority to study at the expense of time with family and friends?
3. Does my employment provide adequate experience? Do I use my employment to gain experience?
4. Have I discussed my plans with a supervisor or sympathetic consultant paediatrician? Do others feel I have the aptitude for paediatrics?
5. Can I accept constructive criticism from those who want to help me?

You must understand that in any endeavour, obstacles and conflict are inevitable. In your efforts to overcome these factors, at some stage you will experience the pain of present limitation. The only way to overcome the limitation is to *push through* the limitation towards your objective.

Goal-setting

If you fail to plan, plan to fail.

Once you have made up your mind to become a paediatrician, you must chart a course towards this ultimate goal. This means intelligent goal-setting. Goal-setting is not easy. To be effective it requires constant review and change. Goal-setting involves *writing out the steps* it will take to accomplish your mission. It may take 5 months, it may take 10 years, but the mission must be broken down into smaller units so that you know what you are to achieve in each area every day, week, month.

Goal-setting will allow you to plan your time for study most effectively. Service commitments, domestic demands and social obligations are the main factors affecting study time. Organise your working time to your greatest advantage by sensibly reviewing your commitments. Ensure that realistic time periods are allotted. Decide an order of priority in their execution and then do it! A small amount of time used at the start of the day reviewing what tasks need to be done pays off in time saved for studying. Remember always to differentiate between *important* tasks and *urgent* tasks.

Here are some guidelines for setting goals:

1. **Set specific goals.** Specific goals are much more productive than general goals which merely stress 'doing your best'.
2. **State goals positively.** For example, set aside 2 hours every evening to study Nelson's textbook. Effective goals need a positive mental image of yourself achieving what you want or being what you want to become. You cannot picture a negative goal.
3. **Set challenging goals.** Psychologist Edwin Locke found that 'the higher the level of intended achievement [that is, the higher the goal], the higher the level of performance'.
4. **Set measurable goals.** Goals need to be measurable in terms of *what* is achieved and when it is achieved. A goal of 'increasing performance in the long case' is not measurable. Rather a goal of 'completing 20 long cases within 3 months' is measurable.
5. **Set realistic and achievable goals.** A goal must not be too difficult, otherwise you will not want to try. But it must not be too easy—there is no challenge. State what results can be realistically achieved, given your resources. For a medical student to say 'My goal is to be professor of paediatrics within 12 months' is unrealistic. 'My goal is to be professor of paediatrics in 20 years' is a more realistic goal, especially if the student sets down the intermediate goals.
6. **Set tangible goals.** Some of your goals will be intangible. You can accomplish these intangible goals by achieving related tangible ones. The goals you set should always be tangible. For example, if you lack self-confidence, the intangible goal of 'achieving greater confidence' is not measurable. How will you know when you have enough confidence? Setting specific, tangible goals fostering development of confidence will be effective (e.g. 'I speak up at grand rounds').
7. **Make sure goals include behavioural changes.** You must set goals of becoming, of developing whatever characteristic you lack before you achieve your tangible goal. You cannot expect to become proficient in short cases if you continue to avoid doing them. You need to alter your behaviour.

8. **Write out your goals in present tense.** Written goals ensure that you clearly describe what you want and that you commit yourself to its accomplishment. Written goals need to be in the positive, present tense so that your mind accepts them. Written goals force you to *establish* **priorities**, for often two very desirable goals will come into conflict. Prioritise your values to determine which is the most important.

9. **Vividly imagine your goals.** Develop the habit of several times a day vividly imagining yourself achieving your goal.

10. **Write down the benefits of reaching your goals.** Writing down the benefits of reaching your goals improves motivation and desire.

11. **Write out a plan to reach your goal.**

12. **Write out a list of obstacles** that hinder you in reaching your goals. Listing the obstacles that hinder goal achievement allows you to focus on what needs to be done: 'A problem stated is a problem half-solved'.

13. **Set short-term and long-term goals.** Set time-priority goals: a 5-year plan, a 1-year plan, a daily 'to do' list. Every day, write down the six most important things that need to be done. Rank the six items with the hardest first down to the easiest last. Start on number 1. If interrupted, take care of the interruption and return to finishing number 1. Check off each item as it is completed and carry over into the following day those that were not accomplished. Every night make out a new list for the next day.

14. **Set goals to maintain a balanced life.** True happiness can be reached only by living a balanced life. To ensure a balanced life, set goals in the following areas: physical, mental/career, spiritual, financial, family and social.

The secret of success lies in establishing a *clearly defined goal*, writing it down, and then hammering it into your subconscious mind with unrelenting practice—daily rehearsal with words, images and emotions as if you had already accomplished it.

Affirmation

Destiny is not a matter of chance, it is a matter of choice—it is not a thing to be waited for, it is a thing to be achieved.

W. Bryan

An affirmation is a positive statement describing what you want to be, have or do. The constant repetition of positive thought day in and day out displaces stored negative thoughts in your subconscious mind. In the words of Benjamin Franklin, 'Little strokes fell great oaks'. Here are a few guidelines for constructing affirmations.

1. **Use the first person, 'I'.**

2. **State affirmations positively.** 'I will not be afraid when I perform in long cases' is not as effective as 'I enjoy the challenge and sense of achievement I feel when I perform in long cases'.

3. **State affirmations in the present tense.** Even though you know it is not true yet, affirmations need to be worded in the present tense. Therefore state 'I am a paediatrician, rather than 'I will be a paediatrician' and see yourself *already in possession of your goal*.

4. **State affirmations with emotion.** The more feeling you can generate when repeating the affirmations, the more effective they will be.

5. **Write out affirmations.** Write down your affirmations on 3 × 5 cm cards and carry them with you (in your pocket, wallet etc) and place them in areas where

you will see them (e.g. study desk, bathroom mirror, dressing table, dashboard). Repeat them throughout the day, especially first thing upon awaking and before going to sleep.

Self-talk

We can do anything we want to do if we stick to it long enough.

Helen Keller

Another application of affirmation is self-talk. You are constantly having an internal dialogue with yourself about events that are occurring in your internal and external environment. The self-talk has a very strong effect on emotions and behaviour. It usually happens subconsciously but with practice you can learn to listen to it and control it. Most of the inner dialogue is negative, e.g. 'I can't do it. I'm not good enough. I'll mess it up. It's too hard. There is no point going on. They'll think that I'm stupid and useless' and so on. Negative self-talk creates pressure.

Candidates in a pressure situation, such as being unable to answer a question in the long case, may react in the following ways:

1. Magnify the obstacles and underestimate their own resources.
2. Think irrationally and feel the examiners dislike and are 'out to get' them.
3. Visualise the outcome they fear or do not want to happen and not concentrate on what they want to achieve.
4. Try too hard with 'do nots' and 'must nots'.
5. Worry about criticism, rejection by others and embarrassment.

Self-defeating thoughts are difficult but not impossible to control. Some of the strategies used are given below.

1. Repeating negative thoughts *aloud* as soon as they come to mind helps some individuals get rid of them.
2. Thought-stopping. As soon as you are aware of negative thoughts, say 'STOP!', 'CANCEL!' and/or imagine a red light or the word 'STOP!', and then focus on something else such as your breathing. Another technique is to wear an elastic band around the wrist, and to pull and flick it each time a self-defeating thought comes to mind.
3. Being aware that everyone has negative thoughts, particularly in pressure situations, helps to lessen their impact.
4. If you fight negative thoughts, you concentrate on them and make them worse. You need to *replace* them with positive thoughts.
5. Encouraging negative thoughts to go through your mind and then allowing them to pass out may also get rid of them (e.g. saying to yourself 'Come on, I'm waiting for you').
6. Asking yourself questions such as 'Why am I doing this?', 'What's my plan?', 'What do I have to do now?', 'What's the worst thing that can happen?' may also reduce self-defeating thoughts.
7. You can stop undesirable self-talk by taking a few slow deep breaths and thinking positive affirmations. For example, say to yourself 'Take a few deep breaths, relax and take control', 'You can do it!', 'Relax and flow', 'Slow down', 'I perform better under pressure'.

As James Rohn states, 'Don't say "If I could, I would". Say, "If I can, I will"'.

Visualisation

Men's natures are alike; it is their habits that carry them far apart.

Confucius

Visualisation or mental rehearsal is the technique of picturing the results you would like to see happen, and using these images to focus all your energies on attaining your goals. Visualisation reinforces affirmations. Visualisation becomes several times more effective when three or more senses (sight, smell, touch, taste, hearing) are involved in the process. There are two aspects to visualisation: one is picturing a future desired result as being already in existence (e.g. picturing yourself seeing your name on the 'pass' list for an exam, being congratulated by your colleagues, friends and spouse and then savouring the emotions of joy and happiness you feel). The other is mentally rehearsing a physical act, the actual process or performance (e.g. picturing yourself going through a perfect short case). There are slightly different guidelines for each form of visualisation.

Research has shown that the subconscious mind cannot differentiate between a real event and one which is vividly imagined. When you repeatedly imagine something with feeling, your subconscious mind accepts these images as reality, storing these images for future use. When in a future situation similar to the one you have visualised, your subconscious mind with its stored information will go to work for you, helping you to live out the event as near to the one in your vivid mental rehearsal as possible. Capture the feelings of success. Clearly picture yourself in conclusion enjoying the rewards of your success.

An important requirement of practising mental rehearsal of an actual process is that the *mental images must involve movement*; that is, they should be mental images of actions rather than static postures. Recall the moment of your best performance or the best segment of a performance (e.g. long-case introduction). You must actually see yourself going through the *complete action*, and the *timing* of the images you create should be as close as you can make it to the duration of the actual event. The best test of a visualisation is that after mentally rehearsing the activity three or four times you should be able to run through it effortlessly. At this stage, choose a single word which accurately describes or names the event or action you are rehearsing. You can use this 'trigger word' to elicit a replay of what you mentally rehearsed whenever you want to use it. For example, just before a cardiac short case, you could close your eyes momentarily, repeat your trigger word 'cardiac short case' and replay the rehearsed mental image to prime yourself.

Not only will proper mental rehearsal enhance your ability, it can also be superior to actual physical practice because the mental rehearsal will be letter perfect, whereas the actual performance is often filled with errors that can lead to bad habits or discouragement. The perfect visualisation will eliminate any potential bad habits. You will later go through the performance physically *in the same perfect manner* as you have visualised.

Apply the technique as follows. Lie down as still as possible and let your eyelids close and relax completely by concentrating on your breathing. As you exhale mentally repeat the word 'calm'. As you do, generate the feeling of calmness and imagine the 'calm' flowing through you. When you are deeply relaxed, mentally see, feel and experience yourself as dynamic, confident, competent and successful, an individual of superior ability. Don't just watch this mental movie, *become* this individual. Think the thoughts, feel the feelings and experience yourself as this peak performer *as if it is an already accomplished fact!* Remain with your mental movie for 10–15 minutes, then focus your attention on your breathing. If you are doing this visualisation before sleep, mentally repeat the word 'drowsy' as you exhale and let the associated sensations deeply relax you. To return to full alertness, see yourself slowly climbing five steps. While climbing, suggest to yourself that at the top you'll feel relaxed, revitalised and alert. When you reach the top step, open your eyes, breathe in deeply and stretch. For maximum benefits, this technique should be practised *twice daily* (once in the morning upon awaking, and then just before going to sleep). It is best to *set aside a specific time* each day for practice.

It is crucial that you practise this reprogramming exercise *consistently* because establishing a new conditioned, stimulus-response (thinking, feeling and acting differently) needs *continuous* reinforcement of the programming in your subconscious. Your subconscious mind becomes so familiar with *seeing and feeling* yourself being the 'successful you' that in time you'll find yourself actually behaving this way. This technique should be used each day and night until you've experienced a satisfactory change (usually takes between 21 and 90 days).

Mental toughness

> Surrounded by a forest of enemy spears—enter deeply and learn to use your mind as a shield.
>
> *Morihei Ueshiba*

Mental toughness is the ability to consistently perform at your best during the heat of competitive battle despite adversity. It is the capacity to handle and thrive in stressful situations. Some tips for developing mental toughness are:

1. **Learn** everything you can about individuals who have overcome adversity and succeeded.
2. **You do not need to experience** a setback to get ahead.
3. **Provide solution-oriented feedback** when problem-solving.
4. **Expect the unexpected**—stretch yourself beyond your comfort zone. Expect the best, but plan for the worst.
5. **Strengthen your abdomen.** According to sports psychologist James Loehr, 'The foundation of mental toughness is grounded in the physical. You want to develop a tremendous capacity for absorbing physical stress'. Your abdomen determines your posture and breathing, and supports your lower back. To strengthen your abdomen, do 100 abdominal crunches daily.
6. **Practise interval training** by contrasting periods of stress with rest and recovery. Aim to exercise your body for 30 minutes daily, using the interval training principle. For example, if you are a jogger, run fast and then slowly.
7. **Develop performer skills.** Acting 'as if' you feel a certain way, such as confident, causes biochemical changes in your body. Physically relax, breathe and hold for about five heartbeats between each inspiration and expiration until your mind is calm. Recall a positive emotionally loaded memory and get fully associated with it, then magnify it many times and step into it. Repeat with a second positive memory, then see and feel yourself facing the impossible and succeeding. Open your eyes and perform your task. Remember 'Practice makes the impossible possible'.
8. **Practise winning rituals.** Establish a consistent schedule of eating, exercising and studying. Highly ritualised routines will enhance your effectiveness when so much of your life is out of control.

Failure

What if you do all the right things and still fail? Remind yourself that you can never really fail if you refuse to accept 'failure'. Failure is a temporary setback and is never final until you accept it as such. Hemingway said that 'man can be defeated but not destroyed'. Defeat is not the end of the world. Every failure carries with it the seed of an equivalent or greater success.

The main reasons for failure are the following:

1. Difficulty comprehending questions.
2. Succumbing to the 'stress' of physical confrontation.
3. Fatigue.
4. Relying on luck rather than planned preparation. Remember that luck is where preparation meets opportunity.
5. Inadequate teaching and training in paediatrics.
6. Lack of aptitude for paediatrics.

Turn each defeat to your advantage by examining how and why you have been unsuccessful and determine that you will never be defeated in the same way again. You need to ask yourself honest questions about the following:

1. Your attitude and approach.
2. Whether or not your experience was adequate to allow you to deal with the examinations.
3. Whether or not you studied sufficiently, sought the necessary experience and avoided distractions during your training.
4. Whether or not your training is of the required standard.

If your training is inadequate, then what is your plan to overcome this? To formulate your plan you need to answer the following questions:

1. Am I going to sit again?
2. How am I going to get the missing experience?
3. Do I require more intensive study?
4. Is this the correct career for me?
5. What are my motives for doing paediatrics?
6. Do I need to seek help from a trusted senior colleague or clinical psychologist?

In this way, failure becomes an opportunity for growth, 'a teacher', and by reframing it in positive and beneficial terms you become more resourceful. Instead of seeing your experiences as random events, use each and every one of them. Even the most boring or demeaning occurrence can serve you by allowing you to take control. Likewise, the most demanding or stressful event is also an opportunity to learn. As Nietzsche said, 'that which does not kill you only makes you stronger'.

Behavioural and developmental paediatrics

Long cases

Anorexia nervosa

The eating disorders anorexia nervosa (AN) and bulimia nervosa (BN) are potentially lethal pathological conditions, and two of the leading bio-psychosocial developmental disorders amongst adolescents, particularly females, in countries with Western culture. They occur predominantly in countries where there is abundant food, where the ultimate sought-after physique is a slim one and where society is orientated to achievement. Eating disorders are 10–20 times more common in females than males in adolescence, but only three times more common in females than males in pre-pubertal children. AN affects around 0.5–1% of adolescent females in the USA, while BN affects around 1–5%.

AN involves an inability to maintain a body weight that is normal for the patient's age and height, or failure to gain weight when growing, with fear of gaining weight and disturbed perception of body weight and/or shape, and endocrine complications of malnutrition such as amenorrhoea.

The aims of this long-case section are as follows:

- To give an overview of current management strategies employed in treating children and adolescents diagnosed as having AN (by correctly interpreted criteria of ICD-10 [World Health Organization: ICD-10 *Classification of mental and behavioural disorders: clinical descriptions and diagnostic guidelines*, 1992] or DSM-IV [American Psychiatric Association: *Diagnostic and standard manual of mental disorders*, 4th edn, 1994]). This section predominantly follows the DSM-IV manual.
- To suggest a directed examination technique for detecting salient physical findings, and to guide the ordering of appropriate investigations which will enable accurate diagnosis of AN and its common complications.
- To give clear guidelines regarding need for hospitalisation and a review of the mechanisms of the irreversible, life-threatening complications of AN.

This long case deals exclusively with AN. The long case can be challenging but offers a wide discussion base regarding management. As AN is the third most common chronic illness in adolescent girls in Australia, the UK and the USA, there are always long-term patients available in hospitals where examinations are held.

Background information

The eating disorders are developmental disorders, which involve pathological solutions to developmental challenges. There is increasing evidence of a strong biological predisposition to anorexia nervosa. The eating disorders are psychiatric disorders, representing a common pathway for expressing developmental difficulties at certain ages. They are chronic and ego-syntonic conditions (i.e. patients do not see the behaviour as a disorder but as part of their self), where the patient has distorted perceptions about food and body image that interfere with normal functioning and involve the establishment of a range of unhealthy behaviours. Although many texts have described disturbed parent–child relationships as often underpinning the development of eating disorders, current research does not support abnormal parent interactions as aetiological. There is no single aetiology for eating disorders. It has been postulated that recurrent exposure to 'ideally thin' body images can lead to body dissatisfaction; this has yet to be proved. Sometimes a conversion to vegetarianism is an early sign of an eating disorder developing. For many adolescents, overall self-esteem is linked directly to body esteem.

Risk factors that create susceptibility for the development of eating disorders include:

- Occurrence of eating disorders, substance abuse or affective disorders, in other family members.
- Obsessional, perfectionist personalities with negative self-evaluation.
- Co-morbid clinical problems such as depression, anxiety, obsessive-compulsive disorder, post-traumatic stress disorder (including child abuse, particularly sexual abuse), substance use disorders.

Other risk factors include being involved in ballet or athletics, or having insulin-dependent diabetes mellitus (IDDM)—a chronic illness that causes a significant life stress, involves special attention to diet, is associated with increased risk of depression and anxiety (which themselves are risk factors for AN), and involves challenges and stresses in the parent–child relationship.

Trigger factors may include adolescence itself, with its concomitant developmental strivings, identity definition and need for independence, or traumatic life events such as recent loss of loved family member or animal, move to new school, starting high school, move to new home, family disruption (marital discord, domestic violence, divorce), a fight with a close friend, being picked on at school.

Perpetuating factors include, most importantly, the biological effects of being underweight and undernourished (from sustained caloric malnutrition and self-starvation), which include the classic psychological responses of food obsession, depressed mood, food-related rumination and aberrant food-related behaviours. Inadvertent positive reinforcement can occur if the patient was initially overweight, and the initial weight loss was greeted with support for dieting efforts. Parents' accidental tacit agreement by complying with demands of the eating-disordered child (buying diet foods, allowing vigorous exercise schedules) can reinforce the evolving 'anorexic identity'.

As these behaviours persist, becoming habitual, they evolve into a defence system against awareness, or resolution, of the causal developmental difficulties. The eating-disordered behaviours, or self-perpetuating compulsions, express the repressed thoughts of the affected adolescent, including fear of growing up (delay in growth and puberty, and amenorrhoea in AN, help this), negative feelings (anger, fear, loneliness, sadness, worry), desire for competition and achievement (using food restriction and controlling weight), feeling of control (refusing food despite hunger), and rebelliousness (refusing to eat despite insistence by family they do so).

AN is very much a misnomer. These patients are *not* anorexic; they have normal appetites. They just exert their control, as mentioned above, by refusing to take notice of their (initially) ordered physiology. If a child or adolescent labelled as having AN does complain of anorexia, and does not have body image distortion, then that patient needs to be assessed for an organic problem such as inflammatory bowel disease or occult malignancy (for the differential diagnosis of AN, see the short-case approach to weight loss in Chapter 8, Gastroenterology).

History

Ideally the history should be taken from the patient and the parent, but the logistics of an examination situation makes it prudent to take the history from one or other predominantly; the history from the parent will (hopefully) not be as divorced from reality as that of the patient. The examiners need to know that the candidate appreciates the need to get the contrasting histories from both parties, in order to have a comprehensive overview of the dynamics of the patient and their family unit.

Presenting complaint

This should be the reason for current admission: often a critical drop in weight, constant vomiting, safety concerns (e.g. self-harm), hypothermia, serious electrolyte abnormalities or circulatory failure.

Current status

Behavioural symptoms: the A to F of AN

1. **A**ctivity: exercise (compulsive, at unusual hours, solitary, not part of competitive sport, prolonged duration, long-distance running, sit-ups or stomach crunches a favourite), constant movement, standing rather than sitting.
2. **B**ody image: negative comments (unhappy with thighs, abdomen, hips), frequent weighing of self, not happy with new lower weight, chooses baggy clothes to hide weight loss. Ask 'What do you think about your weight? Are you average, skinny, or overweight? What would be a healthy weight for you?' Document how large the patient judges his or her body to be.
3. **C**ognitive aspects: rigid thought processes, impaired judgment, obsessive thoughts, rigid beliefs (e.g. cannot eat this food with that food; cannot eat after specified time, such as 6 pm, as will not digest food).
4. **D**rug aspects: use of laxatives, diet pills, diuretics, stimulants, thyroxine, cigarette smoking, IDDM patients withholding insulin.
5. **E**ating behaviour: missing meals, eating very slowly (e.g. cuts peas in half), hiding food, feeding her or his food to pets, feigning eating (e.g. pushing food around plate), avoiding social events involving eating, vomiting after meals.
6. **F**ood intake: types of eating—restrictive (eating less), selective (limiting intake to a range of preferred foods), restrained (controlling type and amount of foods); refusal to eat foods perceived as fattening (e.g. meat, dairy products, fat, carbohydrates); high intake of water, diet drinks, vegetarian foods; claims 'allergy' to various foods; immediate guilt after eating (may induce vomiting, or exercise excessively).

Physical symptoms of AN

1. Weight loss, rate of weight loss, fluctuations in weight, lowest weight, highest weight, current weight, body mass index (BMI).
2. Amenorrhoea, oligomenorrhoea.

3. Lethargy, weakness.
4. Constipation (including pretending to have this to obtain laxatives).
5. Hair and skin: hair loss, dry skin, purplish skin peripherally, oedema.
6. Circulation: dizziness, lightheadedness, near-syncope, palpitations.

Physical symptoms of refeeding
1. Fullness, bloating.
2. Chronic abdominal pain (superior mesenteric artery syndrome: compression of superior mesenteric bundle and third part of duodenum as protective fat pad gone). This is very rare, and is only mentioned here for completeness.
3. Refeeding syndrome with cardiac failure and delirium. This is generally associated with low phosphate.

Complications of AN
1. Acute: rhythm disturbances, irritable bowel syndrome, oesophagitis.
2. Chronic (may be irreversible): growth deceleration, pubertal arrest, bone loss.
3. Potentially fatal: severe hypokalaemia, arrhythmias, congestive heart failure.

Current management of AN
1. Multidisciplinary team: members (e.g. paediatrician, physician specialising in adolescents, psychiatrist, psychologist, dietician, occupational therapist, physiotherapist, social worker, nurse, teacher, art therapist); degree of engagement with patient (against wishes perhaps) and parents; degree of success so far; whether the team addresses issues adequately in the opinion of patient/parents.
2. Procedures of management program: usual measurements made (how patient is weighed: e.g. in underwear with gown; whether bladder scan is done (to subtract volume of urine from weight) or urine specific gravity checked (to detect water loading); whether there is a target weight known by patient; how height is checked; how often blood tests are performed; whether bone density is checked and how often; whether calcium supplements are given.
3. Refeeding: whether this is currently occurring; success or otherwise; symptoms noted by the patient previously. This is given as nasogastric feeding in medically unstable patients.

Co-morbid psychiatric diagnoses
Ask about any psychiatric diagnoses made, especially mood disorders and anxiety disorders. AN is associated with very high rates of co-morbid psychiatric illness, with between 30% and 50% of children having major depression and around 30% having anxiety disorders, including obsessive compulsive disorder (OCD), so the candidate must remember to look for this in the history.

Past history of AN

Initial symptoms, investigations and management before diagnosis, diagnosis (when, where, how), subsequent investigations and management, progress of disease, hospitalisation details (frequency, duration, usual treatment), complications of disease, specialists and therapists involved (child psychiatrist, paediatrician, psychologist), outpatient or other clinics attended, any recent change in symptoms or management.

Social history

Disease impact on patient

Growth, development, self-image, independence, requests for transfer to adult care, compliance with management program, schooling (attendance, performance, teacher awareness of disorder, peer interactions), employment prospects, effects on activities of daily living, co-morbid pathology issues including depression.

Disease impact on parents

Marriage stability, depression, denial, guilt, fears for the future.

Disease impact on siblings

Sibling rivalry, hostility, support, similar disordered thoughts developing.

Social supports

Social worker, community nurse, extended family, close friends, AN 'social network' (this is usually a negative support, disseminating pro-AN ideation).

Coping

Who attends with patient, who supervises eating, confidence with management, parents' main concerns, degree of understanding of disorder, expectations for future, understanding of prognosis (by patient and parent).

Access

To local doctor, paediatrician, psychiatrist, psychologist, hospital.

Family history

Other members with AN, whether other siblings are demonstrating similar disordered thoughts, other family members with any psychiatric diagnoses.

Immunisation

Routine.

Examination for anorexia nervosa

The approach given in Table 5.1 assesses patients with AN for disease severity and current status. It looks specifically at the classic findings in AN, but omits the various negative findings that would be relevant in a patient in whom the diagnosis was only suspected but not yet proven (for a differential diagnosis for AN, see short case on weight loss in Chapter 8, Gastroenterology).

Investigations

Most centres treating AN patients have an initial work-up that involves, as a minimum, several blood tests—full blood count and film (to detect anaemia, neutropenia), urea and electrolytes (to check for hypokalaemia), magnesium, phosphorus, liver function tests (especially transaminases, albumin, protein), thyroid function tests (low T_3, euthyroid sick syndrome)—and an ECG (to detect arrhythmias, Q-Tc abnormalities). Other investigations which may be helpful in ongoing monitoring include amylase isoenzymes (high salivary isoamylase with vomiting), red blood cell B_{12} levels, serum zinc, FSH, LH and oestradiol (useful measures of malnutrition in post-pubertal females) and bone density studies (for osteopenia, osteoporosis).

Table 5.1 Examination for anorexia nervosa	
1. Introduce self **2. General inspection** Parameters • Weight • Height • Head circumference Percentiles • Weight age versus height age • Weight for height (quantitate) Sick or well, cachectic, depressed affect, nasogastric tube **3. Demonstrate fat and protein stores** Subcutaneous fat: mid-arm, axillae, subscapular, suprailiac Muscle bulk: biceps, triceps, quadriceps, glutei **4. Skin** Pallor, acrocyanosis Yellowish hue (from hypercarotenaemia) Petechiae—limited to SVC distribution (vomiting) Dry, scaling Dermatitis artefacta (e.g. cigarette-burns, other self-injury) Excoriated acne Hypertrichosis—lanugo-like, fine downy hair Eczematous scaling around mouth, elbows, knees, genitals, anus (zinc deficiency)	**5. Head and neck** Hair: loss of discrete areas (trichotillo-mania), thinning, brittle, pluckable Eyes: conjunctival pallor (anaemias), cataract Palate: scarring from self-induced vomiting Teeth: erosion of enamel (purging) Contour of lower face: prominent salivary glands (bulimic features) **6. Upper limbs** Hands: Russell's sign (calluses, scars or erosions over dorsal surface of hands, especially metacarpophalangeal joints, with self-induced vomiting) Nails: bitten, brittle Pulse: bradycardia, irregular (atrial arrhythmia) Blood pressure: hypotension—check for postural drop **7. Chest** Tachypnoea (metabolic acidosis) Subcutaneous emphysema (with pneumomediastinum) **8. Abdomen** Scars (dermatitis artefacta), Tanner staging—pubertal delay **9. Lower limbs** Muscle bulk, pretibial oedema **10. Other** Urinalysis: high specific gravity (dehydration) Temperature chart: hypothermia (PCM)

PCM = protein calorie malnutrition; SVC = superior vena cava.

Monitoring of disease

Not many routine tests are done in AN.

1. Routine clinic visits

Patients are seen weekly to monthly until they have recovered weight and are eating normally. Note target weight, weight, triceps skin-fold thickness (shows high degree of correlation with percentage of body fat), height (used to calculate the body mass index—BMI), biochemistry, menstrual history.

2. Documentation of disease progression

Progression is documented at intervals of 6 months to 1 year. The following may be done: bone density checked using DEXA (dual energy X-ray absorptiometry) machine; gonadotropin levels (low); follicle-stimulating hormone (FSH); luteinising hormone (LH); oestradiol (low); pelvic ultrasound (ovarian shrinkage, few follicular cysts).

Management

In this age of evidence-based medicine, AN remains a condition with significant morbidity (potential mortality), but in which until recently there has been little high-level evidence to support any particular form of intervention that could be said to approach a 'gold standard'. There are now three large published randomised controlled trials of Maudsley Family Therapy to demonstrate efficacy for adolescents less than 19 years old with a duration of illness of less than 3 years. Treatment is now manualised with 20 sessions over 12 months. There is also 5-year follow-up data to demonstrate the ongoing efficacy of this treatment. Most management plans in the past have been based on opinions of experts, in the form of consensus guidelines. What is known is as follows: early intervention is more efficacious than later intervention; younger patients do better than older; requirement for hospitalisation is a negative prognostic sign; involvement of the family is crucial. The various forms of management currently offered are described below.

Hospitalisation

Most patients with AN manage to avoid admission to hospital. However, there are a number of parameters used in assessing the need for hospitalisation. Those who are admitted for stabilisation should ideally be admitted to a specialised child and adolescent eating disorders unit, as found in most tertiary referral centres. Indications for serious consideration of admission are as follows (mnemonic **POLICE WT**, police weight):

P **P**ostural hypotension (drop in systolic pressure of over 20 mmHg, from lying to standing)
O **O**bvious (over 5%) dehydration
L **L**oss of over 30% of pre-morbid weight
I **I**ntractable vomiting
C **C**irculatory failure (hypotensive (BP <70/40), bradycardic (<45 bpm), slow capillary return)
E **E**lectrolyte abnormalities (hypokalaemia, hyponatraemia, hypernatraemia)

W **W**orrying ideation (parasuicidal, depression, self-harming)
T **T**emperature low (hypothermia: <35.5°C)

(The figures used above for observations, including BP (in mmHg) <70/40, HR <45 beats per minute and temperature <35.5°C, are consensus figures from the Society of Adolescent Medicine.)

Most management programs for AN involve a multidisciplinary team, which may include paediatric psychiatrists, paediatric psychologists, paediatricians, adolescent physicians, nurses, dieticians, occupational therapists, physiotherapists, social workers, teachers and art therapists. The parents must be engaged with the plan, which is not usually problematic. Engagement of the patient, however, can be difficult, as it not infrequently conflicts with the patient's agenda. Most management plans deal directly with ongoing, perpetuating issues, and do not delve into the precipitating reasons for the development of the disorder. An important aspect seems to be externalising the eating disorder, separating the thoughts attributable to the perpetuation of the disorder and its associated behaviours per se, and the thoughts of the patient. Healthy eating is promoted and optimised physical health is discussed, which includes a healthy weight. Educational needs have to be provided, and normalisation of interactions with the (non-AN) peer group are encouraged. The most difficult aspect is getting the patient to relinquish the eating-disordered lifestyle and achieve a normal non-AN (healthy) lifestyle. No medication has been found effective in overcoming AN, although, as bone density is adversely affected in AN, calcium supplementation is appropriate.

One of the main problems is that until a critical weight is re-established, eating disorder–controlled thought processes predominate, and it is non-contributory to discuss target weights with a patient with severe protein calorie malnutrition. It can take many months to reach an appropriate lean body mass and weight.

Monitoring parameters

A target weight must be calculated for the patient, knowing their height (measured with a stadiometer), pre-morbid weight, their current weight (many units weigh patients in their underwear wearing a gown, checking for hidden weights and performing an ultrasound of the bladder to subtract the volume of urine), their previous maximum weight and their minimum weight, and their Tanner staging. The target weight will need ongoing revision, until epiphyseal fusion. When patients become aware of the exact numerical alteration required in their weight, they have an uncanny ability to produce that number when on the scales (even if assisted by hidden weights in their underwear). For this reason, many units do not specify the target weight, but merely indicate whether there has been a gain or loss, and the degree of that change.

Refeeding

Any appeal that food may have had has usually gone by the time a patient with AN commences refeeding; previous positive feedback from the smell and taste of food are almost eradicated by severe weight loss and food deprivation. Hence, initially achievable intake goals are small. Gradually the intake is increased, weekly. The patients may well complain of fullness and bloating; these feelings eventually resolve. A very rare complication of refeeding is the superior mesenteric artery syndrome, where the patient complains of chronic abdominal pain and feeling full after a meal, and then vomiting can occur; this is due to compression of the superior mesenteric bundle and the third part of the duodenum, as they are no longer protected by the fat pad around the bundle, the fat pad having disappeared.

Bone disease

Patients with AN have low bone density, increased bone fragility, and increased risk of fractures, including stress fractures. Patients should have their bone density measured by dual energy X-ray absorptiometry (DEXA). DEXA assesses the femoral neck, the lumbar spine and the forearms, and can also assess body composition—the body's proportion of bone mineral (calcium), lean body mass (muscle) and fat. Low bone density is caused by inadequate nutrient intake, specifically calcium, plus low hormone levels including oestrogen (which is anabolic to bone, especially in the spine). Oestrogen supplementation, however, is not helpful in restoring bone, and it can also mask a return to reproductive health (with a return of periods), and is not recommended.

Most units prefer patients to have three or four dairy serves a day, and do not use calcium supplementation.

Prognosis

Unlike adults with AN, children and adolescents with AN recover well in around two-thirds of cases, around one-third recover partially, and about 5% have chronic AN. There is a small mortality rate, usually due to suicide or secondary to the metabolic, electrolyte or cardiac derangements of AN. There have been some studies indicating that long term, adolescents who have had eating disorders are at increased risk of chronic fatigue, chronic pain, poor sleeping, anxiety disorders and suicide attempts.

Attention deficit hyperactivity disorder (ADHD)

Introduction

In the USA, ADHD is diagnosed in 3–10% of children and 1– 6% of adults. In 1999 the Center for Disease Control and Prevention identified ADHD as a serious public health problem. Children diagnosed with ADHD can have social and academic impairments and low self-esteem. Having ADHD is associated with increased risk of smoking cigarettes, substance abuse and encountering police officers. The rate of medication treatment for ADHD has increased in the last decade. In 1997, over 2 million children in the USA were treated with stimulants. Up to a third of children diagnosed as having ADHD do not respond to stimulants or cannot tolerate them due to adverse side effects. There has been an expansion in the number of non–stimulant medications that have been used in ADHD recently, plus wider use of longer-lasting stimulant medications.

The aims of this long-case section, as well as of the subsequent short-case section, are as follows:

- To give a practical guide to the management of children diagnosed as having ADHD (by correctly interpreted criteria of ICD-10 [World Health Organization: ICD-10 *Classification of mental and behavioural disorders: clinical descriptions and diagnostic guidelines*, 1992] or DSM-IV [American Psychiatric Association: *Diagnostic and standard manual of mental disorders*, 4th edn, 1994]). This section predominantly follows the DSM-IV manual.
- To enable diagnosis of conditions which can be misinterpreted as ADHD (a common pitfall in the heyday of ADHD diagnosis).
- To enable the candidate to define not only that symptoms are present (to fulfil criteria) and to exclude relevant differential diagnoses, but also to define the developmental predicament—which areas of development are 'handicapped' because of ADHD self-control problems.
- To provide clear guidelines regarding the use of stimulants including dosage and timing recommendations, side effects, contraindications and appropriate follow-up.
- To enable the candidate to articulate a long-term management program based on routine regular visits to the paediatrician, developmental and mental health optimisation and a plan to eventually get the child off medication (akin to epilepsy management). The candidate needs to understand that ADHD is usually lifelong neuropathology, hence there needs to be a long-term management structure such as we would regard as routine for other chronic conditions such as diabetes or CF.

Background information

Few diagnostic labels have caused as much controversy and divergence of opinion within the medical fraternity as ADHD. The incidence of diagnosis still varies widely between countries: as previously noted, it is very commonly diagnosed in the USA but remains an infrequent diagnosis in the UK. In some countries paediatricians doubt whether ADHD exists as a distinct entity. There is still uncertainty as to whether ADHD represents the dysfunctional end of a continuum of normal temperamental characteristics or whether it represents a discrete qualitatively different biological or psychological condition. The name for this behavioural syndrome has changed over the years, from labels that were unpopular with parents ('minimal brain damage') to 'minimal brain dysfunction', 'hyperkinetic child syndrome', 'minimal cerebral dysfunction', 'psycho-organic syndrome of childhood', to attention deficit disorder (ADD) and finally ADHD, which has been the most widely accepted term.

There is no single diagnostic test for ADHD. The DSM-IV manual sets out the criteria, grouped under the following headings:

- Symptoms of inattention that are maladaptive and inconsistent with developmental level.
- Symptoms of hyperactivity-impulsivity that are maladaptive and inconsistent with developmental level.
- Some symptoms causing impairment have been present before age 7.
- Some impairment from the symptoms present in at least two settings (e.g. at school and at home).
- Clear evidence of clinically significant impairment in social or academic functioning.
- The symptoms must not occur exclusively during, or be better accounted for by, a pervasive developmental disorder, a psychosis or another mental disorder.

The criteria set out in DSM-IV should be fulfilled, at the very least, before a diagnosis of ADHD is entertained. In the age of evidence-based medicine, some cynics note that the criteria used in the DSM-IV are described using terminology that is not entirely succinct; the words 'often' and 'some' figure strongly in the criteria, although they are not concise quantitative or even qualitative terms, but the meaning they impart is integral in the determination as to whether the criteria are met. The cynics then question how the condition can be diagnosed accurately using such non-specific terms within the diagnostic criteria. As for the exclusion criteria, accurate appraisal of child-hood psychiatric diagnoses is outside of the scope of most paediatricians.

It would be overly simplistic to equate the symptoms of ADHD with the disability or problems experienced by the child with ADHD, or to equate successful symptom control with successful treatment. A two-step approach can be followed. The first step is to confirm that the symptoms are present to fulfil the criteria and to exclude differential diagnoses. The second step is to assess the child's development and ask whether the symptoms are a problem. It only becomes a disorder if the symptoms lead to developmental delays, or problems in other areas such as learning, social development, self-esteem, mental health, fine motor abilities and organisational skills. The candidate needs to define the developmental predicament: which areas of development are impacted on by the self-control problems seen in ADHD.

The aetiology of ADHD is likely to be multifactorial, a combination of genetic, biological and environmental aspects. Twin studies suggest 75% of the cause of ADHD is genetic. Parental ADHD increases the risk of ADHD in the child eightfold. Researchers have been trying to find a candidate gene for ADHD. The most recognised gene association is the 7-repeat allele of the D4 dopamine receptor gene (DRD4*7);

agonists at the D4 receptor site include dopamine, adrenaline, and noradrenaline. Independent of parental ADHD, exposure to cigarettes and alcohol *in utero* increases the risk of ADHD.

Parents and health workers can get 'hung up' on whether a child has ADD or ADHD. This differentiation is unimportant. The hyperactivity in a child's condition does not alter the principles behind treatment. The hyperactivity in ADHD refers more to restlessness and increased minor motor function rather than 'swinging from the trees'. The condition does not refer to 'naughty children'. Children who destroy your office are not demonstrating the hyperactivity to which the 'H' in ADHD refers.

ADHD may be regarded as a spectrum disorder. Children with ADHD have varying degrees of the different characteristics that make up the condition, which include inattention, impulsivity, overactivity, insatiability, disorganisation and social clumsiness.

One of the difficulties of diagnosis is that all children can have the characteristics, comprising the diagnostic criteria, to some degree. Most 3-year-olds could comfortably meet all the criteria. The difficulty is in determining when these characteristics become pathological or at the extreme end of normal development. These characteristics may lead to difficulties in learning, social interaction and behaviour. The home environment may accentuate the severity of subsequent symptoms and difficulties with which children and their families have to deal. Poor parenting skills are not the cause of true ADHD but they may well exacerbate matters.

For the strict clinical diagnosis of ADHD, refer to the ICD-10 and DSM-IV criteria. Confusion in the diagnosis can result from difficulty in differentiating other disorders that can cause inattention and hyperactivity and in identifying co-morbid diagnoses. A comprehensive differential diagnosis is listed in the short-case section. It includes the normal, active preschool child, autistic spectrum disorder, conduct disorder, oppositional defiant disorder, reaction to social problems/environment (poor parenting skills, disruptive family dynamics), expressive language disorders, hearing impairment and epilepsy syndromes (e.g. childhood absence epilepsy).

Co-morbid diagnoses include the following:

- Specific learning difficulties (SLD).
- Conduct disorder (repetitive, persistent pattern of behaviour where the basic rights of others or major age-appropriate societal norms or rules are violated; see DSM-IV).
- Oppositional defiant disorder (ODD, a pattern of negativistic, hostile, defiant behaviour; see DSM-IV).
- Poor fine motor and gross motor function.
- Expressive language delay.
- Autistic spectrum disorders.

It has been hypothesised that there is a delay in maturation of inhibitory processors in the brain; this presents a useful working model of this condition. A loss of inhibition could explain decreased ability to concentrate, impulsive behaviour and motor hyperactivity. Children with ADHD have similar problems to children with frontal lobe deficits (problems with executive functions). A delay in functional cortical maturation of the frontal lobes has been hypothesised, with some support from some preliminary research studies of noninvasive functional MRI (fMRI) and quantitative EEG (QEEG), although these tests are not useful clinical tools at present.

The frequency of diagnosis varies between countries. In some states of the USA, over 25% of boys are taking stimulant medication for ADHD. In Australia, it has been estimated to affect between 1 and 5% of the population. Difficulty arises in diagnosis because the condition is considered as a delay in maturation of normal learning processes. Poor short-term memory, lack of concentration, impulsiveness and hyperactivity are all normal in a child at 3 years of age. By age 5–7, however, these characteristics are usually controlled. This is the reason why many kindergarten and primary school teachers describe these children as immature. Approximately 95% of children will be capable of controlling these characteristics by 5–7 years of age. Although parents, teachers and health professionals seem quite comfortable with the concept of a spectrum of developmental *motor* function (some normal children walk at 10 months, others at 18 months), any apparent delay within the spectrum of the (normal) development of *learning* engenders great concern. It should help to remember that the brain is continually growing, doubling in size in the first 12 months of life, with neuronal growth occurring throughout adolescence and adult life. Obviously this growth and development will not occur at the same rate in all children.

Children with ADHD tend to have selective concentration. They can become obsessive in concentration if the situation or task interests them, such as a videogame or television, but are unable to concentrate on a task of no specific interest. These children have difficulty concentrating in a group situation. It is as if they are unable to filter information coming into the brain from sight, hearing and/or touch; they may be unable to differentiate, for example, between the teacher talking, the birds singing outside and little Johnny dropping his pencil in the classroom. All this sensory information appears to be presented to the brain at the same level of importance. In a mature learning system the brain is able to sift and differentiate, excluding useless information and only processing what is important at the time.

Parents will often describe their child with ADHD as bright, but lacking concentration and persistence in a task. Children with ADHD tend to have poor organisational skills, be argumentative and impulsive, tend not to read body language well and make poor eye contact. Some will be said to display poor 'eye–hand coordination'; cynics also dislike, and question the usefulness of, this term, pointing out that most of the central nervous system is interposed between the eye and the hand. These children may have difficulty with reading and writing. If one considers the sensory–motor processing required for these two functions, it is not surprising. Most parents will report that these children respond well to a one-on-one learning situation.

The age at diagnosis often reflects the difficulty these children are having, and the likely difficulty the physician will experience in their management. They may present in the early years of schooling with poor behaviour, lack of concentration, fidgetiness and impulsiveness. These characteristics may be described by teachers as immature behaviour. For some children this leads to poor school performance and loss of self-esteem, worsening general behaviour. Other children's problems are not recognised until they reach secondary school, when poor organisational skills result in decreased work performance and subsequent loss of self-esteem. The workload is difficult because they have not obtained the basic building blocks/foundations in their education. In this situation, some children may present with depression or symptoms of chronic lethargy. Disruptive behaviour in the classroom may develop as an avoidance technique.

History

Presenting complaint.

Reason for current admission/presentation for the examination.

Current symptoms

1. *Inattention:* failure to attend to details, careless mistakes in school work, difficulty sustaining attention in tasks or play activities, not seeming to listen, not following through on instructions, failing to finish school work, difficulty organising tasks, avoiding tasks requiring sustained mental effort, losing things necessary for tasks, easily distracted, forgetful in daily activities. Note duration.
2. *Hyperactivity:* fidgeting, squirming in seat, leaving seat when should be seated, running or climbing excessively, 'on the go', talking excessively.
3. *Impulsivity:* blurting out answers before questions completed, difficulty awaiting turn, interrupting or intruding on others.
4. *Comorbid problems:*
   - Symptoms of *conduct disorder*: aggression to people or animals (e.g. bullying, using a weapon, cruelty to animals or people), destruction of property (e.g. lighting fires), deceitfulness, theft, violation of rules.
   - Symptoms of *oppositional defiant disorder*: negativistic, hostile, defiant behaviour—losing temper, arguing with or defying adults, deliberately annoying people, blaming others for mistakes, touchy or easily annoyed by others, angry, spiteful.
   - Learning disabilities: difficulties at school, writing, reading, spelling, arithmetic.
   - Minor motor problems: clumsiness, ball-game skills.

Past history

Previous therapies tried, previous medication tried, past medical investigations (e.g. serum ferritin, psychometric testing, audiology, EEG).

Birth history

Pregnancy complications, gestational age, mode of delivery, Apgar score, resuscitation required, birth weight, need for oxygen, nursery care, neonatal period, any intracranial pathology (e.g. neonatal encephalopathy in term baby, intraventricular haemorrhage in premature infants, periventricular leukomalacia, hydrocephalus).

Developmental history

Age at which milestones achieved.

Family history

Any family history of ADHD or specific learning difficulties (SLD).

Current management

Usual medication at home, stimulants (e.g. dexamphetamine, methylphenidate) used currently or previously, other drugs (e.g. antidepressants, clonidine), dosage regimen, side effects noted (e.g. stimulants may cause decreased appetite, insomnia, rebound moodiness, irritability or hyperactivity), any therapies (e.g. occupational therapy), school issues (e.g. any school assistance, where the desk is positioned in the classroom—hopefully not next to a hyperactive twin, or at the back where the teacher cannot see the child), psychosocial interventions (e.g. behavioural therapies, educational tutoring), professionals seen (e.g. local doctor, psychologists, paediatricians, psychiatrists), activities to promote concentration and self-discipline (e.g. martial arts), alternative therapies tried (e.g. homeopathic preparations), educational CD-ROMs.

Social history

Impact of condition on parents, siblings, friends, children in their class at school, family financial situation (e.g. private health insurance, cost of stimulant medications, visits to multiple professionals, government benefits received), social supports (e.g. social worker, extended family, respite care, ADHD parent groups).

Understanding of problems and prognosis

By parents, degree of education regarding ADHD, consideration of ongoing stimulant medication into adulthood, realistic career/occupational choices (e.g. not wise to try for air traffic controller).

Examination

See short-case section.

Teacher report

A report from the teacher outlining the child's academic and social strengths and weaknesses can be extremely useful in further assessment of the child's performance. Allowing the teacher to write a freehand report gives useful information, and gives the physician insight into the teacher's understanding of the child's problems. Teacher reports are necessary for clinical diagnosis, and are an extension of examination, rather than additional investigations.

Rating scales

These are also an extension of the examination. The most widely used scales in the USA are the Connors rating scales, which include a parent–teacher questionnaire, and a teacher questionnaire. Other scales include the child behaviour checklist (CBCL), teacher rating form (TRF) and youth self-report (YSR) described by Achenbach and Edelbrock, and the Rowe behavioural rating inventory scale, described by Rowe and Rowe.

Diagnosis of ADHD

There is no single diagnostic test for ADHD. For the diagnosis to be made documentation is required of specific impairing symptoms of the disorder in at least two settings, according to the criteria set out in the current ICD-10 and DSM-IV diagnostic manuals. These criteria act as a guide as do the various ADHD rating scales (see below) for parents, teachers and child. A thorough clinical history is essential. The history may enable the exclusion of differential diagnoses (especially social causes) and the inclusion of co-morbid conditions. The examination can be very rewarding in excluding ADHD impersonators (see the short-case section). Several evaluation tools can be used, but *no* test commonly employed by school-based psychologists (such as the Wechsler Intelligence Scales) can distinguish children with ADHD from normal children, with any reliability.

Educational audiology assessment

An educational audiology assessment allows documentation of auditory processing and may reveal difficulties with short-term auditory processing and hearing in association with loud background noise. A standard audiology assessment is of limited assistance.

Educational psychology assessment

Assessment by an educational psychologist is essential. This may well reveal that the child has a normal or high IQ. It will also help to identify children with specific learning difficulties and/or a low IQ, will assess difficulties with concentration and spatial orientation, screen for ADHD characteristics and help to exclude conditions such as autistic spectrum disorder. The Wechsler scale WISC-III gives full IQ, verbal and performance IQ scores and factors for freedom from distractibility plus speed of information processing.

Diagnostic interviews

These are not recommended but are mentioned for completeness. These semi-structured interviews are used particularly in a research setting. They include the Diagnostic Interview for Children (DISC-2C and DISC-2P), child and parent versions, Diagnostic Interview for Children and Adolescents (DICA), and the Child Assessment Schedule (CAS). (Acronymophilia has been and continues to be rampant in scales and interviews concerned with ADHD.)

Vigilance testing

Again, note that these tests are not recommended. They aim to indicate an objective measurement for sustained attention. They include the Connors continuous performance test (CCPT) and the vigil continuous performance test. The main problem is lack of standardisation or comparability.

EEG

It is not uncommon for children with ADHD and/or learning difficulties to have non-specific changes on EEG; these are in no way diagnostic or useful. However, an EEG will be useful if absence epilepsy is suggested by the presentation and needs to be excluded.

Ophthalmology evaluation

Standard eye examination is important to exclude visual deficits. In specific subgroups of children further assessment of eye tracking and visual processing may be useful.

Miscellaneous investigations

Suspicion of other diagnoses should lead to the relevant investigations to exclude these (e.g. DNA probe for fragile X syndrome, serum ferritin for iron deficiency, serum lead levels for lead toxicity, EEG [as above] for suspected absence epilepsy, overnight oxygen saturation or formal sleep studies for obstructive sleep apnoea impersonating ADHD).

There are a number of neurophysiological and brain imaging techniques that have been used in evaluating ADHD which remain experimental at this stage. They include neurometrics (brain maps derived from 16 to 32 electrodes positioned in a grid formation on the scalp); positron emission tomography (PET), which measures glucose metabolism in areas of the brain concerned with attention processes; single-photon emission computed tomography (SPECT), which measures cerebral blood flow (one study showed hypoperfusion of caudate and frontal lobes); and magnetic resonance imaging (MRI). None of these, however, has established sensitivity or specificity, and none is recommended.

Management

Correct diagnosis is essential for appropriate management. It is important to establish that drug therapy is not the only option for treating this condition, although stimulant medication has been proved more effective than any form of behavioural therapy. Adolescent patients may gain sufficient understanding of their difficulties that they do not require drug treatment, but rather develop strategies to cope. There are children who will not respond to basic behavioural management/assisted teaching techniques without the use of medication.

A child with ADHD can have significant problems with communication, which may be exacerbated by the family's behaviour. Some households have the television turned on most of the day, and during dinner the children are asked to be quiet so that Dad can listen to the news. Significant improvement in behaviour can be achieved simply by asking the family to turn the television off during dinner. Encouraging parents to learn how to communicate with, rather than talk at, their children, is important. While obvious to most physicians, this can be a startlingly new concept to many families. Adolescent patients in particular should not have a television in the bedroom. This will only lead to more reclusive behaviour and reinforce poor communication skills. One approach is to turn the television off after 6 p.m. and encourage the parents to help children with their homework or alternatively play family games, which promote communication and learning to take one's turn. Simple techniques such as these can be effective in changing the child's behaviour. Most social skills and behaviour are learned at home, not at school.

School strategies (educational management principles)

School difficulties are almost universal in children with ADHD. Specific problem areas may include mathematics, reading, writing or abstract thinking. Parents and teacher should be aware that these children may have difficulty with loud background noise. Short-term auditory processing is difficult, and the children need to be brought back on task. Instructions should be short, direct and repeated. Eye contact with the child is important when giving instructions. These children perform best in small classes. Teachers who have a firm, fair, consistent teaching style will find that the student copes better. Some children with significant problems may need the assistance of an integration aide. Children with poor fine/gross motor coordination may need the assistance of occupational or physical therapy. Some children will have speech difficulties requiring speech therapy.

Tutoring on a one to one basis can help these children significantly. A good tutor can liaise with the teacher to document specific deficiencies in the child's knowledge base. It is important to ensure that for each child the proper foundation stones for their education are laid. This will enable them to go to the next step. As these children succeed, their self-esteem will improve markedly.

The areas of difficulty in the classroom can be divided into eight groups as follows, with three sample suggestions for each area:

1. *Inattention.* Maximise attention by: (a) seating the child at front of class near a good role model; (b) breaking longer assignments into smaller sections so the child can see an endpoint to the work, and master material within his or her attention span; (c) pairing written instructions with oral instructions.

2. *Impulsiveness.* Counter this by: (a) complementing positive behaviour and increasing immediacy of rewards; (b) using time out for misbehaviour, avoiding lecturing or criticism; (c) supervising carefully at transition times.

3. *Motor activity.* Reduce overactivity by: (a) allowing the child to run errands that involve movement; (b) allowing the child to stand at times during schoolwork; (c) providing breaks between academic tasks.

4. *Socialisation.* Improve this by: (a) giving frequent praise to appropriate behaviour; (b) encouraging cooperative learning tasks with other children; (c) encouraging the child to take up an activity with supervised socialisation (e.g. sporting groups, scouts).

5. *Academic skills.* Overcome learning difficulties by: (a) organising remedial assistance for specific problem areas; (b) if mathematics is a problem, allowing calculator, and providing additional time for maths; (c) if written language is weak, allowing nonwritten project submissions (using a tape recorder or a word processor).

6. *Mood.* Increase self-esteem by: (a) setting easily obtainable goals initially, then increasing difficulty of tasks; (b) assisting the child to feel his or her contributions to the class are significant; (c) providing reassurance and encouragement.

7. *Compliance.* Increase compliance by: (a) seating child near teacher; (b) ignoring minor misbehaviour and reinforcing good behaviour; (c) recognising positive behaviour of a child seated nearby.

8. *Organisational planning.* Help child to follow instructions by: (a) checking homework assignments written down in homework diary; (b) encouraging neatness but not criticising sloppiness; (c) encouraging the child to use notebooks with dividers and folders to organise schoolwork.

There are many CD-ROMs available which help these children to improve their skills in mathematics, spelling, reading and abstract writing. Computerised learning techniques provide audiovisual reinforcement and allow the child to learn in a more efficient manner and can be graded to the child's current ability.

Ideally, before considering drug therapy, the above matters should be addressed. If the child is not responding to these techniques, then medication may be considered. While drugs are not a panacea in the management of a child's condition, if used appropriately they can be very helpful. Children require close supervision if medication is to be used; as the brain is continually developing, the response to medication may vary over time.

Medication

If drugs are used in a child with ADHD, the paediatrician (the candidate) managing the child needs to ensure that the drugs have treated the symptoms successfully. However, symptom treatment does not mean that the development will suddenly normalise. There is more to management than just knowing the drugs used and their side effects. The candidate should be able to delineate how the educational, social, behavioural and emotional problems are currently being managed to rehabilitate the child.

Stimulants

These are the mainstay of treatment for ADHD. Controversy remains as to whether they can cause long-term growth suppression. It is established that they do not result in substance abuse disorders during treatment, and their use may protect against developing substance abuse later in life. Stimulants may be short-acting (3–6 hours), intermediate-acting formulations with extended release (ER) (6–8 hours), or long-acting (8–12 hours) which can be given once daily.

Short-acting: dexamphetamine, methylphenidate (MPH)

The most widely used are dexamphetamine and MPH. Dexmethylphenidate is the d-isomer of MPH and a newer preparation; it is more active than the l-isomer, has fewer side effects, requires half the standard MPH dose and lasts 4–6 hours. Dexamphetamine's mechanism of action involves increasing extracellular synaptic dopamine, inhibiting noradrenaline reuptake and exerting weak effects on the serotonin system. Its average duration of action is 5 hours and its half-life is 3–6 hours. MPH's mechanism is thought to involve selective binding of the presynaptic dopamine transporter (DAT) in striatal and prefrontal areas, with the effect of increasing extracellular dopamine levels, as does dexamphetamine. MPH also acts on the noradrenaline system by blocking the noradrenaline transporter; its average duration of action is around 3 hours and its half-life is 2–4 hours. The stimulant effect commences between 30 and 60 minutes after taking the dose. Both medications have similar side-effect profiles, and in head-to-head trials neither appears to have an advantage over the other; each works in around 70% of children diagnosed with ADHD. In children with co-morbid psychiatric disorders, stimulants may worsen the symptoms of the condition, especially in those with tic and mood disorders.

Dexamphetamine: dose range 0.2–1.0 mg/kg/day (usually 0.3–0.7 mg/kg/day; maximum 40 mg/day)

MPH: dose range 0.25–2.0 mg/kg/day (usually 0.3–0.7 mg/kg/day; maximum 60 mg/day)

The side-effect profiles for both drugs are similar: anorexia, weight loss (often 1–2 kg in the first three months), emotional lability, tics, insomnia, social and emotional withdrawal and occasional psychotic reaction. Most side effects are dose-related. Both drugs have a good safety record.

Neither drug is recommended in patients with marked anxiety, motor tics or a family history of Tourette's syndrome. It is suggested that at first the dose is small (say a morning dose of 5 mg), gradually increasing every 3–4 days to help reduce unwanted side effects. Generally medication is best given two or three times a day. An afternoon dose at 3 p.m. often helps older children with their homework. Suggested dose times are with breakfast (7–8 a.m., to achieve therapeutic levels while in class during the morning), lunch (around 12 noon, to achieve therapeutic levels in class during the afternoon, often a smaller dose than at breakfast), and immediately after school (3–4 p.m., a smaller dose than at lunch, to avoid the phenomenon of rebound hyperactivity as that dose wears off; later or higher doses can lead to insomnia).

Intermediate-acting (6–8 hours): sustained-release MPH, mixed salts amphetamine (ER)

These were developed because many children and adolescents do not like taking multiple daily doses of any drug; also, they dislike having attention drawn to them when they may have to go to the school office for their medication. A sustained-release MPH was developed lasting 6–8 hours, but problems with this include limited dosing (only one strength of tablet) and erratic absorption in many patients. A newer form of MPH comprises capsules with 50% immediate-release and 50% sustained-release beads. There is a mixed salts amphetamine preparation (75% d-isomer, 25% l-isomer) that lasts up to 8 hours; this is not available in Australia, but is used in the USA.

Long-acting (8–12 hours): extended-release MPH, mixed salts amphetamine (ER)

These can be given once daily. MPH is available as a once-daily encapsulated formulation made up of immediate-release beads that provide 30% of the dose and extended-release beads that provide 70% of the dose. Capsules are taken whole or can be sprinkled on food. A further preparation of extended-release MPH uses an osmotic time-release mechanism, with an outer layer that contains 22% of the MPH. This produces a peak plasma concentration at 1–2 hours, and the rest of the drug is released gradually from the core of the tablet; in total this preparation lasts 10–16 hours.

Long-acting dexamphetamine spansules, lasting 8–10 hours (again, not available in Australia, but used in the USA), provide immediate release of drug, followed by a more even release than sustained-release MPH, with a longer-lasting effect than the latter. A combination of two salts of amphetamine and two salts of dexamphetamine is available as an extended-release once-daily formulation. This can be taken whole or can be sprinkled on food, and mimics twice-a-day dosing with a biphasic release of short-acting and longer-acting beads.

Non-stimulants

Atomoxetine

This is a highly selective inhibitor of the presynaptic noradrenaline transporter, and is considered a first-line drug as it is as effective as the stimulants. Its efficacy is based on three double-blind, placebo-controlled studies. It can be used when parents are opposed to stimulant medication. Animal studies show that it increases extracellular noradrenaline and dopamine levels in the prefrontal cortex. There have been no serious adverse effects reported. It is metabolised by cytochrome P450 2D6; drugs that inhibit this (such as SSRIs) can increase levels and side effects of atomoxetine. Adverse effects include decrease in appetite, nausea, vomiting, fatigue, sedation, dizziness, mood swings and decreased growth velocity.

Clonidine (an alpha-2 noradrenergic agonist)

A second-line option, clonidine is not as effective as stimulants in ADHD, but can be useful if there is a co-morbid tic disorder. It can cause loss of appetite, and sedation. Clonidine has been used for years, despite concerns about its efficacy and safety, to reduce impulsive behaviour, aggressive tendencies and oppositional-defiant symptoms. It has been used in combination with stimulants as it allows a lower dosage of these medications to be used; there have been sporadic reports of death from this combination, however. One side effect of clonidine is drowsiness for 60–90 minutes, approximately 30 minutes after taking the tablet, which excludes its use as a morning dosage in children. The duration of behavioural effects is 3–6 hours (oral preparation). In the USA, a patch form is available, which can last 5 days. In patients in whom drowsiness is not a problem it may be useful in a twice-daily dosage. Nocturnal dosage with the side effect of drowsiness counteracts the insomnia that occurs with the stimulants dexamphetamine and methylphenidate patients, and can help in ADHD patients with primary sleep problems. Tics are not uncommon in children with ADHD and can increase when they receive stimulant medication; clonidine can be useful in the management of tics. Low doses are used in ADHD (1–3 micrograms/kg/dose). These dosages rarely affect blood pressure. Parents must be told all the significant side effects of clonidine, including the cardiotoxicity of overdosage, and the uncommon but recognised complication of sudden discontinuation, which results in rebound hypertension. Other side effects include depression, dry mouth, hypotension (rare), confusion (with high doses) and local irritation with the transdermal form. Parents must be fully informed as to all the potential side effects of this alpha-2 noradrenergic agonist, including the several reports of death associated with the use of clonidine together with stimulants.

Tricyclic antidepressants (TCAs): imipramine, desipramine

These are second-line options. TCAs have been widely used in patients with ADHD, the likely mechanism of action being on catecholamine reuptake. They may have potential benefits in children with ADHD and comorbid mood disorders, anxiety disorders, and tic disorders, but they have major potential cardiotoxicity. Children who have not been coping well with ADHD can develop low self-esteem and depression. Rather than initiate antidepressant medication, it is preferable to address the specific problems of the child. If co-existing depression, sadness or anxiety are severe, then antidepressants may be warranted, and they may clarify thinking and improve concentration. For ADHD without depression, antidepressants are rarely justified. As with clonidine, overdosages may be cardiotoxic (heart block and rhythm disturbances which, rarely, can be fatal). There have been reports of sudden, unexpected death in four children treated with desipramine. The author has encountered children admitted to paediatric intensive care units after an overdose of (inadvertent poisoning by) antidepressants prescribed for 'ADHD' in children as young as 3 years old has been taken by the patients themselves or by their friends or siblings, because no drug safety precautions were taken in the home. Antidepressants are much less popular with patients and parents than stimulants. Parents must be fully informed as to all the potential side effects of TCAs, including the cardiotoxicity.

Bupropion

Another second-line option, this is an antidepressant that has indirect dopamine agonist and noradrenergic effects. It can be used for ADHD with co-morbid depression. Its main side effects include insomnia, irritability and drug-induced seizures, particularly in adolescents with bulimia (in whom, thus, it is contraindicated). It is being used to help cocaine addicts who have ADHD and, in another formulation, is useful to help nicotine addicts stop smoking. It could be useful in an adolescent with ADHD with substance abuse who smokes.

Venlafaxine

This is a serotonin/noradrenaline reuptake inhibitor, another second-line drug, which has mainly been used to treat depression and anxiety disorders in adults. More recently there has been interest in using it to treat adult ADHD with co-morbid mood disorders. One study showed monotherapy with venlafaxine to be as efficacious as combined stimulant and antidepressant treatment. This study was in adults and cannot be generalised to children, but is mentioned for completeness.

Prognosis

If ADHD can be considered a delay in the normal maturational processes of a developing brain, then there is an analogy with the maturational delay in nocturnal enuresis; as occurs in children with nocturnal enuresis, the problem may continue into adulthood. Many children either grow out of their ADHD or as adults learn to cope with the specific characteristics that cause them difficulty. As the condition is dynamic rather than static, children with this condition require regular review. It is not appropriate to prescribe medication and see the child once or twice a year for renewal of the prescription. It is more appropriate to follow them on a minimum three-monthly basis to assess both social and academic progress.

During adolescence, which is often a difficult time for any child, patients may require more frequent follow-up. It is not uncommon for the adolescent patient to require a decrease in stimulant dosage. Always ask about HEADS: **H**ome, **E**ducation, **A**lcohol, **D**rugs, **S**ex. Assessment of drug effect/side effects/compliance is critical, along with assessment of sleep patterns, growth/eating habits and blood pressure if taking medication.

Children with ADHD and co-morbid conduct disorder represent a poor prognostic group. It is not uncommon for these children to leave school at an early age. Children with poorly controlled conduct disorder have a high probability of being in trouble with the law by the age of 21 years (in reality, it is usually much earlier). Sometimes the best that can be achieved for these children is the teaching of life skills. They are often not candidates for stimulant medication as it is usually abused with other drugs or sold for money. Principles for life skills include the teaching of budgeting, communication skills and organisational skills. If taught to budget, then these children are less likely to resort to unlawful means of obtaining money. Good communication skills may allow them to cope within the workforce and can increase the likelihood of establishing a stable relationship with a spouse.

Alternative treatments

The management of children diagnosed as having ADHD can be an emotional minefield. Parents at the end of their tether will try many and varied treatments, and any suggested 'cure' or quick fix will invariably lead some parents to try unorthodox treatments suggested by 'practitioners' of no fixed ability, representing a range of 'therapies'. Challenging this approach may damage the doctor–patient/parent relationship. While unusual 'therapies' can 'work' in children who do not really have ADHD, the fact remains that stimulants are the most effective treatment, but as long as there are desperate parents, there will be charlatans who will make money from treatments that have no scientific basis. Most alternative treatments are 'justified' by the suggestion that drug therapy will not be necessary; universally their theoretical justification is inconsistent with current scientific knowledge. Included within the many non-traditional approaches are: optometric training, tinted lenses, megavitamins, patterning, kinaesthesiology, homeopathic substances to counter 'allergens' and sound therapy. Most of these therapies have not undergone controlled clinical trials, and their use is based on anecdotal testimony. The disadvantages to these approaches include high cost, wasting valuable time, delay in commencing recognised treatments, damage to self-esteem caused by suggestions that the child's eyes, brain or ability to handle food are abnormal.

Diet has been suggested as a cause of ADHD. To date many diets have been tried without success. The picture here is somewhat cloudy as there are some children who appear to become hyperactive when exposed to certain food dyes or preservatives. This phenomenon is seen in normal children as well as in children with ADHD, but the behavioural changes are somewhat exacerbated in children with ADHD. Most parents are aware of changes in their child's behaviour when exposed to these foods (e.g. tomato sauce, chocolate and various types of 'junk food'). Rather than adopting specialist restrictive diets, the best approach is to keep a simple food diary to identify the particular culprit and then restrict this from the diet. Despite some mythology about sugar (quote from one parent 'He can't have sugar, it sends him hypo! He had it once, he went mad for a week!'), sugar is never the culprit.

Autistic disorder (autism)

Children with autism demonstrate impairment in three areas: reciprocal social interaction, communication, and repetitive, restricted, stereotyped behaviours and interests. There is a range from mild eccentricities to severe developmental disabilities; in view of the qualitative and quantitative differences in symptomatology, autism is now often termed 'autistic spectrum disorder' (ASD), including classic autistic disorder and its milder 'variants'—Asperger's syndrome and pervasive developmental disorder–not otherwise specified (PDD-NOS). This section deals with classic autistic disorder, and although it alludes to the conditions under the ASD umbrella, it does not discuss them.

The aim of this long-case section is as follows:

- To give a practical guide to the management of children diagnosed as having autistic disorder/autism (by correctly interpreted criteria of ICD-10 [World Health Organization: ICD-10 *Classification of mental and behavioural disorders: clinical descriptions and diagnostic guidelines*, 1992] or DSM-IV [American Psychiatric Association: *Diagnostic and standard manual of mental disorders*, 4th edn, 1994]). This section predominantly follows the DSM-IV manual, and discusses the classic autistic disorder. It does not cover the milder 'variants' of autistic disorder, such as Asperger's disorder/syndrome (intellectual ability within the average range, and, superficially at least, normal early language development: there are a multiplicity of varying criteria for this depending on which 'authoritative' source is read) or pervasive developmental disorders (PDD) in the DSM-IV. The term 'autistic spectrum disorder' (ASD) is widely used now to encompass autistic disorder, Asperger's disorder, atypical autism and pervasive developmental disorder–not otherwise specified (PDD-NOS), but it does not appear in the DSM-IV. Within the PDD classification in DSM-IV are included Rett disorder and childhood disintegrative disorder.
- To enable diagnosis of conditions which can be misinterpreted as autism (which can be a pitfall in the environment of increased diagnoses of 'ASD').
- To clarify which potential aetiological factors have some evidence, and which do not but receive adverse publicity, to counter much misinformation in the lay press.
- To give clear guidelines regarding therapies for which there is evidence of efficacy and therapies for which there is insufficient evidence to support their use. Autism is an area in which 'complementary' and 'alternative' medical therapies (CAM) are widely used. While parents appreciate their doctor's support for their use of their chosen CAM, it is also important to caution them against therapies which could have significant detrimental effects on their child's health (and on their finances).

Background information

Autism is known to be a more heterogeneous disorder than was appreciated a decade ago. In keeping with other behavioural diagnoses, there has been much controversy and divergence of opinion within the medical fraternity as to the classification of autism and its milder variants and associated pervasive developmental diagnoses. The prevalence of classic autism is 1 in 1000, and of ASD is around 2 in 1000. There seems to have been a rise in prevalence, partially due to changed criteria that include milder forms within the spectrum of autism, partially due to increased recognition by both the public and professionals, and perhaps also a true rise in prevalence. There is no single diagnostic test for autism. The DSM-IV manual sets out the criteria for autism disorder grouped under headings as follows:

- Symptoms of impaired social interaction. These can include impaired non-verbal behaviours (e.g. eye-to-eye gaze), failure to develop peer relationships, lack of seeking to share (e.g. interests) and lack of emotional reciprocity.
- Symptoms of impairment in communication. These can include delay in development of spoken language, impaired ability to initiate or sustain a conversation (in those with adequate speech), stereotyped use of language and lack of make-believe play.
- Symptoms of repetitive behaviours and stereotyped behaviour patterns. These can include preoccupation with restricted patterns of interest, inflexible adherence to specific rituals, stereotyped repetitive motor mannerisms and persistent preoccupation with parts of objects.

- Delays of abnormal functioning in at least one of the following areas, with onset before 3 years: (a) social interaction, (b) language as used in social communication or (c) symbolic or imaginative play.
- Disturbance not better accounted for by Rett disorder or childhood disintegrative disorder.

The criteria set out in DSM-IV should be fulfilled before a diagnosis of autism is entertained.

Aetiology

Autism can be the endpoint of a number of disorders: fragile X syndrome, tuberous sclerosis, Angelman's syndrome and Down syndrome can cause children to have symptomatology that fulfils the criteria of DSM-IV. Under 25% of autistic children have a demonstrable recognisable aetiologic disorder. Twin studies demonstrate a significant genetic component. Monozygotic twins have 60% concordance for classic autistic disorder, and up to 90% for ASD. Dizygotic twins and siblings have a 10% concordance for classic autism, and 30% for other developmental issues including personal/social issues as well as speech and language delays. Over the decades many theories have attempted to explain the thought processes apparent in autism. In terms of cognitive explanations, there are currently three main theories, discussion of which is beyond the scope of this section: 'executive dysfunction' (inability to plan, inability to inhibit socially inappropriate responses, inability to flexibly shift attention), 'weak central coherence' (inability to integrate pieces of information into a meaningful whole) and 'lack of theory of mind' (lack of the ability to attribute feelings and belief systems to others and appreciate they are different to one's own).

Some more famous pieces of misinformation about autism deserve mention. Despite several controversial claims in the lay press, extrapolated from an article in 2001 in the journal *Medical Hypotheses*, it is clear that *there is **no** causative association between thiomersal and autism*. Thiomersal was a mercury-containing preservative once used in multiple-dose vaccines. It has now been removed from vaccines, and is therefore no longer an issue (indeed, the prevalence of autism increased in Denmark after cessation of thiomersal-containing vaccines). Similarly, an article in *The Lancet* in 1998 proposed an association between autism and MMR vaccine. It is now clear that *there is **no** causative association between autism and the administration of the MMR vaccine*. There have been many spurious claims regarding theories of causation of autism over the last few years, which, like the MMR belief, seemed to endure well after they have been debunked effectively in medical and scientific literature. Hypotheses on aetiology lead to hypotheses on treatment. Hence, claims for various treatment modalities have had similar levels of credibility (e.g. secretin), but persist (see below). As autism is without cure, and parents will explore any avenue that might help their child, it is not surprising that many parents of children with autism have tried many unproven therapies and may not follow rational advice.

History

Presenting complaint

Reason for current admission/presentation for the examination.

Current symptoms

1. *Impaired social interaction*: impaired non-verbal behaviours (level of eye contact, cuddling family members, hugging, facial expressions, body posture, gestures used), any friends of similar age, any attempts at sharing of interests, enjoyment,

achievements, show-and-tell at preschool, showing toys to friends and family, bringing or pointing out objects of interest, any demonstration of empathy, social or emotional.

2. *Impaired communication:* current level of spoken language, ability to converse with another, quality of language, any unusual patterns of speech quality and content, including echolalia, repetition, pronoun reversal and semantic pragmatic language disorder.

3. *Behaviour patterns:* preferring own company, tendency to be loner, 'in his own world', wandering aimlessly, preoccupation with specific areas of interest (e.g. able to talk only about *Star Wars*). Depends not on the presence of special interests but on the level of handicap from the time spent with and intrusion on routines and family members. For the less able, may involve primary sensory stimulation: e.g. fascination with noises, lights, patterns, movements of objects or part objects. The underlying deficit is a lack of reciprocity in social interaction, communication and imagination.

4. *Most problematic behaviours* at present (e.g. rituals, anxiety, aggression, self-injury) and impact of these on family, educational facility (e.g. special school), therapists, carers.

5. *Comorbid problems:*
   - Symptoms of ADHD-like behaviour (see long case on ADHD).
   - Symptoms of *oppositional defiant disorder:* negativistic, hostile, defiant behaviour—losing temper, arguing with or defying adults, deliberately annoying people, blaming others for mistakes, touchy or easily annoyed by others, angry, spiteful.
   - Symptoms of *conduct disorder:* aggression to people or animals (e.g. bullying, using a weapon, cruelty to animals or people), destruction of property (e.g. lighting fires), deceitfulness, theft, violation of rules.
   - Sleep disorders.
   - Learning disabilities: difficulties at school, writing, reading, spelling, arithmetic.
   - Minor motor problems: clumsiness, ball-game skills.
   - Coexistent epilepsy: details of seizures (see the long case on seizures in Chapter 13, Neurology; 7–14% of children with autism have epilepsy).

Past history

Any illnesses predating first features of autism (e.g. meningitis, encephalitis, other intracranial pathology, head injury). Details of past history of coexistent diagnoses (e.g. tuberous sclerosis complex). Symptoms leading to the diagnosis may include symptoms referrable to the following:

- *Language delay:* e.g. not responding to name, no babbling, no pointing or waving by 12 months, no sharing of interest in objects, no single words by 16 months, appeared deaf, no spontaneous (non-echolalic) phrases/word combinations by 24 months, loss of words, language.
- *Lack of social interaction:* e.g. not smiling socially, very 'independent', treating others as object rather than person, lacking or only superficial interest in other children, lack of or restricted eye contact, seeming to be in 'own world', seeming to 'tune out', lack of cuddling, no development of expected social skills.
- *Behavioural issues:* e.g. temper tantrums, uncooperative, overactive, lining things up, obsessions with certain things (such as water, wheels, mechanical devices), odd motor movements, not playing with toys, unusual attachments to objects, refusal to wear anything but favourite outfit (e.g. dressing exclusively as Batman every day for many months), preoccupations, unusual sensory reactions, toe walking.

Previous therapies tried, previous medication tried, past medical investigations (e.g. serum ferritin, chromosomal analysis, psychometric testing, audiology, EEG).

Birth history

Pregnancy complications, gestational age, mode of delivery, Apgar score, resuscitation required, birth weight, need for oxygen, nursery care, neonatal period, any intracranial pathology (e.g. neonatal encephalopathy in term baby, intraventricular haemorrhage in premature infant, periventricular leukomalacia, hydrocephalus).

Developmental history

Age at which all major milestones achieved, especially speech and language acquisition, and personal social interaction (25% of children with autism demonstrate regression in language and socialisation skills before 18 months of age).

Family history

Any family history of ASD (recurrence is 10–20% in subsequent siblings). Genetic risk for second child with autism is 5%. Genetic risk for broader spectrum of ASD is greater.

Immunisation

Is immunisation up to date? Do parents have any concerns regarding possible aetiological link? Timing of immunisation and noting first symptoms (there will of course be temporal coincidence as the timing of some immunisations may well coincide within a few months of the noting of symptoms).

Current management

Usual routine at home, any medications used (e.g. selective serotonin reuptake inhibitors (SSRIs), stimulants used (e.g. dexamphetamine, methylphenidate) currently or previously, other drugs for ADHD-like symptoms (e.g. antidepressants, clonidine), dosage regimen, side effects noted (e.g. stimulants may cause decreased appetite, insomnia, rebound moodiness, irritability or hyperactivity), any therapies (e.g. occupational therapy), school issues (e.g. which sort of school, any school assistance, where the desk is positioned in the classroom), psychosocial interventions (e.g. behavioural therapies, educational tutoring), professionals seen (e.g. local doctor, psychologists, paediatricians, psychiatrists), activities to promote concentration and self-control (e.g. relaxation or exercise), alternative therapies tried (e.g. homeopathic preparations), educational CD-ROMs.

Social history

Impact of condition on parents, siblings, friends, children in same class at school, family financial situation (e.g. private health insurance, cost of stimulant medications, visits to multiple professionals, government benefits received), social supports (social worker, extended family, respite care, autism associations).

Understanding of problems and prognosis

By parents, degree of education regarding autism, realistic long-term plans for care/career/occupational choices.

Examination

See the short-case section. Most children with autism have entirely normal physical appearance, other than macrocephaly in around 25%. A recognisable aetiological disorder is associated in under 25% of cases with ASD (e.g. tuberous sclerosis, fragile X syndrome). Others may have minor abnormalities of uncertain significance such as on EEG or brain scan.

Diagnosis of autism

There is no pathognomonic sign, no definitive biologic marker and no diagnostic laboratory test for autism. To make the diagnosis, specific impairing symptoms of the disorder must be documented according to the criteria set out in the current ICD-10 and DSM-IV diagnostic manuals. Multidisciplinary teams are involved in the diagnosis of autism in Australia, the UK and the USA. They comprise a range of professionals that usually includes a doctor (paediatrician or psychiatrist), psychologist, speech therapist, occupational therapist and social worker. A thorough neurological and general medical examination must be performed (as per the short-case approach).

Several evaluation tools can be used. Autism may be suspected by routine developmental surveillance (see below). The next step involves a number of autism-specific screening tests (see below). The traditional tool for developmental screening, the Denver-II (DDST-II, formerly the Denver Developmental Screening Test–Revised), is regarded as being insensitive and lacking in specificity. Similarly the Revised Denver Pre-Screening Developmental Questionnaire (R–DPSDQ) is not recommended for primary-care developmental surveillance.

There is a wide differential diagnosis for the ASDs. In children with neurogenetic disorders autistic behaviour can be a prominent aspect of their medical condition. The most common of these disorders are fragile X syndrome, which comprises less than 5% of autism, and tuberous sclerosis, which comprises less than 3% autism (but 8–14% of autism with epilepsy). Smith-Magenis, Cohen's and Joubert's syndromes have specific association. Other genetic disorders, (e.g. Down syndrome or Angelman's syndrome) may be associated with ASD because of their cognitive involvement. Chromosomal abnormalities have been described in 5–9% of patients with ASD. The prevalence of intellectual impairment with autism is around 50–75%. Rett syndrome, which also always has autistic disorder, is the only ICD-10 psychiatric disorder defined by aetiology.

The differential diagnoses are listed in the short-case section.

Screening tests and diagnostic instruments

Routine developmental surveillance

This uses instruments such as the following:

- Ages and Stages Questionnaire, 2nd edition (ASQ).
- BRIGANCE Screens.
- Child Development Inventories (CDI).
- Parents' Evaluation of Developmental Status (PEDS).
- Pervasive Developmental Disorder Screening Test (a parent completed survey of the early features of ASD).

Autism-specific screening tests

These include:

- Checklist for Autism in Toddlers (CHAT; administer at 18 months).
- Modified Checklist for Autism in Toddlers (M-CHAT; administer at 24 months).
- Autism Screening Questionnaire (for children age 4 and over).
- Social Communication Questionnaire (SCQ; there are two of these, one for those under 6 years, the other for those 6 years or over).

- Developmental Behaviour Checklist (DBCL; administer at age 4 or older).
- Australian Scale for Asperger's Syndrome (for older verbal children).
- Social Responsiveness Scale, a questionnaire to aid diagnosing broader spectrum of ASD, including Pervasive Developmental Disorder

Diagnostic parental interviews
- Gilliam Autism Rating Scale (GARS).
- Parent Interview for Autism.
- The Pervasive Developmental Disorders Screening Test (PDDST).
- Autism Diagnostic Interview–Revised (ADI-R).
- Diagnostic Interview for Social and Communications Disorders (DISCO), which takes a developmental framework.

Diagnostic observation instruments
- Childhood Autism Rating Scale (CARS).
- Autism Diagnostic Observation Schedule (ADOS).
- Screening Tool for Autism in Two-Year-Olds.

Investigations

Blood tests
1. High-resolution chromosomal analysis (karyotype).
2. DNA probe for fragile X syndrome (3–25% of fragile X syndrome children have ASD).
3. Specific genetic testing for Rett syndrome (caused by MeCP2 mutation; gene map locus Xq28, Xp22), Angelman's syndrome (due to deletion of maternally inherited 15q11–q13), or Smith-Magenis syndrome (due to deletion of a portion of 17p11.2), if clinically indicated.
4. Serum lead levels for lead toxicity (especially if there is a history of pica, or living in an old house with lead-containing paint).
5. Serum amino acids to detect phenylketonuria (PKU).

Urine test
Metabolic screen (if initiated by presence of suggestive clinical findings, such as cyclic vomiting, lethargy, early seizures, dysmorphic or coarse features, intellectual impairment).

Neurophysiological testing
1. Audiology is required to exclude impaired hearing as a contributing cause of speech delay.
2. EEG is not a routine requirement, but if a seizure has occurred, it may be indicated.

Ophthalmological assessment
Formal assessment by a paediatric ophthalmologist is appropriate to exclude any unrecognised visual impairment which could contribute to restriction of eye contact.

Other
Often many more tests than the above are ordered. There is inadequate evidence to support the following (which may well be requested by parents): routine EEG, routine neuroimaging, coeliac disease serology, allergy testing, immunological studies, hair analysis, testing for micronutrients such as vitamins and trace elements, heavy metal screen, thyroid function tests, non-selective screening for mitochondrial disorders,

intestinal permeability studies, stool analysis, urinary peptide levels—the list can go on and on. Many obscure investigations may be sent to the Great Plains Laboratory in Kansas; what to do with the results, if some are abnormal, remains unclear.

Educational psychology assessment

Assessment by an educational psychologist may be useful. This may reveal that the child has a normal or high IQ. It can help identify children with specific learning difficulties and/or a low IQ. The Wechsler scale WISC-III gives full-scale IQ, verbal and performance IQ scores.

Teacher's report

A report from the special school teacher, aide or regular school teacher outlining the child's academic and social strengths and weaknesses can be extremely useful in further assessment of the child's performance. Allowing the teacher to write a free-hand report gives useful information, and gives the physician insight into the teacher's understanding of the child's problems.

Management

Prognosis depends on intellect and the establishment of functional communication by the age of 5 years.

Management can be divided into seven groups of headings, with the mnemonic **SPECIAL**.

S   **S**chool-based special education (for children over 3 years)
P   **P**harmacotherapeutic intervention
E   **E**ducation of, and support for, parents
C   **C**ommunity supports
I   **I**ntervention
A   **A**lternative treatments
L   **L**earning / Links: useful websites

School-based special education

For most children with autism, education authorities assess the particular level of additional teaching/support required to optimise their education. Many public schools have special education development units that cater for children with autism.

Pharmacotherapeutic intervention

In autism, an effective medical treatment has yet to be found for the core problems involving language and social cognition, although the atypical antipsychotic agent risperidone does show some promising effects in improving social relatedness, and managing interfering, stereotyped and repetitive behaviours. Its use should be limited to associated psychiatric problems of aggression, self-injury, hyperactivity, anxiety or stereotypes.

Irrespective of which drug is used, informed consent should be obtained regarding potential benefits and potential adverse side effects. Safe storage of medication in the home is essential. Careful and regular review must be carried out to monitor response, and carers, school teachers and general practitioners must be kept apprised of any change in, or new addition to, the therapeutic armamentarium.

Four main groups of behaviours may show a positive response to medication:

1. ADHD-like behaviours

Here, the same medications may be tried as are used in ADHD:

- The stimulants dexamphetamine and methylphenidate have poorer response rates and greater side effects in those with intellectual disability and autism. Side-effect profiles are similar, with anorexia, weight loss (often 1–2 kg in the first 3 months), emotional lability, tics, insomnia, social and emotional withdrawal, and occasional psychotic reaction. Most side effects are dose-related. Both drugs have a good safety record. Neither is recommended in patients with marked anxiety, motor tics or a family history of Tourette's syndrome (see the long case on ADHD for discussion).
- Atomoxetine and amitriptyline have a noradrenergic pathway effect and are often better for impulsiveness and aggression. These drugs have a different side effect profile to that of stimulants.
- The antihypertensive clonidine, to reduce impulsive behaviour, aggressive tendencies and oppositional-defiant symptoms. Low doses are used in autism, as in ADHD (1–3 micrograms/kg/dose), and rarely affect blood pressure. Parents must be told all the significant side effects of clonidine, including the cardiotoxicity of overdosage, and the uncommon but recognised complication of sudden discontinuation, which results in rebound hypertension (again, see the long case on ADHD for discussion).

2. Ritualistic/compulsive behaviours

- Selective serotonin reuptake inhibitors (SSRIs) such as fluoxetine, sertraline, fluvoxamine and paroxetine, have been used in treating repetitive behaviours and aggression. Abnormalities of serotonin function have been noted in patients with ASD, and there is dysregulation of serotonin in obsessive-compulsive disorder. Although these drugs are selective, they can still cause *serotonin syndrome*, from an excess of serotonin. Symptoms may include aggression, agitation, autonomic dysfunction, tremor, sweating, chills, restlessness, confusion, impaired coordination, fever, hyperreflexia, myoclonus, coma, and, very rarely, death. SSRIs are much safer than tricyclic antidepressants as regards cardiac side effects; tricyclics can cause prolongation of corrected QT interval, which can lead to fatal arrhythmias, but SSRIs have lower cardiotoxicity. SSRIs may cause behavioural activation (which can lead to an increase in impulsive self-harm) or a switch to hypomania.
- Respiridone (see point 4 below).

3. Sleep disturbances

The types of problems noted in autism include dyssomnias (problems with initiating sleep, maintaining sleep, excessive sleepiness) and parasomnias (problems with arousal, partial arousal, sleep stage transitions), disoriented awakening. One medication that has proved useful is melatonin.

4. Difficult behaviours (e.g. aggression, self-injury, temper tantrums)

- If aggression is related to impulsivity, then stimulants may be useful.
- If aggression is related to anxiety, then SSRIs or mood stabilisers (e.g. carbamazepine, sodium valproate) may be useful.
- If aggression is intractable, then the newer atypical antipsychotic drugs (e.g. risperidone) may be useful. Risperidone blocks postsynaptic dopamine and serotonin receptors. Side effects may include increased appetite, mild fatigue (usually short-lived), tremors, and upon discontinuing this drug after long-term use (over six months) mild, reversible withdrawal dyskinesias. Children receiving risperidone may show improvements in disruptive behaviours (including aggression, self-abuse,

temper tantrums), plus improvements in degree of irritability, social withdrawal, hyperactivity and inappropriate speech.

Education of, and support for, parents

In Australia, there are autism associations in each state and territory. In the USA, there are national and regional parent support organisations such the Autism Society of America. Similar parent support organisations exist in most countries and can be a good source of information and very beneficial to families. Parents must be warned about misinformation, particularly from Internet sources, regarding aetiology (e.g. alleged association with MMR) and management (e.g. alleged miracle cures). Parents should be provided with reliable and relevant information, specifying useful websites (see 'Links', below).

Community supports

The amount of community support the family of an autistic child requires depends on the family's situation (e.g. there may be close relatives nearby, friends, neighbours, church groups), as well as the supports and therapies available at the local educational facility. There are many agencies serving children with autism; government-run education departments may offer specified amounts of aide time (several hours) per week. In Australia, all children with a diagnosis of autism (but not ASD) are eligible to receive a carer's allowance. Also, families can obtain allied health therapies through the Medicare Enhanced Primary Care program.

Intervention

There is adequate evidence to support the short-term and medium-term benefits of early intervention. Intervention should begin as early as possible. Early interventions may take place in the child's home, in preschools with support, in special playgroups and in child-care facilities, and are individualised. The time required is around 15–25 hours of specific therapy per week: the National Initiative for Autism Plan in the UK recommends that 15 hours a week should be available to all; some have suggested 40 hours is required, but this adds financial constraints without definite benefit. Early intervention may include behaviour management strategies, early developmental education, communication therapy, speech therapy, occupational therapy, physiotherapy, structured social play and much parent training. Once the child is old enough to enter the school system, it is essential to find the best educational facility available for that child's intellectual ability, language, communication and socialisation skills, and safety (many parents wish to avoid schools on main or busy roads, or near bodies of water).

Alternative treatments

The management of children with autism can be an emotional minefield. Parents at the end of their tether will try many and varied treatments, and any suggested 'cure' will invariably lead some parents to try unorthodox treatments. Challenging this approach may damage the doctor–patient/parent relationship. As long as there are desperate parents, there will be people who make money from treatments with no scientific basis. Included within the many non-traditional approaches are three examples listed below. The disadvantages to these approaches may include cost, wasting valuable time, delay in trying recognised treatments and potential public health issues (e.g. refusing to get child immunised for fear of autism).

Diet has been suggested as a cause of autism. To date many diets have been tried (e.g. gluten-free) without success. As many children with autism have restricted diets as a result of their self-imposed eating routines, their parents appreciate sensible guidelines on healthy eating. This advice should be the same as for any child, including avoiding caffeinated drinks and excessive fruit juice, and encouraging the intake of adequate water, fibre and fresh foods.

The following are some examples of alternative treatments for autism that have insufficient evidence to support them:

- *Chelation with dimercaptosuccinic acid (DMSA):* oral preparation for lead poisoning. The hypothesis is that exposure to heavy metal accumulation from vaccines/environment may be causing autism. No randomised controlled trials exist investigating chelation and autism.
- *Vitamin B$_6$ with magnesium.* Vitamin deficiencies were found in disturbed children in one study in 1979. B$_6$ is a coenzyme in several metabolic processes, including neurotransmitter synthesis. Early studies in 1980s suggested positive behavioural response; there are methodological flaws in all studies.
- *Gluten-free diet.* The hypothesis is that gluten (and casein) are absorbed through a 'leaky gut' and form exorphins that mimic opioids that affect the brain; constant exposure leads to less endogenous opioid released during social interaction. Studies show no association between autism and coeliac disease or gluten challenge and behaviour. A gluten-free diet can further isolate already socially handicapped patients and families.

Learning/Links: useful websites

The following may be useful both for candidates and for parents of children with autism:

<www.autism-society.org>, <www.mrc.ac.uk>, <www.firstsigns.org>, <www.dbpeds.org>, <www.autismaus.com.au>, <www.health.state.ny.us/nysdoh/eip/autism>, <www.nas.org.uk>, <www.rcpsych.ac.uk/college/faculty/niasa.htm>.

Short cases

Child suspected of having ADHD

The lead-in here could be: 'This child does not seem to concentrate at school', 'This boy has trouble paying attention', or 'The parents are worried he has ADHD. Could you assess please?'

Remember that ADHD has no single diagnostic test; the diagnosis is based on criteria, many of which can apply to a multitude of conditions, both normal and abnormal (see the long case). All the DSM-IV criteria can be met by a normal 3-year-old, hence the reluctance to diagnose ADHD in children under 6 years.

Just as 'all that wheezes is not asthma', so 'all that is inattentive and/or hyperactive is not ADHD'. Furthering that analogy, if all wheezing were treated simply with bronchodilators, then diagnoses such as inhaled foreign body would be missed and the treatment would not work. Similarly, if all inattentiveness, impulsiveness or hyperactivity were treated simply with stimulants, diagnoses such as obstructive sleep apnoea, iron deficiency and lead intoxication would be missed and the stimulants would not work.

Given that so many conditions can present with inattention and hyperactivity, a fairly comprehensive mnemonic may help: **A**CCURATE **D**IAGNOSIS **H**IGHLY **D**ESIRABLE contains the vast majority of diagnoses or problems that must be excluded, or taken into consideration, before ADHD is diagnosed. These conditions can mimic ADHD or can coexist with ADHD. Most have been encountered by the author. Several causes listed may seem far-fetched (e.g. faking ADHD just to get government benefits, or to get dexamphetamine to sell): these will be relevant in the real world, rather for the examination format, and are noted for completeness.

A	**A**utistic spectrum disorder/**A**norexia nervosa (overactive to lose weight)
C	**C**erebral palsy (CP), various aetiologies/**C**erebral tumour (e.g. frontal lobe tumour)
C	**C**onduct disorders
U	**U**rea cycle disorders
R	**R**eaction to social problems: divorce/marital discord
A	**A**buse (physical/sexual)
T	**T**eratogens in utero (crack, cocaine, heroin, methadone)/**T**ourette's syndrome (tic disorder)
E	**E**xpressive language disorder
D	**D**eafness/**D**iencephalic syndrome (thin infants with third ventricle/hypothalamic tumours)
I	**I**mpaired vision
A	**A**lcohol—fetal alcohol syndrome (FAS)/**A**lcoholic parents
G	**G**lobal developmental delay (intellectual impairment; various aetiologies)
N	**N**eurofibromatosis type 1 (NF-1)
O	**O**bstructive sleep apnoea/**O**bsessive-compulsive/**O**ppositional defiant disorders
S	**S**mall for gestational age (SGA; various aetiologies)
I	**I**ron deficiency
S	**S**yndromes: fragile X, Williams, Sotos', Down
H	**H**ydrocephalus/**H**ead injury (post-traumatic syndrome)/**H**aemorrhage (IVH in ex-premmie)
I	**I**ntrauterine disorders: infections (TORCH)/teratogens (crack, cocaine, heroin, methadone)
G	**G**raves' disease/hyperthyroidism/**G**overnment benefits (faking ADHD to obtain benefits)
H	**H**ypothyroidism (can cause a more 'dreamy' sort of inattention)
L	**L**ead intoxication
Y	**Y**oung/inexperienced parents (unrealistic expectations; e.g. 15-month-old referred!)
D	**D**epression/**D**rug acquisition (pretending child has ADHD to get dexamphetamine to sell)
E	**E**pilepsy: childhood absence epilepsy ('petit mal') or temporal lobe absences
S	**S**ickness in sibling (handicap)/parent/caregiver; reactions to psychiatric/medical diagnoses

I **I**atrogenic (e.g. phenobarbitone/long-acting beta-2-sympathomimetics/antihistamines)

R **R**eaction to food/food additives (e.g. caffeine, red colourings, certain preservatives, cheeses)

A **A**ttention seeking/**A**cting out

B **B**right but bored (i.e. gifted and curious)

L **L**earning disability (e.g. semantic pragmatic disorder)

E **E**nvironmental stressors at school or home (doing poorly in class; chaotic house)

Examination

The examination is to detect (exclude) any of the above diagnoses. It comprises a combined neurological, developmental and dysmorphic assessment, plus growth percentiles, vision and hearing.

1. Growth parameters

Head circumference (increased with hydrocephalus, decreased with brain injury), weight (decreased with anorexia nervosa, thyrotoxicosis, small for gestational age [SGA], syndromes [e.g. FAS], height (decreased with SGA). In adolescents, note Tanner staging (delayed in anorexia).

2. Upper limbs

Nails (koilonychia), palmar creases (iron deficiency), pulse (slow in hypothyroid, anorexia; fast in hyperthyroidism, or with sympathomimetic side effects), blood pressure (low in anorexia, or secondary to clonidine treatment; high in some cases of neurofibromatosis, and with stimulant side effects; important baseline measurement before commencing on stimulant medication). Check for tremor (hyperthyroidism). Note any involuntary movements (e.g. tics, either from primary tic disorder mimicking ADHD, or side effect from stimulants, clonidine) or abnormal posturing (CP).

3. Dysmorphology examination (head and neck)

Minor features associated with ADHD/SLD: epicanthic folds, hypertelorism, low-set ears, malformed pinnae (e.g. jughandle ears), high-arched palate. Significant features associated with fragile X (prominent ears, elongated face)/Williams syndrome (elfin face, large mouth, up-turned nose)/FAS (short palpebral fissures, smooth to absent philtrum). Note that some minor features (e.g. epicanthic folds) also occur in syndromes (Williams, FAS).

4. Head

Look for shunt (hydrocephalus), scars (surgery for trauma/tumours), bony defects (encephalocoele).

5. Eyes

Vision, visual fields, external ocular movements, conjunctival pallor (iron deficiency).

6. Ears

Note any hearing aids, check eardrums, check hearing (irrespective of result, comment on need for formal audiology).

7. Speech

Evaluate quality, content (impression of whether age-appropriate) as examination proceeds, and mention this later.

8. Mouth

Check for angular cheilosis or pale tongue (iron deficiency), and size of tonsils (OSA).

9. Neck

Check for goitre.

10. Skin

Look for neurocutaneous lesions: café-au-lait spots (NF-1), hypopigmented macules (tuberous sclerosis), vascular malformation in trigeminal distribution (Sturge-Weber syndrome).

11. Neurological examination

Look for any evidence of brain injury or other cerebral pathology. Examination is best commenced with the gait, followed by the motor system. During the neurological examination, certain so-called 'soft' signs (minor motor anomalies, such as asymmetry, e.g. positive Fog test) may be noted. These are not infrequent in children diagnosed as having ADHD or learning disorders, but are in no way diagnostic of any condition and should not be thought to influence in any way the diagnosis of ADHD. Soft signs resolve with developmental maturation and are common in young children; they tend to persist in clumsy children who are developmentally immature. Many children diagnosed as having ADHD have associated motor problems, including developmental coordination disorder (DCD) (clumsiness).

12. Developmental assessment

Gross motor, personal–social, fine motor adaptive, language. Check spoken language (chat about an area of interest for that child). A specimen of handwriting could be useful, as poor legibility may indicate poor fine motor organisation. Regarding gross motor assessment, most normal children can hop by 5 years, skip by 6 and (by report from parent) ride a bike without training wheels by 7. Also, a tennis ball is very useful to test a child of an appropriate age. A child can usually throw a ball to the examiner's (your) hand by age 4, catch a tennis ball bounced to his/her hands by 5½ years, catch a ball in the air with the hands (when thrown to child's hands) by 6 years, move to a ball to catch it by 7½, and catch a ball in a container by 8½.

Mention to the examiners that there are standardised tests that may be useful, both to identify ADHD and to note co-morbid pathology. These include behaviour rating scales, psychometric profiles (e.g. Wechsler scales), reading test booklets, drawing tests such as the draw-a-person test (which gives an indication of general intelligence and also of any graphomotor disability), and the kinetic family drawing test (a drawing of the child's family with each person doing something, which can reveal underlying psychopathology).

13. Side effects of treatment

If the child has already been labelled as having ADHD, and is on medication such as dexamphetamine, methylphenidate or clonidine, then evidence of any side effects of these drugs should be sought as included above (check the blood pressure, note any tics). See the long case on ADHD for discussion of management.

Child with possible autism/autistic spectrum disorder (ASD)

The approach given here can be used for a short-case approach to a child suspected of having autism or autistic spectrum disorder (ASD), or to guide the examination of a child with autism who presents as a long case.

The differential diagnosis for autism/autistic spectrum disorder is broad. The mnemonic used here is **DIFFERENT CHILD**.

D	**D**eafness (hearing loss alone, or combined with visual impairment [can cause poor eye contact, stereotypic head nodding, hand/finger flapping])/**D**isordered mood (bipolar or unipolar mood disorders)/**D**own syndrome
I	**I**ntellectual impairment (any cause)
F	**F**ragile X syndrome
F	**F**etal (intrauterine) TORCH infections
E	**E**xpressive language disorder
R	**R**ett syndrome (females almost exclusively)
E	**E**lective mutism
N	**N**euro-degenerative conditions/**N**eurocutaneous conditions (other than tuberous sclerosis, which has the strongest association, ASD also has been associated with neurofibromatosis type 1 [NF-1], and hypomelanosis of Ito)/**N**eglect (or abuse)
T	**T**uberous sclerosis complex (TS)
C	**C**erebral palsy/**C**erebral tumour/**C**hildhood schizophrenia
H	**H**yperactivity with attention deficit disorder/'**H**appy puppet' syndrome (Angelman's syndrome)
I	**I**nborn errors of metabolism (presenting with encephalopathy)
L	**L**andau-Kleffner syndrome (acquired epileptic aphasia with frontal epilepsy)
D	**D**isintegrative disorder

Examination

A suggested order for the examination is as follows:

1. Introduce self to parent and patient

Note child's degree of eye contact (ASD children classically avoid eye contact), gain an impression of hearing ability, note quality of speech. Decreased vocalisation occurs in severe ASD, hearing impairment and Rett syndrome. In girls, look for any unusual pattern of respiration, such as periods of hyperventilation or breath-holding and midline hand wringing (Rett). Observe how the child interacts with the surroundings. Note any compulsive replacement of any objects moved by the child to their exact original positions (ASD).

2. Quality of movement and posture

In females, note any Rett features (e.g. tortuous wringing of hands, flapping, pill-rolling, rocking body movements, jerky truncal ataxia). Note any features suggesting cerebral palsy (e.g. hemiplegic posturing, choreoathetoid movements).

3. Growth parameters

Head circumference (decreased with intrauterine TORCH infections; deceleration on progressive centiles in Rett syndrome).

4. Dysmorphology examination (head and neck)

Note any features associated with fragile X (prominent ears, elongated face).

5. Eyes

Vision, visual fields, external ocular movements (particularly important in children who are not demonstrating any eye contact), fundi: retinopathy (TORCH), grey flat retinal lesions (TS).

6. Ears

Look for hearing aids, check eardrums, check hearing (irrespective of result, comment on need for formal audiology).

7. Speech

Evaluate quality and content (impression of whether age-appropriate). Return to this later.

8. Skin

Hypopigmented macules (TS), café-au-lait spots (NF-1).

9. Full neurological examination

Look for any evidence of brain injury, or other cerebral pathology. Examination is best commenced with gait, followed by the motor system. This must include inspection of the back, looking for scoliosis (Rett, cerebral palsy, fragile X). During the neurological examination, certain so-called 'soft' signs (minor motor anomalies, such as asymmetry e.g. positive Fog test) may be noted. These are not infrequent in children diagnosed with coexistent learning disorders, but are in no way diagnostic of any condition and should not be thought to influence in any way the diagnosis of autism. Soft signs resolve with developmental maturation, and are common in young children. They tend to persist in clumsy children who are developmentally immature. Many children diagnosed with coexistent behavioural disorders have associated motor problems, including developmental coordination disorder (DCD)—clumsiness.

10. Developmental assessment

Gross motor, personal–social, fine motor adaptive. Be aware that the Denver-II lacks specificity (see the long case). Check spoken language (chat about an area of interest for that child, such as trains, wheels). The draw-a-person test is a good clinical measure of IQ/conceptual development. Reading age can be clinically estimated by testing the length of word the child can read. In autism reading recognition is frequently better than comprehension. A specimen of handwriting can be useful, as poor legibility may indicate poor fine motor organisation. Regarding gross motor assessment, most normal children can hop by 5 years, skip by 6 and (by report from parent) ride a bike without training wheels by 7. Also, a tennis ball is very useful to test a child of an appropriate age. A child can usually throw a ball to the examiner's (your) hand by age 4, catch a tennis ball bounced to his/her hands by 5½ years, catch a ball in the air with the hands (when thrown to child's hands) by 6 years, move to a ball to catch it by 7½, and catch a ball in a container by 8½.

Mention to the examiners that there are various levels of assessment for autism. These can be listed under the headings routine developmental surveillance, autism-specific screening tests, diagnostic parental interviews and diagnostic observation instruments (see the long case for more detail).

The diagnostic criteria as noted in the DSM-IV should be mentioned to demonstrate the candidate's knowledge.

1. Mention that there are three main areas: (a) impairment in social interactions, (b) impairment in communication and (c) repetitive behaviours and stereotyped behaviour patterns, with a total of at least six items from (a), (b) and (c): at least two from (a) and one each from (b) and (c).
2. Mention the other criteria of delays in abnormal functioning before the age of 3, in at least one of the following areas: (a) social interaction, (b) language used as social communication or (c) symbolic or imaginative play.
3. Mention that the disturbance is not better accounted for by Rett's syndrome or childhood disintegrative disorder.

11. Side effects of treatment

If the child has already been diagnosed with autism, and is on medication such as dexamphetamine or risperidone, then evidence of any side effects of these drugs should be sought (check the blood pressure, note any tics). See the long case for discussion of management.

12. Investigations

After the candidate has completed the physical examination, the examiners may ask which investigations might be appropriate. This depends upon the individual child, as there may be features (e.g. dysmorphism) that will direct this. See the long case for a list of investigations that may be found useful when contemplating autism as a diagnosis.

6

CHAPTER

Cardiology

Long case

Cardiac disease

This chapter deals with problems that are likely to be discussion areas in the long-case section. Cardiac long-case patients may have complex cyanotic heart disease, or heart disease and other medical problems either causally related, as in Noonan's syndrome or congenital rubella, or as a complication of their heart disease or its treatment (e.g. hemiparesis with cyanotic heart disease).

There have been many advances on several fronts in cardiology recently:

- Noninvasive diagnostic modalities have expanded.
- Transoesophageal echocardiography (TEE) has evolved from biplane to multiplane imaging that can be used on patients weighing only 1500 g, and is used to assist intraoperative management of particular cardiac lesions.
- Intracardiac echocardiography is now used to confirm device positioning in cardiac catheter laboratories.
- Tissue Doppler echocardiography (TDE) analyses systolic and diastolic myocardial motion, and may be useful for assessing preclinical cardiomyopathy.
- The myocardial performance index (MPI), which uses Doppler flow information to measure systolic time intervals, can assess biventricular cardiac function.
- Cardiac magnetic resonance imaging (CMRI) is now recognised as the best modality to evaluate the relationship of the heart and great vessels to the other intrathoracic structures, and can provide three-dimensional sets of data through time, making CMRI the imaging choice for Marfan's and Turner's syndromes, with its superior imaging of aortic aneurysms and coarctation.
- Cine MRI is developing rapidly as a standard clinical tool as data acquisition times decrease.

Clinical electrophysiology advances include:

- The development of three-dimensional electroanatomic mapping of arrhythmias, which has improved the catheter-based approaches to atrial flutter and other post-surgical tachycardias (related to the incision).
- Smaller pacemakers and thinner pacing leads that can be used, even in premature infants, in treating bradyarrhythmias.
- Miniaturisation of implantable cardioverter defibrillators (ICDs), for managing children with life-threatening tachyarrhythmias, prolonged QT syndromes or Brugada syndrome, as early as one month of age.

- Improved pacemaker programmability.
- Sustained tachycardias, such as supraventricular tachycardia (SVT) or ventricular tachycardia (VT) are now managed routinely with catheter ablation techniques in any child with a life-threatening arrhythmia which is amenable to ablation.

Interventional cardiac catheterisation has become the routine treatment (replacing surgery) for many lesions, including pulmonary and aortic valvuloplasty, stenting of recurrent postoperative coarctation of the aorta, occlusion of systemic to pulmonary collateral arteries (as in pulmonary atresia), device closure of secundum atrial septal defect (ASD), and coil embolisation of patent ductus arteriosus (PDA).

Advances in genetics and understanding of embryogenesis include recognition that completely different genes can cause identical cardiac defects (e.g. genetic heterogeneity of atrioventricular (AV) canal: autosomal dominant forms with loci at chromosomes 1q and 3p, but also associated with trisomy 21). Conversely, it is also now recognised, that 'modifier genes' can change the phenotype leading to different or milder forms of the same condition (e.g. relatives of patients with hypoplastic left heart syndrome (HLHS) may just have a bicuspid aortic valve); such incomplete penetration occurs in conotruncal defects, anomalous pulmonary venous drainage (APVD) and AV canal. Advances in ascertaining the molecular basis of many diseases, including the cardiomyopathies, continue at a remarkable rate.

History

Presenting complaint

Reason for current admission.

Diagnosis

When made (birth, days, weeks or months); where; symptoms at diagnosis (e.g. cyanosis, tachypnoea, poor feeding, failure to thrive, recurrent infection); how (initial investigations: chest X-ray, electrocardiography, echocardiography, angiography).

Initial treatment

1. Surgical (e.g. palliative such as balloon septostomy or shunting procedures, or corrective such as patent ductus ligation).
2. Pharmacological (e.g. digoxin and diuretics) and side effects thereof.

Past history

1. Aetiology (e.g. rheumatic fever, pregnancy complicated by maternal rubella, smoking, alcoholism, or drugs such as lithium, warfarin or phenytoin).
2. Indications for, and number of, previous hospital admissions.
3. Pattern and timing of change in condition (e.g. when cyanosis or heart failure developed, when and how it was controlled).
4. Episodes of infective endocarditis.
5. Other complications of disease (e.g. cerebral thrombosis or cerebral abscess with cyanotic heart disease).

Treatment

1. Past surgery, complications thereof, plans for further operative procedures.
2. Past interventional catheter procedures.
3. Past ablation therapy, pacemaker, or defibrillator placement.

4. Medications, past and present, the side effects of these, monitoring levels (e.g. digoxin), treatment plans for future.
5. Exercise restrictions (may be inappropriately applied by parents).
6. Recommendations for antibiotic prophylaxis for dental procedures; maintenance of dental hygiene.
7. Compliance with treatment.
8. Any need for identification bracelet.
9. Instructions for air travel and high altitude.
10. Any recent investigations monitoring treatment (e.g. Holter monitoring; oxygen saturation).
11. Any recent changes in treatment regimen, and indications for these.

Current state of health

Note any of the following:

- Symptoms of cardiac failure such as fatigue and shortness of breath (in comparison with peers), cough, sweating, poor feeding, recurrent chest infections.
- Cyanosis, squatting with 'Fallot's turns'.
- Episodes suggestive of arrhythmias such as syncope, alteration of consciousness, dizziness, shortness of breath, palpitations in older children (what was the rate: i.e. faster than when usually playing or excited), or a 'funny feeling' in the chest, sweating, nausea, vomiting, or the parents being unable to count the rapid pulse rate, suggesting a tachyarrhythmia.
- Chest pain (e.g. myocardial ischaemia versus musculoskeletal, pleural or pericardial causes) or headache (e.g. polycythaemia in cyanotic heart disease, severe hypertension, cerebral abscess).
- Recent change in condition. Note the temporal relationship between associated symptoms with any tachycardia or palpitation: they should coincide—functional chest pain can be followed by a reflex sinus tachycardia.

Other associated problems

These may either be related to the main diagnosis (e.g. Down syndrome, Marfan's syndrome) or be more general problems (e.g. poor growth, developmental delay, especially involving gross motor abilities, exercise limitations and psychological effects).

Social history

1. Disease impact on child: e.g. growth, development, schooling (academic performance, sports restrictions, teachers' attitudes, peers' attitudes, teasing, amount of school missed and whether schooling is appropriate).
2. Disease impact on parents: e.g. financial situation, financial burden of disease so far, government allowances being received, marriage stability, restrictions on social life, plans for further children, genetic counselling, or at least an awareness of the risks of recurrence, and availability of fetal echocardiography.
3. Disease impact on siblings: e.g. sibling rivalry, effect of family's financial burden.
4. Social supports: e.g. social worker, contact with other families of children with similar problems, break from managing child.
5. Coping: contingency plans (e.g. plan if child develops severe febrile illness); parents' degree of understanding regarding cause, prognosis, exercise restriction, and antibiotic prophylaxis for operations and dental procedures.

6. Access to local doctor, paediatrician, cardiac outpatients clinic (where, how often), other clinics attended.

Family history

Any early cardiovascular death (e.g. hypertrophic cardiomyopathy [HCM]), unexplained death (e.g. long QT syndromes [LQTS]), or arrhythmias (e.g. Wolff-Parkinson-White [WPW] syndrome), any known cardiovascular diagnoses (e.g. cardiomyopathies), any known syndromes (e.g. Marfan's).

Immunisations

Any unnecessary delays, local doctor's attitudes, parents' understanding of importance.

Examination

The physical examination of the cardiac long case includes a full cardiological appraisal (see short-case section of this chapter), plus assessment of associated problems, either aetiologically associated (e.g. findings of syndromal diagnoses such as Down syndrome) or complicating the course of the disease (e.g. hemiplegia).

Management issues

The following covers most areas of management that may be relevant in the long-case context, but use of this section should be tailored to the case you are discussing.

1. General development, growth and nutrition

Most children with congenital heart disease develop normally, but children seen in the examination context often have cyanotic heart disease, congestive heart failure or underlying syndromal diagnoses, all of which may be associated with some degree of developmental delay. Children with cyanotic heart disease or chronic congestive cardiac failure may have delay in their motor milestones. Other children can have prolonged periods of hospitalisation or over-protective family or schooling environments, which can adversely affect social development. Parents should be counselled regarding development. In an otherwise normal child, the degree of delay associated with heart disease is not severe, and provision of a stimulating environment and encouragement of normal schooling should be discussed.

Marked hypoxia can be associated with growth retardation. However, most patients who have Eisenmenger's syndrome with cyanotic heart disease and pulmonary hypertension do not have increased energy requirements or inadequate caloric intake and do not have growth retardation. It takes profound hypoxia to cause growth retardation.

Nutrition is an important issue in general development. Issues to discuss regarding feeding include role of solids, undesirability of fluid restriction, requirements for additional caloric intake, dangers of iron deficiency in cyanosed patients and, perhaps most importantly, support for the mother regarding the above. There is some evidence that more intensive nutritional treatment and early corrective surgery may optimise outcomes in some children with correctable lesions that have previously been associated with poor growth.

2. Prophylaxis against endocarditis risk

Dental procedures and dental care

A high level of dental hygiene should be maintained, and problems such as carious teeth and periodontal disease should be dealt with promptly with appropriate antibiotic cover, and not avoided because of misunderstanding regarding the dangers of dental procedures without prophylaxis. Prophylaxis is usually given as amoxycillin, 1 hour before the procedure, orally, or when anaesthesia is needed, parenterally. The usual oral dose is 3 g for a child over 10 years, and 1.5 g if under 10 years of age. If the patient is allergic to penicillin, then a cephalosporin can be used. All children with congenital heart disease should be given a letter or card to show any dentist or doctor, explaining the need for antibiotic prophylaxis for any dental or similar procedure (e.g. tonsillectomy), including the recommended doses.

Genitourinary and gastroenterological surgery
As enterococci are the usual problem, the recommended treatment should adequately cover these organisms; thus parenteral gentamicin and ampicillin is an appropriate choice.

Prosthetic heart valves
These patients have the highest risk of acquiring endocarditis from any procedure; some units add an aminoglycoside to the usual cover for other valve disease.

Non-cardiac surgery
Generally, it is sensible to consult with the child's cardiologist before any surgical procedure, as the concerns are not only those of bacteraemia, but of acid–base and electrolyte balance and oxygenation. The patient groups of most concern are those with severe congestive cardiac failure, pulmonary hypertension, severe cyanosis or severe outflow tract obstruction. Other children who need careful monitoring are those with conduction disturbances and those with significant arrhythmias. Polycythaemic cyanotic patients must have adequate hydration and intravascular volume maintained, to avoid risks of thrombosis, hypoxia and acidosis.

During any procedure, monitoring of blood pressure, oxygenation (with provision of supplemental oxygen if necessary, although avoid unnecessary oxygen in patients with failure due to left-to-right shunts), arterial pH and electrolyte balance are of paramount importance. Preoperatively, checking of electrolyte levels is mandatory. Digoxin need be stopped only for by-pass operations. Diathermy is contraindicated in patients with pacemakers.

3. Infection
Common infections
Viral upper respiratory tract infections can cause significant problems in children with cardiac failure or cyanosis (e.g. respiratory syncytial virus) because of the effect of hypoxia on pulmonary vascular resistance (especially in Down syndrome).

Gastroenteritis can lead to dehydration and result in thromboses in polycythaemic patients; care must be taken to avoid dehydration. Gastroenteritis can also lead to hypokalaemia in patients taking diuretics, or cause toxicity in patients taking digoxin.

Any febrile illness may precipitate cardiac decompensation via the increase in the body's metabolic needs. Appropriate cultures should always be taken; if subacute bacterial endocarditis is suspected antibiotics are contraindicated until multiple blood cultures have been taken, unless the child is very sick.

Cerebral abscess
Children over 2 years of age with cyanotic congenital heart disease have an increased incidence of brain abscess, the severity of which relates to the degree of hypoxia. They may present with fever, headache, seizures, or focal neurological signs.

Immunisation

There is no contraindication to immunisation, with the exception of associated immune defects (e.g. asplenia, DiGeorge syndrome). Children with heart disease are particularly at risk if not immunised.

4. Social issues

Impact of disease

The young child may be pampered and over-protected. During adolescence, issues such as anxiety regarding contraception, sexual performance and peer approval become important.

Parents tend to over-protect and pamper the child and give the other siblings less attention. Parents should be given adequate education regarding the nature of the defect; they should appreciate the need for antibiotic prophylaxis for dental and other surgical procedures and understand the rationale for treatment, e.g. with digoxin, and be supplied with clear guidelines as to age-appropriate activities and any exercise restrictions (see later). Common problem areas can be anticipated and dealt with before they become a concern.

Siblings receiving less parental attention than expected in a normal family is a commonly encountered problem.

Schooling

The teachers and school nurse need sufficient education regarding the disease to help them understand the most likely type of future employment (e.g. sedentary) for that patient, the symptoms that warrant referral for a medical opinion, and in the case of athletics, whether restrictions apply (see below).

Exercise

Parents and school teachers often ask about exercise. It is a difficult area, and parents' questions must be answered on an individual patient basis. Many units let children set their own levels rather than try to enforce restrictions, but may suggest avoidance of strenuous or competitive sport (and anaerobic exercise) if there is severe pulmonary hypertension, or more than mild aortic stenosis, subaortic stenosis or hypertrophic cardiomyopathy (HCM).

Adolescence

The problems of non-compliance, peer group acceptance, non-participation in sporting activities, decisions regarding future career possibilities, delayed puberty and anxiety related to sexual performance are commonly encountered. Other issues include contraception, pregnancy, genetic counselling (see later), eligibility for life insurance and obtaining a driving licence (if suffering recurrent syncope).

Some teenagers have never had their heart disease explained to them, as it has been discussed only between doctors and parents in the past; this area should be considered.

Pregnancy

Certain conditions are considered contraindications to pregnancy (e.g. severe pulmonary hypertension, severe congestive cardiac failure and severe cyanosis with oxygen saturation below 80%) because of a high risk of maternal and fetal morbidity and mortality. Several other problems (e.g. severe aortic valve disease, cardiomyopathy, hypertension) also carry an increased risk to both mother and fetus. Teratogenic drugs (e.g. warfarin) should be ceased for the pregnancy, fetal echocardiography can be performed to detect congenital heart disease, and, at birth, prophylaxis against endocarditis is given. Breast milk from mothers who are taking warfarin, propranolol or quinidine can produce toxic effects in the baby; digoxin, however, is safe in this respect.

Genetic counselling

Most parents will ask the risk of recurrence. The answer depends on whether the heart disease is the only problem, or whether it is part of a syndromal diagnosis, such as Marfan's or Noonan's syndrome. Most cardiac defects have a multifactorial inheritance, with a recurrence risk of between 1% and 4% if one sibling has the condition, and between 2% and 4% if one parent has the condition; the percentage may be higher in some conditions, such as truncus arteriosus. A notable exception is HCM, which has an autosomal dominant mode of inheritance. Those with syndromal diagnoses will have the recurrence risk of that syndrome. The parents should be advised about fetal echocardiography (available from around 18 weeks' gestation).

Travel

All these children should carry a letter explaining the nature of their heart lesion, their usual medications, and the name of their doctor or usual treatment centre, and have access to a hospital if they have a disease prone to sudden deterioration (e.g. Fallot's 'spells'). An identification bracelet should also be worn. Those with pacemakers in particular should carry written details regarding their unit and its program. Patients with severe congestive cardac failure, severe cyanosis or pulmonary hypertension must avoid high altitudes (e.g. above 1500 m) and require supplemental oxygen to be available during commercial air travel. Hot climates can be a problem in children with polycythaemia, and adequate hydration must be maintained. The child's exercise tolerance must be considered when planning the trip itinerary and should be included in the letter.

5. Specific problems

Drugs

The more common medications prescribed for congenital heart disease include digoxin, diuretics and antiarrhythmics. Most candidates will be fairly familiar with these agents. The candidate should also be familiar with vasodilators. Angiotensin-converting enzyme (ACE) inhibitors (e.g. captopril) are often used in the treatment of cardiac failure, as they reduce afterload (mainly) and preload. Important side effects of captopril include hypotension, renal impairment and hyperkalaemia.

The issues to consider include whether the dose is appropriate, noting any adverse side effects, and whether regular monitoring of levels, and of electrolytes, has been performed. In children with prosthetic valves receiving warfarin therapy, the prothrombin ratio should be checked regularly. Drug interactions can pose problems; these should be considered when changing drugs or adding any new drug to the treatment regimen.

Contraception

The combined oral contraceptive pill is contraindicated in girls with prosthetic heart valves, cyanotic heart disease, pulmonary hypertension, and in smokers. Intrauterine devices are also contraindicated as they are potentially a source of bacteraemia, causing endocarditis. The patient can try a parenteral progesterone, or else must rely on abstinence (somewhat unreliable), barrier methods (somewhat more reliable), with or without spermicidal creams, tubal ligation (for high-risk patients, a preferred method), or male vasectomy (dependent on monogamy). The risks of pregnancy for each patient must be assessed and suitable counselling given.

Specific syndromes: cardiac involvement
For Down syndrome and Turner's syndrome involvement, see Chapter 9.

Marfan's syndrome

This is an autosomal dominant condition caused by defective fibrillin, a protein important to the integrity of connective tissue. The relevant gene (FBN1) has been mapped to chromosome 15q21.1. The cardiac features are the most important and life-threatening aspects of Marfan's syndrome, manifesting in childhood in 25% of those affected. The cardiac involvement is progressive in around one-third of these children. Features include the major diagnostic criterion of dilatation of the ascending aorta with or without aortic regurgitation, and involving at least the sinuses of the valsalva or dissection of the ascending aorta. Minor diagnostic criteria for Marfan's syndrome include mitral valve prolapse with or without mitral valve regurgitation, dilatation of the main pulmonary artery in the absence of another anatomic cause (before age 40), calcification of the mitral annulus (before age 40), and dilatation or dissection of the descending thoracic or abdominal aorta (before age 50).

Parental education regarding the importance of avoiding strenuous exercise and competitive or contact sports is important, and should begin before preschool, placing less emphasis on the importance of sporting activities. Non-strenuous activities should be encouraged (e.g. walking, fishing, golf). The symptoms of aortic dissection must be discussed, including chest pain and syncope. In teenage years, important issues include consideration of beta blockers to slow the progress of aortic dilatation, and counselling to teenage girls about the risks of pregnancy, as rupture of the aorta can occur during pregnancy or at delivery.

Noonan's syndrome (NS)

NS is an autosomal dominant condition, in which 50% of cases are associated with a gene locus at 12q24.1, with mutations in PTPN11, the gene encoding for the non-receptor type protein, tyrosine phosphatase SHP-2. Almost all patients with NS have some cardiac defect, particularly a dysplastic (and often stenotic) pulmonary valve, which is more common with a PTPN11 mutation, or hypertrophic cardiomyopathy (HCM), which affects around 20–30% of NS children, but is less common with a PTPN11 mutation. The ECG frequently shows left-axis deviation and a dominant S wave over the praecordial leads, even in NS patients with no known cardiac disease; the cause for this is not known. Phenotypic features of NS include dysmorphic facial features, short stature, webbed neck and skeletal anomalies (see short case on dysmorphism).

NS patients with dysplastic pulmonary valves can have rapid progression of pulmonary valvular obstruction and may require review more frequently than for non-NS pulmonary valve lesions. Also, NS-associated valve obstruction is more likely to require surgical intervention. Balloon valvoplasty is usually unsuccessful in abolishing the obstruction, and simple valvotomy may be inadequate. Often complete excision of the valve, resection of the right ventricular outflow muscle, and occasionally an outflow tract patch may be needed. Atrial septal defects (ASDs) and pulmonary artery branch stenoses may coexist with valvular pulmonary stenosis. Other infrequent findings with NS include ventricular septal defects (VSDs) and tetralogy of Fallot.

HCM in NS does not have a clearly defined natural history. HCM can become progressive in infancy, or may not develop or be recognised until late in childhood. Symptomatic HCM in NS can lead to sudden cardiac death, even in infancy.

Treatment is as for non-syndromic HCM. Some children with NS and HCM have required cardiac transplantation. Relief of symptomatic obstruction surgically can be effective in older children.

NS can be mimicked by three other conditions with NS-syndrome-like facies:

- Cardio-facial-cutaneous syndrome (cardiac lesions: pulmonary valve stenosis; atrial septal defects); hyperkeratosis, haemangiomata, icthyosis.
- **LEOPARD** syndrome (**L**entigines, **E**CG abnormalities [axis deviations, unilateral or bilateral hypertrophy, conduction abnormalities], **O**cular hypertelorism, **P**ulmonary stenosis, **A**bnormalities of genitalia, **R**etardation of growth, and **D**eafness).
- Neurofibromatosis–Noonan's syndrome.

Chromosome 22q11 deletions: neural crest-associated conotruncal defects

Deletion of chromosome 22 is the commonest chromosome deletion affecting 1 in 4000 live births. The deletion most commonly spans three megabases of DNA and contains almost 30 genes. A wide variety of cardiac defects are described in patients with microdeletions in band 11 of the long arm of chromosome 22 (22q11 deletions). The acronym **CATCH-22** (**C**ardiac defects, **A**bnormal facies, **T**hymic hypoplasia and T-cell deficiency, **C**left palate, **H**ypoparathyroidism and **H**ypocalcaemia) can be used as an aide-mémoire for those with such deletions. Other findings include renal anomalies, developmental delay and late onset psychiatric problems. CATCH-22 encompasses the findings in most (but not all) children with DiGeorge's syndrome (DGS), Shprintzen's velocardiofacial syndrome (VCFS) and conotruncal anomaly face syndrome (CTAFS). These children may be born with duct-dependent complex cyanotic heart disease. Around one-third of children with non-syndromal conotruncal cardiac defects have 22q11 deletions as well. Deletions of 22q11 have also been identified in children with various forms of familial, and sporadic, congenital heart disease.

Note that similar phenotypic characteristics may occur in association with microdeletions on chromosomes 5, 10 and 17, as well as 22. The 22q11-deletion-associated cardiac defects include **T**runcus arteriosus, **T**etralogy of fallot, **T**ricuspid atresia with d-malposition of the aorta (three Ts); **A**ortic arch interruption, **A**trial septal defect, **A**berrant right subclavian artery (three As); **P**ulmonary atresia and ventricular septal defect, **P**ulmonary valve absence, and **P**atent ductus arteriosus (three Ps). Deletions of 22q11 can also be seen in isolated heart disease (e.g. found in 30% of interrupted aortic arch, 20% of truncus arteriosus and 8% of tetralogy of Fallot).

Dysmorphic facial features include a myopathic facial appearance, unusually shaped ears, long nose with a broad bridge, small mouth, micrognathia, short upward slanting palpebral fissures, and cleft or high palate (may be accompanied by hypernasal speech).

With any patients with these anomalies, genetic assessment and counselling is warranted, with chromosomes and fluorescence in situ hybridisation (FISH) for the 22q11 microdeletion. The parents should be tested for 22q11 deletion, and must be educated as to the associated problems (e.g. problems with the palate, immunodeficiency, learning difficulties, developmental delay), the likelihood of further syndromal traits developing and the risk of transmitting the deletion to their offspring (50%). The patient should have blood taken to check for hypocalcaemia, and abdominal ultrasound to assess renal anatomy.

Supraventricular tachycardia(SVT)

The commonest sustained tachyarrhythmia in children, SVT is caused mainly by an accessory atrioventricular connection (AAVC) in those under 12; in teenagers atrioventricular node re-entry tachycardia may be a cause. Those with AAVCs often have 'orthodromic' tachycardia with antegrade conduction down the atrioventricular (AV) node and retrograde conduction up the AAVC (the right way down the right path, the wrong way up the wrong path). Some patients have an AAVC that conducts in an antegrade fashion as well (giving 'antidromic' tachycardia, with retrograde conduction either up the AV node or the AAVC).

Wolff-Parkinson-White (WPW) syndrome is a combination of pre-excitation on surface ECG and episodic SVT, whether orthodromic or antidromic. In WPW the ECG shows a short PR interval and wide QRS complex. During episodes of tachycardia the ECG develops either a narrow QRS tachycardia with a retrograde P wave after the QRS (orthodromic SVT) or a wide QRS (antidromic SVT). Children with WPW can develop atrial flutter, and also have a small risk of sudden cardiac death from extremely fast atrial tachycardias (e.g. atrial flutter or atrial fibrillation being conducted down the AAVC producing ventricular tachycardia [VT] or ventricular fibrillation [VF]).

Treatment modalities for acute SVT include vagal manoeuvres (e.g. Valsalva, blowing up balloons with nose occluded, application of icepack to face, doing a 'headstand', carotid body massage), IV adenosine (the preferred IV drug, given rapidly and can be increased incrementally) or IV propranolol, digoxin, procainamide, or amiodarone. Adenosine is the treatment of choice in the haemodynamically unstable child; if unsuccessful, or there is difficult venous access, synchronised cardioversion (0.5–1.0 joule per kg) can be used. Verapamil is best avoided; IV verapamil is contraindicated in infants, in whom it can be lethal because it can produce AV block.

For long-term treatment, radiofrequency (RF) catheter ablation has a success rate of around 90–95%. RF ablation comprises delivery of a high-frequency (500 kHz), low-energy electric current to the relevant cardiac area by an intracardiac catheter. This raises the temperature and burns the arrhythmia substrate. Risks of RF catheter ablation include inadvertent AV block and cardiac perforation; these are both very rare, the overall complication rate for RF ablation being below 4%.

Long-term pharmacologic treatments usually involve beta blockers or digoxin (however, digoxin is contraindicated in those with WPW, as it can precipitate arrhythmias by enhancing AAVC conduction). For more difficult to control cases, other useful agents include flecainide, procainamide, sotalol and amiodarone.

Long QT syndrome (LQTS)

Children with arrhythmias (e.g. sick sinus syndrome, severe bradycardia, complete AV block), congestive cardiac failure, myocarditis or anthracycline cardiotoxicity, or those on certain medications (e.g. several antiarrhythmics [especially quinidine], some antibiotics, diuretics [by causing acute/chronic hypokalaemia], promotility agents, [cisapride]) have an increased risk of developing LQTS, and subsequent 'torsades de pointes' (twisting of points) ventricular tachycardia, which can present with Sudden death, Syncope or Seizures (the three Ss).

Recent molecular breakthroughs are unravelling the congenital forms of LQTS: the autosomal dominant Romano-Ward syndrome has at least six distinct genotypes; and the autosomal recessive Jervell and Lange-Nielsen syndrome with its associated sensorineural hearing loss has at least two genotypes. More than 50 mutations in four cardiac ion (sodium or potassium) channels on the myocyte have been delineated; medications implicated in causing LQTS affect these same channels. Studies correlating the genotype to clinical features have shown that a person known to have a disease-related mutation can still have a normal corrected QT interval on ECG and, conversely, people with a prolonged corrected QT interval may not carry the disease-related gene.

This suggests the ECG lacks sensitivity and specificity for identifying children carrying the mutation. Symptomatic LQTS can be triggered by physical activity (e.g. swimming), intense emotions, or awakening, all of which cause adrenergic arousal.

Any child (with cardiac disease in particular) who is due to commence any of the drugs known to trigger LQTS must have an ECG to measure the corrected QT interval (Bazett's formula: QT (corrected) = QT/square root of the R-R interval; QT is measured from the start of the Q to the end of the T), which should be less than or equal to 0.46. If greater than this, avoid all drugs known to precipitate LQTS. Not all LQTS can be detected on a standard resting ECG; exercise ECG will unmask the 5–10% of those with the LQTS gene who have absent QT prolongation at rest. As untreated LQTS has a mortality rate of around 50%, appropriate therapy should be commenced quickly once the diagnosis is made. Treatment options include beta blockers (reduces mortality to less than 5%), implantation of a pacemaker and/or defibrillator, or a left cervicothoracic sympathetic ganglionectomy.

LQTS should be sought/excluded in any child with breath-holding attacks, seizures precipitated by emotion or exertion, all initial afebrile seizures, unexplained syncope and congenital deafness.

Brugada syndrome

Described in 1992, this is an inherited cardiac disease causing ventricular tachy-arrhythmias in patients with structurally normal hearts, presenting with syncope or cardiac arrest, and a strong family history of syncope or sudden death. It is inherited as autosomal dominant. It has a characteristic ECG pattern: right bundle branch block (RBBB) and ST elevation in V1 to V3; some patients with normal resting ECGs can have the classic changes induced by giving ajmaline, an antiarrhythmic medication. A cardioverter defibrillator can be implanted to prevent any life-threatening arrhythmias.

Myocardial disease

Dilated cardiomyopathy (DCM)

The most common form of cardiomyopathy, DCM, has been extensively researched at the molecular level, identifying at least six genes for autosomal dominant familial DCM, and at least two genes for X-linked DCM (these genes encoding structural proteins of cardiac muscle, including dystrophin, delta sarcoglycan and cardiac actin). Other genes are involved in metabolic causes, such as deficiencies of enzymes need for myocardial fatty acid oxidation. Symptoms may be those of CCF, palpitations, chest pain, exercise intolerance or syncope; signs include hypotension, weak peripheral pulses and hepatomegaly, with investigations showing cardiomegaly (CXR), arrhythmias (ECG), dilatation of the left ventricle and left atrium (echocardiography).

Treatment options include controlling CCF with antifailure therapy, including beta blockers (especially carvedilol), controlling arrhythmias with antiarrhythmics, minimising the risk of thromboembolism with anticoagulants and antiplatelet drugs and, for those more refractory to treatment, a ventricular assist device or transplantation. Approximately one-third recover fully, one-third die and one-third are left with cardiac dysfunction.

Hypertrophic cardiomyopathy (HCM)

Inherited as an autosomal dominant trait most often, HCM's penetrance is incomplete in early childhood, increasing with age. Over 100 mutations have been identified in genes that account for HCM, which encode sarcomeric proteins (e.g. alpha-tropomyosin, beta-myosin heavy chain, cardiac troponin T, essential myosin light chain, myosin light chain regulatory subunit, myosin-binding protein-C). Particular mutations determine prognostic factors, including risk of early death. HCM is occasionally transmitted as mitochondrial disorder (i.e. maternally inherited).

Symptoms include failure to thrive, CCF, cyanosis, dyspnoea, fatigue with exercise, chest pain, syncope and palpitations. Signs include systolic murmur (increased by exercise, standing, straining; decreased by squatting), extra heart sounds (S3 and S4) and mid-diastolic rumble (mitral flow murmur with severe mitral regurgitation). Investigations show cardiomegaly (CXR), right and left ventricular hypertrophy (RVH and LVH) in infants, LVH and abnormal Q waves in older children, LQTS in infants or older children, or arrhythmias (ECG), asymmetric septal hypertrophy and concentric hypertrophy (echocardiography). Other tests may include gated technetium-99m labelled blood pool scan (assess ejection fraction), thallium perfusion scan (regional perfusion abnormalities) and positron emission tomography (regional metabolic abnormalities). In children under the age of 4, metabolic studies are warranted to exclude secondary causes of HCM (e.g. Pompe's, Noonan's or Beckwith-Wiedemann syndromes; mitochondrial disease), which are more common than primary HCM in that age group.

Treatment includes beta blockers (e.g. propranolol, atenolol) or calcium channel blockers (e.g. verapamil, nifedipine) for those who are symptomatic (note: verapamil excluded in infants under 12 months, or in those with major conduction disturbances), and consideration of the same treatment for asymptomatic children with a worrying family history. Disopyramide may be used if the other drugs are unsuccessful. Children with lethal, refractory arrhythmias may be treated with amiodarone. Endocarditis prophylaxis is important. Active sports participation is exceedingly unwise.

Surgery is an option for failed medical therapy, to ease subaortic obstruction; the Morrow operation (myotomy/myectomy) can relieve symptoms and prolong life. Cardiac transplantation is a further option for high-risk patients. Another treatment described is dual-chamber permanent pacing, but this is controversial.

Congestive cardiac failure (CCF)

Angiotensin-converting enzyme (ACE) inhibitors (e.g. captopril) are very useful in lowering afterload and have been shown to decrease mortality in adults; usually started in hospital due to risk of initial dose hypotension and worsening of any unrecognised renovascular pathology. Diuretics (e.g. combined low-dose loop and thiazide diuretics) give rapid symptomatic relief. Digoxin is still widely used; it acts as an inotrope, but its use remains controversial and in adults it does not increase survival in CCF. Beta blockers (e.g. metoprolol, carvedilol) are also used increasingly in carefully graduated doses. Growth hormone has been used in a small number of patients (e.g. pre-transplant) and has been associated with improved indices on echocardigraphy, increased exercise capacity and decreased myocardial oxygen consumption.

There are surgical forms of circulatory support other than transplantation. External left ventricular support devices and second generation implantable devices have been developed, which provide prolonged mechanical unloading, and can be used in myocarditis. These surgical support methods can act as a 'bridge' to transplantation, or a 'bridge' for biding time until the myocardium recovers in cases of myocarditis with acute cardiogenic shock. Advances in technology of axial flow impeller pumps is producing smaller devices (e.g. the Jarvik 2000 impeller pump, smaller than a finger, but capable of a flow of 3 litres per minute). Another procedure for end-stage disease is partial left ventriculectomy and mitral valve replacement/repair (the Batista operation). This has been successful in children with DCM.

Research into preventing apoptosis is proceeding with potential gene therapy targets including the genes coding for caspase enzymes, and the bcl-2 gene which can prevent programmed cell death of ventricular myocytes.

Cardiac transplantation

Transplantation is now a well-established procedure for infants and children with severe congenital heart disease with ventricular failure or end-stage cardiomyopathies, and survival rates continue to improve: 90% at 1 month, 85% at 1 year, 75% at 5 years and 65% at 10 years. For transplantation to be considered, generally the life expectancy is below 1 or 2 years, and/or quality of life is very poor. Prognosis is worse for those under 1 year of age and those with assistive devices. Survivors of childhood cancer with cardiomyopathy due to anthracyclines represent a growing number of potential recipients, as do babies requiring primary transplantation for hypoplastic left-heart syndrome.

The major problem is finding suitable donors, who must be ABO compatible. For combined heart-lung transplantation the requirements are ABO and CMV compatibility plus donor-recipient chest size compatibility within 10%. The main immunosuppressive drugs used include the antiproliferatives (azathioprine [AZA], sirolimus or mycophenolate mofetil [MMF], which increasingly is replacing AZA in many centres), the calcineurin inhibitors (cyclosporin [CSA] or tacrolimus [TRL]) and steroids. Most centres have a triple immunosuppression protocol involving one agent from each group.

Allograft rejection occurs to a moderate or severe degree in most children, with the risk of rejection being highest in the first six months, and remains the most common cause of mortality in the first 3 years post-transplant. Risk factors for rejection are older age at transplant, CMV, gender mismatch or a previous episode of rejection. Rejection can be asymptomatic, but severe acute rejection can cause tiredness, poor appetite, nausea, poor feeding, abdominal pain, weight gain or fever. Haemodynamically significant rejection is associated with an increased mortality rate. However, there is no blood test proven to screen accurately for rejection; in most centres, endomyocardial biopsy is the diagnostic gold standard. Infections remain a significant cause of morbidity. Early infections (up to a month after transplant) are usually bacterial or fungal; intermediate (2–6 months after transplant) infections are often viral (e.g. Epstein-Barr virus [EBV], cytomegalovirus [CMV]); and late infections include viruses (EBV, varicella) and fungi (e.g. *Aspergillus* genus).

The commonest long-term side effects are related to immunosuppression:

- **Coronary artery disease** in up to 75% examined by intravascular ultrasound 5 years after transplant. Symptoms can include presyncope, syncope, exercise intolerance, chest pain (rare due to cardiac denervation). This form of chronic rejection is an accelerated graft vasculopathy that presents at a median of 6 years. To assess risk, coronary angiography can be done 1–2 yearly and, if positive, infers severe disease. Other imaging studies can be used: myocardial perfusion scanning, dobutamine stress echocardiography and MRI studies. It may lead to requirement for retransplantation.
- **Hypertension** in up to 60% at 5 years; more in those on steroids and CSA; less with CSA alone; least with TRL alone. Aggressive treatment is required, usually with an ACE inhibitor or the calcium blocker diltiazem. For those with relevant congenital heart pathology, evaluation for residual pathology (e.g. residual coarctation) is required; check renal function yearly; may need nuclear scans to calculate glomerular filtration rate (GFR).

- **Neoplasia** in 20%, most commonly lymphoproliferative diseases, at 6 months to 6 years after transplantation.
- **Abnormal renal function** in up to 25% at 5 years. With longer survival, a small number of patients are developing end stage renal disease (ESRD) and then have renal transplant; increased use of MMF and sirolimus (no renal toxicity) may allow decreased use of CSA and TRL and thus less nephrotoxicity.
- **Osteoporosis** probably occurs in 100%: steroids and calcineurin inhibitors decrease bone formation and increase bone destruction; steroids decrease calcium absorption. Supplemental calcium and vitamin D are recommended; yearly bone density (DEXA) scanning is useful.

Other long-term issues include psychological issues (up to a third of children have behavioural problems at 5 years post-transplant: neurocognitive and neuropsychiatric support are important), noncompliance in adolescents and altered lifestyle requirements (need to get routine exercise—3–4 times a week, for at least 30 minutes, stop smoking, maintain a heart-healthy diet avoiding saturated fats and cholesterol).

Telemedicine

Advances in telecommunications technology, with the widespread introduction of integrated services digital network (ISDN) lines, allows transmission of echocardiogram images from peripheral to tertiary centres, with a paediatric cardiologist interpreting the transmitted images and guiding the performance of the scan to ensure that the best possible views are obtained. This approach has been used successfully in many countries. The defects that must be correctly diagnosed early include those causing cyanosis, obstructive lesions of the left and right heart and total anomalous pulmonary venous drainage (TAPVD), the latter providing the greatest diagnostic difficulty. The other two lesions that can be difficult to diagnose are coarctation of the aorta (obtaining good aortic arch views can be challenging) and patent ductus arteriosus (if present, ascertaining how much it contributes clinically).

Cardiac imaging

Positron emission tomography (PET) scanning is being used to assess the cross-sectional functioning of the myocardium after significant cardiac insults related to coronary artery problems such as in Kawasaki disease, corrective surgery for congenital heart disease (coronary occlusion can complicate the arterial switch procedure for transposition of the great arteries) and coronary arteriopathy seen in cardiac transplantation (here, there may be few clues; chest pain does not occur as the heart is denervated). Cardiac PET studies can assess regional substrate metabolism, chemical recognition (of receptors and enzymes) and regional blood flow. It can accurately differentiate between areas that can be reperfused (so-called 'stunned' areas) and infarcted areas from irreversible ischaemia.

Short case

The cardiovascular system

One of the most common examination cases, a cardiac case is expected to be performed extremely well. A slick, complete examination, followed by a logical, relevant differential diagnosis and sensible interpretation of chest X-rays and electrocardiograms are all minimum requirements.

Introduce yourself. Stand back and give a brief general description of the child. Note any dysmorphic features (Down, Turner's, Noonan's, Williams, Marfan's, Alagille syndromes) and general growth parameters (in particular failure to thrive or short stature). Then fully expose the child's chest. Look for any scars (so as not to miss a Blalock shunt which may be associated with an absent radial pulse on that side) or chest asymmetry. Pick up the child's hands, check the fingernails for clubbing and splinter haemorrhages, and check the toenails. Feel the radial pulse, noting the rate, amplitude and character; lift the arm up to detect hyperdynamic pulsation (e.g. aortic incompetence). Note the respiratory rate at this stage (left ventricular failure). Feel both radial pulses and femoral pulses: absent femoral pulses, with normal or increased brachial pulses, suggest coarctation (brachiofemoral delay is found only in adults with coarctation.) Next, ask to measure the blood pressure in both upper limbs. Usually the examiners will give the values, but at other times you may be given a sphygmomanometer to measure it yourself. Check the jugular venous pressure (JVP) in older children, by sitting them at 45 degrees in the standard manner.

Look at the conjunctivae for pallor and the sclera for icterus (haemolysis associated with artificial valves). Look at the tongue and state whether the patient is cyanosed; if uncertain, comment on the need to look again in natural daylight, if the room is artificially lit. Avoid saying 'pink' or 'blue': say 'not cyanosed' or 'cyanosed'. Check the teeth for caries for risk of subacute bacterial endocarditis (SBE). So far, the examination should have taken less than 2 minutes.

Now, turn your attention to the chest. If not already done, check for scars and asymmetry carefully. At this point, lay the child down on the examination bed. Look for the apex beat and then palpate for it. Describe the location (make a show of counting down the intercostal spaces) and the quality of the impulse. Beware dextrocardia if the apex appears elusive. After the apex, feel the parasternal border and substernal region, for heaves, suprasternal and supraclavicular regions for thrills, and feel over the pulmonary area for palpable closure of the pulmonary valve (i.e. 'palpable S2').

By the time auscultation is performed, a short list of possibilities should have been formulated, based on previous findings, by considering the following points, as you proceed.

1. Cyanotic or acyanotic.
2. Heart failure or not heart failure.
3. Peripheral findings (pulses, blood pressure, JVP).
4. Praecordial findings.

Auscultation should commence at the apex, with the diaphragm of the stethoscope initially and then the bell (for diastolic murmurs). Listen at the apex, work across to, and up, the parasternal border, and listen over pulmonary and aortic areas. Listen to each component of the cardiac cycle carefully. Note the intensities of S1 and S2 and whether S2 splits normally with respiration. Listen for added sounds and then systolic and diastolic murmurs. Note radiation of any murmurs to axillae or carotids. Next, sit the child up and listen to any murmur's variation with this change in position. Listen with the child in full expiration for the subtle early diastolic murmur of aortic incompetence.

Listen to the back for radiation of any murmurs and for any pulmonary adventitious sounds (inspiratory crackles with left ventricular failure; variable findings with coexistent chest infection in Kartagener's primary ciliary dysmotility syndrome). Lay the child down again and examine the abdomen for hepatomegaly (congestive cardiac failure), pulsatile liver (tricuspid incompetence) and splenomegaly (SBE).

Then, feel for ankle oedema. Request the urinalysis for blood (SBE) and the temperature chart (SBE). If SBE does appear likely, request an ophthalmoscope to detect Roth spots.

Give a succinct differential diagnosis based on your clinical findings, and only after this should you request the chest X-ray and ECG.

You do not have to give a specific diagnosis immediately; this is fraught with danger. If, for example, you are sure that a patient has valvular aortic stenosis, you should say so, but if there is any uncertainty, it is prudent to give as a diagnosis 'left ventricular outflow tract obstruction' (LVOTO) and then proceed to delineate which of the various causes of LVOTO (supravalvular, valvular or subvalvular) is most likely and why.

Similarly, if a child is cyanosed and has a confusing array of murmurs, you do not have to give an anatomically correct diagnosis. It is better to start in general terms, such as: 'This child has complex cyanotic congenital heart disease'. If you have a reasonable idea of the likely anatomical diagnosis, say so, but if not, it is sensible to take each murmur in turn and give a brief differential diagnosis of each (provided these are relevant to a child with cyanotic congenital heart disease). When the chest X-ray and ECG have been examined, the precise diagnosis may become apparent.

Additional manoeuvres may be needed to clarify suspected diagnoses. The Valsalva manoeuvre is useful in identifying hypertrophic cardiomyopathy (HCM) as it increases the intensity of the murmur (via increased intrathoracic pressure, decreased venous return and hence decreased intracardiac volume and more severe LVOTO), and in mitral valve prolapse, where the murmur is also increased and the systolic click is heard earlier. Innocent systolic outflow tract murmurs decrease in intensity in response to the Valsalva manoeuvre.

Exercising the child is especially useful in bringing out a tricuspid diastolic murmur in an atrial septal defect (ASD); this is most easily achieved by having the child do several sit-ups. In patients with ventricular septal defects (VSDs) and ASDs, the appearance of a mid-diastolic murmur suggests a pulmonary blood flow at least twice that of the systemic circulation, and in patients with mitral or tricuspid incompetence, such a murmur suggests at least a moderate degree of regurgitation.

With any findings strongly suggestive of a specific diagnosis, make a point of going beyond simple diagnosis of the said lesion, and be aware of clinical signs indicating the severity of that lesion. For example, with a ventricular septal defect, assess the size of the shunt, as outlined above; with pulmonary stenosis, assess the severity by the timing of the peak of the murmur, associated presence or absence of a click, movement of S2 with respiration, and clinical signs of right ventricular hypertrophy.

With an infant or fractious toddler, the approach is different, and the order may need to be completely rearranged. Distant observation is very important, noting size, colour, respiratory rate and perfusion. It is appropriate to tell the examiners that you are going to start with auscultation while the baby is quiet; if the baby does become restless, a breast or bottle may be a life saver. With a very uncooperative child, the key is to do what you can, while you can, without becoming angry or overtly frustrated. Your approach to this is just as important as your differential diagnosis or ECG interpretation.

One final point concerns correct coinage in cardiac cases. Do not use abbreviations when presenting your finding or in your discussion: do not say 'VSD', say 'ventricular septal defect', and say 'electrocardiogram', not 'ECG'.

Figure 6.1 shows the major points as outlined above. A more comprehensive listing of possible findings on cardiovascular examination is given in Table 6.1.

Figure 6.1 The cardiovascular system

1. Introduce self

2. General inspection
Position patient: lying down
Well or unwell
Growth parameters
Dysmorphic syndromes
Scars
Chest asymmetry
Respiratory rate

3. Upper limbs
Nails
Clubbing
Pulses
Blood pressure

4. Head and neck
Jugular venous pressure
Eyes
- Conjunctival pallor (anaemia)
- Scleral icterus (fragmentation haemolysis with artificial valves)
Lips: cyanosis
Tongue: cyanosis
Teeth: caries

5. Chest
Inspect
Scars
Symmetry
Apical pulsation
Palpate
- Apex position (beware dextro-cardia) (count down the ribs)
- Heaves (parasternal, substernal, apical)
- Thrills (suprasternal, supra-clavicular)
- Liver (palpate edge and measure span by percussion)
- Enlarged (RVF)
- Pulsatile (tricuspid incompetence)
- Spleen: enlarged (SBE)

6. Lower limbs
Inspection
- Clubbing (if not already done)
- Splinter haemorrhages (if not done)
Palpation
- Ankle oedema (RVF)

7. Other
Urinalysis: blood (SBE)
Temperature chart (SBE)
Fundoscopy for Roth spots if SBE seems likely

8. Investigations
After presenting a differential diagnosis, request CXR / ECG

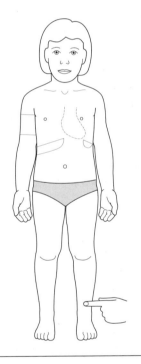

RVF = right ventricular failure; SBE = subacute bacterial endocarditis.

Table 6.1 Additional information: possible findings on cardiovascular examination

General observations

Height
- Short (Down, Noonan's, Turner's; heart disease causing failure to thrive, e.g. large atrioventricular canal)
- Tall (Marfan's; check arm span if you suspect this)

Weight: failure to thrive (congenital rubella, severe heart disease, cyanosis or congestive cardiac failure)

Head circumference: small (congenital rubella)

Dysmorphic syndromes: Down, Noonan's, Marfan's, Turner's, Williams, Alagille, neurofibromatosis type 1

Scars
- Median sternotomy (all open heart corrections)
- Lateral thoracotomy (e.g. coarctation repair, pulmonary artery banding, ligation of PDA or vascular ring, pulmonary artery reconstruction, shunts)
- Groin (cardiac catheters)

Chest asymmetry
- Left chest prominence (chronic right ventricular hypertrophy)
- Right chest prominence (dextrocardia with chronic ventricular hypertrophy)

Respiratory rate: tachypnoea with left ventricular hypertrophy

Upper limbs

Nails: check both hands and both feet
- Clubbing (cyanotic heart disease, SBE, suppurative lung disease—e.g. Kartagener). Note any differential clubbing (e.g. clubbed toes, normal fingers in Eisenmenger's syndrome with patent ductus)
- Splinter haemorrhages (SBE)

Pulses
- Rate, amplitude, character (lift arm to detect hyperdynamic pulsation of AI) and rhythm
- Radial (both sides, for radioradial delay)
- Brachial and femoral together (for brachiofemoral delay in older adolescents)
- Femorals (both sides): reduction of one femoral only is not due to coarctation, but to local trauma (cardiac catheter)

Blood pressure

Both upper limbs

All four limbs if any suggestion of coarctation

Jugular venous pressure (sit child at 45 degrees): elevated in right ventricular failure

---

AI = aortic incompetence; PDA = patent ductus arteriosus; SBE = subacute bacterial endocarditis.

Chest X-ray and electrocardiography

At the completion of the cardiac short case, it is customary to request the accompanying chest X-ray and electrocardiogram.

Chest X-ray (CXR)

When describing a CXR, first note the name and date, and then which side is marked right (the position of the gastric air bubble on the left can help unless there is complete situs inversus) to avoid the embarrassment of missing dextrocardia twice (once clinically and then again on the CXR). Then comment on the centring and penetration of the film, and the degree of inspiration. The cardiac diameter should be measured and compared to chest width at the level of the right hemidiaphragm (cardiothoracic ratio); normally this ratio is less than 50% (but up to 55–60% in neonates).

Next, the cardiac contour can be assessed, particularly for the size of the pulmonary artery and the position of the aortic arch. Then, the lung fields should be evaluated, with particular emphasis on pulmonary vascularity (see below). Finally the bony structures are assessed, especially for rib notching in children with possible coarctation.

In children with cyanotic heart disease, a major clue is whether the pulmonary vascularity is increased or decreased.

Increased pulmonary vascularity occurs in the following:

1. Truncus arteriosus.
2. Total anomalous pulmonary venous drainage (TAPVD).
3. One condition of 'textbook interest', rarely seen outside the neonatal period nowadays, is transposition of the great arteries (TGA).

Decreased pulmonary vascularity occurs in the following:

1. Pulmonary atresia.
2. Tricuspid atresia.
3. Ebstein's anomaly.
4. Tetralogy of Fallot: 25% of these have a right-sided aortic arch.
5. Another cause is critical pulmonary stenosis associated with a right-to-left shunt in the neonatal period, but this again is more of 'textbook interest'.

Electrocardiography

Start by determining the rate (roughly; do not waste time), rhythm and then the axis. Next, systematically look at the P waves, the P-R interval, then the QRS complexes, the S-T interval and finally the T waves. Several patterns give important clues to the diagnosis. The age of the child must always be taken into consideration. The following lists outline several important points regarding age-related changes and clues to certain diagnoses.

Axis
1. Birth: +60 to +180 degrees.
2. 1 year: +0 to +100 degrees.
3. 10 years: +30 to +90 degrees.

Right-axis deviation (RAD)—i.e. axis at +90 to +180 degrees (after infancy)—is often associated with right ventricular hypertrophy, whereas left-axis deviation (LAD) has numerous causes including atrioventricular canal, tricuspid atresia and conduction anomalies.

Definitions of ventricular hypertrophy
Right ventricular hypertrophy
1. R greater than S in V1 after 1 year.
2. Upright T wave over right praecordial leads after 1 week of age.
3. sV6 greater than 15 mm at 1 week.
4. sV6 greater than 10 mm at 6 months.
5. sV6 greater than 5 mm at 1 year.

Left ventricular hypertrophy
1. sV1 + rV6 greater than 30 mm to 1 year.
2. sV1 + rV6 greater than 40 mm after 1 year.

Causes of atrial hypertrophy
Right atrial hypertrophy (RAH) is seen in the following:
1. Tricuspid atresia.
2. Complex congenital heart disease.

Table 6.2 Electrocardiographic findings and associated pathologies

If the finding is	Think of
Prolonged P-R interval	Endocardial cushion defect Ebstein's anomaly Acute rheumatic fever Congenital block (maternal SLE)

Partial RBBB
  with LAD
  with RAD
  with RAH, delta waves
	
	Ostium primum ASD
	Ostium secundum ASD
	Ebstein's anomaly

Complete RBBB	Post-ventriculotomy
LAD	Endocardial cushion defect Tricuspid atresia Hypertrophic cardiomyopathy Inlet VSD

RAH
  without RVH
 	
  with axis over 90 degrees
	Ebstein's anomaly
	Tricuspid atresia (LAD)
	Pulmonary atresia with intact septum
	Truncus arteriosus
	Tetralogy with large VSD

Deep Q waves	Hypertrophic cardiomyopathy Transposition of great arteries Anomalous left coronary artery

ASD = atrial septal defect; LAD = left axis deviation; RAD = right axis deviation; RAH = right atrial hypertrophy; RVH = right ventricular hypertrophy; VSD = ventricular septal defect.

3. Hypoplastic right heart.
4. Ebstein's anomaly.
5. Pulmonary atresia.

Left atrial hypertrophy (LAH) is seen in the following:
1. Mitral valve disease.
2. Cardiomyopathy.
3. Large patent ductus arteriosus.

QRS and Q wave abnormalities
Prolonged QRS is seen in the following:
1. Bundle branch block (especially postoperatively).
2. Ventricular hypertrophy.
3. Others: digoxin therapy; hyperkalaemia; hypothyroidism.

Q waves occur in the following circumstances:
Normal in leads II, III, aVf, V5, V6, and abnormal in other leads. Think of:
1. Hypertrophic cardiomyopathy.
2. Congenitally corrected transposition.
3. Anomalous left coronary artery.

Particularly large Q waves occur in:
1. Septal hypertrophy.
2. Infarction.

Specific diagnosis by ECG

Although a pathophysiological approach is of course preferable to a mnemonic or list in cardiology, ECGs do lend themselves to the latter. Table 6.2 is one such list, but rather than rote-learning this, the candidate should endeavour to understand the pathophysiology and always consider the ECG in the context of the clinical findings.

Endocrinology

Long cases

Congenital adrenal hyperplasia

Background information

Congenital adrenal hyperplasia (CAH) refers to a number of inherited defects in adrenal steroidogenesis. The most common of these is 21-hydroxylase deficiency (21-OHD), which is caused by a range of mutations in one gene—the CYP21 gene on chromosome 6p21.3, which codes for 21-hydroxylase. The end result is a lack of cortisol (and usually aldosterone) synthesis by the adrenal cortex. This leads to increased adrenocortical stimulation by hypothalamic corticotropin-releasing hormone (CRH) and pituitary adrenocorticotropic hormone (ACTH), which induces adrenal glandular hyperplasia, hence the term CAH. This long case deals with the common form of CAH due to 21-OHD.

CAH can present in two forms: early onset (classic) and late onset (non-classic). The CAH heterozygote carrier rate has been estimated at around 1.5% for classic CAH and at around 10% for non-classic CAH. The incidence of 21-OHD is 1:10,000 to 1:15,000 live births.

The majority (up to three-quarters) of patients with CAH have the classic salt-losing form and can develop adrenal insufficiency in the early weeks of life, which can be lethal. This is due to a lack of adequate aldosterone production to maintain normal sodium balance. A further result of the excess adrenal stimulation in CAH is synthesis of adrenal sex hormone precursors and their by-products. This variably leads to andro-genisation of females in utero, or to virilisation of either sex later in childhood.

Females with classic early-onset CAH are born with ambiguous genitalia. The degree of virilisation of the external genitalia is scored by the Prader scale (see the short case on ambiguous genitalia in this chapter). Males with classic early onset CAH appear normal at birth, but then deteriorate with adrenal insufficiency after 2–3 weeks. Females with late onset CAH may present with clitoromegaly, early development of pubic hair, increased growth rate, gynaecological problems such as oligomenorrhoea, abnormal menses, infertility, hirsutism and acne. Males with late onset CAH may develop early penile growth, pubic hair, increased growth rate and increased musculature.

Deficiency of cytochrome P450 enzyme 21-hydroxylase causes 90% of CAH cases. Ten types of mutation in CYP21 account for more than 90% of affected cases, although well over 60 have been described, with more than half involving nucleotide substitutions. Inherited as autosomal recessive, CAH demonstrates a heterogeneous phenotype, with concordance between phenotype and genotype. The Human Gene Mutation Database, Cardiff (<www.hgmd.org>) lists all known mutations.

Macro-deletions, comprising a quarter of CAH cases, always cause a severe salt-wasting form. Patients with classic salt-wasting CAH possess two mutant alleles that obliterate 21-OH activity (CYP21 deletion). Those with a splice mutation in intron 2 have significantly diminished 21-OH activity as well as salt-wasting.

Patients with simple virilising CAH tend to have one severe mutant allele and one moderate mutant allele. The latter can include the point mutation Ile172Asn in exon 4, which permits about 2% of normal enzyme activity.

The majority of cases with non-classic CAH have two mildly compromised alleles; many are associated with a valine-to-leucine missense mutation at amino acid position 281 (termed Val281Leu) in exon 7, which permits around 50% of normal enzyme activity. Other missense mutations that can cause non-classic CAH include Pro453Ser and Pro30Leu.

Genotyping of CYP21 can be useful in establishing the requirement for gluco-corticoid and mineralocorticoid replacement. In over 90% of cases, phenotype correlates with genotype. Many children with CAH are compound heterozygotes. These children tend to present with clinical features more in keeping with the less deleterious allele.

Diagnosis

CAH can be diagnosed at different ages, as follows.

Prenatal diagnosis of CAH with 21-OHD

Only performed in mothers with a previously affected child with CAH, prenatal diagnosis of CAH with 21-OHD is possible by determining amniotic fluid (AF) hormone levels, by means of human leukocyte antigen (HLA) typing of chorionic villus cells or AF cells, or through molecular genetic studies of chorionic cells or AF cells. The latter is preferred, analysing DNA for CYP21B, C4 and HLA class I and II genes. Currently most centres analyse fetal P450c21B genes from chorionic villus cells (obtained at 8–9 weeks) or amniocytes, as well as karyotyping. For accurate diagnosis, correct molecular genetic analysis of the index case is needed, along with molecular genetic analysis of the parents, with the parents' hormone profiles. De novo mutations occur in around 1% of patients with CYP21B mutations.

Neonatal diagnosis of CAH with 21-OHD

This may follow neonatal screening. Screening occurs in nearly 20 states in the USA. The sample is taken (ideally) between days 2 and 3 of life, 17-OHP levels are analysed and those above cutoff levels have diagnostic testing: false negatives are very rare; false positives can occur in premature, small-for-gestational-age or very unwell infants. In classic 21-OHD, 17-OHP serum levels are markedly elevated. Levels of 17-OHP are normally high in the first 2–3 days after birth, then fall in healthy babies by day 3, but levels rise in those affected by 21-OHD. In affected infant girls, serum testosterone may be elevated, and in infants of either sex androstenedione is elevated.

Presentation at 1–4 weeks

Neonates with 21-OHD may present with ambiguous genitalia (affected girls) or adrenal crisis (especially affected boys) between 1 and 4 weeks. Diagnosis of patients with symptoms of classic CAH is by elevated serum 17-OHP (and in those with ambiguous genitalia, ultrasound of the abdomen and genital tract: for more details see the short case on ambiguous genitalia in this chapter).

Non-classical forms of 21-OHD

Patients presenting with the non–classical forms of 21-OHD usually manifest with androgen excess (late onset). If the basal 17-OHP level is unconvincing, further investigation using the ACTH stimulation test can be considered. The level of serum 17-OHP should show a significant rise 60 minutes after an intravenous bolus of ACTH. The cortisol is also measured: the 17-OHP–cortisol ratio will be elevated .

CAH due to 11 beta-hydoxylase deficiency

Patients with CAH due to 11 beta–hydroxylase deficiency (11β-OHD) may present in a similar way to 21-OHD, with virilisation of the affected female fetus. These patients, however, can also present with hypertension, due to accumulation of salt-retaining aldosterone precursors. Paradoxically, some infants with 11β-OHD are transiently salt losers and become hypertensive at a later stage. They also have mildly elevated 17-OHP levels and can easily be misdiagnosed as 21-OHD unless a careful urine steroid analysis is performed by gas chromatography. 11β-OHD represents around 8% of CAH cases.

Other forms of CAH

Patients with other forms of CAH (<2% of CAH patients) may present at various ages. For discussion, see the short case on ambiguous genitalia in this chapter.

History

Presenting complaint

Reason for current admission.

Initial diagnosis

1. Initial symptoms
   Neonate—ambiguous genitalia, adrenal insufficiency, vomiting, seizures (from hyponatraemia or hypoglycaemia); near-death episodes resembling SIDS have been reported.
   Older child—symptoms associated with virilisation, recurrent sinus or pulmonary infections (from poor response to stress of infection).
   Adolescent—syncope or near syncope, hypotension (21-OHD); hypertension (11β-OHD); tempo of onset (developing over days, weeks or months before diagnosis).
2. Immediate pre-diagnosis symptoms
   Symptoms of *adrenocortical failure*: e.g. lethargy, disorientation (cortisol lack), salt craving (aldosterone lack), weakness, anorexia, vomiting, weight loss (lack of cortisol and aldosterone).
   Symptoms associated with *virilisation*: e.g. girls—clitoromegaly, increased pigmentation of genital skin, pubic hair, increased height, abnormal menses, hirsutism, acne, oligomenorrhoea; boys—increased penile growth, increased pigmentation of genital skin, pubic hair, increased height, increased muscle growth.

3. Where, when and how the diagnosis was made, length of hospital stay, education given, any treatment of mother with steroids while embryo in utero, treatment in hospital, treatment at discharge.

Progress of disease

1. Details of subsequent hospitalisations (frequency, indications, usual length of stay, usual outcome).
2. Complications of disease: e.g. need for corrective genital surgery, episodes of adrenal crisis, abnormal growth and development, psychosexual developmental aspects (for example, girls with male type play, physical aggression, low interest in babies or maternal nurturing behaviours; increased incidence of lesbian relationships), inadequately treated hyperandrogenism, hypoglycaemic reactions.
3. Complications of treatment: e.g. overtreatment with steroids causing deceleration of linear growth, too much fludrocortisone causing hypertension, degree of control (number of episodes of adrenal crisis).
4. Monitoring of disease: how often seen in clinic, usual investigations performed, how often seen by local doctor.
5. Changes in management: e.g. usual increases in steroid dosage on sick days.
6. At what age was the patient administering his or her own steroids?
7. Compliance: e.g. previous refusal to take steroids in teenage males.

Current status

1. General health: lethargic or energetic.
2. Current medications: type (e.g. hydrocortisone, fludrocortisone, salt supplement, antiandrogens dose), regimen, (how much, when, given by whom, modifications with intercurrent illness), salt craving (not enough fludrocortisone), hypertension (too much fludrocortisone), compliance with treatment.
3. Adrenal insufficiency: how often, what symptoms (e.g. vomiting, lethargy, crying, convulsions, near-syncope, syncope, loss of consciousness), usual precipitants, anticipatory strategies for prevention, response.
4. Hypoglycaemia: any episodes, any suggestion of this (e.g. sweating, pallor, tremulousness, hunger, headache, odd behaviour, lethargy, crying, bad temper, lack of coordination, dizziness, vomiting, convulsions, loss of consciousness).
5. Symptoms attributable to virilisation: acne, increased linear growth, amenorrhoea.
6. Other problems: e.g. adolescent self-image, compliance problems.

Social history

1. Impact on child: self-image, reaction of school friends, effects (e.g. virilisation), coping with taking steroids, amount of school missed.
2. Impact on siblings: sibling rivalry, risk of CAH.
3. Impact on parents: family finances, employment, concern regarding future complications, genetic counselling.
4. Social supports: parents groups, access to social worker, government benefits obtained.
5. Coping: who attends the clinic with the patient, level of education of child and parents, contingency plans for intercurrent illnesses or severe adrenal crisis causing loss of consciousness, access to local doctor, paediatrician, hospital.

Family history

Record details of other affected members.

Immunisation

List all routine immunisations.

Examination

For a neonate, see the short case on ambiguous genitalia and for an older child the short case on precocious puberty (in this chapter). The main areas to focus on are sequential growth parameters and pubertal development (Tanner staging), pigmentation and blood pressure.

Management

All patients with CAH, regardless of type, require treatment with glucocorticoids. These replace cortisol (which is deficient) and provide negative feedback, suppressing ACTH secretion. This then prevents continued adrenal stimulation, inhibiting excess androgen production (as 17-OHP is not available as a substrate for excess androgen production; this prevents virilisation). Patients with the salt-losing form also require mineralo-corticoid replacement to normalise the sodium balance associated with aldosterone deficiency. In the past, surgical procedures directed at correcting virilised genitalia have been performed in the US and UK, but not in Australia. This is now a very controversial area, as previous surgical approaches have led to some loss of clitoral sensation. The overall principles of treatment are given below.

Control of steroid requirements

Glucocorticoids

The usual preparation used is oral hydrocortisone (this is the preferred hormone because cortisone is only active after conversion to hydrocortisone in the liver). It is given at a dosage of 10–20 mg/metre squared per 24 hours, in three divided doses, as hydrocortisone has a short half-life of 90–120 minutes. The usual doses are: for infants, 2.5–5 mg three times a day; for children, 5–10 mg three times a day. The morning dose is given as early as possible to blunt the early morning corticotropin release. The dose can be adjusted according to symptoms, signs, weight and height velocity, and tests (serum 17-OHP and plasma renin activity, PRA).

Mineralocorticoids

These are required for patients with disturbed electrolyte regulation (salt losers) and elevated PRA. The usual preparation used is fludrocortisone acetate (also called 9 alpha-fluorocortisol; fluorination at the 9 alpha position enhances all biological actions of corticosteroids), given at a dosage of 0.05–0.3 mg daily. The dose can be adjusted according to blood pressure and PRA.

Additional salt supplementation (6 mmol/kg/day sodium chloride) may be required. This is necessary in almost all cases occurring in the first three months of life and should be given throughout the first year in very hot climates.

Non–salt-losing CAH

Non–salt-losing CAH, especially in boys, may lead to a bone age more than 5 years in advance of their chronological age when these patients are first diagnosed. Starting glucocorticoid therapy can slow growth and bone maturation towards normal rates. Almost inevitably, treatment of such children with hydrocortisone precipitates the onset of true puberty. This is how it happens. Before treatment with hydrocortisone, the elevated androgens exert a 'maturing' effect on the hypothalamus, but gonadotropin secretion is suppressed by the androgens. When the androgen levels are suddenly suppressed by the hydrocortisone treatment, gonadotropins are released from the pituitary gland. This form of precocious puberty must then be managed with a long-acting luteinising hormone-releasing hormone (LHRH) analogue, in combination with hydrocortisone and fludrocortisone.

Most non–salt-losers do in fact excrete excessive salt in the urine, even though they are asymptomatic or nearly so. If they have high PRA levels, they should be treated with fludrocortisone.

Other potential approaches to treatment

The combination of an antiandrogen (blocking androgen effects) and an aromatase inhibitor (blocks conversion of androgen to oestrogen) may require a lower dose of hydrocortisone. Adrenalectomy has been advocated to eliminate the problem of inadequate adrenal androgen suppression. Synthetic blockers of corticotropin-releasing hormone and corticotropin receptors could achieve pharmacological adrenalectomy.

Prevention of acute complications

Adrenal crises can be averted by anticipatory strategies. All patients with CAH need extra steroid cover for stress: this includes any acute medical condition (such as gastroenteritis, other viral illnesses), any surgical procedure requiring an anaesthetic, and any significant orthopaedic injury (such as a major fracture). Treatment may include hydrocortisone 25–100 mg parenterally (IM or IV), repeated 4–6 hourly until recovery from the acute aspect of the illness: triple the usual dose for 2 days, then double the usual dose for 3 days.

Optimum growth and development

Timely diagnosis of CAH may prevent precocious puberty leading to short stature. Adequate education of patient and parents is essential to ensure compliance with recommended treatment. It should be explained to parents that the doses of hydrocortisone and fludrocortisone must be adjusted to be correct for each child and that correct doses allow normal growth, normal response to stress and illness, and normal pubertal development. Parents must be made aware of the dangers of too little or too much hydrocortisone and fludrocortisone: too little hydrocortisone leads to ongoing pituitary stimulation and ongoing overproduction of androgens, while too little fludrocortisone leads to salt craving and low blood sodium; too much hydrocortisone leads to slowed growth, and too much fludrocortisone leads to high blood pressure. They need to know that the normal hydrocortisone dose should be tripled at the start of any illness and that if the child needs surgery for any reason, they must inform both the anaesthetist and the surgeon that extra hydrocortisone is needed to cover that stressful procedure.

Psychological support

The treating paediatrician should ensure adequate access to appropriate social supports. In females who were born with ambiguous genitalia, who have had surgical correction for virilised external genitalia as a neonate, or who have virilisation, issues regarding sexuality may need to be discussed. Surgery should be avoided between the ages of 2 and 12 years as far as possible. Girls should not be subjected to repeated genital examinations. Clinical photography should be banned.

The following basic principles are important:

1. Discourage use of the disease for manipulation.
2. Minimise the number of days off school.
3. Involve child in management of his or her CAH as appropriate to age and ability.

4. In times of 'adolescent rebellion', support and encourage; never resort to threats.
5. Identify and treat negative family responses to CAH, including overindulgence, overanxiousness, neglect and disinterest, resentment and overcontrolling parents.
6. When the initial diagnosis is made, be aware of depression in patients, siblings and parents, and counsel accordingly.

For the purposes of the long case, the usual problem is that of a noncompliant adolescent. Unfortunately, it is in adolescence—the least receptive time of the patient's life—that it is crucial to avoid serious complications. For a teenager, immediate peer acceptance, which may involve nights out at parties or hotels, far outweighs the long-term benefits of adequate steroid replacement. Most teenagers with CAH require additional emotional support, which may be achieved through attendance at discussion groups or talking one-on-one with a clinical psychologist. Problems affecting adolescents can be foreseen and discussed with the parents before they occur. Generally, parents should be encouraged to emphasise the positive aspects of adequate control, to explain the need for increased steroid dosage during illness, and to be supportive and avoid chastisement during rebellious episodes. By 18 years of age, most adolescents will be more responsible in caring for their CAH.

Social supports

All families of children with CAH should have access to an experienced social worker. The disease represents a significant financial burden for many families and the social worker can make them aware of the various government benefits to which they may be entitled. Contact with CAH groups will allow access to many helpful people and ideas.

Routine follow-up

Children with CAH should be seen every 3 to 4 months. On each occasion, the child's growth (height and weight percentiles), Tanner staging, blood pressure and evidence of any complications should be documented, and then managed accordingly. Investigations should include serum 17-OHP, PRA and electrolytes. Bone age should be checked annually.

Types of corticosteroids

The examiners will expect you to be familiar with the various types of steroids and their equivalents. Table 7.1 is a brief guide; refer to the latest *MIMS*, *British National Formulatory* or equivalent publication for the names of the various preparations available.

Table 7.1		
Steroid	**Relative glucocorticoid activity**	**Relative mineralocorticoid activity**
Hydrocortisone (cortisol)	1	1
Cortisone acetate (11-deoxycortisol)	0.8	0.8
Prednisone	4	0.8
Prednisolone	4	0.8
Methylprednisolone (6 alpha-methylprednisolone)	5	0.5
Fludrocortisone (9 alpha-fluorocortisol)	10	125
Betamethasone (9 alpha-fluoro-16 beta-methylprednisolone)	25	0
Dexamethasone (9 alpha-fluoro-16 alpha-methylprednisolone)	25	0

CAH prenatal diagnosis and intervention

This area may be mentioned in the long case discussion. Prenatal treatment of CAH attributable to 21-OHD by administration of corticosteroids (dexamethasone) to the mother is most commonly performed in females with a previously affected child. Informed consent must be obtained from the parents before prenatal treatment is contemplated. There are possible maternal adverse effects with CAH, the genital outcome is variable and there may be long-term effects on children that are presently unknown. Masculinisation of the external genitalia begins at 6–7 weeks' gestation; if treatment before this suppresses the fetal pituitary–adrenal axis it could prevent ambiguous genitalia. Of reported cases where prenatal treatment has occurred, it was successful in three-quarters of them (one-third normal genitalia, two-thirds mildly virilised) and unsuccessful in a quarter.

Maternal complications from dexamethasone have included features of Cushing's syndrome, marked weight gain, irritability, mood swings, hypertension and significant striae with permanent scarring. These adverse effects occurred in about one-third of women treated until delivery; of these women, one-third would not undergo such treatment again in a future pregnancy. The diagnostic tests (DNA for CYP21B, C4 and HLA class I and II genes; analysing fetal P450c21B genes from chorionic villus cells) are obtained at 8–9 weeks' gestation. This means that treatment has to be commenced (at 5 weeks) before it is known what sex the fetus is (at 9 weeks) and whether the fetus has CAH. If the fetus is a male or an unaffected female, maternal treatment can be ceased. This means that eight mothers and babies will have to be treated to prevent the disease in one baby, as only one in eight will be an affected female.

Mothers who have previously had some medical conditions themselves—such as psychiatric diagnoses, hypertension or diabetes—should not be treated. If mothers do opt for treatment, the usual dose is 20–25 mcg/kg/day in two or three divided doses, started no later than the ninth week of gestation. Maternal monitoring must continue throughout pregnancy, including serum oestriol to determine adequacy of fetal adrenal suppression and fasting blood sugar monthly. The efficacy and safety of this treatment are yet to be defined adequately.

Management of acute adrenocortical insufficiency (adrenal crisis)

Candidates can thoroughly explore their understanding and practical application of the underlying pathophysiology of CAH through discussion of a hypothetical presentation of the long-case patient with CAH in adrenal crisis.

Adrenal crisis is most commonly seen with an intercurrent illness. Precipitating stresses include febrile illnesses, vomiting and diarrhoea, surgery or anaesthesia. Symptoms are attributable to cortisol deficiency (lethargy, disorientation), aldosterone deficiency (acute dehydration and collapse, salt craving, diarrhoea), or deficiency of both (nausea, vomiting, weight loss, muscular weakness).

Signs include shock, dehydration, muscular weakness, hypotension, decreased pulse pressure (dehydration, decreased vasomotor tone). Examination should include a finger-prick blood glucose level. Hypoglycaemia occurs from decreased gluconeogenesis. Investigations should include diagnostic pre-treatment blood and urine chemistry—decreased serum sodium and chloride, along with increased urinary Na loss, increased serum K, raised blood urea, low blood glucose, acidosis on blood gas. An ECG may demonstrate low-voltage, wide PR interval, peaked T waves from hyperkalaemia due to lack of aldosterone. Plasma renin activity (PRA) is elevated in mineralocorticoid deficiency and ACTH is elevated. Electrolyte abnormalities take a few days to develop and may not be present in acute crisis.

Immediate management

1. Assess and secure airway, breathing, circulation (the ABCs).
2. Insert IV cannula, take blood as above.
3. Restore circulating volume with infusion of normal saline (isotonic, 0.9%) with added glucose to make up to 5% glucose. Start with a 20 mL/kg bolus. Correct hypoglycaemia. Aim to replace fluid and electrolytes over next 24–48 hours.
4. Give bolus hydrocortisone IV (or IM if IV access is difficult):
   Dose under 2 years—25–50 mg.
   Dose 2–5 years—50–100 mg.
   Dose over 5 years—100–200 mg.
   Repeat hydrocortisone dose 6-hourly. Although both cortisol and aldosterone are low, only cortisol is needed during acute treatment. Avoid corticosteroids with negligible mineralocorticoid activity (e.g. dexamethasone) during resuscitation.
5. Hyperkalaemia may need correction with insulin and glucose.
6. Treat precipitating stress: sepsis, trauma.

Diabetes mellitus

There have been a number of recent advances in the knowledge, understanding and management of type 1 diabetes (insulin-dependent diabetes mellitus, IDDM).

- The incidence of IDDM is rising worldwide, and it is presenting at a younger age.
- The use of genetically engineered human insulins has enhanced care.
- Development of insulin analogues, both rapidly acting (lispro and aspart) and long-acting (insulin glargine), has expanded management options.
- Insulin infusion pumps are being used more in children than previously.
- Devices for continuous glucose measurement have been developed.
- There have been advances in understanding the interplay between genetic suscept-ibility and environmental factors in the pathogenesis.
- It is now recognised that the presence of diabetes-related autoantibodies in young children is a major risk factor for developing IDDM in the future.
- Cure is achievable with islet transplantation and new immunosuppressive regimens, but no treatment has been found, as yet, to prevent IDDM.

Diabetic children and adolescents represent a large and readily available group of patients who are frequently suitable as long cases. They may have problems related to inadequate control of their disease, compliance with treatment (especially adolescents), prevention of complications, difficult-to-manage behavioural problems, associated coexistent diseases such as autoimmune thyroid disease or coeliac disease, or other underlying chronic illnesses such as cystic fibrosis or beta-thalassaemia major.

Background information

IDDM affects 1 in 1000 children (and 1 in 400 by adolescence). Incidence increases with age. The main genetic factor determining susceptibility to IDDM lies within the major histocompatibility complex (termed IDDM1). There is an association with certain HLA haplotypes: more than 90% of patients with IDDM have HLA-DR3 and/or HLA-DR4 (class II antigens located on the short arm of chromosome 6, at 6p21); 55% have a DR3/DR4 combination, most commonly DR4-DQ8/DR3-DQ2

(1 in 5 in families of diabetics versus 1 in 25 of the general population). DR3/DR4 heterozygosity is seen most frequently in children who develop IDDM under 5 years of age. One non–HLA gene is recognised as contributing to around 10% of the family aggregation of IDDM: this is termed IDDM2 and is situated on chromosome 11p5.5. This locus maps to a variable number of tandem nucleotide repeats (VNTR) of the insulin gene. Different sizes of the VNTR are associated with a risk of IDDM, the long form of VNTR being associated with protection from IDDM. At least 17 inherited susceptibility loci for IDDM are known.

Sibling studies have shown that approximately two-thirds of the susceptibility to developing IDDM is linked to the HLA system. Compared to the proband, identical twins have a 40–50% chance of developing diabetes, HLA identical siblings have a 15–20% risk, HLA haploidentical siblings a 5–8% risk, and non-identical siblings only a 1–2% risk. The role of viral agents in the aetiology has been discussed for years. Children with congenital rubella have a far greater incidence than the general population: this is the only environmental trigger conclusively associated with IDDM. Other environmental factors (e.g. cow's milk protein) continue to be studied. Recent reports suggest some increased risk from early ingestion of cereal or gluten.

IDDM is associated with other autoimmune-type diseases (such as Hashimoto's thyroiditis, Addison's disease, primary ovarian failure, vitiligo) and with coeliac disease. However, the role of autoantibodies in the pathogenesis of IDDM has not been established. IDDM is considered a T-cell-mediated disease; islet tissue from patients with recent-onset IDDM shows insulitis, with an infiltrate made up of CD4 and CD8 T-lymphocytes and macrophages (and anti-C3 treatment in mice can prevent IDDM).

The development of IDDM in relatives of IDDM patients can be predicted by detecting islet-related antibodies; detection of two or more autoantibodies (GADA, IA-2, or insulin autoantibodies) has a positive predictive value of more than 90%.

Diagnosis

Type 1 diabetes can be diagnosed in children as follows:

- Patients with the 'classic' symptoms of IDDM, namely the triad of polydypsia, polyuria and weight loss despite polyphagia, are diagnosed by having a random blood sugar level (BSL; the commonly used term for plasma glucose level) above 11 mmol/L. Some units recommend a level of 14 mmol/L, but in practice the diagnosis is usually clear cut, and the level much higher than either figure.
- Asymptomatic patients require two criteria: a fasting BSL above 7.8 mmol/L, plus a 2-hour post-prandial BSL above 11 mmol/L. Alternatively a formal oral glucose tolerance test (GTT) demonstrating a sustained elevation in BSL above 11 mmol/L at 2 hours is required, as well as a similarly elevated intervening value taken between the time the glucose load (which is 1.75 g/kg, up to 75 g) is given and the 2-hour value. Again, this is fairly theoretical, as doubtful cases requiring a GTT for diagnosis are very rare.

History

Presenting complaint

Reason for current admission.

Initial diagnosis

1. Initial symptoms: e.g. early symptoms preceding the classic triad, lack of weight gain, nocturia, behaviour change, altered school performance, changed vision (blurring), tempo of onset (developing over days, weeks or months pre-diagnosis).

2. Immediate pre-diagnosis symptoms: polydypsia, polyuria, weight loss despite polyphagia.
3. Symptoms associated with ketoacidosis: e.g. vomiting, abdominal pain, clouding of consciousness.
4. Where, when and how the diagnosis was made, length of hospital stay, education given, treatment in hospital, treatment at discharge.

Progress of disease

1. Details of subsequent hospitalisations (frequency, indications, usual length of stay, usual outcome).
2. Complications of disease: e.g. eye problems with cataracts, retinopathy, joint problems with limited joint mobility (LJM), severe hypoglycaemic reactions.
3. Complications of treatment (e.g. fat atrophy or hypertrophy, insulin allergic reactions); degree of control (number of episodes of ketoacidosis, frequency of hypoglycaemic symptoms).
4. Monitoring of disease: how often seen in clinic, usual investigations performed, how often seen by local doctor.
5. Changes in management: e.g. increase in insulin administration from daily to twice daily, twice daily with additional short/ultra-short-acting or basal bolus regimen, use of insulin pump, altered dosages due to occult nocturnal hypo-glycaemia, changeover from human insulin to analogues.
6. At what age did the patient begin to administer his or her own insulin.

Current status

1. General health: lethargic or energetic.
2. Insulin type, dose, regimen (which sort, how much, when, given by whom, where, rotation of sites; modifications with raised BSL, sporting activities, intercurrent illness or dining out), compliance with treatment.
3. Diet prescribed (whether portions/exchanges used, glycaemic index, recom-mended foods), diet actually taken, alcohol intake (adolescents), involvement of dietician, any restrictions (adhered to or not).
4. Hypoglycaemia: how often, what symptoms (e.g. sweating, pallor, tremulous-ness, hunger, headache, odd behaviour, lethargy, crying, bad temper, lack of coordination, dizziness, vomiting, convulsions, loss of consciousness, early morning headaches after nocturnal 'hypo', restless sleep); usual precipitants; anticipatory strategies for prevention of 'hypos'; response to 'hypos' such as taking fast-acting sugars (e.g. glass of orange juice with added sugar, glass of lemonade, jelly beans) followed by a small protein and complex carbohydrate snack (e.g. bread, biscuits); ever any need for intramuscular glucagon? (*Note*: if no 'hypos' have occurred, BSL may have been too high.) Any evidence of 'hypoglycaemia unawareness'?
5. Control: hypoglycaemia (see above); hyperglycaemia (e.g. any nocturia, polyuria, blurred vision, weight loss, excessive weight gain, disturbance of menstrual periods in postpubertal girls); BSL readings (usual levels, when performed, how often, by whom, response to high level); usual HbA$_{1c}$ levels; urine testing (how often, what indications); amount of school missed in the last few months, vaginal thrush, other infections such as pilonidal sinus, infected ingrown toenail.
6. Other problems: e.g. adolescent self-image, compliance issues.

Social history

1. Impact on child: self-image, reaction of school friends, coping with giving insulin, dietary restrictions, exercise, amount of school missed.
2. Impact on siblings: sibling rivalry, risk of diabetes.
3. Impact on parents: family finances, employment, concern regarding future complications, genetic counselling.
4. Social supports: Diabetes Association, access to social worker, government benefits obtained.
5. Coping: who attends the clinic with the patient, level of education of child and parents, contingency plans for intercurrent illnesses or severe hypoglycaemia causing loss of consciousness, access to local doctor/paediatrician/hospital.
6. Peer pressures, risk-taking behaviours.

Family history

Other affected members, other autoimmune diseases (e.g. thyroid disease).

Immunisation

Influenza vaccine (recommended).

Associated diseases

Autoimmune (e.g. thyroid disease), underlying chronic illness (e.g. cystic fibrosis, congenital rubella).

Examination

See short case on diabetes.

Management

This involves the use of insulin, diet and regular exercise with the following aims:

1. Control of BSL: maintaining close to normoglycaemia; see below.
2. Prevention of acute complications: e.g. hypoglycaemia, ketoacidosis.
3. Ensuring optimum growth and development.
4. Maintaining normal lifestyle.
5. Adequate education of patient and parents.
6. Early detection and treatment of associated disease (e.g. Hashimoto thyroiditis).
7. Provision of psychological support and counsel.
8. Ensuring adequate access to appropriate social supports.
9. Reducing long-term complications by maintaining good metabolic control.
10. Regular screening for complications and early intervention when they appear (ACE inhibitors for hypertension or proteinuria, etc).
11. No readmissions with IDDM.

Age-specific aspects of control

The expectations at different ages vary. There are three groups:

1. **Infants to preschoolers.** The main goal is to avoid hypoglycaemia and preserve cognitive function (in line with the findings of the Diabetes Control and Complication Trial [DCCT]). The acceptable range for BSLs at this age is between 6 and 15 mmol/L, and the HbA_{1c} between 8.0 and 9.5 gm%.

2. **School-age to puberty**. Again, avoidance of hypoglycaemia is a top priority. Acceptable ranges: BSL 4–10 mmol/L; HbA$_{1c}$ 8.0 gm%.
3. **Adolescence**. Acceptable ranges: BSL 4–8 mmol/L; HbA$_{1c}$ as low as possible. It may be that postpubertal control is more important than prepubertal; this is unclear.

Insulin therapy

Average dosage requirements are as follows:

1. 'Honeymoon' period: 0.5 units/kg/day (or less).
2. Preadolescent: 1.0 unit/kg/day.
3. Adolescent: 1.0–2.0 units/kg/day (increase with pubertal growth spurt and reduce later when growth has finished).

The 'honeymoon' period, which tends to commence about 2 weeks after diagnosis, occurs in about two-thirds of newly diagnosed patients (especially older boys); the nadir of insulin requirements is at an average of 13 weeks post-diagnosis.

Traditionally insulin has been given 30 minutes before a meal. The newer ultra-short-acting insulin analogue (insulin lispro) can be given with, or just after, the commencement of a meal. It has become apparent since the development of insulin lispro that the short-acting insulins may also be effective if given *with* the meal.

Candidates should be familiar with the various insulin regimens. These include:

1. Daily (longer-acting only, or mixed short and longer).
2. Twice daily (see below).
3. Twice daily with additional short or ultrashort.
4. Basal bolus (three pre-meal short or ultra-short, plus longer in evening; only used in motivated adolescents).
5. Premixed (biphasic) insulin (only used for noncompliance, or inability to mix insulin).
6. Insulin pumps.

The most common regimen is a twice-daily dosage based on the 'two-thirds/one-third' rule. The total daily insulin dosage is divided up as follows:

- *Two-thirds* is given in the *morning* (before breakfast).
- *One-third* is given in the *evening* (before dinner).

And for each time it is given:

- *Two-thirds* is given as *longer-acting* (intermediate) insulin.
- *One-third* is given as *short-acting* insulin.

This may give insufficient control (which may well be the case in the complicated long-case patient). Most newly diagnosed diabetics are started on the twice-daily regimen, although some very young patients may require only intermediate or long-acting insulin.

Types of insulin/insulin analogue

The examiners will expect you to be familiar with the various types of human insulin, the types of insulin analogues and their durations of action. The following is a brief guide, noting the action after subcutaneous (SC) injection; refer to the latest *MIMS* or equivalent publication for the names of the various preparations available.

Standard human insulins
Short-acting (clear) insulins (regular/soluble insulin)
1. Onset at 30–60 minutes.
2. Peak effect at 2–5 hours.
3. Total duration of 6–8 hours.

Intermediate-acting insulins (longer acting than regular/short)
These include isophane insulins, semilente and lente preparations.

1. Action of *isophane* insulins (complexed to fish protamine), after SC injection:
   a. Onset at 1–2 hours.
   b. Peak effect at 4–12 hours.
   c. Total duration of 16–24 hours.
2. Action of *semilente* insulins (complexed with zinc, amorphous), after SC injection:
   a. Onset at 1–2 hours.
   b. Peak effect at 4–8 hours.
   c. Total duration of 12–16 hours.
3. Action of *lente* insulins (complexed with zinc in two forms, amorphous (30%) and crystalline (70%), after SC injection:
   a. Onset at 1–2.5 hours.
   b. Peak effect at 6–12 hours.
   c. Total duration of 12–24 hours.

Long-acting insulins
There are two types of long-acting insulins, ultralente preparations (complexed with zinc; crystalline form only, thus longer-acting) and protamine zinc insulins.

1. Action of *ultralente* insulins, after SC injection:
   a. Onset at 2–4 hours.
   b. Peak effect at 6–30 hours.
   c. Total duration of 24–36 hours.
2. Action of *protamine* zinc insulins, after SC injection:
   a. Onset at 4–8 hours.
   b. Peak effect at 16 hours.
   c. Total duration of 36 hours.

Biphasic insulins
These are premixed preparations of short-acting insulin (comprising 25–30%, depending on the preparation) and intermediate-acting insulin (making up 70–75%).
   Action after SC injection:

1. Onset at 30 minutes.
2. Peak effect at 1–12 hours.
3. Total duration of 16–24 hours.

Insulin analogues
These can replicate the basal and prandial aspects of insulin replacement more accurately than human insulins. Appropriate use of insulin analogues allows more flexibility in timing of meals, snacks and exercise. Also, the occurrence of hypoglycaemia is less common with analogues.

Ultra-short-acting insulin analogues (insulin lispro, insulin aspart)

An ultra-short-acting analogue can be very useful in toddlers, as it can be given after food. It may improve management compliance with adolescents, and it can reduce nocturnal hypoglycaemia. It can be given as an additional dose during illness or when eating extra food. Disadvantages can include the rapid fall in blood sugar, which is especially a problem in toddlers. It does not suit all patients.

1. Onset at 5–15 minutes.
2. Peak effect at 30–120 minutes.
3. Total duration of 3.5–6 hours.

Long-acting insulin analogue (insulin glargine)

This is produced by substituting glycine for asparagine at position A21 of the insulin molecule, and by adding two arginine molecules at position B30; this produces a molecule that precipitates in the subcutaneous tissue at the injection site, forming a depot from which the analogue is released slowly.

1. Onset at 2–4 hours.
2. There is little peak effect: this is a 'peakless basal insulin'.
3. Total duration of 20–24 hours.

Newer insulin analogues

Insulin glulisine is an ultra-short-acting analogue with a similar profile to insulin lispro and insulin aspart. Insulin detemir is a long-acting analogue. It has a shorter time-action profile than insulin glargine and requires twice-daily injections. It has lower variability of absorption than intermediate-acting human insulins.

The glycaemic index (GI)

This measures how rapidly a foodstuff can raise the blood sugar. Glucose is the fastest carbohydrate available except for maltose. Glucose is given a value of 100; other carbohydrates are rated compared to glucose. Faster-acting carbohydrates have higher numbers and are useful to alleviate hypoglycaemia and to cover brief periods of exercise. Slower-acting carbohydrates are useful to prevent nocturnal hypoglycaemia, and for prolonged periods of exercise.

Other points about insulin

1. Ultra-short-acting insulin analogues do not suit all children; they may cause very sudden falls of BSL which can be dangerous in toddlers.
2. Insulin given intramuscularly has a higher peak and shorter duration than when given subcutaneously.
3. Insulin absorption varies with the site of the injection: it is best when injected into the abdominal wall, followed by upper limbs, and then lower limbs.
4. Insulin should not be injected into an area which is going to be exercised, so if playing tennis, inject into abdomen, but if doing sit-ups, inject into thigh.
5. Lipohypertrophy can occur when the same site is used repeatedly for injection. This can be avoided by ensuring rotation of injection sites.
6. Lipoatrophy is now of historical interest. It was due to impurities in the preparation, leading to local immune complex formation. This has been eliminated with the development of genetically engineered human insulin and insulin analogues. It was managed by injecting around the periphery of the atrophied area, aiming towards the central portion.

Specific problem areas

Intercurrent illness

Insulin must be given irrespective of illness, and adequate portions must be kept up (a portion contains 15 g carbohydrate), so that in the absence of recurrent vomiting an input of half a portion every hour is a fair guide, in conjunction with regular BSL measurements (2-hourly). If the BSL is above 15 mmol/L, then checking for ketonuria, avoidance of carbohydrates, maintenance of low-calorie fluids, and a stat dose of 20% of the usual daily insulin dose are appropriate. Some units recommend giving 20% of total daily requirements as short-acting insulin regularly, every 6 hours, and stopping the longer-acting insulin temporarily (for the duration of the illness). If there is recurrent vomiting or ketonuria, the BSL should be checked hourly, and admission to hospital may be appropriate. Note that ketonuria by itself does not indicate whether the patient is responding to the management. This is because the dipstick test actually measures acetoacetate and acetone, and as acidosis improves, beta-hydroxybutyrate is converted to acetoacetate, which suggests, incorrectly, that there is a lack of response, as the 'positive' test persists.

Insulin allergy

This has been virtually eliminated by recombinant human insulin and insulin analogues. Historically 3–5% of children with IDDM had clinical evidence of allergy, ranging from local reactions at the site of injection to anaphylaxis.

Insulin resistance

This has been virtually eliminated by the use of recombinant human insulin and insulin analogues, as with allergy above. It was due to development of IgG antibodies against insulin.

Hypoglycaemic episodes

The best treatment for hypoglycaemia is prevention, which is essentially anticipation of likely provoking circumstances, such as prolonged exercise (remember that low BSL readings can occur many hours after exercise).

Symptoms of a hypoglycaemic episode (e.g. tremor, hunger, sweating, pallor, confusion, headache) without access to a glucometer, or a BSL reading below 3 mmol/L, should be treated immediately. Fast-acting sugars should be given (e.g. half a glass of lemonade, four jelly beans, or two sugar cubes: each of these approximates half a portion) if consciousness is not impaired.

All family members should be instructed in intramuscular glucagon administration, in case loss of consciousness occurs. Generally, it takes 10 minutes or so before the child starts to feel better, so a delay of this duration should not prompt further amounts of fast-acting sugar to be given, which would result in hyperglycaemia.

If a meal is due within 30 minutes of such an episode, it should be given early. If not, then additional food should be given as a complex carbohydrate (e.g. a slice of bread or a banana).

Occult nocturnal hypoglycaemia can occur in association with early morning high blood sugar readings; this is believed to be due to the effect of insulin wearing off. Isophane insulins may peak around 1 a.m, thus a very low BSL can occur at this time, but by 6 or 7 hours later the BSL may be elevated. Endocrinologists no longer believe in the 'Somogyi phenomenon'. Nocturnal BSLs must be checked before attributing high early morning readings to insufficient evening insulin dosages. The importance of this is to recognise that the insulin dose should be decreased in the evening and not increased inappropriately by trying to 'chase' the hyperglycaemia.

All children with IDDM should have an identification bracelet stating that they are diabetic, their usual insulin requirements, the name of their usual doctor and the hospital they attend. If found unconscious, which will usually be due to a 'hypo', this will allow glucose to be administered. Hypoglycaemia-induced convulsions are common. Parents are advised to position the child appropriately, call an ambulance and administer IM glucagon. After any 'hypo', the patient and parents should ask why this particular episode happened.

Alternative modes of insulin delivery

Insulin pumps

These supply a basal infusion of insulin, with increases given at meal times. Generally, most patients have been disappointed by this method. Children under 12 may have technical difficulties operating these pumps themselves.

There is also a risk of superficial skin infections and abscesses at the infusion sites, plus a risk of ketoacidosis if insufficient short-acting insulin is infused or of hypoglycaemia if the converse occurs. The pumps can work well in an older, highly motivated adolescent, but after 6 months or so, initial metabolic improvement tends to fade.

Both ultra-short-acting insulin analogues can be administered by continuous infusion. A meta-analysis comparing analogues with standard human insulin found that analogues led to a small but significant reduction in glycosylated haemoglobin (HbA_{1c}) levels and less hypoglycaemia.

Insulin pens

These are popular with diabetic adolescents, as they allow insulin to be given easily and discreetly, particularly when dining out, or at other social outings.

Diet

Normalisation of diet is important. The usual caloric requirements are 1000 kilocalories plus 100 kilocalories per year of life: 50% of this should comprise carbohydrate, approximately 35% protein and 15% fat. Generally, the child can be given what he or she normally eats, with some degree of modification and adjustment of insulin dosage. The diet is planned using glycaemic index (GI) principles. There are few absolute restrictions. High carbohydrate, high fibre and low fat are preferable. The concept of 'portions' or 'exchanges' is less important than the use of the GI. The former terms describe set amounts of carbohydrate. One 'portion' contains 15 g carbohydrate, which is equivalent to 60 kilocalories. (This is not universal; in some diabetic clinics, the size of a portion is 10 g carbohydrate.)

The diabetic diet is planned with the help of a dietician, with the daily requirements divided usually into three main meals and three snacks. Some units use the concept of a 'traffic light' division of foods, namely foods that can be eaten relatively freely ('go', or green light foods such as meat, fish, black coffee, clear soups), some that can be eaten in moderation ('caution', or amber light foods such as bread, milk, cereals, pasta), and finally those which should be avoided in excess ('stop', or red light foods such as chocolate, raw sugar, soft drinks, cakes).

Exercise

Exercise promotes glucose entry into cells and increases the number of insulin receptors. The positive effects of exercise include increased cardiovascular fitness and increased utilisation of glucose at the same insulin dosage. Exercise also allows certain normally 'red light' foods to be consumed, such as chocolate bars or lollies, due to the increased caloric needs.

The only difficulties are the additional considerations about diet and insulin (which are dealt with easily), and that certain groups of patients should not engage in strenuous exercise, namely those with BSL readings above 20 mmol/L, significant ketonuria, significant retinopathy, and hypertension.

During acute exercise, if the BSL readings remain within the normal range or fall, this suggests fairly good control. If the BSL levels remain above normal but the patient feels unwell, this suggests poor control. It is much easier to manipulate food intake than to modify the insulin dose; it may be necessary, during strenuous exercise, to have fast-acting carbohydrates frequently.

Monitoring and control

Home BSL monitoring

The glucometer is used at least twice daily to record the BSL in a log book, which all diabetics should keep. It is useful for decisions regarding altering dosages of insulin, in particular longer-acting insulin. The goals are for a preprandial BSL of 4.0 to 10.0 mmol/L (in adolescents and older, between 4.0 and 8.0 mmol/L) and a postprandial value of below 10 mmol/L. Some units recommend checking BSL readings 2 hours after breakfast and dinner, and using the results to alter short-acting insulin if needed.

Certain patients can be a problem in terms of the accuracy of their BSL recordings. Beware the 'dumb cheat' who does the test but fakes the results (the solution here is to use a memory glucometer), and the 'smart' cheat, who does not do the test, and cannot do it if asked because he does not know how.

Glycosylated haemoglobin (HbA$_{1c}$)

This is a useful indicator of metabolic control over the preceding 6 weeks to 3 months. The HbA$_{1c}$ levels are as follows: normal, 4–6%; excellent control, 7–8%; good control, 8–9%; unacceptable, 9–10%; bad, >10%.

Usually the child does the test at home, on special blotting paper, and posts the sample to the hospital every 3 months.

Glycosylated albumin (fructosamine)

Like HbA$_{1c}$, this gives an indication of recent diabetic control, but over the preceding 2–4 weeks.

Urine tests

Urine should be free of ketones and have glucose below 1% for 80–90% of the time. It is important to check that the test tablets or dipsticks are not out of date and spoiled. Urine should be tested for glucose and ketones when the BSL is above 15 mmol/L.

Some centres measure quantitive 24-hour urine glucose excretion every 3–4 months as an additional means of assessing control (maximum excretion less than 7% daily dietary carbohydrate is a reliable index of satisfactory control).

Routine follow-up

These children should be seen every 3–4 months. On each occasion, the child's growth (height, weight, percentiles, maturation) and evidence of any complications should be documented (see the short case in this chapter for method of examination) and then managed accordingly. Proteinuria is checked for with dipstick testing, and if positive, a 24-hour urinary protein collection is performed. Fixed proteinuria suggests significant nephropathy. Microalbuminuria above 20 micrograms in 24 hours is predictive of development of chronic renal failure within 10 years. (*Note*: 1–2% of normal children have microalbuminuria.)

The other important clinical point is regular eye examination by an ophthalmologist, annually if postpubertal. Recommendations vary for prepubertal children. Routine investigations should include the following.

Initially

1. Antimicrosomal and antithyroglobulin antibodies.
2. Baseline blood urea, creatinine, electrolytes.
3. Urine microalbumin levels.
4. Baseline blood cholesterol, triglycerides, low and high density lipoproteins.

Yearly

1. Blood urea, creatinine and electrolytes (5 years after onset).
2. Urine microalbumin levels.
3. Blood cholesterol, triglycerides, low- and high-density lipoproteins.
4. Thyroid function tests, including TSH (15% of patients with IDDM develop Hashimoto's thyroiditis, and a third of these develop hypothyroidism).
5. Anti-endomysial and tissue transglutaminase antibodies for coeliac disease (occurs in 3–5% of patients with IDDM).

Complications

Complications generally are divided into microvascular, macrovascular and 'other'. Despite the advances in insulin treatment, over 50% of patients with childhood-onset IDDM will still develop complications such as incipient nephropathy and background retinopathy within 12 years of IDDM. If the glycaemic control in the first 5 years is suboptimal, this shortens the time lapse before complications occur. All children who have had diabetes for 5 years, or are adolescents, should be screened for complications.

Microvascular complications

Risk factors for the development of microvascular complications include long duration of IDDM, poor control of BSL, family history of complications of IDDM, and associated medical problems, such as hypertension.

Retinopathy

This occurs to some degree in 90% or more of patients within 15 years of the onset of their IDDM. The most common lesions seen are 'background' lesions, which include microaneurysms, retinal haemorrhages (named according to appearance: dot, blot and flame), hard exudates, cottonwool spots (retinal nerve fibre infarcts) and venous calibre changes (loops, beading). Background retinopathy can be seen in up to one quarter of adolescent patients. More advanced lesions of 'proliferative' retinopathy occur in 40% of IDDM patients after 20 years of disease, but are uncommon in adolescence. These changes include signs of neovascularisation, fibrous proliferation, haemorrhage into the vitreous (which can cause sudden visual loss or retinal detachment secondary to fibrosis and traction), and can lead to glaucoma (obstruction to aqueous humour from vascular overgrowth).

Severe loss of vision occurs within 5 years in 50% of those with untreated proliferative retinopathy. The other form of retinopathy, maculopathy, causes central visual loss, mainly due to oedema and hard exudate formation at the macula. Retinopathy is documented with colour or red-free retinal photography and the severity assessed with fluorescein angiography. The treatment for early background retinopathy is maintenance of near normoglycaemia, there being some evidence that institution of improved glucose control can actually reverse some of the changes. The treatment used for both proliferative retinopathy and maculopathy is laser photocoagulation: panretinal for the former and focal for the latter. Photocoagulation can reduce the rate of visual loss by half.

Screening for retinopathy should occur annually after 5 years of IDDM in a prepubertal child, after 2 years of IDDM in an adolescent, and as required if there are any symptoms. Smoking must be discouraged, because it accelerates vasculopathy.

Nephropathy

Up to 40% of IDDM patients will eventually develop end-stage renal failure. A microvasculopathy affecting the glomeruli (diffuse or nodular glomerulosclerosis) is the cause of the depressed glomerular filtration rate (GFR). The first sign of this process is microalbuminuria of over 20 micrograms/minute. Intermittent microalbuminuria or 'borderline' levels (7.6–20 micrograms/minute) increase the chance of nephropathy. Once proteinuria is persistent and easily detected, there has already been a reduction in the GFR, which is an ominous sign. There is a 95% occurrence of retinopathy in newly uraemic diabetics, on the basis of the same pathological process, microangiopathy, afflicting both the glomerulus and the retina. This association has been called the 'renal-retinal syndrome'. A clinical point worth remembering is that eye status should be reviewed when any patient develops evidence of renal impairment, such as proteinuria.

Nephropathy is accelerated by hypertension, and control of the blood pressure will decrease the amount of proteinuria and slow the rate of fall in the GFR. Angiotensin converting enzyme (ACE) inhibitors delay progression to/of nephropathy. The renal function can be monitored by plotting 1 divided by serum creatinine versus time. Once end-stage renal failure occurs, the treatment options include renal transplantation (or combined renal-pancreatic transplantation), peritoneal dialysis, haemodialysis or haemofiltration.

Screening for nephropathy should occur annually after 5 years of IDDM in a prepubertal child, and after 2 years of IDDM in an adolescent. Smoking must be discouraged.

Neuropathy

There are several forms of this.

1. Symmetric distal neuropathy predominantly affects sensory neurons, causing paraesthesia or pain, but can also involve the motor system.
2. Autonomic neuropathy can lead to postural hypotension, arrhythmias (due to denervation hypersensitivity to catecholamines), gastroparesis and impaired response to hypoglycaemia, and may be associated with painless myocardial infarction.
3. Carpal tunnel syndrome, due to the neuropathy affecting the median nerve (often the ulnar nerve is involved as well).
4. Mononeuropathy, which particularly affects cranial nerves.

All of these are infrequent in the paediatric age range. However, nerve conduction studies demonstrating subclinical peripheral nervous system involvement and evidence of sensory neuropathy are not uncommon in adolescent diabetics. The underlying pathology is thought to be a combination of polyol pathway abnormality and microangiopathy affecting the vasa vasorum, leading to axonal loss and segmental demyelination.

Macrovascular complications

Coronary atherosclerosis

Coronary artery disease is common in IDDM patients, the prevalence increasing with the duration of the disease. The extent of involvement of coronary vessels also tends to be greater (triple vessel disease more common), and it is more common in women. Clinical disease is rare in the childhood and adolescent population.

Peripheral vascular disease

Atherosclerosis is accelerated in IDDM. Peripheral vascular disease, like coronary arterial disease, is rare in the paediatric population, so that problems such as digit ischaemia are unlikely to be encountered.

Other: limited joint mobility (LJM)

Thought to be due to glycosylation of periarticular tissues, limited joint mobility occurs in approximately 40% of children with IDDM. It is a painless condition that does not cause any significant disability in its early form. It affects the hands (metacarpophalangeal, proximal and distal interphalangeal joints, initially of the fifth, then the more medial fingers), wrists, elbows, spine (cervical and/or thoracolumbar) or other large joints. There seems to be a correlation between LJM and retinopathy, with an increased risk of microvascular disease developing in patients with LJM.

Psychological support

This is a complex area on which entire books are written. The basic principles are as follows.

1. Discourage use of the disease for manipulation.
2. Minimise the number of days off school.
3. Involve children in the management of their own disease as appropriate for their age and ability.
4. In the time of 'adolescent rebellion', give support and encourage; never resort to threats.
5. Identify and treat negative family responses to diabetes, including overindulgence, overanxiousness, neglect and disinterest, resentment, and overcontrolling parents.
6. When the initial diagnosis is made, be aware of depression in patients, siblings and parents and counsel accordingly.

For the purposes of the long case, the usual problem is that of a noncompliant adolescent. Unfortunately, it is most important to avoid serious complications in adolescence, at exactly the least receptive time of the patient's life. For a teenager, immediate peer acceptance, which may involve nights out at parties or hotels, far outweighs the long-term benefits of near normoglycaemia. Most diabetic teenagers require additional emotional support, which may be achieved through discussion groups or by one-on-one talks with a clinical psychologist. The problems for adolescents can be foreseen and discussed with the parents before they occur. The ones who fare worst tend to be females, or those with family disharmony, another chronic medical condition or pre-existing learning problems.

Generally, it may help to emphasise to the parents the positive aspects of improved control, to explain the requirements for increased insulin during growth spurts, to provide support during rebellious episodes and to avoid chastisement. By 18 years of age, most adolescents will again be more responsible in caring for their diabetes.

Social supports

All families of patients with IDDM should have access to an experienced social worker. The disease represents a significant financial burden for many families and the social worker can make them aware of the various government benefits to which they may be entitled. These may include child disability allowance (CDA), isolated patients travel and accommodation scheme (IPTAS) if the patient lives more than 200 km from the hospital, program of aids for disabled people (PADP: scripts for needles, syringes, glucometer, if the patient has a Health Care Card). Diabetes Australia provides access to many helpful people and ideas, including attendance at diabetic camps and the use of the National Diabetes Syringe Scheme (NDSS).

Pre-diabetes screening and intervention

Screening

Islet-cell antibodies may be detected in (future) patients with beta cell autoimmunity months or years before IDDM declares itself clinically. Islet-cell antibodies include antibodies against insulin (insulin autoantibodies, IAA), plus non–beta-cell-specific proteins such as glutamic acid decarboxylase (GAD) and tyrosine phosphatase (IA-2).

Prevention

Many agents have been trialled to prevent IDDM; none has succeeded as yet. There continues to be an enormous amount of research in this area, which is beyond the scope of this book. There is a wealth of information about screening and prevention of IDDM available on the Internet.

Acute management of diabetic ketoacidosis (DKA)

This is an area where the candidate's discussion of a hypothetical presentation of the long-case patient with DKA can explore thoroughly his/her understanding and practical application of the underlying pathophysiology of DKA.

The principles of treatment can be divided into five main areas, the 'diabetic pentathlon':

1. Water and sodium replacement.
2. Potassium replacement.
3. Correction of acid-base imbalance.
4. Insulin administration.
5. Prevention of treatment complications.

The first four areas should be well known to candidates and are not discussed here in detail. The fifth area, which can generate the most questions, is discussed briefly below.

Some complications

Cerebral oedema

Subclinical cerebral oedema occurs frequently in children with DKA. Many children fall asleep during treatment, but failure to rouse easily or onset of headache should raise suspicion of cerebral oedema (or hypoglycaemia, so checking BSL is mandatory). This typically occurs 2–24 hours after starting treatment, especially around 6–12 hours. Once clinically apparent, the mortality rate approximates 90%.

Other causes of depressed level of consciousness include: acidosis; hypoglycaemia; any rapid change in osmolality, serum sodium, serum glucose or pH; hyponatraemia; hypernatraemia; hyperosmolality; hypoxia; hypothermia; hypovolaemia; neuroglycopenia. A cerebral CT scan should be considered if depressed level of consciousness does not respond to colloid, or if it occurs during treatment.

Risk situations include hypernatraemia (serum sodium >160 mmol/L) on presentation, hyponatraemia developing during treatment or hyponatraemia failing to correct during treatment, first presentation with DKA, poor control and children under 5 years of age. Warning features are headache, deterioration in consciousness, irritability, with later (ominous) signs of hypertension, bradycardia and dilated pupils. On occasion, there may be a presentation of polyuria, secondary to diabetes insipidus, which can be misdiagnosed as osmotic diuresis.

Prevention strategies include slow correction of fluid and glucose abnormalities, and nursing children with the head elevated. Active treatment includes 20% mannitol, 0.5 g/kg IV statim, repeated every 15 minutes, decreasing rate of fluid administration, and intubation and hyperventilation.

Hypoglycaemia (BSL <3 mmol/L)

This can present as an altered consciousness state, thus being confused with cerebral oedema. Treatment is with a bolus of 10% glucose (2 mL/kg), plus decrease in insulin infusion rate.

Hypokalaemia (serum potassium <3 mmol/L)

This is a potential cause of cardiac arrhythmia and death.

Short cases

Ambiguous genitalia

This is an uncommon, but exceedingly important, case. The inability to determine the sex of a newborn immediately at birth is one of the most difficult clinical problems. Some causes are life-threatening (congenital adrenal hyperplasia, CAH). A comprehensive approach is essential and, after the diagnosis is made, issues of sex of rearing give candidates much scope for fielding interesting questions. To understand this area, some background embryology is worth reviewing, as are pathways of steroid hormone synthesis. The latter are discussed in the long case on CAH (in this chapter); the former is outlined below. This problem is also termed 'intersex' by some.

There are five groups of babies:

1. Masculinised (virilised) females, previously called female pseudohermaphrodites (46 XX).
2. Undermasculinised males, previously called male pseudohermaphrodites (46 XY).
3. True hermaphrodites, who have both testicular and ovarian tissue (usually 46 XX, can be 46 XY, or mosaics).
4. Mixed gonadal dysgenesis (e.g. 45 XO/46 XY or more commonly, 46 XY).
5. Dysmorphic syndromes (e.g. Beckwith's syndrome).

The most common scenario of these is a masculinised female with CAH.

There are two groups of babies which can be mistakenly labelled as having 'ambiguous genitalia'. The first group are premature female infants with unusual genital appearance; these apparent genital abnormalities are transient. The second group have perineal anatomy that is abnormal, but which is not due to any endocrine problem. They have anatomical anomalies that are not within the range of normal sexual differentiation, such as significant defects in caudal embryogenesis, which can be associated with complete aplasia of the genital tubercle such that neither penis nor clitoris are present. These babies do not have an intersex condition; they have anomalies of the perineum unaffected by hormones. They are mentioned here for completeness.

There is a scoring system for the degree of masculinisation of the external genitalia described by Prader, numerically graded from 0 to 5. Prader 0 refers to normal female anatomy. Prader 5 refers to normal male anatomy. The numbers in between describe the transition from the embryological default outcome of female towards masculinity imposed by exposure to androgens. Prader 1 refers to an enlarged phallus, Prader 2 an enlarged phallus with visibly separate openings of urethra and vagina, Prader 3 refers to an enlarged phallus with a single urogenital sinus opening, and Prader 4 enlarged phallus with hypospadias.

Until 7 weeks' gestation the internal genital tracts are bipotential in both XX and XY embryos. In both, genital ducts are the wolffian (mesonephric) duct and the müllerian (paramesonephric) duct. In a normal male, the wolffian duct transforms into the epididymis, vas deferens and seminal vesicles. In a normal female, the müllerian duct transforms into the uterus, fallopian tubes and upper portion of the vagina.

If the SRY (sex-determining region on the Y chromosome) gene is present (as in a normal male), the ambisexual gonad will develop into a testis. By 8 weeks' gestation, the Sertoli cells in the testis produce müllerian inhibiting substance/anti-müllerian hormone (MIS/AMH) and the Leydig cells produce testosterone and other androgens. The müllerian duct regresses between 8 and 12 weeks, due to MIS/AMH. Concurrently between 8 and 12 weeks' gestation, androgens transform the genital primordium into normal male external genitalia. Testosterone is converted by 5-alpha-reductase into dihydrotestosterone. Dihydrotestosterone causes the genital tubercle to develop into the penis with the male urethra opening at the tip, the outer labioscrotal folds to fuse into the midline scrotal raphe, forming the scrotum, and the urogenital sinus to differentiate into the bladder and the prostatic urethra. From 12 weeks until full term, enlargement of the phallus to normal penile size occurs. All external virilisation is due to androgens.

If the SRY gene is absent (as in a normal female) the bipotential gonad will develop into an ovary. Lack of testosterone and MIS/AMH leads to regression of the wolffian duct and preservation of the müllerian ducts. In the absence of androgens, the genital tubercle and the urethral plate form the clitoris and short female urethra, the labioscrotal folds remain unfused to become labia majora, and the vaginal plate, part of the posterior wall of the urogenital sinus, canalises, so forming the lower vagina.

Sexual differentiation of the brain occurs between 15 and 25 weeks' gestation.

Examination for ambiguous genitalia

1. General examination

Skin: hyperpigmentation (CAH).
Syndromal diagnosis: head, heart, hands (e.g. Beckwith; see short-case approach to dysmorphic child in Chapter 9).
Hydration: assess for dehydration secondary to vomiting (CAH).
Blood pressure: elevated in CAH due to 11 beta-hydroxylase deficiency.

2. Abdomen/pelvis/genitalia

Inspect for Prader grading of virilisation of external genitalia:
Prader 0: Normal female
Prader 1: Enlargement of phallus (looks more like clitoris; abnormal exposure to androgens beyond 8 weeks' gestation)
Prader 2: Enlargement of phallus, vagina and urethra openings separate
Prader 3: Enlargement of phallus, urogenital sinus (single opening)

Prader 4: Enlarged phallus with hypospadias

Prader 5: Normal male

Inspect scrotum:

- Fused, absent gonads (must exclude XX with CAH).
- Bifid, bilateral gonads present (undervirilised XY; true hermaphrodite with bilateral ovotestes rarely).
- Bifid, maldeveloped, bilateral gonads placed high (undervirilised XY, true hermaphrodite with ovotestes rarely, or XY gonadal dysgenesis [dysplastic testes]).

Examine midline cleft/urogenital sinus:

- Gently open cleft/sinus; confirm impression of Prader stage. Skin tags with purplish tinge implies hymen present.

Palpation for gonads:

- Gonads palpable bilaterally, can be brought to base of scrotum (almost certainly testes and almost certainly male; bilateral ovotestes in true hermaphrodite rare).
- Gonads palpable bilaterally but placed high (undervirilised XY, true hermaphrodite with ovotestes rarely, or XY gonadal dysgenesis [dysplastic testes]).
- Gonads palpable bilaterally but asymmetrical position/descent (true hermaphrodite with a testis on one side, and an ovotestis on the other, or mixed gonadal dysgenesis with a testis one side and a streak ovary with a hernia on the other).
- Single gonad palpable (almost certainly testis; other may be ovary, streak gonad [mixed gonadal dysgenesis] or ovotestis [true hermaphrodite]).
- Gonads impalpable bilaterally (cannot predict gonadal status).
- Rectal examination should be mentioned; little finger can palpate cervix and confirm a uterus.

At the completion of physical assessment, give a differential diagnosis, followed by a list of investigations appropriate for that patient. A suggested list for each follows.

Differential diagnosis

Virilised female

1. Congenital adrenal hyperplasia (CAH)—deficiency of:
   - **21-alpha-hydroxylase** (converts progesterone $\rightarrow$ **de**oxycortisone [DOC]; 17OH progesterone $\rightarrow$ 11 deoxycortisol).
   - **11-beta-hydroxylase** (11 deoxycortisol $\rightarrow$ cortisol; 11 deoxycorticosterone $\rightarrow$ corticosterone).
   - **3-beta-hydroxysteroid-dehydrogenase** (pregnenolone $\rightarrow$ progesterone; 17OH pregnenolone $\rightarrow$ 17OH progesterone; **de**hydro**epi**androsterone [DHEA] $\rightarrow$ androstenedione; androstenediol $\rightarrow$ testosterone).
2. Androgen exposure in utero (maternal androgens):
   - Progesterone.
   - Medroxyprogesterone.
   - 19 nortesterones.

Testicular failure (undervirilised males)

1. Enzymatic—incomplete deficiency of:
   - **20,22 desmolase** (cholesterol → pregnenolone).
   - **lipoid adrenal hyperplasia** due to deficiency of steroid acute regulatory protein (StAR).
   - **3-beta-hydroxysteroid-dehydrogenase** (pregnenolone → progesterone; 17OH pregnenolone → 17OH progesterone; DHEA → androstenedione; androstenediol → testosterone).
   - **17-alpha-hydroxylase** (pregnenolone → 17OH pregnenolone; progesterone → 17OH progesterone).
   - **17,20 lyase** (17OH pregnenolone → DHEA; 17OH progesterone → androstenedione).
   - **17-beta-hydroxysteroid-dehydrogenase 17βHSD/17 ketosteroid reductase** (DHEA → androstenediol; androstenedione → testosterone)
   - **5-alpha-reductase** (testosterone → dihydrotestosterone, DHT)
2. Anatomic:
   - 46 XY pure gonadal dysgenesis (usually appear female).
   - 46 XY mosaic (45 X/46 XY) or isochromosome.
3. Partial androgen insensitivity (PAIS)

Investigations

Blood tests

Chromosomes for karyotype, urea and electrolytes, 17OH progesterone, cortisol, ACTH, plasma renin activity (PRA), testosterone, DHT, DHEA, androstenedione.

Provocation tests

HCG stimulation for testosterone or DHT synthesis. Also used to assess ratio of androstenedione to testosterone (elevated in 17βHSD).

Imaging

Pelvic ultrasound.

Specialised tests

Androgen binding studies; androgen receptor gene mutation analysis.

Diabetes

The introduction for this case usually requests examination for complications of diabetes or for assessment of quality of control. The candidate needs to be aware not only of the complications, but also of their time course and relation to glucose control.

It may be another chronic disease process that is causing the diabetes, such as cystic fibrosis or beta-thalassaemia major. This is worth keeping in the back of your mind when initially assessing growth and Tanner staging in particular. Thus, it is relevant to scan for thalassaemic facies and hyperpigmentation, or clubbing and cough, although usually the patient will only have type 1 diabetes. Other associations may be readily apparent, such as Friedreich's ataxia, Wolfram syndrome (features of which are known by the acronym **DIDMOAD**: **D**iabetes **I**nsipidus, **D**iabetes **M**ellitus, **O**ptic **A**trophy, **D**eafness), Cushing's syndrome.

Examination

Begin by introducing yourself. Have the child adequately undressed to allow a complete examination: this usually means fully undressed down to underwear in younger children, but not necessarily in older children. Assess weight and height parameters, and percentile charts. Poor growth can be due to inadequate insulin dosage or poor compliance, associated impaired thyroid function or coexistent chronic disease. Assess pubertal status, hydration and whether the child looks sick or well. Look for any intravenous lines and read labels on any intravenous fluid being administered.

Pick up the child's hands. Look for any cutaneous infection or trophic changes, and carefully inspect fingertips for prick marks indicating regular blood glucose testing. Assess for limited joint mobility (LJM) by asking the child to hold his/her hands in the 'prayer' position, and looking for lack of apposition of palmar aspects of the fingers (when positive, this is called the cathedral sign). If there is evidence of LJM, go on to extend the distal and proximal interphalangeal joints (normally extend to 180 degrees), the metacarpophalangeal joints (normally extend to 60 degrees), the wrist (normally extends to 70 degrees) and the elbow (at least 180 degrees). Note the colour of the palmar creases; they may be pigmented due to coexistent Addison's disease, or underlying thalassaemia major with haemosiderosis.

Next, take, or request, the blood pressure (hypertension with nephropathy, postural hypotension with autonomic neuropathy or dehydration in ketoacidosis, hypotension with Addison's disease).

Examine the eyes. Look carefully for squint, cataract, contact lenses (or nearby glasses). Check the visual acuity in each eye, and then the eye movements (for neuropathy). Check the pupillary reactions and the red reflex, and assess the retinae for diabetic retinopathy, of which there are three groups:

1. Background lesions include microaneurysms, retinal haemorrhages, hard exudates, cottonwool spots (small retinal infarcts), venous beading.
2. Proliferative lesions include new vessel networks (arising from peripheral vessels or from vessels overlying the optic disc), vitreous haemorrhage, retinal detachment.
3. Maculopathy, which is rare, includes oedema and hard exudate deposition. Also look for optic atrophy (DIDMOAD).

Examine the mouth for ketotic breath and oral candidiasis, and to assess hydration. Then inspect for goitre, palpate the thyroid gland, assess movement with swallowing and auscultate if there is thyroid enlargement (associated autoimmune thyroid disease). Next, in girls, assess breast development (for delayed puberty).

The abdomen is then inspected for injection sites, fat atrophy or hypertrophy, any distension (associated coeliac disease) and pubertal status. Palpate the liver for hepatomegaly (from glycogen if 'overinsulinised' or fat if 'underinsulinised'), and, in boys, note the size of the testes (for pubertal delay). Mention looking for perineal candidiasis in girls, but this does not need to be performed.

The legs are then assessed for injection sites on the thigh, any associated fat atrophy or hypertrophy, and the lower legs for necrobiosis lipoidica diabeticorum. Look at, and between, the toes, for trophic changes or candidiasis. Finally, check for peripheral neuropathy: check the reflexes at the knee and ankle, and then examine for light touch, vibration and position sense.

Request urinalysis for glucose, ketones, protein or blood, and also the temperature chart for any infection that may have precipitated the presentation.

At this stage, the examiners may ask if there is anything further that you wish to do. Here, you can request a hearing test (DIDMOAD) and examine the ears, nose, throat and chest for any underlying infection. Finish by giving a succinct summary of the relevant findings and an overall assessment of disease control. You may then express interest in seeing the child's medication chart for insulin dosages, and the daily recordings of blood glucose levels before the current admission.

Figure 7.1 summarises the examination for diabetes.

Short stature

This particular case covers more clinical ground than most and requires a very structured routine. The one outlined here proved successful both in practice cases and in the examination. It comprises four parts:

1. Observation.
2. Measurements.
3. Manoeuvres.
4. Systematic relevant examination.

Observation

Firstly, listen carefully to the patient's age in the introduction. Then, stand back and look for any evidence of an obvious diagnosis (e.g. Turner's or Noonan's syndrome), any dysmorphism, any disproportion (skeletal dysplasias, rickets), and visually assess the pubertal status. Comment on your findings.

Measurements

Next, measure the patient yourself. Stand the child against a wall, position the head and heels appropriately, record the height and measure the lower segment (LS), i.e. from pubic symphysis to the ground. Then calculate the upper segment (US) by subtracting the LS from the total height. Work out the US:LS ratio. Normal values at various ages are given in Table 7.2.

Table 7.2 Normal upper segment to lower segment ratios	
Birth	**Ratio**
Birth	1.7
3 years	1.3
8 years or more	1.0

If the US:LS ratio is high, it suggests short lower limbs (e.g. skeletal dysplasias, hypothyroidism). If the US:LS ratio is low, it suggests a short trunk (e.g. vertebral irradiation, scoliosis) or a short neck (e.g. Klippel-Feil syndrome).

Next, measure the child's arm span, and compare this to the total height. The normal arm span minus height values at various ages is given in Table 7.3. A short arm span can occur with skeletal dysplasias, and an apparently long arm span with a short neck, trunk or legs.

Measure the head circumference and request the weight. Request percentile charts, progressive measurements (if not given) and calculate the height velocity (be aware of the normal range and nature of percentile charts). Request birth parameters (for intrauterine and chromosomal causes), parents' heights and onsets of puberty (for familial maturational delay).

Figure 7.1 Diabetes

1. Introduce self

2. Position patient
Initial inspection standing, then lying,
  adequately undressed

3. General inspection
Parameters
Weight
Height
Percentiles
Well or unwell
Hydration
Intravenous lines
Tanner staging

4. Hands
Fingertip pricks
Trophic changes
Cutaneous infections
Limitation of joint mobility
Pigmented palmar creases (Addison)

5. Blood pressure
Hypertension (nephropathy)
Hypotension (Addison)
Postural hypotension (autonomic
  neuropathy, dehydration)

6. Eyes
Inspection
Squint
Cataract
Contact lenses
Visual acuity
Eye movements
Pupillary reactions
Red reflex (cataracts)
Fundi
Retinopathy
Optic atrophy (DIDMOAD)

7. Mouth
Hydration
Ketotic breath
Oral candidiasis

8. Thyroid
Inspect
Swallowing
Palpate
Auscultation

9. Abdomen
Injection sites
Fat atrophy, hypertrophy
Distension (coeliac disease)
Hepatomegaly

Tanner staging
Perineal candidiasis

10. Lower limbs
Injection sites
Fat atrophy, hypertrophy
Trophic changes
Candidiasis
Necrobiosis lipoidica
Reflexes
Sensation
Light touch
Vibration

11. Urinalysis
Glucose
Ketones
Protein
Blood

12. Other
Hearing (DIDMOAD)
ENT and chest (infection precipitating
  presentation)
Request insulin dosages and
  glucometer readings

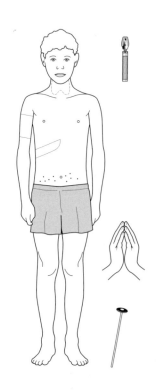

Table 7.3 Normal arm span minus height values	
Age	**Value**
Birth to 7 years	–3 cm
8–12 years	0
14 years	+1 cm in girls

By now, you may well have a good indication of the type of short stature with which you are dealing.

Manoeuvres

Next, a set of manoeuvres can be performed that very rapidly screen for a multiplicity of causes. With each manoeuvre, stand opposite the child and demonstrate, so that he or she will mirror your movements. First, ask the child to put the palms together with the arms out straight and to stand with legs together. This screens for asymmetry (Russell–Silver syndrome). Next, ask the child to hold the arms out straight, with palms forward; assess the carrying angle (increased in Turner's syndrome).

Then, ask the child to touch the tips of the thumbs to the tips of the shoulders. If the thumbs overshoot, there is proximal segment (rhizomelic) limb shortening (e.g. achondroplasia, hypochondroplasia). If the thumbs do not reach the shoulders, there is either middle segment (mesomelic) or distal segment (acromelic) limb shortening. Next, ask the child to hold the palms up; look for simian crease (Down syndrome) and clinodactyly (Russell–Silver syndrome). Ask the child to make a fist and look for a shortened fourth metacarpal (pseudohypoparathyroidism). Examine the back next, for scoliosis and kyphosis, and ask the child to touch the toes, for fuller assessment for scoliosis.

Explain what you are doing as you proceed, so that the examiners will be aware of the significance of the manoeuvres.

For a list of manoeuvres, see Table 7.4.

Examination

The formal physical examination flows well if commenced at the hands, working up to the head, and then downwards: essentially a 'head-to-toe' pattern. Table 7.6 (Additional information) at the end of the section on short stature outlines the findings sought at each point.

At the completion of the comprehensive physical examination, request results of urinalysis (e.g. diabetes mellitus, chronic renal disease) and stool analysis (malabsorption). Finally, summarise your findings succinctly and give a brief differential diagnosis, placing the most likely diagnosis first. (See Figure 7.2.)

Investigations

At this stage, you may be asked what investigations you would perform. Depending on the findings, of course, the answers vary. Generally, a bone age is most useful and, in girls, a chromosomal analysis is always warranted to exclude Turner's syndrome. Other investigations often ordered include thyroid function tests (hypothyroidism), electrolytes, urea and creatinine (chronic renal disease), and tissue transglutaminase antibodies (coeliac disease).

Figure 7.2 Short stature: observation and examination

1. Introduce self

2. General inspection
Position patient: standing, undressed
    adequately to allow examination
    without embarrassment (underwear
    in young children)
Diagnostic facies
Disproportionate stature
Tanner staging
Nutritional status
Skeletal anomalies
Colour
Tachypnoea
Skin

3. Measurements and manoeuvres
See Table 7.4

4. Upper limbs
Structure
Fingertips
Nails
Palms
Pulse
Joints
Blood pressure

5. Head and neck
Head
Hair
Eyes (full examination)
Nose
Mouth and chin
Ears
Hairline
Neck (thyroid)

6. Chest
Tanner staging
Chest deformity
Praecordium
Lung fields

7. Abdomen
Full abdominal examination

8. Genitalia
Tanner staging
Anomalies

9. Gait, back and lower limbs
Inspect lower limbs
Gait (full examination)
Back
Lower limbs neurologically

10. Other
Urinalysis
Stool analysis

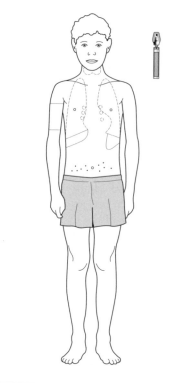

Table 7.5 lists some relatively simple investigations that are often useful in the child with short stature. More common diagnoses appearing in the examination setting include maturational delay and Russell–Silver syndrome.

Aetiologies

The author found the mnemonic **IS NICE** useful to remember the various headings of aetiologies of short stature:

Table 7.4 Short stature: measurements and manoeuvres

A. Measurements
Height
Lower segment (LS)
Calculate upper segment (US) by
   subtracting LS from height
Calculate US:LS ratio
Arm span
Head circumference
Request weight
Assess percentile charts
Calculate height velocity
Request birth parameters
Request parents' percentiles and ages
   at puberty

B. Hands and feet together
To detect:
  • Asymmetry (Russell-Silver)
  • Approximation of shoulders (absent
    clavicles in cleidocranial dysostosis)

C. Arms out straight
To detect cubitus valgus (Turner's,
   Noonan's): over 15 degrees in girls; over
   10 degrees in boys

D. Thumbs on shoulders
To detect:
  • Proximal segment shortening (e.g.
    achondroplasia, hypochondroplasia)
  • Middle segment shortening
    (e.g. Leri-Weill dyschondrostenosis,
    Langer's mesomelic dysplasia)

  • Distal segment shortening
    (e.g. acromesomelic dysplasia)

E. Palms up
To detect:
  • Simian crease (Down, Seckel's)
  • Clinodactyly (Russell-Silver, Down,
    Seckel's)

F. Make a fist
To detect short fourth metacarpal
(pseudohypoparathyroidism, Turner's,
fetal alcohol)

G. Back
To detect:
  • Short neck (Klippel-Feil, Noonan's)
  • Neck webbing (Turner's, Noonan's)
  • Low hairline (Turner's, Noonan's,
    Klippel-Feil)

H. Bend over and touch toes
To detect scoliosis (e.g. Noonan's, Klippel-
Feil)

I. Sit up
To commence systematic physical
examination

I **I**diopathic (constitutional), **I**ntrauterine (small for gestational age [SGA], TORCH, fetal alcohol syndrome [FAS])

S **S**keletal causes (dysplasias, osteogenesis imperfecta), **S**pinal defects (scoliosis, kyphosis)

N **N**utritional (includes malabsorption), **N**urturing (deprivation)

I **I**atrogenic (e.g. steroids, radiation)

C **C**hronic diseases (e.g. chronic renal failure, congenital heart disease, cystic fibrosis, inflammatory bowel disease), **C**hromosomal (e.g. Turner's or Down syndrome)

E **E**ndocrine (e.g. growth hormone deficiency, hypothyroidism, Cushing's syndrome, congenital adrenal hyperplasia, hypopituitarism, IDDM, pseudo-hypoparathyroidism)

Two other lists worth remembering enumerate the conditions that cause short stature and obesity. They are not comprehensive, but are simple to recall.

Table 7.5 Some useful investigations in the child with short stature

Investigation	Indications/relevance
Blood	
Full blood examination and film	Chronic disease, anaemia
Erythrocyte sedimentation rate	Inflammatory bowel disease
Electrolytes, urea, creatinine	Chronic renal disease
Fasting blood glucose	Diabetes
Calcium, phosphate, SAP	Rickets, hypophosphatasia
Liver function tests	CLD, nutritional deficiency
Tissue transglutaminase antibodies	Coeliac disease
Pancreatic isoamylase	Shwachman's syndrome
Thyroid function tests, TSH	Hypothyroidism
Karyotype	Syndromes, e.g. Turner's, Down's
Somatomedin C	Decreased GH deficiency; coeliac disease, Crohn's disease, malnutrition, hypothyroidism, diabetes (poorly controlled)
GH stimulation tests (insulin, GHRH, exercise, clonidine)	GH deficiency
LH, FSH, prolactin, oestradiol, testosterone	Hypogonadism
Dexamethasone suppression test	Cushing's syndrome
Sweat	
Sweat conductivity	Cystic fibrosis
Imaging	
Bone age	Maturational delay, precocious puberty, hypothyroidism, hypopituitarism
Skeletal survey	Skeletal dysplasias
Skull X-ray	Craniopharyngioma
CT or MRI of brain	Intracranial tumour

CLD = chronic liver disease; FSH = follicle-stimulating hormone; GH = growth hormone; GHRH = growth hormone releasing hormone; LH = luteinising hormone; SAP = serum alkaline phosphatase; TSH = thyroid-stimulating hormone.

There are five endocrine causes and five syndromal causes, as follows:

Endocrine
1. Hypothyroidism.
2. Hypopituitarism.
3. GH deficiency.
4. Cushing's syndrome.
5. Pseudohypoparathyroidism.

Syndromal
1. Prader–Willi.
2. Bardet–Biedl.
3. Alström's.
4. Down.
5. Fröhlich's.

Alternative introduction to short stature—endocrine

Occasionally the lead-in for short stature has been: 'This child is short. Would you please examine the endocrine system'. For those who have learned a comprehensive approach such as that previously outlined, this can cause some concern. This should not be the case, as all that is required is some abbreviation of the previous system, with elimination of the irrelevant parts. Remember that assessment for Turner's syndrome is part of an endocrine assessment, as is evaluation for Kallmann's syndrome, septo-optic dysplasia, craniopharyngioma or other central tumour (i.e. do not forget to test the visual fields and perform a gait examination), and rickets.

Table 7.6 Additional information: a comprehensive listing of possible physical findings in children with short stature

General inspection
Diagnostic facies
- Dysmorphic syndromes (e.g. Russell-Silver, Down, Turner's, Noonan's, FAS)
- Endocrine disorders (e.g. GH deficiency, Cushing's syndrome, hypothyroidism)
- Other (e.g. thalassaemia)

Disproportionate stature
- Skeletal dysplasias (e.g. achondroplasia)
- Metabolic bone disease (e.g. rickets)
- Connective tissue disorders (e.g. osteogenesis imperfecta)

Tanner staging
- Advanced (precocious puberty)
- Delayed (maturational delay; chronic illness, e.g. CRF, CHD; endocrine disorders, e.g. hypopituitarism, hypothyroidism)

Nutritional status
- Obese (e.g. endocrine causes, syndromal causes)
- Poor (e.g. malabsorption, under-nutrition, chronic diseases)

Skeletal anomalies
- Asymmetry (Russell-Silver)
- Pectus excavatum (e.g. Noonan's)
- Scoliosis (e.g. Noonan's, Klippel-Feil)

Colour
- Pallor (e.g. thalassaemia, nutritional deficiency, CRF)
- Sallow (e.g. CRF)
- Jaundice (e.g. CLD)
- Cyanosis (e.g. CHD, CF)
- Pigmented (e.g. thalassaemia)

Tachypnoea
- Cardiac (e.g. CCF with large VSD)
- Respiratory (e.g. CF)

Irritability (e.g. coeliac disease)

Skin
- Various rashes related to nutritional deficiencies
- Erythema nodosum (IBD)
- Café-au-lait spots (NF-1, Fanconi's anaemia, Russell-Silver)

Upper limbs
Structure
- Clinodactyly fifth finger (Russell-Silver, Down, Shwachman's, Seckel's)
- Short fourth metacarpal (pseudo-hypoparathyroidism, Turner's, FAS)
- Trident hand (achondroplasia)
- Polydactyly (Bardet-Biedl)

Fingertips: BSL testing (IDDM)

Nails
- Clubbing (CHD, CF, CLD)
- Brown lines (CRF)
- Leuconychia (CLD)
- Short (cartilage hair hypoplasia)
- Hyperconvex (Turner's)
- Hypoplastic (FAS)

Fingers: swollen joints (JIA)

Continued

Table 7.6 *(Continued)*

Palms
- Simian creases (Down)
- Crease pallor (anaemia from nutritional deficiency, CRF)
- Pigmented creases (thalassaemia, long-standing CAH)
- Erythema (CLD)

Wrists
- Swollen (JIA)
- Splaying (rickets)
- Deviation (JIA)
- A-V fistula (CRF)

Pulse
- Bradycardia (untreated hypo-thyroidism)
- Radiofemoral delay (coarctation of aorta with Turner's, NF-1)

Forearms: muscle bulk (malnutrition)

Blood pressure: elevated (CRF, Cushing's, CAH, NF-1, Turner's with coarctation)

Head

Size
- Small (TORCH, syndromes)
- Large (intracranial tumour, toxoplasmosis)

Shape
- Triangular (Russell-Silver)
- Frontal bossing (rickets, thalassaemia)

Consistency: craniotabes (rickets)

Fontanelle
- Large (Russell-Silver, rickets, hypothyroidism)
- Bulging (intracranial tumour with raised ICP)

Hair
- Dry (hypothyroidism)
- Greasy (precocious puberty)

Eyes

Inspection
- Photophobia (cystinosis)
- Hypertelorism (Noonan's, William's)
- Epicanthal folds (Noonan's, William's, Turner's, Down)
- Ptosis (Noonan's, pseudohypoparathyroidism)
- Squint (William's, Prader-Willi, septo-optic dysplasia)
- Nystagmus (septo-optic dysplasia)

Conjunctivae: pallor (CRF, malnutrition, thalassaemia)

Sclerae
- Icterus (CLD)
- Blue (osteogenesis imperfecta)

Cornea: cloudy (rubella)

Visual fields: field defect (intracranial tumour, e.g. craniopharyngioma)

Eye movements
- Upward gaze palsy (pineal tumour)
- Lateral rectus palsy (intracranial tumour with raised ICP)

Cataracts (rubella, Cushing's, treated thalassaemia, IDDM)

Fundi

Papilloedema (intracranial tumour with raised ICP)
- Optic nerve hypoplasia (septo-optic dysplasia)
- Chorioretinitis (TORCH)
- Diabetic retinopathy (IDDM)
- Pigmentary retinopathy (abetalipoproteinaemia)

Nose

Midface hypoplasia (FAS)

Midline dimple (hypopituitarism)

Nasal polyps (CF)

Anosmia (Kallmann's)

Mouth and chin

Central cyanosis (CHD, CF)

Midline defects associated with hypopituitarism
- Cleft lip (repaired)
- Cleft palate (repaired)
- Single central incisor

Delayed dentition (hypothyroidism)

Glossitis (nutritional deficiency)

Facial hair or acne (precocity, Cushing's)

Micrognathia (Russell-Silver, Turner's, Seckel's)

Ears

Low set (Turner's, Seckel's, Noonan's)

Posteriorly rotated (Russell-Silver)

Hairline

Low (Turner's, Noonan's)

Neck

Pterygium colli (Turner's, Noonan's)

Continued

Table 7.6 *(Continued)*

Short (Klippel-Feil)
Scoliosis (Klippel-Feil)
Goitre (hypothyroidism)

Chest
Inspection
- Tanner staging in girls (for precocity or delay)
- Wide-spaced nipples (Turner's)
- Hyperinflation (CF)
- Sternal deformity (Noonan's)
- Rib rosary (rickets)

Palpation
- Praecordium (CHD)
- Ribs for rosary (rickets)

Percuss chest: hyperresonance (CF)
Auscultation
- Lung fields (CF, CCF)
- Praecordium (CHD)

Abdomen
Inspection
- Distension
- Weak muscles (coeliac, nutritional deficiency)
- Ascites (CRF, CLD, nutritional deficiency)
- Hepatosplenomegaly (thalassaemia)

Tanner-staging pubic hair (for precocity or delay)
Operative scars (e.g. Kasai, renal transplant)
Access devices (e.g. Tenckhoff catheter for CRF, access ports in CF)
Striae (Cushing's)
Injection sites (insulin in IDDM, desferrioxamine in thalassaemia)
Palpation
- Abdominal tenderness (Crohn's)
- Hepatomegaly (e.g. nutritional deficiency, IDDM, CF, Shwachman's)
- Splenomegaly (e.g. thalassaemia, storage diseases, CF, CLD)
- Hepatosplenomegaly (e.g. thalassaemia, storage diseases)
- Enlarged kidneys (e.g. polycystic kidneys or hydronephrosis with CRF)
- Transplanted kidney (CRF)

Percussion: ascites (CRF, CLD)
Auscultation: renal artery stenosis (NF-1)
Posterior aspect
- Buttock wasting (malnutrition)
- Perianal fistulae (Crohn's)

Genitalia
Tanner stage genitalia
- Measure penis length
- Measure testes parameters; estimate testes volume
- Advanced stage (causes of long-standing precocity, e.g. CAH)
- Delayed stage (e.g. CRF, thalassaemia, hypopituitarism)

Penile anomalies
- Micropenis (hypopituitarism)
- Hypospadias (Noonan's)

Testicular anomalies: cryptorchidism (Noonan's)

Gait, back and lower limbs
Inspection of lower limbs
- Lower limb bowing (rickets)
- Proximal, middle or distal shortening (bony dysplasias)
- Joint swelling (JIA)
- Injection marks on thighs (IDDM)
- Erythema nodosum (IBD)
- Necrobiosis lipoidica (IDDM)
- Pyoderma gangrenosum (IBD)
- Oedema of dorsa of feet (Turner's)
- Clubbing of toes (CF, CHD)

Palpation: ankle oedema (CCF with CHD, CLD)
Gait—standard examination screening for:
- Long tract signs (IC tumour)
- Peripheral neuropathy (nutritional deficiency, CRF)
- Proximal weakness (Cushing's)

Back
- Scoliosis
- Kyphosis
- Focal spinal shortening (irradiation for malignancy)
- Midline scar (spina bifida)
- Spinal tenderness (Cushing's, rickets)

Lower limbs neurologically
- Long tract signs (IC tumour)
- Neuropathy (CRF, nutritional deficiency)
- Delayed ankle jerk relaxation (hypothyroidism)

Other
Urinalysis
- pH (RTA)
- Specific gravity (CRF)

Continued

Table 7.6   *(Continued)*

- Blood (CRF)
- Protein (CRF)
- Glucose (IDDM, Cushing's)
Stool analysis
- Blood (IBD)
- Pus (IBD)
- Fat globules (CF)

- Fat crystals (coeliac)
- Glucose (IDDM, Cushing's)
Stool analysis
- Blood (IBD)
- Pus (IBD)
- Fat globules (CF)
- Fat crystals (coeliac)

BSL = blood sugar level; CAH = congenital adrenal hyperplasia; CCF = congestive cardiac failure; CF = cystic fibrosis; CHD = congenital heart disease; CLD = chronic liver disease; CRF = chronic renal failure; FAS = fetal alcohol syndrome; IBD = inflammatory bowel disease; ICP = intracranial pressure; IDDM = insulin dependent diabetes mellitus; JIA = juvenile idiopathic arthritis; LS = lower segment; NF = neurofibromatosis; RTA = renal tubular acidosis; SCA = sickle cell anaemia; TORCH = intrauterine infections with toxoplasmosis, other (e.g. HIV, syphilis), rubella, cytomegalovirus, herpes (both simplex and varicella); US = upper segment; VSD = ventricular septal defect.

Tall stature

This is not a common case, but it can appear in the examination setting. The routine outlined is quite comprehensive. Like the short stature case, it comprises four parts:

1. Observation.
2. Measurements.
3. Manoeuvres.
4. Systematic relevant examination.

Observation

Start by noting the child's age in the introduction. This is important for appropriate assessment of the Tanner staging and intellect, which are essential in this case. Introduce yourself to the child and parent. Ask the child which grade he or she is in at school, and note whether the response seems age appropriate (impairment of intellect can occur with Beckwith's or Sotos' syndrome, or with homocystinuria).

Now stand back and inspect for any evidence of a Marfanoid body habitus (e.g. Marfan's syndrome; multiple neuromata syndrome, also called multiple endocrine neoplasia type 2b [MEN 2b]; homocystinuria) or a eunuchoid habitus (e.g. Klinefelter or Kallmann's syndromes), and visually assess the Tanner staging. Note whether the child is wearing glasses (e.g. myopia in Marfan's syndrome or homocystinuria). Note any skeletal anomalies such as asymmetry (e.g. in neurofibromatosis type 1 [NF type 1], Beckwith's, Proteus or McCune-Albright syndrome), pectus carinatum or excavatum (e.g. in Marfan's syndrome or homocystinuria), or scoliosis (e.g. Marfan's syndrome, homocystinuria, NF type 1, Proteus syndrome, Sotos' syndrome), and observe any unusual posturing (e.g. hemiplegia in homocystinuria complicated by a cerebrovascular accident due to thrombotic tendency). Comment on your findings.

Look at the skin for areas of hyperpigmentation, such as café-au-lait spots (in NF type 1, Proteus syndrome, McCune-Albright syndrome) or larger areas (e.g. in sacral area in McCune-Albright syndrome, and epidermal naevi in Proteus syndrome), as well as subcutaneous tumours (numerous types can occur in Proteus syndrome, such as lipomata, haemangiomata and lymphangiomata). Also note whether the child has acne (various causes of precocity).

Measurements

Next, measure the patient yourself. Stand the patient against a wall, position the head and heels appropriately and record the height. Measure the lower segment (LS), i.e. the distance from the pubic symphysis to the ground, then calculate the upper segment (US), which is the height minus the LS. Work out the US:LS ratio. Normal values at various ages are listed in Table 7.2.

If the US:LS ratio is decreased, it suggests that the lower limbs are disproportionately long (e.g. Marfanoid body habitus, eunuchoid body habitus). If the US:LS is normal, this is more in keeping with diagnoses such as familial tall stature or pituitary gigantism.

Next, measure the arm span and compare this to the total height. The normal arm span minus height values at various ages are given in Table 7.3. A long arm span occurs in Marfanoid or eunuchoid patients, or patients with other diagnoses complicated by a shortened trunk, caused by scoliosis (e.g. Sotos') or kyphosis (e.g. pituitary gigantism). Next, measure the head circumference and request the weight.

Request percentile charts, progressive measurements (if not given), and calculate the height velocity (be aware of the normal range and nature of percentile charts for this measurement). Request birth parameters (Beckwith and Sotos' can have large birth weights), parents' heights, percentiles and onsets of puberty (ask age of menarche for women and age when men started shaving).

Manoeuvres

Next a series of manoeuvres can be performed to screen for a number of possible causes of tall stature. With each manoeuvre, stand opposite the child and demonstrate, so that he or she will mirror your movements. First, ask the child to put the palms together with the arms straight, and stand with the legs together. This is to screen for asymmetry (as can occur in Beckwith's syndrome, McCune–Albright syndrome and in NF type 1) and also allows inspection for genu valgum (homocystinuria), genu recurvatum (Marfan's syndrome) and pes planus (Marfan's syndrome). Next, ask the child to bend forward and touch the toes; this is to check for scoliosis (can occur in Marfan's syndrome, homocystinuria, MEN 2b or Sotos' syndrome) or kyphosis (can occur in conjunction with scoliosis in the above diseases, as well as in pituitary gigantism/acromegaly).

Following this, two specific tests that are useful in detecting Marfan's syndrome can quickly be performed. First, test for hyperextensibility: ask the child to try to oppose the thumb to the radius and check extension at the wrists. Second, test for arachnodactyly: ask the child to wrap the fingers of one hand around the other wrist and check if there is complete overlap of the distal phalanx of the fifth finger on the distal phalanx of the thumb (the 'wrist sign'). Then check if the thumb can project beyond the ulnar border of the hand if the thumb is apposed to the palm when making a fist (the 'thumb sign'). If both these tests are normal, then Marfan's syndrome is a less likely diagnosis. If these tests show less mobility than normal, then homocystinuria is more likely.

Finally, ask the child to hold the arms out straight in front with the fingers spread apart and check for tremor associated with hyperthyroidism.

See Table 7.7 for a list of manoeuvres

Examination

Remember, as you proceed, to explain to the examiners what you are doing and why, so that the significance of each manoeuvre will be appreciated. The formal physical examination proceeds from the hands, working up to the head and then downwards, that is, head to toe, as outlined in Figure 7.3. A comprehensive listing of possible findings is given in Table 7.8 at the end of this section.

Table 7.7 Manoeuvres to assess for tall stature

Hands and feet together
To detect:
- Hemihypertrophy (Beckwith's, McCune-Albright, Proteus)
- Unilateral growth arrest (homocystinuria with cerebrovascular accident)
- Genu valgum (homocystinuria)
- Genu recurvatum (Marfan's)
- Pes planus (Marfan's)

Bend over and touch toes
To detect:
- Scoliosis (Marfan's, homocystinuria, Proteus, Sotos', NF-1)

- Kyphosis (with scoliosis, as above, pituitary gigantism)

Extensibility
To detect:
- Hyperextensibility (Marfan's)
- Limitation of extension (homocystinuria)

Arachnodactyly
To detect Marfan's syndrome

Tremor
To detect hyperthyroidism

If the patient appears to be quite clearly Marfanoid, the examination outlined can be substantially abbreviated and can concentrate on the skeleton, eyes and heart. At the completion of your physical examination, summarise your findings succinctly and give a brief differential diagnosis.

Investigations

At this stage you may be asked what investigations would clarify the diagnosis. This, of course, depends on the findings and may include: a slit-lamp ophthalmological assessment if Marfan's syndrome or homocystinuria are possibilities; urine homocystine and blood homocystine and methionine levels if homocystinuria is likely; an electrocardiogram, chest X-ray and echocardiogram if Marfan's syndrome seems likely; plasma somatomedin C concentration and a cerebral CT or MRI scan if a pituitary cause needs to be excluded; and skeletal X-rays if McCune-Albright syndrome is likely (multiple areas of bony fibrous dysplasia) or to confirm and document the degree of scoliosis or kyphosis in patients likely to have Marfan's syndrome or homocystinuria.

Table 7.8 Additional information: details of possible findings in the child with tall stature

Introduction
Impression of mental state: intellectual impairment (homocystinuria, Sotos', Beckwith's, Klinefelter's).

General inspection
Body habitus
- Marfanoid (dolichostenomelia: Marfan's, homocystinuria, multiple neuroma syndrome, i.e. MEN 2b)
- Eunuchoid (Kallman's, Klinefelter's)

Tanner staging
- Delayed (Kallmann's, Klinefelter's)
- Advanced (precocious puberty, virilisation, e.g. adrenal tumour, CAH); wearing glasses (Marfan's, homocystinuria)

Skeletal anomalies
- Asymmetry (Beckwith, NF-1, McCune-Albright, Proteus)
- Pectus excavatum (Marfan's, homocystinuria, MEN 2b)

Continued

Table 7.8 *(Continued)*

- Scoliosis (Marfan's, Sotos', homocystinuria, MEN 2b, NF-1)

Posture
- Hemiplegic (homocystinuria)

Skin
- Café-au-lait spots (NF-1, McCune-Albright, Proteus)
- Subcutaneous tumours, e.g. lipomata, haemangiomata (Proteus)
- Hyperpigmented areas (McCune-Albright, Proteus)
- Acne (virilisation syndromes)

Upper limbs
Arachnodactyly (Marfan's, MEN 2b)
Large hands (Sotos', Proteus, pituitary gigantism)
Nails: thyroid acropathy (hyperthyroidism)
Palms
- Warm, sweaty (hyperthyroidism)
- Pigmented creases (CAH)

Pulse: collapsing (aortic incompetence in Marfan's; hyperthyroidism)
Blood pressure
- Elevated (NF-1, CAH, pituitary gigantism, MEN type 2b with phaeochromocytoma)
- Pulse pressure elevated (aortic incompetence with Marfan's, hyperthyroidism)

Axillae: assess pubertal staging for precocity or delay, apocrine secretion, hair, odour

Head
Size
- Large (Sotos', NF-1)
- Small (Beckwith's)

Shape
- Frontal bossing (Sotos')
- Prominent occiput (Beckwith's)

Hair
Receding frontal hairline (Sotos')
Dry, light, sparse (homocystinuria)
Greasy (CAH)

Face
Asymmetry (Beckwith's, Proteus, NF-1, McCune-Albright)
Fair complexion (homocystinuria)
Malar flush (homocystinuria)

Café-au-lait spots (NF-1, McCune-Albright)
Naevus flammeus (Beckwith's)

Eyes
Inspect:
- Wearing glasses (myopia with Marfan's, homocystinuria)
- Blue irides (homocystinuria)
- Prominent (Beckwith's, hyperthyroidism)
- Exophthalmos (hyperthyroidism)
- Hypertelorism (Sotos')
- Downslanting (Sotos')
- Conjunctival neuromata (MEN 2b)
- Bluish sclerae (Marfan's)
- Lens displacement (up in Marfan's, down in homocystinuria)

Visual acuity
- Myopia (Marfan's, homocystinuria)

Visual fields
- Bitemporal hemianopia (pituitary tumour)
- Homonymous hemianopia (cerebral thrombosis with homocystinuria)

External ocular movements
- Ophthalmoplegia (hyperthyroidism)
- Sixth cranial nerve palsy (intracranial tumour)

Cataracts (homocystinuria)
Fundoscopy
- Retinal detachment (Marfan's, homocystinuria)

Glaucoma (Marfan's, homocystinuria)

Nose
Anosmia (Kallmann's)

Mouth and chin
Lips: prominent (neuromata in MEN 2b)
Tongue
- Big (Beckwith's, pituitary gigantism)
- Nodular (MEN 2b)

Teeth
- Crowding (homocystinuria)
- Separation (pituitary gigantism)

Palate
- High, narrow (Marfan's, Sotos', homo-cystinuria)
- Cleft (Marfan's)

Chin
- Acne (sexual precocity)
- Hair (pubertal staging)
- Prognathism (Sotos', Beckwith's, McCune-Albright)

Continued

Table 7.8 *(Continued)*

Ears
Linear fissures in lobules (Beckwith's)
Punched-out depressions in posterior
    pinnae (Beckwith's)
Large (Proteus, Marfan's)

Neck
Examine for goitre (hyperthyroidism)

Chest
Tanner-stage breasts in girls, hair in boys
Deformity: pectus carinatum or
    excavatum (Marfan's, homocystinuria)
Praecordium: full assessment for Marfan's
    cardiac complications, e.g. aortic
    regurgitation, mitral valve prolapse

Abdomen and genitalia
Inspect:
  • Café-au-lait spots (NF-1, McCune-
    Albright, Proteus)
  • Herniae (Marfan's, homocystinuria,
    Beckwith's)
  • Umbilical scar (repair of exomphalos
    with Beckwith's)

  • Tanner staging of pubic hair
Palpate
  • Hepatomegaly (homocystinuria,
    Beckwith's)
  • Enlarged kidneys (Wilm's tumour in
    Beckwith's)
  • Adrenal mass (tumour; isolated or
    associated with Beckwith's)
  • Tanner staging of genitalia (penis
    size, testicular volume, scrotal
    rugosity)

Lower limbs
Asymmetry (hemihypertrophy with
    Beckwith's, NF-1, Proteus; growth
    arrest with CVA in homocystinuria)
Large feet (Sotos', Proteus, pituitary
    gigantism)
Gait
  • Shuffling gait; like Chaplin's Little
    Tramp (homocystinuria)
  • Hemiplegic gait (homocystinuria with
    CVA)

CAH = congenital adrenal hyperplasia; CVA = cerebrovascular accident: MEN = multiple endocrine neoplasia; NF-1 = neurofibromatosis type 1.

Obesity

There are a number of introductions to the examination of the obese child. These include looking for the underlying cause, assessing the complications of obesity *per se,* and finally, assessing a child for complications of corticosteroid therapy. In the latter case, the child may not be obese, but the structure of the physical examination is similar.

Observation

The first step is to introduce yourself to the child. Note any obvious sleepiness in the response to your questions, which may indicate Pickwickian syndrome (gross obesity, somnolence, hypoventilation with episodes of periodic breathing and cyanosis mainly during sleep, secondary polycythaemia, and right ventricular failure). Note whether the child's reaction seems age appropriate—intellectual impairment with Prader-Willi, Bardet-Biedl (which used to be included in the term Laurence-Moon-Biedl), Fröhlich's or Down syndrome, untreated hypothyroidism, pseudohypoparathyroidism or some storage diseases.

Next, stand back and inspect for evidence of any dysmorphism (Prader-Willi, Bardet-Biedl) or obvious diagnosis (e.g. Cushing's syndrome), note the distribution of

Figure 7.3 Tall stature

1. Introduce self

2. General inspection
Position patient: standing, adequately
    undressed to allow examination
    without embarrassment
Body habitus
Tanner staging
Glasses
Skeletal anomalies
Posture
Skin

3. Measurements
Measure:
- Height
- Lower segment (LS)
- US/LS ratio
- Arm span
- Head circumference

Request weight
Assess percentile charts
Calculate height velocity
Request:
- Birth parameters
- Parents' percentiles and ages of
  puberty

4. Manoeuvres
(See Table 7.8 for findings sought)
Standing with arms and legs together
Touching toes
Tests tor hyperextensibility
Tests for arachnodactyly
Arms and hands outstretched

5. Upper limbs
Hands
Pulse
Blood pressure
Axillae

6. Head and neck
Head (size, shape)
Hair
Face
Eyes (full examination)
Nose
Mouth
Chin
Ears
Neck

7. Chest
Tanner staging
Deformity
Praecordium

8. Abdomen and genitalia
Inspect (e.g. herniae)
Palpate (organomegaly)
Tanner stage genitalia

9. Lower limbs
Inspect
Gait

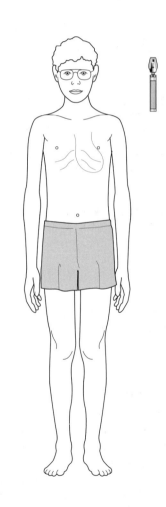

the obesity (truncal in Cushing's syndrome, and fat tends to obliterate the supraclavicular fossae, which are preserved in other cases).

Note the parameters and request the percentile charts. If the child is short, a pathological cause is more likely. There are five well known endocrine causes of a short fat child: Cushing's syndrome, hypopituitarism, hypothyroidism, growth hormone deficiency and pseudohypoparathyroidism (PHPT). If the child is tall, it is more likely to be simple obesity, but can be pathological, e.g. Klinefelter's syndrome.

Take particular note of the size of the hands (small in Prader–Willi syndrome), any glasses (Bardet–Biedl), hearing aid (Alström's syndrome) and the Tanner staging (may appear advanced in simple obesity or in Cushing's syndrome, delayed in hypothyroidism and the syndromal diagnoses).

Examination

After this initial assessment, a systematic physical examination can be performed, looking for most of the more common causes and complications. Depending on the 'lead-in' from the examiners, certain elements of this examination outline may need to be omitted.

The approach given here starts with the hands, followed by checking the blood pressure and then examining the head and neck. When examining the back, ask the child to touch the toes and check for scoliosis or kyphosis; next, ask the child to lie down and examine the abdomen, in particular the genitalia.

Following this, inspect and palpate the lower limbs. Then a series of manoeuvres can be performed to detect orthopaedic complications of obesity, such as slipped capital femoral epiphysis (SCFE) and certain features of Cushing's syndrome, such as proximal myopathy. The child is then returned to the bed for further assessment of the hip joints and lower limbs. Finally, the cardiorespiratory system is examined, having been deferred until now as the findings sought are complications rather than causes. Always request the urinalysis and do not forget to test the hearing if there is suspicion clinically of Alström's or Kallmann's syndrome. If the 'lead-in' is specifically for complications, then this is essentially a cardiorespiratory and lower limb examination, and the order will be somewhat different from the one outlined here. The various findings sought are enumerated in Table 7.9. A summary of the suggested approach is given in Figure 7.4.

Table 7.9 Additional information: details of possible findings on obesity examination

Introduction
Impression of mental state
- Intellectual impairment (PW, B-B, Down, Fröhlich's; hypothyroidism, PHPT, some storage disorders)
- Sleepy (Pickwickian)

General inspection
Growth parameters
Height
- Short (endocrine or syndromal causes)

- Tall (simple obesity, Klinefelter's)
Head circumference: enlarged (intracranial tumour, hydrocephalus with spina bifida)
Percentile charts
Calculate height velocity
Request
- Birth parameters
- Parents' percentiles
Distribution of obesity: central (Cushing's)

Continued

Table 7.9 *(Continued)*

Skin
- Bruising (Cushing's)
- Poor wound healing (Cushing's)
- Café-au-lait spots (McCune-Albright syndrome)

Truncal striae

Tanner staging
- Pseudoprecocity (Cushing's)
- Hypogonadism (syndromes, e.g. PW, B-B, Kallmann's, Fröhlich's)
- Gynaecomastia (Klinefelter's)

Respiratory rate
- Hypoventilation (Pickwickian syndrome)

Head

Shape: prominent forehead and bitemporal narrowing (PW)

Size: large (brain tumour, hydrocephalus with spina bifida)

Hair

Dry, pluckable (hypothyroidism)

Oily (Cushing's)

Face

Cherubic (round, immature face of GH deficiency)

Moonface (Cushing's)

Plethora (Cushing's, or secondary polycythaemia if Pickwickian)

Telangiectasia (Cushing's)

Coarse features (hypothyroidism)

Down syndrome facies

Eyes

Eyebrows: loss of outer third (hypothyroidism)

Almond-shaped eyes (PW)

Squint (PW)

Epicanthic folds (Down syndrome)

Downslanting (Down syndrome)

Visual acuity: impaired (B-B, Fröhlich's, Alström's)

Visual fields: bitemporal hemianopia (pituitary tumour)

Cataract (posterior subcapsular in Cushing's)

Retinae
- Retinitis pigmentosa (B-B, Alström's)
- Papilloedema (pituitary tumour, benign intracranial hypertension in Cushing's)
- Hypertensive retinopathy (Cushing's)

Nose

Anosmia (Kallmann's)

Midline dimple (hypopituitarism)

Mouth and chin

Triangular upper lip (PW)

Central cyanosis (Pickwickian)

Midline defects associated with hypopituitarism or Kallmann's
- Cleft lip (repaired)
- Cleft palate (repaired)
- Single central incisor

Delayed dentition (hypothyroidism)

Oral candidiasis (Cushing's)

Tonsillar size (upper airway obstruction associated with hypoxia and hypercapnia in Pickwickian)

Micrognathia (PW)

Facial hair or acne (Cushing's)

Neck

Goitre (hypothyroidism)

Obliteration of supraclavicular hollow, i.e. supraclavicular fat pads (Cushing's)

Elevated JVP (RVF in Pickwickian)

Abdomen

Striae (Cushing's)

Hepatomegaly (RVF with Pickwickian syndrome),

Adrenal mass (Cushing's syndrome due to adrenal tumour)

Genitalia
- Advanced development of hair or phallus (Cushing's, hypothyroidism)
- Delayed development (hypothyroidism)
- Hypogonadism (PW, B-B, Fröhlich's, Kallmann's, Klinefelter's)

Lower limbs

Inspection
- Small feet (PW)
- Skin: striae, bruises, poor wound healing (can all occur in Cushing's syndrome)
- Limb shortening (with SCFE or avascular necrosis of femoral head)
- External rotation at hip (SCFE)
- Genu valgus or varus (complications)

Measure: limb lengths (for shortening, as above)

Palpate: ankle oedema (RVF in Pickwickian)

Continued

Table 7.9 *(Continued)*	

Manoeuvres	• SCFE (complication of obesity)
Stand child with legs together and	Trendelenberg's test: positive with
reinspect for:	avascular necrosis of femoral head
• Leg shortening (if not measured)	or SCFE.
• External rotation	Lay patient down again for completion of
• Genu valgus or varus	lower limb examination.
Hold arms up against resistance (proximal	
myopathy in Cushing's)	**Lower limbs completion**
Squat (proximal myopathy)	Hip examination: limitation of internal
Walk, looking for limp with:	rotation or abduction (SCFE)
• Avascular necrosis femoral head	Ankle jerks: delayed relaxation
(Cushing's)	(hypothyroidism)

B-B = Bardet-Biedl syndrome; GH = growth hormone; JVP = jugular venous pressure; PHPT = pseudo-hypoparathyroidism; PW = Prader-Willi syndrome; RVF = right ventricular failure; SCFE = slipped capital femoral epiphysis.

Normal puberty

Pubertal development in girls usually commences between the ages of 9 and 13 years, and in boys between 10 and 14 years. During puberty, there is development of the reproductive system and accompanying development of secondary sexual characteristics, as well as an increase in body size, a change in body composition, and acceleration in skeletal growth and muscle mass. It takes between 1.5 and 5.5 years (average 3.5 years) to go through puberty. Most of the changes are sex-specific, although some are common to females and males. The sequence of events tends to be relatively more consistent than the age at which they occur. Rating systems have been devised to indicate the stage a child's pubertal development has reached.

Several terms are invariably used in discussing pubertal development, and these may be confused. Some definitions:

Adrenarche	Maturational increase in adrenal androgen (17-ketosteroid) production as normally occurs at puberty.
Pubarche	Pubic hair development as normally occurs at puberty.
Thelarche	Breast development as normally occurs at puberty.
Gonadarche	Development of pulsatile GnRH and gonadotropin activity resulting in enlarging gonads.
Menarche	First menstrual period.

In the female, the first sign is breast development, then pubic hair development, although occasionally this order is reversed. Development of the uterus and the vagina parallels that of the breasts. The height spurt peaks at approximately breast stage 4 and pubic hair stage 3, at about 1–2 years before menarche, which is quite a late occurrence in the sequence. After menarche, girls tend to grow a further 6 cm, irrespective of age at menarche.

In the male, the first sign of puberty is enlargement of the testes and scrotum, with development of reddening and thickening of the scrotal skin; this is followed by pubarche and later growth of the penis and increase in growth velocity. The height spurt reaches its peak at approximately pubic hair stage 4, which is usually about 2 years after

Figure 7.4 Obesity

1. Introduce self

2. General inspection
Position patient: standing, adequately
  undressed to allow examination
  without embarrassment (underwear
  in younger children)
Dysmorphic features (PW, B-B)
Cushingoid features
Growth parameters
  • Weight
  • Height
  • Head circumference
  • Percentiles
Distribution of obesity
Skin
Tanner staging
Respiratory rate

3. Hands
Small (PW)
Short fourth metacarpal (PHPT)
Polydactyly (B-B)
Scars from removal of additional digit
  (B-B)
Temperature
  • Cool (hypothyroidism)
  • Warm (CO_2 retention in
    Pickwickian)
Pulse
Slow (hypothyroidism)
Bounding (CO_2 retention)
Hypotonic (PW)
Flap (CO_2 retention)

4. Blood pressure
Hypertension (Cushing's, or
  complication of obesity)

5. Head and neck
Head
Hair
Face
Eyes (acuity, fields, lens, retina)
Nose
Mouth and chin
Neck
Throat (tonsillar hypertrophy)

6. Back
'Buffalo hump', i.e. interscapular fat pad
  (Cushing's)
Kyphosis (Cushing's)
Scoliosis (with spina bifida, or
  osteoporosis with Cushing's)

Midline scar (repaired
  myelomeningocoele)
Spinal tenderness (osteoporosis with
  Cushing's)

7. Abdomen
Striae
Hepatomegaly (RVF)
Adrenal mass
Genitalia

8. Lower limbs and manoeuvres
Inspect
Measure
Palpate
Manoeuvres (see text)
Hip examination
Ankle jerks

9. Cardiorespiratory
Full praecordial examination for
  evidence of cor pulmonale:
  • Right ventricular hypertrophy
  • Loud second heart sound

10. Urinalysis
Glucose (PW, Alström's, Cushing's)

11. Hearing
Impaired (Alström's, Kallmann's)

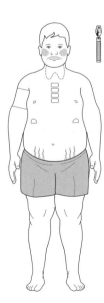

the beginning of pubic hair growth. This is also the time at which axillary hair appears. Deepening, or 'breaking', of the voice tends to be a late occurrence, and can take place very gradually, so it is not, of itself, a reliable index of pubertal development.

Staging

The Tanner staging system is widely used in Australia. The stages (abbreviated) are as follows:

Breast development

Stage 1: Preadolescent.
Stage 2: Breast bud.
Stage 3: Breast and areolae enlarged and elevated, but no separation of their contours.
Stage 4: Areola and papilla form a mound above the contour of the breast.
Stage 5: Mature.

Pubic hair stages (for females and males)

Stage 1: Preadolescent.
Stage 2: Long, fair, straight hair; sparse, mainly along labia or at base of penis.
Stage 3: Darker, coarser, curlier, sparse.
Stage 4: Adult type hair, smaller area covered than in adult.
Stage 5: Adult. Spread to medial surface of thighs.

Genital development in boys

Stage 1: Preadolescent.
Stage 2: Enlargement of scrotum, with reddening and thickening of scrotal skin.
Stage 3: Enlargement of penis, further growth of scrotum.
Stage 4: Further growth of penis and scrotum, darker scrotal skin.
Stage 5: Adult.

Precocious puberty

Sexual development is described as precocious if the onset is before 8 years in girls, and before 9 years in boys. True or central precocious puberty occurs when the hypothalamic control mechanism for puberty (the GnRH pulse generator) is prematurely turned on, leading to early gonadal maturation. Pseudoprecocious puberty, also called incomplete, or peripheral precocity, in contrast, is not due to premature activation of the hypothalamic control system. However, to complicate the picture further, long-standing pseudoprecocious puberty can lead to premature activation of the central GnRH generating mechanism, and thence to true precocious puberty.

True precocious puberty is far more common in girls than in boys. In girls, it is usually idiopathic, whereas in boys, the diagnosis is more often a central nervous system disorder, e.g. intracranial tumour or malformation.

The short-case approach covers a large amount of clinical ground, and requires a very structured routine to enable its completion in the time constraints of the examination. The approach given here is comprehensive and covers most relevant findings for girls and boys.

Examination

The examination essentially focuses on accurate staging of puberty and assessment of growth parameters, followed by evaluation of the central nervous system, the adrenal glands and the gonads. The other signs sought provide further evidence of suspected diagnoses, such as café-au-lait spots and scoliosis in neurofibromatosis type 1 (NF-1).

Commence by introducing yourself to the patient and the parent; note the quality of the child's voice replying, particularly in boys, for deepening of the voice. Next, ask the child to undress as fully as possible without causing her or him undue embarrassment; underwear can be left on for this initial inspection. Visually scan the child and assess the Tanner staging, noting the androgen effects in boys and the oestrogen effects in the girls. Next, assess the growth parameters, commencing with the height. Precocious puberty *per se* can cause tall stature early in its course. Tall stature can also occur in underlying causes such as McCune-Albright syndrome (which can cause central or peripheral precocity), or NF-1 (causes central precocity). Short stature can result from long-standing precocious puberty, but is also a feature of Russell-Silver syndrome and can occur in NF-1 (not a misprint: NF-1 can cause tall or short stature, just as it can cause large or small head circumference), two causes of true precocious puberty. Short stature may also occur in Cushing's syndrome (causes premature pubarche) and in severe hypothyroidism, which causes precocity by an unknown mechanism.

Weight is also important, as obesity can be a feature of hypothyroidism (true precocity) or Cushing's syndrome (premature pubarche). The head circumference may be increased (e.g. in hydrocephalus or intracranial tumours) or decreased, such as in previous severe head injury or in cerebral palsy. Other parameters of importance include arm span and upper segment versus lower segment (US:LS) ratio. The arm span is normally less than height before the age of 8 years. If it is greater than height before this age, it implies that the growth spurt has already occurred. The US:LS ratio for the child's age may be increased in hypothyroidism, or decreased in children with NF-1 who have scoliosis.

Next inspect the skin for any evidence of hyperpigmentation, which can occur in congenital adrenal hyperplasia (CAH), or café-au-lait spots, which can occur in NF-1, McCune-Albright syndrome or Russell-Silver syndrome. Also look for evidence of carotenaemia, which can occur in hypothyroidism, or increased sebaceous gland activity, which occurs with increased androgen secretion. Note any obvious dysmorphic or diagnostic features, such as Russell-Silver syndrome, Cushing's syndrome, McCune-Albright syndrome or NF-1.

The remainder of the examination commences at the upper limbs, initially checking for any asymmetry and then starting with the hands, working up to the head and neck, with particular emphasis on the eyes. Continue with the chest in girls, and to a lesser extent boys (e.g. pubertal gynaecomastia), and the abdomen, with accurate staging of the genitalia in boys. It is important to estimate the volume of the testes, as this is the best indicator of the maturational age. Prepubertal testes are usually less than 3 mL in volume, and the easiest way of measuring the volume is with an orchidometer. A rough approximation is that a prepubertal testis is the size of a small grape. The penile length can be easily measured by using a cottonwool-tipped swab stick: the penis is measured up against the swab stick, with the cottonwool end on the abdominal wall, and the stick is broken at the point where the tip of the glans reaches, so the stick can then be measured accurately on a ruler.

This is followed by examination of the gait, back and lower limbs. The relevant findings sought are set out in Figure 7.5.

Investigations

At the completion of your examination, give a succinct summary and differential diagnosis, followed by a brief list of investigations you feel are appropriate. These investigations depend on the sex of the child and the particular findings in that child, but may include the following.

Figure 7.5 Precocious puberty

1. Introduce self

Quality of voice
- Deep (androgenised)
- Mature female (oestrogenised)
- Higher-pitched child's voice (normal for age)

2. General inspection

Position patient: standing, adequately undressed to allow examination without embarrassment

Visually assess Tanner staging

Boys (androgen effects)
- Male body habitus
- Muscle development
- Hair: facial, axillary
- Axillary odour
- Pubic hair (stage this)
- Increased size of genitalia (stage these formally later)

Girls (oestrogen effects)
- Female body habitus
- Fat distribution
- Breasts (stage these)
- Pubic hair (stage this)

Skin
- Syndromal diagnosis

3. Measurements

Height
- Short (e.g. Russell-Silver, NF-1, hypothyroidism, Cushing's, long-standing precocity)
- Tall (e.g. recent onset precocity, NF-1, McCune-Albright)

Lower segment

US:LS ratio (for age)
- Increased (hypothyroidism)
- Decreased (scoliosis, e.g. with NF-1)

Arm span: greater than height before 8 years infers growth spurt has already occurred

Weight
- Increased (e.g. Cushing's, hypothyroidism)

Head circumference
- Increased (e.g. hydrocephalus, IC tumour)
- Decreased (previous severe head injury)

Assess percentile charts

Calculate height velocity
- Increased (true precocity)

Request parents' percentiles and ages of puberty

4. Upper Limb

Symmetry
Fingers
Palms
Pulse
Blood pressure
Axillae

5. Head and neck

Head (size, scars, shunts)
Hair
Face
Eyes (full examination)
Mouth and chin
Neck

6. Chest

Breasts
Tanner staging in girls
Galactorrhoea (hypothyroidism, pituitary tumour, hypothalamic tumour)

7. Abdomen and genitalia

Liver
- Enlarged (hepatoblastoma producing hCG, in boys)
- Bruit (hepatoblastoma)

Adrenal glands
- Mass (tumour)

Ovaries
- Mass (tumour; mention rectal examination for completeness)

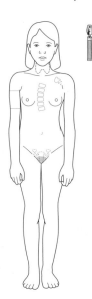

Continued

Figure 7.5 Precocious puberty (*continued*)

Uterus
- Size (stage of development; mention rectal examination for completeness)

Pubic hair
- Tanner staging

External genitalia (boys)
- Tanner staging
- Penis length (measure with swab stick)
- Testicular volume (estimate or request orchidometer, 3 mL or

less is prepubertal)
- Scrotal rugosity

8. Gait, back and lower limbs
Full gait examination to screen for long tract signs (IC tumour, hydrocephalus, head injury)
Back: scoliosis (NF-1)
Full lower limb examination to detect:
- Long tract signs
- Delayed ankle jerk relaxation (hypothyroidism)

Blood tests

1. Baseline LH, FSH, testosterone, oestradiol.
2. GnRH stimulation test (LH and FSH responses).
3. DHEAS (dehydroepiandrosterone sulfate), which may be extremely high in adrenal tumours.
4. hCG (can be produced by various tumours).
5. Thyroid function tests, including TSH level.

Imaging

1. X-ray of left wrist and hand for bone age (the most important investigation). A normal bone age suggests, depending on the clinical picture, premature adrenarche, premature thelarche or ingestion of exogenous sex steroids. An accelerated bone age is more in keeping with central precocity (various causes), adrenal or ovarian pathology (such as tumour) or McCune–Albright syndrome.
2. Skeletal survey for suspected McCune–Albright syndrome.
3. Ultrasound studies of pelvis, testes and adrenal glands.
4. Brain CT or MRI (for various intracranial pathologies, such as hypothalamic hamartoma, pinealoma, hydrocephalus, third ventricular cysts).

Additional information

Details of possible findings on precocious puberty examination are given in Table 7.10.

Table 7.10   Additional information: details of possible findings on examination of precocious puberty

General inspection
Skin
- Hyperpigmentation (CAH)
- 'Coast of Maine' café-au-lait spots (McCune-Albright)
- 'Coast of California' café-au-lait spots (NF-1)

- Carotenaemia (hypothyroidism)
- Dry, cool (hypothyroidism)
- Sebaceous gland activity

Syndromal diagnosis (Russell-Silver, McCune-Albright, NF-1)

Continued

Table 7.10 *(Continued)*

Head
Size
- Large (hydrocephalus, NF-1, IC tumours)
- Small (head trauma, cerebral palsy)
Scars (cranial surgery)
Shunts (hydrocephalus)

Hair
Dry (hypothyroidism)
Greasy (CAH)

Face
Moonface (Cushing's)
Coarse (hypothyroidism)
Asymmetry (Russell-Silver, McCune-Albright)

Eyes
Inspect
- Prominent (hyperthyroidism with McCune-Albright)
- Squint (sixth cranial nerve palsy with IC tumour)
- Lisch nodules (NF-1)
Visual fields
- Bitemporal hemianopia (pituitary tumour)
- Other field cuts such as homonymous hemianopia (IC tumour)
External ocular movements
- Sixth cranial nerve palsy (IC tumour)
- Loss of upward gaze (pineal tumour)
- Ophthalmoplegia (hyperthyroidism with McCune-Albright)
Pupils
- Argyll Robertson pupils (pineal tumour)
Cataracts (Cushing's)

Fundoscopy
- Papilloedema (IC tumour)

Nose
Comedones (androgens)

Mouth and chin
Facial hair (androgens)
Acne (androgens)
Brown pigmentation (Peutz-Jeghers associated with granulosa cell tumours in girls)

Neck
Goitre (hypothyroidism, hyperthyroidism with McCune-Albright)

Upper limbs
Hands together in front
- Asymmetry (McCune-Albright, NF-1, Russell-Silver)
Fingers
- Clinodactyly (Russell-Silver)
Palms
- Pigmented creases (CAH)
- Cool, dry (hypothyroidism)
- Warm, sweaty periphery (hyperthyroidism with McCune-Albright)
Pulse
- Slow (hypothyroidism)
- Collapsing (hyperthyroidism with McCune-Albright)
Blood pressure
- Elevated (e.g. CAH, Cushing's, NF-1)
Axillae
- Hair, odour, apocrine secretion (androgens)
- Freckling (NF-1)

CAH = congenital adrenal hyperplasia; IC = intracranial; NF-1 = neurofibromatosis type 1.

Delayed puberty

Sexual development is described as delayed if the onset of puberty has not occurred by two standard deviations from the mean, namely, 13 years in girls and 15 years in boys. Delay in puberty occurs in any condition where the bone age is delayed; bone age correlates with developmental and pubertal stage, and puberty normally occurs when the bone age is pubertal, irrespective of the chronological age.

Conditions that retard bone growth include chronic malnutrition (e.g. under-nutrition, anorexia nervosa, cystic fibrosis, Crohn's disease), many chronic illnesses (e.g. thalassaemia, sickle cell anaemia, chronic renal failure, cyanotic congenital heart disease, juvenile arthritis, and other severe connective tissue diseases), and several endocrine conditions (e.g. hypothyroidism, growth hormone deficiency, hypopituitarism).

The other diagnosis associated with delay in bone age is 'constitutional delayed puberty', which tends to have a positive family history. In this condition puberty occurs at a bone age of 12 in girls (which usually occurs at a chronological age of 16), and a bone age of 14 in boys (chronological age 18).

Other groups of disorders have normal bone age for chronological age, including syndromal diagnoses (e.g. Klinefelter's, Turner's and Noonan's syndromes) or causes of organic hypogonadism (again several syndromes—Prader-Willi, Bardet-Biedl, Fröhlich's and Kallmann's syndromes—all cause hypothalamic deficiency of gonadotropin-releasing hormone; pituitary tumours causing pituitary gonadotropin deficiency).

Unlike precocious puberty, pubertal delay is far more common in boys. 'Idiopathic' or 'constitutional' delay occurs mainly in boys. There are multiple causes in boys; in girls, causes include the majority of those that can affect boys, but there are some that are quite specific (e.g. Turner's syndrome) or relatively more common in females (e.g. anorexia nervosa, hypothyroidism).

This short-case approach covers as much clinical material as precocious puberty and requires as structured a routine. The approach covers relevant findings in boys and girls.

Examination

The examination focuses on accurate staging of puberty and assessment of growth parameters, followed by evaluation for evidence of chronic disease, syndromal features (e.g. Turner's syndrome, Noonan's syndrome) or certain endocrine disorders (e.g. hypopituitarism).

Begin by introducing yourself to the patient and parent, and note the quality of the child's voice replying, particularly in boys, for lack of deepening (but comment to the examiners that the voice 'breaking' is a late sign and is quite variable, not a reliable indicator of pubertal status). Next, ask the child to undress as fully as possible without causing undue embarrassment; underwear should be left on for this initial inspection. Visually scan the child and assess the Tanner staging, noting the lack of androgen effects in boys or oestrogen effects in girls.

Next, quickly note any obvious dysmorphic features suggesting a diagnosis such as Turner's, Noonan's, Prader-Willi or Bardet-Biedl syndrome, or diagnostic facial features (e.g. thalassaemia). Note the nutritional status, as nutritional deficiency may occur in Crohn's disease, cystic fibrosis and anorexia nervosa, and excessive adipose tissue can occur with several endocrine disorders (e.g. hypopituitarism, hypothyroidism) or in syndromes (e.g. Prader-Willi and Fröhlich). Pallor may indicate a chronic anaemia (e.g. chronic renal failure, sickle cell anaemia or thalassaemia). Also note the body habitus (e.g. eunuchoid habitus: i.e. arm span significantly greater than height, and lower segment greater than upper segment length) suggestive of Kallmann's or Klinefelter's syndrome.

The measurements of height, lower segment, upper segment to lower segment (US:LS) ratio, and arm span should then be carried out (or requested of the examiners), followed by the head circumference. Request the weight and the percentile charts, calculate the height velocity and interpret this appropriately. Finally, ask for the parents' percentiles and ages of puberty. The height and height velocity are especially important, as can be appreciated from the large number of causes of short stature listed in Table 7.6. Measuring the US:LS ratio and the arm span helps to evaluate whether there is any eunuchoid body habitus, which can occur in Kallmann's or Klinefelter's syndrome, and also detects a short lower segment, such as classically occurs in hypothyroidism. The weight is also important in detecting diagnoses such as anorexia nervosa and chronic diseases in thin children, and endocrine and syndromal problems in obese children. Head circumference, if increased, may indicate an intracranial tumour. Always request the percentile charts and do not forget to calculate the height velocity. Finally, requesting the parents' ages of puberty may make a diagnosis of constitutional delay apparent.

The remainder of the examination begins with the hands and proceeds up to the head and neck, with particular emphasis on assessment of any midline defects or visual field loss, and then to the chest, abdomen and finally accurate staging of the genitalia in boys. The volume of the testes should be estimated, as this is the best indicator of the maturational stage. Prepubertal testes are usually less than 3 mL in volume, and less than 2 cm in length. An orchidometer can be requested if you are familiar with its use. Another measurement that may be used is the testicular volume index, which is the average length multiplied by the width of both testes. Prepubertally, it is usually betweed 1.0 and 1.4 cm^2.

Finally, request the urinalysis.

The procedure is outlined in Figure 7.6. A detailed listing of possible findings is given in Table 7.11 at the end of the section on delayed puberty.

Investigations

At the completion of the physical examination, the examiners may ask which investigations you would perform. These of course depend upon the physical findings, but the following list covers some of the more useful investigations. Note that the various causes of hypogonadism are often divided into two groups, based on the gonadotropin levels: patients with primary hypogonadism (primary hypofuncton of testis or ovary) have high gonadotropin levels, and are said to have 'hypergonadotropic' hypogonadism, while those with gonadal hypofunction secondary to lack of pituitary gonadotropic hormones (on the basis of hypothalamic or pituitary disease) have 'hypogonadotropic' hypogonadism.

Blood tests

1. Baseline luteinising hormone (LH), follicle-stimulating hormone (FSH), testosterone, oestradiol.
2. GnRH stimulation test (LH and FSH responses).
3. Provocative testing for growth hormone release (with exercise, insulin induced hypoglycaemia, arginine infusion or levodopa).
4. TRF stimulation testing (prolactin and TSH responses).
5. Thyroid function tests.
6. Karyotype (especially for Turner's syndrome and testicular feminisation in girls, Klinefelter's syndrome in boys).
7. Full blood count and film (for chronic anaemias).
8. Electrolytes, urea and creatinine (for renal failure).

Imaging

1. X-ray of left wrist and hand for bone age (the most important investigation).
2. Brain CT scan or MRI (for intracranial pathologies, such as craniopharyngioma).

Figure 7.6 Delayed puberty

1. Introduce self
Quality of voice
- High pitched (prepubertal)

2. General inspection
Position patient: standing, undressed
  (consider leaving underwear on to
  avoid embarrassing the child)
Visually assess Tanner staging
Boys (lack of androgen effects)
- Male body habitus
- Muscle development
- Facial or axillary hair
- Body odour
- Pubic hair (stage this)
- Size of genitalia (stage these
  formally later)
Girls (lack of oestrogen effects)
- Female body habitus
- Fat distribution
- Breasts (stage these)
- Pubic hair (stage this)
Dysmorphic features
Body habitus
Nutritional status
Pallor

3. Measurements
Height
- Lower segment
- US/LS ratio
Arm span
Weight
Head circumference
Percentiles
Calculate height velocity
Request parents' percentiles and ages
  of puberty

4. Upper limbs
Hands
Fingertips
Nails
Palms
Pulse
Forearms
Blood pressure
Axillae

5. Head and neck
Head
Hair
Eyes (full examination)
Nose
Mouth and chin
Ears
Hairline
Neck

6. Chest
Breasts
Sternal deformity
Lung fields
Praecordium

7. Abdomen
Inspection
Palpation
- Hepatomegaly
- Splenomegaly

8. Genitalia
Tanner stage genitalia
- Measure penis length
- Measure testes parameters;
  estimate testes volume
Penile anomalies
- Micropenis (Kallmann's,
  hypopituitarism)
- Hypospadias (Noonan's)
Testes anomalies
- Cryptorchidism (Klinefelter's,
  Kallmann's, Noonan's)

9. Gait and lower limbs
Inspection
Gait
Lower limbs
  neurologically

10. Other
Urinalysis
Low specific gravity
  (CRF, diabetes
  insipidus with
  septo-optic
  dysplasia)
Glucose (IDDM)

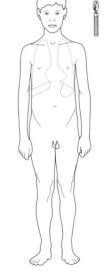

Table 7.11 Additional information: details of possible findings on delayed puberty examination

General inspection

Dysmorphic features (various syndromes—Turner's, Noonan's, P-W, B-B)

Body habitus: eunuchoid (Kallmann's, Klinefelter's)

Diagnostic facies (e.g. Turner's, Noonan's, thalassaemia)

Nutritional status
- Poor (anorexia nervosa, Crohn's disease)
- Excess adiposity (hypothyroidism, P-W, B-B, Fröhlich's, hypopituitarism)

Pallor (thalassaemia, SCA, CRF)

Measurements

Short stature
- Constitutional delay
- Chronic malnutrition (undernutrition, CF, Crohn's disease)
- Chronic illness (thalassaemia, SCA, CRF, cyanotic CHD, juvenile arthritis)
- Endocrine disorders (hypothyroidism, growth hormone deficiency, hypo-pituitarism, severe IDDM)
- Syndromes (Turner's, Noonan's, P-W, B-B, Fröhlich's, Kallmann's)

Normal stature (excludes most of the above)
- Primary gonadal failure (dysplastic, e.g. Klinefelter's; absent, e.g. congenital anorchia, or removal due to gonadal tumour; dysfunction, e.g. testicular feminisation, or rarer forms of congenital adrenal hyperplasia)
- Anorexia nervosa
- IDDM

Tall stature
- Kallmann's (can cause tall or short stature)
- Klinefelter's

US:LS ratio
- Increased (hypothyroidism)
- Decreased (Klinefelter's, Kallmann's)

Arm span
- Over 4 cm more than height (eunuchoid habitus, e.g. Kallmann's)

Weight
- Decreased (chronic illnesses, malnutrition; see above)
- Increased (endocrine disorders, syndromes; see above)

Head circumference
- Increased (intracranial tumour)

Height velocity
- Decreased (chronic illnesses, chronic malnutrition, endocrine disorders)
- Normal (constitutional delay, primary gonadal failure)

Upper limbs

Hands
- Small (P-W)
- Polydactyly (B-B)

Fingertips: BSL testing (IDDM, thalassaemia, CF)

Nails
- Clubbing (CHD, CF, Crohn's)
- Brown lines (CRF)
- Hyperconvex (Turner's)

Palms
- Crease pallor (chronic anaemias, CRF)
- Crease pigmentation (thalassaemia)

Pulse
- Bradycardia (untreated hypo-thyroidism)
- Absent femorals (Turner's with coarctation)

Forearms: muscle bulk (malnutrition)

Blood pressure: elevated (CRF, Turner's with coarctation)

Axillae: lack of apocrine secretion, hair or odour (confirm delay)

Head

Midline scar (repaired frontal encephalocoele)

Hair

Dry (hypothyroidism)

Eyes

Inspection
- Hypertelorism (Noonan's)
- Epicanthal folds (Noonan's, Turner's)
- Ptosis (Noonan's)
- Squint (septo-optic dysplasia, P-W)
- Nystagmus (septo-optic dysplasia)

Conjunctival pallor (thalassaemia, CRF, malnutrition)

Visual acuity: diminished (pituitary tumour, IDDM, B-B)

Continued

Table 7.11 *(Continued)*

Visual fields: bitemporal hemianopia (craniopharyngioma, pituitary tumour)
External ocular movements: sixth cranial nerve palsy (intracranial tumour)
Cataracts (IDDM)
Fundi
- Papilloedema (raised ICP, craniopharyngioma)
- Optic nerve hypoplasia (septo-optic dysplasia)
- Optic atrophy (raised ICP, craniopharyngioma)
- Diabetic retinopathy
- Retinitis pigmentosa (B-B)

Nose
Anosmia (Kallmann's)
Midline dimple (hypopituitarism)
Nasal polyps (CF)

Mouth and chin
Central cyanosis (CHD)
Midline defects associated with hypopituitarism
- Cleft lip (repair)
- Cleft palate (repair)
- Single central incisor
Delayed dentition (hypothyroidism)
Glossitis (malnutrition)

Ears
Low set (Turner's, Noonan's)

Hairline
Low (Turner's, Noonan's)

Neck
Pterygium colli (Turner's, Noonan's)
Goitre (hypothyroidism)

Chest
Breasts
- Tanner staging in girls

- Gynaecomastia (Klinefelter's)
- Well developed but with no pubic or axillary hair (testicular feminisation)
- Wide-spaced nipples (Turner's, Noonan's)
Sternal deformity (Noonan's)
Hyperinflation (CF)
Percuss for hyperresonance (CF)
Auscultate: chest (CF); praecordium (CHD)

Abdomen
Inspection
- Tanner staging of pubic hair
- Injection sites (IDDM, thalassaemia)
- Scars (CF-meconium ileus; CRF-peritoneal dialysis, renal transplant; Crohn's disease surgery)
- Venous access port (CF)
- Perianal disease (Crohn's)
Palpation
- Hepatomegaly (thalassaemia, CF, IDDM, malnutrition, chronic active hepatitis)
- Splenomegaly (thalassaemia, CF with portal hypertension)

Gait and lower limbs
Inspection
- Injection marks on thighs (IDDM)
- Erythema nodosum (IBD)
- Necrobiosis lipoidica (IDDM)
- Oedema of dorsa of feet (Turner's)
- Clubbing of toes (CF, CHD)
Gait, screening for:
- Long tract signs (IC tumour)
- Peripheral neuropathy (CRF, nutritional deficiency)
Lower limbs neurologically
- Long tract signs (IC tumour)
- Neuropathy (CRF, nutritional deficiency)
- Delayed ankle jerk relaxation (hypothyroidism)

B-B = Bardet-Biedl syndrome; CF = cystic fibrosis; CHD = congenital heart disease; CLD = chronic liver disease; CRF = chronic renal failure; IBD = inflammatory bowel disease; ICP = intracranial pressure; IDDM = insulin dependent diabetes mellitus; P-W = Prader-Willi syndrome; SCA = sickle cell anaemia.

Thyroid disorders

These are not uncommon cases, but there are a number of possible introductions that may be used, including examining the neck, the thyroid (specified) or the eyes, or examining for causes of irritability, nervousness or even cold intolerance. Probably the most common introduction is to examine the neck. The approach outlined below is for children beyond infancy; in infants, the approaches for congenital hypothyroidism or hyperthyroidism are somewhat different and are discussed at the end of this section.

Most cases will have an autoimmune thyroid disease, such as Graves' disease or Hashimoto's thyroiditis. These may be associated with other autoimmune diseases, such as insulin-dependent diabetes mellitus (IDDM), Addison's disease, and less commonly hypoparathyroidism, pernicious anaemia, vitiligo and hypogonadism.

Graves' disease comprises three components, namely a hyperfunctioning goitre, an ophthalmopathy and a dermopathy. The ophthalmopathy comprises exophthalmos (due to infiltration of orbital contents, excluding the eyeball, by inflammatory cells) and the findings of sympathetic overactivity, which are found in hyperthyroidism irrespective of cause. The dermopathy usually occurs over the dorsal aspect of feet or legs, and is termed pretibial myxoedema.

Hashimoto's disease, or autoimmune thyroiditis, includes chronic lymphocytic thyroiditis and primary myxoedema. Most patients with this diagnosis are initially euthyroid but eventually become hypothyroid. A small percentage are initially hyperthyroid, and may have ophthalmopathy: this is called 'Hashitoxicosis'.

The approach outlined assesses for the presence of autoimmune thyroid disorders, as well as associated autoimmune diseases. It also assesses for other underlying diagnoses, causing hyperfunction (e.g. toxic adenoma) or hypofunction (e.g. endemic cretinism, fetal iodine deficiency or haemosiderosis from thalassaemia).

Examination

Begin by introducing yourself to the child and the parent. Note any hoarseness in the child's voice when he or she replies (hypothyroidism in older children), and ask the child which school he or she attends and which grade, for an impression of mentation (slow in hypothyroidism, restless in hyperthyroidism).

Next, stand back and inspect the child for any obvious signs associated with hyperthyroidism (such as exophthalmos, tremor) or hypothyroidism (such as short stature, thyroidectomy scar, yellow skin discolouration due to carotenaemia, facial myxoedema). Note the height and weight parameters, and request the percentile charts. Hyperthyroidism is associated with tall stature and decreased weight, while hypothyroidism is associated with short stature and increased weight.

If the child is short, or hypothyroidism seems likely, then the US:LS ratio should be measured to see if it is increased. Now, ask the child to sit on a chair for examination of the neck. Inspect the neck from all angles, noting any redness overlying the thyroid region (thyroiditis) and any obvious swelling. Note the size, shape and symmetry of any swelling, and confirm it is the thyroid gland by obtaining a glass of water and having the child swallow a small amount. Do not be tempted to rush in and palpate before careful inspection during swallowing. The thyroid is best palpated from behind in the first instance, with the child's chin lowered and the head slightly inclined towards whichever side is being examined, to relax the overlying sternomastoid muscle.

The palpation of the thyroid gland itself should be along similar lines to that of any lump (after first checking with the child that it is not exquisitely tender). Note the site, size, shape, symmetry (symmetrical enlargement is the rule in thyrotoxicosis), surface (smooth in thyrotoxicosis, irregular in multinodular goitre), consistency and mobility (any degree of fixation to surrounding structures suggests malignancy). Tenderness is present in subacute thyroiditis (de Quervain's; very rare in children) or acute suppurative thyroiditis. Thyrotoxicosis may be accompanied by a thrill, due to the increased vascularity of the gland, which can be felt by lightly laying your hand over the lateral lobes; this needs to be differentiated from transmitted carotid pulsation. Also note that if the carotid pulsation cannot be felt on one side, this may be due to malignancy surrounding the artery. Check for involvement of draining lymph nodes (in malignant thyroid tumours) and distortion of normal anatomy (such as a retrosternal goitre displacing the trachea).

Next, check for retrosternal extension of thyroid enlargement by percussing across the upper portion of the manubrium sterni (e.g. from right to left) to assess for any retrosternal dullness. Next, auscultate for any bruits (a systolic bruit can accompany a thrill in thyrotoxicosis).

Finally, assess for any direct effects on other neighbouring structures, by quickly checking the child's eyes (for Horner's syndrome due to involvement of the cervical sympathetic chain in malignant thyroid disease) and the voice (for hoarseness due to malignant involvement of the recurrent laryngeal nerve). Then check for Pemberton's sign of thoracic inlet obstruction (due to retrosternal thyroid enlargement), by asking the child to raise both arms fully and checking a few seconds later for facial plethora and distended jugular veins, and note any evidence of inspiratory stridor. Ask the child to take a big breath in, through an open mouth, to check more formally for stridor.

Only when the thyroid gland itself has been fully evaluated should the examination proceed to look for signs of hyperfunction or hypofunction; a suggested format is as follows.

The examination flows well if you start at the neck and then move to the head (in particular the eyes). Make a point of thoroughly inspecting the eyes from all angles, especially from above, over the child's forehead. Next examine the upper limbs (these aspects can be checked with the child sitting on a chair), followed by a series of manoeuvres and then the lower limb examination, the praecordium and lung fields (looking for complications such as congestive cardiac failure), and then the abdomen. Finally request the temperature chart, urinalysis, and, depending on the findings so far, check the child's development and/or the hearing, and/or test for signs of hypo-parathyroidism (essential if a thyroidectomy scar is present). It can be difficult to assess a child who is being treated for either problem, as many expected signs, such as a slow pulse, are not present and this may fluster the inexperienced candidate. Should this happen to you, try to remain calm and simply perform a comprehensive examination, looking for all the signs mentioned, until it becomes apparent whether hypofunction or hyperfunction is the problem, and then proceed with a more directed assessment. For a summary of the examination, see Figure 7.7.

Investigations

At the completion of your examination, the investigations worth mentioning are as follows.

Hyperthyroidism

Blood tests
1. Thyroid function tests, including thyroid-stimulating hormone (TSH) level.
2. Thyroid autoantibodies found in Graves' disease, including the following:
   • Thyroid-stimulating immunoglobulin.

- TSH-binding inhibiting immunoglobulin.
- Exophthalmogenic immunoglobulin.
- Dermopathy-associated immunoglobulin.
3. Other autoantibodies found in associated diseases:
  - Pancreatic islet cell antibody.
  - Adrenal cell antibody.

Figure 7.7 Thyroid disorders

1. Introduce self
Mentation

2. General inspection
Position patient: standing for initial
   inspection, then sitting
Obvious signs of:
  - Hyperthyroidism
  - Hypothyroidism
Parameters
  - Height
  - US/LS (if short or suspect
    hypothyroidism)
  - Weight
  - Percentile charts
  - Height velocity
Skin

3. Neck—thyroid gland
Examine with patient sitting
Inspection for goitre
Swallowing
Palpation (from behind)
Percussion (for retrosternal extension)
Auscultate for bruit (+)
Assess direct local effects
Check for Horner's syndrome and for
   hoarse voice (if possibility of
   malignancy)
Pemberton's sign (for retrosternal
   extension)

4. Head
Hair
Face
Eyes (full examination)
Mouth

5. Upper limbs
Hands
Fingertips
Nails
Palms

Pulse
Manoeuvres for hyperthyroidism
  - Hands out
  - Take pulse with arm elevated
  - Proximal strength
Blood pressure

6. Lower limbs
Inspection
Manoeuvres
Power
Reflexes
Sensation

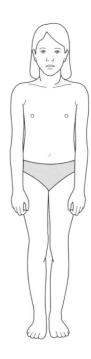

Imaging
Radionuclide scanning.

Hypothyroidism

Blood tests
1. Thyroid function tests, including TSH.
2. Thyroid autoantibodies found in Hashimoto's disease, including the following:
   - Antithyroglobulin antibody.
   - Antimicrosomal antibody.
3. Other autoantibodies found in associated diseases:
   - Pancreatic islet cell antibody.
   - Adrenal cell antibody.

Imaging
1. Bone age.
2. Radionuclide scan.
3. Cranial CT or MRI if a pituitary lesion is suspected.

Thyroid disorders in infants

The most common scenario is a baby with hypothyroidism, although a neonate with hyperthyroidism may occasionally be encountered. Transient neonatal thyrotoxicosis is usually due to transfer of thyroid autoantibodies across the placenta. In these cases, the examination can proceed in the same order as that outlined for the older child, but with much more emphasis on assessing lack of weight gain, and also watching the baby feed. These children are usually tremulous, irritable and do not gain weight; sweating and tachycardia are prominent. The nappy of such a baby should be checked, as diarrhoea is the rule. After assessing the baby with hyperthyroidism, remember to ask to examine the mother for manifestations of Graves' disease.

Congenital hypothyroidism is not uncommon, although screening has afforded most infants prompt diagnosis and treatment. The examination of the infant with suspected hypothyroidism commences with general inspection, after taking particular note of the age of the baby. Inspection may reveal jaundice, somnolence, respiratory difficulties (noisy respirations, apnoeic episodes due to large tongue), delayed separation of the umbilical cord, umbilical hernia, protruberant abdomen, peripheral cyanosis, oedematous extremities and genitalia. The growth parameters are usually normal at this early stage. Next, inspect the head and neck. Note the facial features: the hairline may reach a long way down on the forehead; the eyes seem far apart; the eyelids swollen; palpebral fissures narrowed; the nose broad with a depressed nasal bridge; the mouth open and the tongue large. The neck may appear short and thick, with increase in adipose tissue (above the clavicles and between the neck and the shoulders). In an older infant, there is a delay in the development of the teeth. Now, palpate the hair, which may be coarse and brittle. Feel the head; the scalp may be thickened and the fontanelles wide open. Look at the conjunctivae for pallor. Look in the mouth with a spatula for a lingual thyroid. Next, with the infant lying prone on the mother's lap, look for a goitre; this is best palpated with the baby in this position. Following this, examine the heart and the abdomen, in the standard fashion, looking for evidence of cardiomegaly, constipation and oedema of the external genitalia. Perform a gross motor developmental assessment, to evaluate for delay and hypotonia. Finally, request the temperature chart (for hypothermia) and ask to watch the child feed; there may be disinterest in feeding, poor effort and choking episodes. Remember to ask to examine the mother for hyperthyroidism in neonates with a goitre (transplacental delivery of antithyroid medication).

The most useful investigations are thyroid function tests, including TSH level, and a thyroid scan, to differentiate between dyshormonogenesis and ectopic or absent thyroid tissue.

Table 7.12 gives detailed possible findings on examination of a child with a thyroid disorder

---

Table 7.12 Additional information: details of possible findings on examination of a child with a thyroid disorder

Introduce self
Quality of voice: hoarse (–)
Mentation
- Impaired (–)
- Irritable (+)

General inspection
Obvious signs associated with:
- Hyperthyroidism (e.g. exophthalmos, tremor, sweating, nervousness)
- Hypothyroidism (e.g. short stature, coarse facies, thyroidectomy scar)
- Associated autoimmune diseases (e.g. Addison's, vitiligo)
- Causes of hypofunction (thalassaemia)
Tanner staging
- Precocity (–)
- Delay (–)
Skin
- Yellow tinge (–)
- Vitiligo (autoimmune association)
- Hyperpigmentation (Addison's, thalassaemia)
- Pretibial myxoedema (Graves')

Hair
Dry (–)
Alopecia (autoimmune association)

Face
Flushed, sweaty, anxious (+)
Coarse, bloated, yellow (–)
Rodentoid features (thalassaemia)
Hyperpigmented (Addison's)

Eyes
Inspection (from above and from side)
- Exophthalmos (Graves')
- Thyroid stare (+)
- Lid lag (+)
- Lid retraction (+)

- Strabismus (fetal iodine deficiency, exophthalmic ophthalmoplegia)
- Nystagmus (fetal iodine deficiency)
Conjunctivae
- Pallor (hypothyroidism per se or secondary to thalassaemia; associated pernicious anaemia)
- Oedema, inflammation (in exophthalmos)
Cornea (ulceration in exophthalmos)
Visual fields: bitemporal hemianopia (pituitary tumour causing hypothyroidism)
Extraocular movements: muscle paresis in exophthalmos (in order)
- Inferior oblique (first affected)
- Adductors (muscles of convergence: medial, superior, inferior recti)
- Lateral rectus
- Test for lid lag (+)
Lens: cataracts (associated IDDM)
Retina
- Optic atrophy (with exophthalmos)
- Diabetic retinopathy (associated IDDM)

Mouth
Pigmented buccal mucosa, gums (Addison's)
Lingual thyroid (–)
Poor dentition (–)

Upper limbs
Hands
- Dry, cool, puffy (–)
- Peripheral cyanosis (–)
- Peripheral neuropathy (–)
- Tremulous, warm, sweaty (+)
Fingertips: prickmarks from BSL testing (IDDM)

Continued

Table 7.11 *(Continued)*

Nails
- Onycholysis (+)
- Thyroid acropathy (+)

Palms
- Erythema (+)
- Crease pallor (-, pernicious anaemia)
- Crease pigmentation (Addison's, thalassaemia)

Pulse
- Slow (–)
- Rapid (+)
- Ectopic beats (+)
- Atrial fibrillation (+)
- Collapsing pulse (+)

Manoeuvres for hyperthyroidism
- Hands out in front (tremor)
- Take pulse with arm elevated (collapsing pulse)
- Test proximal muscle strength (proximal myopathy)
- Reflexes (brisk)

Blood pressure
- Decreased (Addison's)
- Wide pulse pressure (+)

Lower limbs
Inspection (standing)
- Onycholysis (+)
- Acropathy (+)
- Pseudohypertrophy (–)
- Pretibial myxoedema (Graves')
- Injection sites on thighs (IDDM)

Manoeuvres
- For hyperthyroidism: squat and stand (proximal myopathy)
- For hypothyroidism: gait (normal and heel-toe)
- High stepping (peripheral neuropathy)
- Ataxia (endemic cretinism)
- Spasticity (endemic cretinism)

Kneel on chair to test ankle jerks (delayed relaxation)
Neurological examination (on bed)
Power
- Proximal myopathy (+)
- Generally decreased (–)

Reflexes
- Brisk (+, endemic cretinism)
- Slow relaxation (–)

Sensation: diminished (demyelinating neuropathy in hypothyroidism)

BSL = blood sugar level; IDDM = insulin dependent diabetes mellitus.
If a finding is related to hyperthyroidism it is marked with a plus sign (+), and if to hypothyroidism, with a minus sign (–).

Gastroenterology

Long cases

Inflammatory bowel disease

In the last few years there has been an increase in the number of therapies for inflammatory bowel disease (IBD). Standard treatments have been predominantly *anti-inflammatory* (aminosalicylates [mesalamine, sulfasalazine], antibiotics [metronidazole, ciprofloxacin], nutritional therapy [nasogastric or oral]), *immunosuppressive* (6-mercaptopurine [6-MP], azathioprine [AZA], methotrexate [MTX] or cyclosporine A [CSA]), or *both* (corticosteroids). More recently immunotherapeutic *biologic agents* have been developed including anti-tumour necrosis factor alpha (anti-TNFα) antibodies (infliximab, CDP571), and TNF fusion protein (etanercept). *Non-biologic agents* being researched including granulocyte colony-stimulating factor (GCSF) and growth hormone (GH).

Progress has been made in understanding the basic pathophysiology of IBD. It is apparent that genetic, immunologic and environmental factors interact to produce IBD. A specific disease-associated gene, *Nod-2* (also called *CARD 15*) has been described in some patients with Crohn's disease (CD). *Nod-2* codes for an intracellular molecule involved in inflammatory response to bacterial peptidoglycans; this supports the concept of enteric flora being important in pathogenesis.

Patients with Crohn's disease (CD) and ulcerative colitis (UC) are often used as long cases. Both diseases are commonly complicated by extraintestinal manifestations, including arthralgia, erythema nodosum, uveitis and sclerosing cholangitis. Either may present with these extraintestinal features years before IBD is diagnosed. Both may require surgical intervention at some stage in their course. All candidates should be familiar with the differentiating features between the two. Candidates should know the medications used to induce remission and those used to maintain remission in each condition.

History

Presenting complaint

Reason for current admission.

Gastrointestinal symptoms

Interval/current: weight loss, growth, abdominal pain (site, interference with sleep, precipitation by eating), anorexia, nausea, vomiting, odynophagia or dysphagia (oesophageal CD), diarrhoea, urgency, tenesmus, incontinence, rectal bleeding, fistulae (CD, usually enterocutaneous), perirectal disease (CD).

Extraintestinal symptoms

Interval/current: rashes (e.g. erythema nodosum [more in CD], pyoderma gangrenosum [more in ulcerative colitis, UC]), mouth involvement (e.g. aphthous ulcers), liver involvement (e.g. chronic active hepatitis), joint disease (e.g. arthralgias, spondyloarthropathies), visual problems (e.g. uveitis), vascular complications (e.g. vasculitis), renal tract involvement (e.g. nephrolithiasis), hypertension, myocarditis, pericarditis, fever, pubertal delay, neurologic problems (e.g. peripheral neuropathy), haematological disease (e.g. anaemia), musculoskeletal weakness (e.g. vasculitic myositis, steroid-induced myopathy), pancreatitis, extraintestinal neoplasia (e.g. lymphoma), amyloidosis, thromboembolic disease (e.g. cerebral, retinal).

Past history

Initial presentation, symptoms, when, where and how diagnosed, response to treatment, subsequent course, doctors involved, clinics attended, previous hospitalisations, past surgery, previous complications of disease and treatment, coexistent congenital immunodeficiencies (e.g. common variable immunodeficiency, neutrophil disorders), previous misdiagnoses (e.g. avoidance of food, thinness and pubertal delay as in anorexia nervosa, joint disease as in juvenile arthritis, severe perirectal disease as in child sexual abuse).

Treatment

Drugs, nutritional therapy (elemental and parenteral), surgical, alternative medicine, side effects of treatment (e.g. steroids), past courses of antibiotics (*Clostridium difficile* colitis).

Social history

1. Impact on child
Problems of chronic disease: energy levels, behavioural problems, chronic hospitalisation, altered self-image, school absence, depression, feeling of missing out due to disease exacerbations and energy levels, initial denial of interference with life, frustration, anger about physical symptoms (pain, diarrhoea, faecal incontinence), altered appearance, unpleasant and demanding treatments, lack of independence, lack of control of choices of activities (school, leisure, employment, sport), isolation, cigarette smoking (exacerbates CD), steroid effects, short stature, delayed sexual development (adverse effects on socialisation, self-esteem), effect on overall quality of life, perception of long-term effects on peer group recognition, whether and when desired transition to adult care, refusing counselling (not 'cool').

2. Impact on family
Financial burden of multiple hospitalisations, surgical procedures, parents' worries (how disease will affect future, problems at school, medication side effects, guilt), conflicts with parents (concerning eating habits and compliance with medication), siblings' worries (being kept ignorant of disease and treatment, jealousy of attention and overprotection of patient).

3. Social supports
Social worker, parent support groups, psychologist (IBD has one of the highest effects on mental health of chronic diseases in children), online 'chat groups' for teenagers.

Family history

Inflammatory bowel disease, ankylosing spondylitis, rheumatoid arthritis.

Examination

The salient findings sought on physical examination are listed in Figure 8.1.

Investigations

Investigations to clarify the diagnosis and those to assess disease activity are undertaken concurrently, so they are listed together here. In 10–15% of cases, it is not possible to differentiate CD from UC; these patients have 'indeterminate' colitis (an interim diagnosis).

Stool

Mainly to differentiate other causes of symptoms.

1. Microscopy (fresh specimen) for cysts, ova, parasites.
2. Culture for bacteria (e.g. *Campylobacter,* enteropathogenic *E. coli, Shigella*).
3. *Clostridium difficile* toxin.
4. Alpha-1-antitrypsin level (screen for protein loss from bowel).

Blood

1. Full blood count (leucocytosis found in two-thirds of CD).
2. ESR/CRP (elevated in 90% of CD).
3. Liver function tests (liver dysfunction as part of IBD; low albumin, total protein from protein-losing enteropathy).
4. Vitamins: folate (serum and red cell), vitamin B_{12} (ileal disease), vitamins A, D, E and prothrombin time for vitamin K (fat malabsorption).
5. Minerals: calcium, magnesium, phosphate, iron, ferritin, zinc, copper, selenium.
6. Electrolytes, urea and creatinine (associated renal disease).
7. Serology for *Yersinia* species (*enteropathica* and *pseudotuberculosis*) to exclude this as a diagnosis. *Yersinia* colitis can present with erythema nodosum and arthralgia, as can CD.
8. Perinuclear anticytoplasmic antibodies (pANCAs) to neutrophil proteins may be elevated in UC. Not tested routinely.
9. Anti-*Saccharomyces cerevisiae* (ASCA) antibodies may be present in CD (more sensitive and specific with elevated pANCA). Not tested routinely.
10. Antibodies to *E. coli* (outer membrane porin C antibodies), anti-OMPC. Presence of these may correlate with diagnosis of IBD. Not tested routinely.

Imaging

1. Plain abdominal X-ray, erect and supine (may see evidence of incomplete bowel obstruction with distended bowel loops and air/fluid levels in CD).
2. Barium meal and follow through (may identify terminal ileal disease in CD).
3. Double-contrast barium enema (may identify rectal and colonic disease in CD and UC).
4. Chest X-ray (to help detect tuberculosis, a well-known cause of chronic bowel inflammation).
5. Abdominal and pelvic ultrasound and CT scanning. These may be useful in

Figure 8.1 Inflammatory bowel disease

1. General inspection
Weight
Height
Percentiles
Tanner staging
Nutritional status (muscle bulk, subcutaneous fat, peripheral oedema)
Pallor
Jaundice
Cushingoid appearance
Abdominal scars and stoma
Joint swelling (especially lower limbs)
Skin rashes (erythema multiforme, erythema nodosum, pyoderma gangrenosum)

2. Upper limbs
Clubbing (especially CD)
Palmar crease pallor (anaemia from dietary deficiency, iron loss in gut, folate malabsorption, vitamin B_{12} malabsorption, chronic disease, or side effects of salazopyrine)
Arthritis (wrists, elbows)
Palpable epiphyseal enlargement (vitamin D deficiency)

3. Head and neck
Cushingoid facies
Conjunctival pallor (anaemia)
Conjunctivitis
Scleral icterus (sclerosing cholangitis, chronic active hepatitis)
Iritis
Corneal xerosis or clouding (vitamin A deficiency)
Cataracts (if on steroids)
Aphthous stomatitis

4. Abdomen
Scars
Stoma
Striae (if on steroids)
Tenderness
Mass (matted loops or abscess)
Hepatomegaly (sclerosing cholangitis, chronic active hepatitis)
Ascites (protein deficiency, protein-losing enteropathy in CD)
Enlarged kidneys (hydronephrosis in CD from ureteral compression by inflammatory mass or fibrosis)

Fistulae (CD)
Gluteal wasting
Perianal disease (anal fissures, fistulae, abscesses, anal tags)
Rectal examination (blood, pus on glove)

5. Lower limbs
Joint swelling (knees, ankles)
Tibial bowing (vitamin D deficiency)
Erythema nodosum, pyoderma gangrenosum
Toe clubbing

6. Stool and urine
Stool
• Inspection for blood, pus
• Analysis for white cells reducing substances
Urinalysis
• Urinary tract infection (recurrent in CD with enterovesicular fistulae)
Calculi: oxalate (CD), urate (UC)

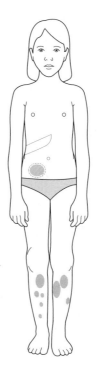

CD = Crohn's disease; UC = ulcerative colitis.

delineating intra-abdominal masses (e.g. solid lesions or bowel loops), including abdominal or pelvic abscesses.

6. Gadolinium-enhanced magnetic resonance imaging (MRI). Advances in MRI technology including use of intravenous gadolinium has improved intestinal image resolution: CD shows transmural enhancement of colon, and bowel wall thickening of terminal ileum or proximal small bowel; UC shows mucosal enhancement and submucosal sparing extending proximally from the rectum. Cheaper and more pleasant than endoscopy.

7. Radio-labelled white blood cell scan (useful if mid-small bowel pathology suspected but not able to be found using conventional evaluations).

8. Bone age (assessment of growth delay in CD).

9. Bone density assessment (DEXA).

Endoscopy

Sigmoidoscopy, colonoscopy and ileoscopy. In active UC, the mucosa is oedematous, hyperaemic and friable. In CD, aphthous or serpiginous ulcers may be seen, as well as erythema and 'skip' lesions, and an appearance like cobblestones.

Newer developments in adults include video-capsule endoscopy, in which the patient ingests the capsule, and the images are transmitted to a belt-worn recorder, allowing an ambulatory and prolonged (e.g. 8-hour) examination, which is especially useful for assessing areas where upper endoscopy or colonoscopy cannot reach. There is no 'paediatric' capsule yet, but children over 10 may be able to swallow the capsule. In Australia, the Health Insurance Commission has approved capsular endoscopy for children over 10 years of age. Any procedure (e.g. colonoscopy, barium enema) may precipitate fulminant colitis in those with severe disease.

Other

1. Mantoux test (to help exclude tuberculosis).
2. Urine culture (to detect urinary tract infection, which can be recurrent in CD with fistulae between gut and bladder).

Management

Short-term aims include induction and maintenance of clinical and histologic remission, improvement in overall quality of life and prevention of complications. Longer-term aims include preventing relapses, normalising growth and pubertal development, maintaining bone mass and minimising need for surgery. These therapeutic aims are based on early aggressive therapy, including use of newer biologic agents. Earlier use of potent agents, previously considered 'third line', may be more effective than awaiting resistance to treatment. When evaluating new therapies, remember that a placebo response rate over 30% has been noted in IBD.

The Paediatric Crohn's Disease Activity Index (PCDAI) and quality-of-life measures are recognised as useful in assessing response to therapies. The PCDAI gives a score out of 100, based on well-being, abdominal pain, number of bowel movements with or without blood, weight, linear growth, physical findings and laboratory indices (haematocrit, ESR, albumin): 0–10 indicates remission, 10–30 mild to moderate disease, and over 30, severe disease. No equivalent index exists for children with UC. For quality-of-life aspects in children over 10 years old with IBD, the IMPACT questionnaire, a validated and age-specific set of short questions, has proved useful.

Crohn's disease (CD)

No medication alters the long-term outcome of CD. Corticosteroids are the most efficacious drugs in achieving *remission*, but relapse is common. In the past, around 20% of patients have become steroid-dependent, and 20% steroid-resistant. Corticosteroids have no proven value in *maintenance* therapy, so should be used only for short-term treatment, preferably for no longer than 3 months.

Remission: corticosteroids, infliximab, nutrition, immunomodulators

The best agents for remission in CD are currently prednisolone (for moderate to severe disease), budesonide (potent steroid control-released in the small intestine and right colon), and the biologic agent infliximab (for refractory disease, steroid dependency or fistulising disease)

Patients with mild disease are followed up regularly, but may not require steroids. In moderate CD, corticosteroids can induce a remission in around 70% of patients with small bowel disease. Steroids are given orally (prednisolone, methylprednisolone, budesonide) or intravenously (hydrocortisone, methylprednisolone).

Controlled ileal release budesonide is useful in treating active ileal and ileocaecal disease and can also delay relapses. Budesonide may have fewer side effects and less adrenal suppression than prednisolone. Severe hypokalaemia and benign intracranial hypertension have been described in children receiving oral budesonide.

Steroid side effects relate to dose and duration, and can include bone loss. This can occur rapidly, within weeks of commencing treatment, and is not prevented by alternate-day treatment. Effective preventative therapies established in adult patients include calcium supplements, vitamin D and calcitriol.

Lack of response to steroids may be due to presence of strictures or, less commonly, complications such as an abscess or fistula. Treatment may involve bowel rest (TPN in hospital or at home, or elemental diet by nasogastric infusion) or surgery. Surgery in CD tends to be conservative, being limited to dealing with emergencies (perforation, obstruction, massive haemorrhage, toxic megacolon), relieving less urgent problems (fistulae), resecting very localised disease and preserving bowel.

Infliximab (anti-TNFα antibody) is effective in active and fistulising CD. Pro-inflammatory cytokines such as TNFa are involved in the pathogenesis of CD. Infliximab, an anti-TNFa monoclonal antibody, neutralises these cytokines, stopping inflammation. It can induce a clinical remission and mucosal healing within weeks, with a response rate of over 80% (both clinical and endoscopic) in moderate to severely active treatment-resistant CD in patients already receiving immunosuppressive treatment. It is given initially at 0, 2 and 6 weeks. It can maintain remission if given every 8–12 weeks. Around 20% of patients develop antibodies (human-antichimaeric antibodies [HACAs]) to infliximab, which limits its effectiveness; HACAs can be induced after one or several infusions. The clinical effect of infliximab appears to be improved when a patient is also taking one of the other immunomodulating drugs such as AZA or 6-MP.

Enteral nutritional therapy can be used to induce remission in patients with active CD involving small bowel (with or without proximal colonic disease) who have growth failure or intolerable steroid side effects. As a primary management, it can lead to remission in up to 80% of patients, but relapse rates are high, so it is more often used as an adjuvant therapy to avoid malnutrition or micronutrient deficiencies (e.g. folate, vitamin B_{12}, fat soluble vitamins [A, D, E, K], iron, calcium, magnesium, zinc), and to optimise growth.

Nutritional interventions have been used widely in Europe, with steroid use diminishing accordingly. Both elemental and polymeric diets can lead to improved scores of disease activity, healing histologically, and down-regulation of pro-inflammatory cytokines. Severely malnourished patients may require overnight nasogastric tube feeds with elemental formulae or polymeric preparations; lactose-intolerant patients need lactase supplements; patients with strictures may find a low-residue diet helpful; patients with severe terminal ileal disease should have a low-oxalate diet and decreased dietary fat. There are now formulae with anti-inflammatory cytokines, prebiotics and pro-biotics, but there is insufficient evidence to support their use as yet. Total parenteral nutrition (TPN) can be used where other therapies fail, but it is more expensive and no more impressive than enteral feeding with elemental or polymeric formulae. Home TPN and home enteral nutrition are widely used in the USA in patients with CD.

Immunomodulator drugs such as 6-MP, AZA (which is metabolised to 6-MP, the active agent) or MTX may be required by patients with CD who are steroid-dependent or have Cushingoid side effects. In particular 6-MP has been shown useful as initial treatment in children with moderate to severe CD.

Maintenance of remission: immunomodulators, infliximab, 5-ASAs

Immunomodulator drugs such as AZA and 6-MP may be indicated for maintenance therapy for CD, prophylaxis after surgery in CD, and perianal CD. AZA and 6-MP have a slow onset of action (3–4 months) so need to be combined with nutritional therapy or steroids until their effect is seen. Duration should be over years, as there is a high relapse rate if AZA or 6-MP are stopped within first year. Bone marrow suppression can occur (in 2–5% of patients) at any time. If using AZA or 6-MP, it is useful to know the patient's thiopurinemethyltransferase (TPMT) status. TPMT is the enzyme that cata-lyses the conversion of 6-MP to 6-methylmercaptopurine (6-MMP). If there is a deficiency of TPMT, then 6-MP can be metabolised along an alternate pathway to 6-thioguanine (6-TG), which is toxic and can cause bone marrow depression: that is, low TPMT means high 6-TG levels and high risk of leukopenia. Higher 6-MMP levels correlate with hepatotoxicity in adults. Aminosalicylates and methotrexate inhibit TPMT activity and can increase 6-TG levels.

MTX may be indicated for the treatment of steroid-dependent chronically active CD when AZA or 6-MP fails (after 4 months), or if the patient is intolerant of AZA or 6-MP. MTX may be given in low-dose oral form (oral bioavailability is complete with low doses and decreases if higher doses given) or intramuscularly. Low-dose MTX side effects include nausea (in about 40%), anorexia, stomatitis, diarrhoea, headache, dizzi-ness, fatigue and altered mood, and can be reduced by giving supplemental folic acid therapy. Pulmonary toxicity (especially interstitial pneumonitis) can occur at any time and with any dose.

Infliximab (anti-TNFα antibody) can maintain remission if given every 8–12 weeks. Infliximab is very expensive. Side effects include an increased risk of infection (e.g. tuberculosis), autoimmune disease and malignancy (e.g. lymphoproliferative).

5-ASAs (5-aminosalicylates: mesalazine [also called mesalamine], olsalazine, balsalazide) and their role in CD have become controversial, as many controlled studies have shown little effect. For primarily small bowel disease, the 5-ASAs may be bene-ficial, but for any patient with oesophagitis, gastritis or duodenitis, other medications are likely to be required. For symptomatic colonic disease, treatment may include aminosalicylates.

Antibiotics such as metronidazole and ciprofloxacin have been used in patients with colitis that is unresponsive to aminosalicylates, and in those with perianal disease and fistulae, although there are no controlled data to show they are efficacious.

Newer treatments aim to block destructive mucosal responses or decrease levels of antigens in the gut lumen. These include biologic treatments aimed at TNF (CDP571, a more humanised anti-TNF antibody than infliximab), intercellular adhesion molecules, integrins and probiotics (live organisms such as *Lactobacillus* species) that alter gut flora. For very severe CD, bone marrow ablation and stem cell transplantation are being investigated.

Ulcerative colitis (UC)

In UC medical management is successful in preventing relapses and surgical management is curative. *Remission* in UC is usually achieved with corticosteroids for moderate to severe disease, and with 5-ASAs for mild to moderate disease. For severe refractory disease, intravenous CSA can be a useful 'rescue' therapy, avoiding immediate surgery. *Maintenance of remission* in UC can be achieved by immunomodulators (AZA/6-MP, MTX) for moderate to severe disease, 5-ASAs for mild to moderate disease, and oral CSA for refractory disease.

Mild disease

Patients with mild disease look well and produce two to five stools per day. Management usually comprises steroid enemas, one twice a day initially, if urgency is severe (proctitis). As the disease settles, this can decrease to one nightly for 2 weeks or until settled fully. Topical mesalazine is also used in topical left-sided UC and this can reduce the relapse rate if used prophylactically (e.g. twice a week). The main problem with enemas is compliance. Oral steroids may be required. When parents see the Cushingoid effects of oral steroids, they start to comply with the enemas. The volume of the enemas is 50–100 mL, retained for half an hour.

5-ASAs can treat the acute situation and are also valuable prophylactically. Treatment is usually lifelong (for the life of the colon). Sulphasalazine comprises sulphapyridine linked to 5-aminosalicylate (5-ASA) by an azo bond which is broken by colonic bacteria; 5-ASA, the active component, is released directly to the colon. The 5-ASAs are enteric-coated and deliver the drug to the small and large bowels. The most common problems encountered with sulphasalazine are related to the sulpha part (rashes, bone marrow depression), whereas 5-ASAs can cause nephrotoxicity.

Moderate disease

Patients with moderate disease have rectal bleeding and urgency, are slightly unwell and have static weight. They require systemic corticosteroid therapy for a few months. Aminosalicylates are also used. A combination of steroid and sulphasalazine brings the condition under control quickly in most cases and hopefully surgery can be avoided. Alternate-day steroids tend not to work in these children.

Severe disease

Children with severe disease may be very unwell, have abdominal pain and anaemia, and are hypoproteinaemic. However, children with severe pancolitis may have few constitutional symptoms but very severe disease. The rare 'toxic megacolon' can present requiring hospitalisation for intravenous steroids, bowel rest and TPN.

Cyclosporine (CSA) can be used as a 'rescue' treatment for severe UC to avoid emergency colectomy. The response is within 2–3 weeks, but this only postpones colectomy; despite clinical remission in around 80%, most will need colectomy within a year. CSA may allow time to educate families regarding acceptance of this treatment. CSA is a peptide which blocks interleukin-2 production by T helper cells. Side effects of CSA are frequent, including paraesthesiae in about 25% of patients, hypertrichosis, hypertension, renal insufficiency and tremors. CSA can be used only where blood levels of CSA can be determined readily.

The colon needs to be removed. Indications for emergency surgery include gastrointestinal haemorrhage (UC is the second leading cause of massive gastrointestinal blood loss in children), intestinal perforation, fulminant colitis or toxic megacolon. Emergent operative treatment usually comprises total abdominal colectomy, with an end ileostomy, subsequent proctocolectomy, and then ileoanal reconstruction.

Removal of the colon and rectum is curative for the intestinal manifestations of UC. Extraintestinal disease, however, continues despite colectomy. A total colectomy with endorectal removal of rectal mucosa and an ileoanal sphincter-saving anastomosis (an endorectal pull-through procedure, ERPT) with some variant of pouch reservoir, is performed commonly, and preserves continence in 90–98% of children, with an expected four to six stools per 24 hours after the first postoperative year. During this procedure all rectal mucosa is removed to avoid the risk of malignant change. To preserve sphincter function, most surgeons leave the distal 4–5 cm of rectal muscle layer intact, and remove *only* the rectal mucosa; this also decreases the rate of inadvertent injury to the pelvic sympathetic and parasympathetic nerves responsible for sexual function.

There are several reservoir options with the ERPT, including J-, S- and W-shaped pouches fashioned from the terminal ileum. Pouchitis, presenting with loose bloody stools, urgency and frequency, develops in 30–40% of those undergoing this procedure. Pouchitis is associated with an increase in extraintestinal manifestations of UC. It may be treated with metronidazole. A repeat endoscopy within 3 months is suggested by some units.

Pubertal delay
Management of pubertal delay involves obtaining adequate remission and maintaining this. Reduction of intestinal inflammation and caloric supplementation to reverse malnutrition are important. It is well described that surgical intervention, in UC particularly, can be associated with the onset of puberty. Pubertal delay is thus a relative indication for surgery. Escalating therapy using biologic agents or immunomodulators can be considered to maintain remission through puberty. Many adolescents are psychologically upset by pubertal delay and many units use sex steroid therapy in these patients. In boys with IBD, testosterone for 3–6 months can have very positive effects on virilisation, growth and psychological well-being, although there are no controlled trials of testosterone use. In girls with IBD, ethinylestradiol can be used for a similar period of time.

Metabolic bone disease
Bone disease can occur in IBD as a result of malnutrition; calcium homeostasis and bone growth are of paramount importance. It is now recognised that peak bone mass (PBM) is the main determining factor in the risk of developing osteoporosis later in life, and over 90% of PBM is acquired during childhood and adolescence. Calcium supplementation is effective in preventing bone disease. It is controversial as to whether bisphosphonates have any role in paediatric patients.

Malignant potential (UC only)
Once a child has had the disease for 8–10 years, the general risk of colon cancer is 1% per year, and by 20 years may be up to 25%. After 8 years of disease, yearly colonoscopy and biopsy are recommended, with further colonoscopies if the child is symptomatic between visits.

If carcinoma is found, the treatment is colectomy. If carcinoma in situ is found, the treatment is colectomy. If dysplasia is found, colonoscopy should be repeated in 3 months and, if found again, colectomy is recommended.

If a child has continuous disease, or a frequently relapsing course, the risk of malignancy is greater than in those with less severe disease.

Chronic liver disease (CLD)

The prognosis for children with end-stage CLD has improved markedly: liver transplantation (LTx) now has over 90% survival with good quality of life. CLD provides many issues for discussion. There is a crisis in donor supply for LTx, and the long-term consequences of immunosuppression remain of concern.

The causes of CLD can be divided into three groups: cholestatic diseases, metabolic diseases and chronic hepatitis (various forms).

Cholestatic diseases

Extrahepatic biliary atresia (EHBA)

This is the most common form of liver failure in children, and the main indication for LTx. It is of unknown cause. There is destruction of extrahepatic and intrahepatic bile ducts causing cholestasis, fibrosis and cirrhosis, with clinical correlates of jaundice and failure to thrive. Initial treatment is the Kasai portoenterostomy, a palliative procedure, which involves removal of the fibrosed biliary tree and forming a roux-en-Y anastomosis, and which leads to biliary drainage in around 30% of affected children. Management includes low-dose antibiotics to prevent cholangitis and nutritional support. Recurrent cholangitis, cirrhosis and portal hypertension inevitably occur, making LTx a requirement.

Alagille syndrome

This is an autosomal dominant multisystem disorder with intrahepatic biliary hypoplasia, plus facial, cardiac, renal, skeletal and ocular anomalies. The genetic defect is on the jagged I gene on chromosome 20. The disorder presents with jaundice, pruritis and failure to thrive. Fifty per cent of patients regain normal liver function by adolescence. For those who progress to cirrhosis and portal hypertension, or have intractable pruritis and poor overall quality of life, LTx is required.

Progressive familial intrahepatic cholestasis disorders (PFIC)

These are due to defects on chromosomes 2 (PFIC 2), 7 (PFIC 3), and 18 (PFIC 1) with abnormalities in bile salt transport, and are hence characterised by pruritis and jaundice. There is a low serum gamma glutamyltransferase (GGT) in PFIC 1 and 2, and a high GGT in PFIC 3.

Metabolic disease

WATCH this is not missed (mnemonic).

Wilson's disease (WD)

This is the most common cause of fulminant liver failure in children over 3 years. It is an autosomal recessive disorder of copper metabolism in which the liver cannot excrete this metal into the bile. The WD gene ATP7B is located on *13q14.3*, and encodes a copper-transporting P-type ATPase: there are more than 200 disease-causing mutations of this gene. Initially there is copper accumulation in the liver, then excess copper spills over into the brain (basal ganglia), kidneys, bones and cornea (Kayser-Fleischer rings). Investigation findings include low serum copper and caeruloplasmin, and raised urinary copper. It is rare for WD to present before 3 years. Neurological features present in WD in adolescence. WD is managed with penicillamine, zinc and pyridoxine, chelating copper which is excreted in urine. One-third of patient die if untreated. LTx is required if the patient is unresponsive to penicillamine or has advanced liver failure with coagulopathy and encephalopathy. WD liver disease does not recur after LTx, which provides an effective phenotypic cure, converting the copper kinetics of a homozygous child to that of a heterozygote.

Alpha-1-antitrypsin (AT) deficiency

This is the most common inherited cause of CLD to present in the neonatal period and the most frequent metabolic diagnosis requiring LTx. It presents with cholestasis, failure to thrive and vitamin K–responsive coagulopathy. It is diagnosed by low serum levels of AT, followed by phenotype (protease inhibitor type [PI type]) determination—PIZZ (homozygous AT deficiency) or PISZ (compound heterozygous). AT is the main blood-borne inhibitor of neutrophil proteases (elastase, cathepsin G, proteinase 3). AT is encoded by a gene (PI) located at 14q32.1. The pathogenesis of liver disease (entirely different from that of lung disease) is from retention of a mutant alpha-1-antitrypsin Z (ATZ) molecule in the endoplasmic reticulum (ER) of liver cells. No specific therapy for AT-deficiency CLD exists. Protein replacement therapy is only for the emphysema of AT deficiency, there being no evidence that low-serum AT levels play a role in CLD. Just over one-third of patients need a LTx, just under one-third recover and one-third get cirrhosis.

Tyrosinaemia type 1

This is an autosomal recessive disorder in which there is a deficiency of fumaryl acetoacetase, which prevents metabolism of tyrosine. Toxic metabolites accumulate and damage the liver, kidneys, heart and brain. The abnormal gene is located on 15q23–q25. The disorder presents in infants with acute liver failure and in older children with CLD. It is diagnosed by finding succinylacetone in the urine, and increased plasma tyrosine, phenylalanine and methionine.

Management of chronic tyrosinaemia includes a low-protein diet (to reduce tyrosine), vitamin D and 2-(2-nitro-4-trifluoromethylbenzoyl)-1,3-cyclohexenedione (NTBC), which prevents the formation of toxic metabolites, reverses biochemical and clinical effects, allows hepatic regeneration and almost eliminates the risk of hepatocellular carcinoma (HCC). If NTBC fails, LTx is required. Also, LTx is required if HCC (rising alpha-fetoprotein, liver nodularity on ultrasound, CT or MRI) is suspected.

Cystic fibrosis(CF)

See the long case on this disorder. It is the most common indication for LTx in older children. CF liver disease does not recur after transplant.

Hereditary fructose intolerance (HFI)

This is an autosomal recessive disorder. The abnormal gene is located on 9q22.3 and codes for fructose-bisphosphate aldolase, which catalyses the cleavage of D-fructose-1, 6-bisphosphate to glycerone phosphate and D-glyceraldehyde 3-phosphate. Most cases present with neonatal hypoglycaemia and lactic acidosis. The disorder can cause failure to thrive, cirrhosis, gastrointestinal bleeding, ongoing hypoglycaemia attacks later in life, vomiting, seizures, proximal renal tubular acidosis and an aversion to sweets and fruit, and is characterised by an absence of dental caries. It is treated by avoiding fructose, and avoiding fasting, particularly during febrile episodes. Investigations may show fructosaemia, hyperbilirubinaemia, hypophosphataemia, hypermagnesaemia, glycosuria, phosphaturia, bicarbonaturia and high urinary pH. It does not require LTx, as medical treatment is successful.

Chronic hepatitis

All forms of progressive liver disease can lead to the common end point of cirrhosis with portal hypertension. Cirrhosis can be compensated or uncompensated, the latter occurring when the liver loses its synthetic function and develops complications as outlined below.

Autoimmune liver disease is the commonest liver disease in older children, but an uncommon cause of liver failure. Most respond to (first line) prednisolone or azathioprine, or (second line) cyclosporine A or tacrolimus. LTx is reserved for failure to respond to these, or fulminant hepatic failure. Autoimmune hepatitis can recur after LTx.

With chronic hepatitis B or C, affected children are usually asymptomatic carriers who very slowly develop cirrhosis and portal hypertension (and hepatocellular carcinoma) over 20–30 years. They rarely need treatment in childhood. Hepatitis B and C can recur after LTx.

Cirrhosis is technically a histological diagnosis, usually associated with blood tests showing elevated transaminases, alkaline phosphatase, gammaglutamyl transferase, and prothrombin time, and decreased serum albumin, calcium and phosphate (secondary to rickets), and haemoglobin. On imaging, ultrasound may show echogenic liver, splenomegaly and oesophageal varices, and endoscopy may show gastric and oesophageal varices.

Complications of cirrhosis are as follows, mnemonic **HEPATIC**.

H	**H**epatorenal syndrome, **H**epatopulmonary syndrome, **H**ypersplenism.
E	**E**ncephalopathy, **E**sophageal varices.
P	**P**ortal hypertension, **P**rotein calorie malnutrition.
A	**A**scites.
T	**T**hrombosis of portal vein.
I	**I**nfection (spontaneous bacterial peritonitis).
C	**C**oagulopathy, **C**arcinoma (hepatocellular, many years later).

History for CLD

Presenting complaint

Reason for current admission, length of stay in hospital, management changes that have occurred since admission, the indications for the types of investigations that have been done, the specialists that have been involved. In particular, look for any suggestion of incipient liver failure, any discussion of liver transplantation as a future or current option.

Past history (including initial presentation)

Initial symptoms (e.g. jaundice, pale stools, dark urine, gastrointestinal tract bleeding, pruritus), age at diagnosis, where diagnosed, initial treatment, response to treatment, subsequent course, doctors involved, clinics attended, previous hospitalisations, past liver biopsies, past complications of disease (e.g. haematemesis, ascites), or its treatment (e.g. rashes or marrow suppression with penicillamine in WD, or Cushingoid effects in CAH treated with steroids, cyclosporine side effects in LTx patients).

Gastrointestinal symptoms (interval and current)
Appetite, nausea, vomiting, haematemesis, melaena, steatorrhoea, acholic stools, weight loss, abdominal pain.

Other symptoms
1. General health: lethargy, weakness.
2. Related to diagnosis: respiratory symptoms in CF, neurological problems in Wilson's disease.
3. Related to complications: bruising (vitamin K deficiency), ataxia (vitamin E deficiency).

Treatment
Drugs, surgery, side effects of treatment, monitoring of treatment, alternative medical therapies.

Social history

Problems of chronic disease, especially in older children, e.g. behavioural problems, the effects of chronic hospitalisation, dietary restrictions, treatment side effects, effect of disease on siblings and school friends, school absence, depression.

Family history

Thorough family history (including distant relatives who died in infancy of unknown causes, e.g. galactosaemia, tyrosinaemia), as many diseases are autosomal recessive in inheritance (e.g. CF, WD).

Examination for CLD

Figure 8.2 shows complications (only) of CLD. For the approach to the examination for the aetiology (e.g. KF rings and neurologic assessment for WD), refer to the short-case section in this chapter.

Investigations

These are outlined in the short-case section on jaundice. It is always worth discussing with the examiners the previous investigations in which you are particularly interested, showing your understanding of the significance of each. Furthermore, you must specify which investigations are important at present, which are likely to be important in future management, and how often these should be checked. This may seem obvious, but is often not considered until the examiners put you 'on the spot', which is not optimal.

Principles of management of CLD

General

Monitor weight, serum albumin, serum bilirubin (total and conjugated), prothrombin time. Psychosocial support is important.

Nutrition

Deficiencies in nutrients are common in CLD. Patients require a high energy (120–150% of recommended daily amount), moderately high-protein intake (3–4 g/kg/day) for growth. Branched chain amino acid enriched formulations have been shown to be clearly advantageous in providing nutritional support and are the formulae of choice. Branched

Figure 8.2 Chronic liver disease

1. General inspection
Jaundice (note depth)
Unwell (end-stage disease)
Well (compensating at present)
Mental state (encephalopathy)
Peripheral stigmata of CLD
- Spider naevi
- Bruising, bleeding
- Scratch marks
- Xanthomata
Evidence of rickets (vitamin D
    malabsorption)

2. Hands
Leuconychia
Clubbing
Palmar erythema
Xanthomata (between fingers and on
    extensor surfaces)
Asterixis (liver failure)
Wrists: epiphyseal widening (vitamin D
    deficiency)

3. Head and neck
Eyelid xanthomata
Conjunctival xerosis (vitamin A
    deficiency)
Scleral icterus
Corneal xerosis, clouding or
    opacification (vitamin A deficiency)

4. Chest
Sternal deformity (vitamin D
    deficiency)
Rib rosary (vitamin D deficiency)

5. Abdomen
Prominent abdominal wall veins
Ascites
Splenomegaly (portal hypertension)
Hepatic bruit (HCC can have this)
Haemorrhoids

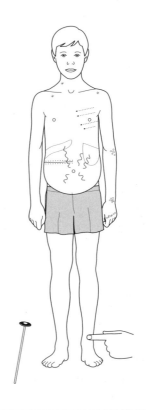

chain amino acids are metabolised in the periphery and do not require the liver for metabolism. Consider enteral feeding if the child is anorectic. Nocturnal nasogastric enteric feeding may be needed: parents can do this at home. Decreased bile flow leads to diminished intraluminal bile acids, and fat malabsorption. Provision of adequate essential fatty acids, fat soluble vitamins (A, D, E, K), zinc, iron and calcium is important. If enteral feeding is not tolerated due to ascites, variceal bleeding or recurrent hepatic complications, TPN may be needed.

Salt and water retention/ascites

Development of ascites is a poor prognostic sign. Management is by sodium restriction (less than 2 mmol/kg/day) and salt restriction to 0.3 to 0.5 g/day. Aim for negative salt balance to lose water. A loss of 100 to 150 mEq of salt will result in a loss of 1 litre (1000 g) of water. Aim for 250 g weight loss per day. Spironolactone (aldosterone antagonist) may be used; salt-poor albumin and frusemide may be needed. An abdominal tap may be diagnostic with infected fluid, but is otherwise of little value. If acute renal failure or hepatorenal failure supervene, haemodiaysis or haemofiltration may be necessary.

Encephalopathy

This can be difficult to detect, presenting with vague symptoms of lack of energy, drowsiness and regression in school work. The mainstays of therapy are decreasing the nitrogenous load to the bowel and reducing the bacterial production of ammonia in the colon. Review precipitating factors such as infection, large gastrointestinal bleed, excessive protein intake, electrolyte imbalance and diuretics. Restrict protein (to 2 g/kg/day); consider substitution with branch-chained amino acids. Use oral lactulose and neomycin.

Portal hypertension, varices and variceal haemorrhage

Oesophageal varices inevitably develop with portal hypertension. They can be evaluated endoscopically. Some centres suggest prophylactic sclerotherapy; this is a controversial point, and most centres do not recommend it. An acute episode of variceal bleeding can be life threatening, requiring intensive-care management, intravenous fluids and blood products, and therapy with intravenous vasopressin, octreotide or glypressin to reduce portal pressure. Once the patient is haemodynamically stable and the diagnosis has been confirmed by endoscopy, band ligation or sclerotherapy can be performed. Should these fail, balloon tamponade with a modified Sengstaken-Blakemore tube and intravenous vasopressin for 24–48 hours are useful. Complications of balloon tamponade can include pulmonary aspiration, oesophageal rupture and suffocation.

Endoscopic sclerotherapy has been replaced by band ligation, which ablates varices successfully in 70–100% of cases, has rebleeding rates of 15–30%, has fewer complications than sclerotherapy, except for dysphagia, which is more common with band ligation. In some children, bleeding may be controlled by insertion of a transjugular intrahepatic portosystemic stent shunt (TIPSS), which has success rates of 80–100%: complications include occlusion of stent, development of encephalopathy and infection. TIPSS can be used to control portal hypertension in children with compensated CLD, such as in some children with CF.

Avoid splenectomy if possible. As well as the risk of infection after splenectomy, it may lead to increased bleeding from removal of good collateral vessels from the splenic capsule (azygos system) that bypass the lower oesophageal junction vessels. Haemorrhage can be exacerbated by deficiency of vitamin K–dependent factors, thrombocytopenia secondary to hypersplenism and circulating fibrinolysins.

Coagulopathy

An adequate dose of vitamin K (2–10 mg/day) is needed. Fresh frozen plasma, cryoprecipitate and platelets (for hypersplenism) may be required during bleeding episodes.

Pruritus

Pruritus associated with CLD may cause significant morbidity and may be intractable in children with biliary hypoplasia. Ursodeoxycholic acid is widely used and is the treatment of choice. Often more than one drug is required, including rifampicin, cholestyramine, phenobarbitone, ondansetron and naltrexone.

Drugs

Certain drugs should be avoided in children with CLD. These include phenytoin, sulphonamides, erythromycin and paracetamol.

Sepsis

Infections are common in CLD, especially ascending cholangitis and bacterial peritonitis, and can precipitate encephalopathy, or acute or chronic liver failure.

Other non-transplantation treatment options

There are several areas where there have been recent advances. Replacement of a deficient abnormal end product can be achieved, such as in patients with abnormal biosynthesis of bile acids, by oral administration of primary bile acids. Depletion of the substance stored is another strategy, as used in neonatal iron storage disease with chelation and antioxidant mixtures. Metabolic inhibitors may be used, such as NTBC in tyrosinaemia. Enzymes can be induced, such as with the use of phenobarbitone in Crigler-Najjar syndrome type II. Substrates can be restricted in the diet, as with galactose in galactosaemia. Molecular manipulation can be achieved, such as by inhibition of polymerisation of alpha-1-antitrypsin. Future treatment may incorporate gene therapy and receptor-based targeted enzyme replacement therapy.

Liver transplantation (LTx)

LTx is associated with a survival of 90% at 1 year and 80% at 5 years, and can be used as treatment for a multiplicity of liver diseases, many of which were considered incurable a decade ago. Recent improvements in LTx include refinements in immunosuppression, technical advances in the transplantation process, the use of reduced, split and living related donor organs, and improved management of infectious complications.

Timing of transplantation

The timing of LTx depends upon a variety of factors and may be hastened by any of the following:

1. History of life-threatening variceal haemorrhage.
2. Development of (a) hepatorenal state; (b) hepatic encephalopathy; (c) refractory ascites; (d) reduction in psychosocial development; (e) intractable pruritus; (f) severe metabolic bone disease; (g) diminished quality of life.

Assessment occurs in specialist liver units, with preparatory education and counselling of the child and family, a multidisciplinary team that may include a psychologist and a play therapist (especially for children under 2 years), intensive nutritional support, completion of routine immunisation (especially hepatitis A and B) before commencement of immunosuppression, and management of CLD complications.

Indications for LTx

As noted above, indications for LTx include failure of hepatic synthetic function, poor quality of life (e.g. intractable pruritis, lethargy, anorexia, recurrent infections), intractable malnutrition or failure to thrive, refractory ascending cholangitis, hyperammonaemia from certain inborn errors of metabolism (IEMs), encephalopathy, oesophageal varices from portal hypertension, and hypersplenism.

Specific diseases requiring LTx, in order of decreasing frequency, include:

1. Extrahepatic biliary atresia (EHBA): over 50% of LTx.
2. IEMs (10–15% of LTx) include AT deficiency, CF, galactosaemia, glycogen storage diseases (GSDs) type IA and IV, mitochondrial functional defects (e.g. defects of fatty acid beta-oxidation), some organic acidaemias, tyrosinaemia, urea cycle defects and WD.
3. Acute hepatic necrosis (around 10%).
4. Cirrhosis from chronic active hepatitis or primary biliary cirrhosis (under 10%).
5. Cholestatic liver disease, other than EHBA (under 5%).
6. Primary hepatic malignancy (2%).

The only absolute contraindication to LTx is irreversible extrahepatic disease (e.g. HIV, irreversible brain damage, incurable malignancy).

The following requirements must be met for a cadaveric donor for LTx:

1. Brain death prior to circulatory arrest.
2. Absence of sepsis, HBsAg and HBeAg, HIV, malignancy, drug abuse, liver or gall-bladder disease, chronic hypertension.
3. Liver enzymes, serum bilirubin within three times normal values.
4. No period of hypoxia (PaO_2 <60 mmHg) or hypotension (over 2 hours).
5. Absence of more than minimal pressor support to maintain normal blood pressure and peripheral perfusion.
6. To match a recipient, the suitable donor must have ABO compatibility with the recipient. Sex and HLA type compatibility are not necessary.

There have been many technical innovations in the LTx process. These include reduction hepatectomy (cutting an adult liver down, in an anatomic fashion, to fit one child, which wastes some of the adult liver), followed by the development of split-LTx (one donor liver offered to two recipients, usually an adult and a child) and then living related LTx (where the left lobe [occasionally the right lobe] or left lateral segment is removed from the parent/adult liver).

Complications of LTx

Rejection occurs most often in the first 3 months after transplant; it is less common in children under 6 months and in those receiving a living donor graft. The liver allograft is an 'immunologically privileged' organ, because rejection, especially if steroid sensitive, has no adverse effect on graft survival or even function. Further, some studies show rejection itself may benefit patient survival. It seems that some rejection may be protective of graft function: a controlled amount of immune activation seems necessary (perhaps to delete clones of the recipient's lymphocytes that can damage the graft). Most late graft losses are related to immunosuppression: either too much leading to sepsis, post-transplant lymphoproliferative disease (PTLD), lymphomas or other de novo tumours, or too little leading to graft loss, which is often a result of noncompliance (especially in teenagers). Chronic rejection is becoming rare, which some attribute to increased use of tacrolimus. Increased awareness of the adverse effects of immunosuppression are channelling interest to achieving just the right amount of immunosuppression: enough to prevent damaging rejection, but without the risks of unnecessary over-immunosuppression.

Graft rejection (60%)
* Late acute rejection can occur anywhere from 1 month to several years post-LTx.
* Chronic rejection (also known as 'ductopaenic rejection') with loss of over 50% of bile ducts, occurs 6 weeks to 6 months after LTx and can lead to biliary strictures

and cholangitis. Treatment may include optimising immunosuppression, dilatation of strictures.
- Autoimmune hepatitis can develop irrespective of initial disease process. It can occur months to years after LTx. It is treated with the addition of azathioprine and prednisolone to the immunosuppressive regimen.

Infection (50%)
- Earlier infections (up to one month after LTx) tend to be bacterial or fungal. Intra-abdominal and line infections are the most common early causes. Bacterial and fungal infections can be secondary to technical complications such as vascular thrombosis, bile leaks, strictures. Fungal sepsis, especially aspergillosis, can be seen with re-operation, bowel perforation and long stays in intensive care: prophylaxis is with antifungal agents such as itraconazole and fluconazole, or newer drugs (e.g. the caspofungins) and the lipid complex formulation of amphotericin (less nephrotoxic).
- Later infections (2–6 months after LTx) tend to be viral (e.g. cytomegalovirus [CMV], Epstein-Barr virus [EBV], herpes varicella-zoster virus [HVZ]) and have been reduced by prophylactic courses of ganciclovir, acyclovir and CMV hyper-immunoglobulin. Still later infections (>6 months) may be viral or fungal. Common respiratory viruses (adenovirus, parainfluenza, influenza) can produce necrotising pneumonitis.

Biliary complications (20%)
These can occur anywhere from 6 weeks to 6 years post-LTx and may present with cholangitis. There may be extrahepatic strictures (anastomosis site) or intrahepatic strictures (due to ischaemia). Treatment may include percutaneous balloon dilatation, surgical revision or retransplantation.

Hepatic vascular compromise (<10%)
This may be due to hepatic artery, hepatic vein or portal vein stenosis or occlusion. Hepatic artery thrombosis can lead to urgent retransplantation, biliary leaks, peritonitis, relapsing septicaemia, biliary strictures. Portal vein stenosis can cause portal hypertension. Treatment may include ballooning, stenting, surgical reconstruction or retransplantation.

PTLD (EBV-driven B cell proliferation) (5–25%)
This spectrum of disease ranges from lymphohyperplasia to true lymphoma, and may occur 3–12 months post-LTx. It can present with lymphadenopathy. Risk factors include: (a) primary EBV infection after transplant; (b) young age; (c) EBV-negative recipient of EBV-positive donor; (d) CMV infection; (e) significantly immunocompromised children. The evolution of PTLD can be monitored by serial EBV polymerase chain reaction (PCR) determinations in peripheral blood: a rising EBV PCR is sensitive for PTLD. It may be treated by decreasing or stopping immunosuppression (usually successful, but this increases risk of LTx rejection), and starting ganciclovir, acyclovir and CMV hyperimmunoglobulin (has high levels of EBV antibodies). More recent therapies include anti-CD20 monoclonal antibodies (e.g. rituximab), and injection of in-vitro expanded autologous EBV-specific cytotoxic T cells. Mortality is around 20%; this has decreased due to EBV viraemia surveillance.

Long-term toxicities of calcineurin inhibitors (CNIs)—CSA and tacrolimus
Nephrotoxicity remains the most serious complication of CNIs. Glomerular filtration rate (GFR) is the best way to monitor its development. Early renal impairment can be

reversible, and the dose of CNI can be reduced, but at some stage renal impairment can become irreversible. Hypertension that requires therapy occurs in around 20–30% of LTx recipients, and can be compounded by steroid use. Other effects include neuro-toxicities and hyperlipidaemia. Some alternatives to CNIs have been used to address this problem, including the addition of either mycophenolate mofetil or sirolimus.

Recurrence of original disease
The conditions most likely to recur are autoimmune hepatitis, viral hepatitis and sclerosing cholangitis.

Bowel perforation
This is a feared complication, with high mortality. Previous abdominal surgery increases the risk. As the most common indication for LTx is EHBA with a failed Kasai, many children have a predisposing risk for perforation.

Improved outcomes

Improved immunosuppression has contributed to the improved outcomes of LTx. The main agents used, other than corticosteroids, are the calcineurin inhibitors (CNIs) tacrolimus (TRL, previously called FK506) and cyclosporin (CSA). Both inhibit the production of cytotoxic T-lymphocytes and interleukin 2 (IL-2), and have similar side effects, although the former is more potent and does not cause hirsutism or gum hyperplasia. Levels of both TRL and CSA may be decreased by concomitant use of anticonvulsants and antituberculous drugs, and may be increased by calcium channel blockers, antibiotics (macrolides and quinolones) and antifungals. TRL is usually combined with steroids alone, whereas CSA is often combined with a third agent, such as mycophenolate mofetil or azathioprine (AZA). TRL is interesting in that its phar-macokinetic patterns retain the characteristics of the age of the donor, not the recipient. Most children may be weaned to a single immunosuppressive agent. Most units now focus on minimisation of long-term maintenance immunosuppression, with steroid withdrawal as the first step. Some adult LTx protocols avoid steroids entirely and use either polyclonal or monoclonal antibody therapy , instead of steroids, given with TRL or CSA.

Evaluation for complications may include serial LFTs, tissue sampling, and imaging including Doppler ultrasonography for vascular patency, magnetic resonance imaging (MRI) and percutaneous transhepatic cholangiography (PTC).

Long term, there is significant improvement in nutritional status after LTx, with weight, fat stores, and muscle mass (protein) recovering within 12 months and, of more importance, maintenance of psychosocial development, normal intellectual functioning, normal (if delayed) puberty, growth spurts with normal final height, and participation in age-appropriate activities. Renal dysfunction occurs in around 30% of cases. Malignancy remains the long-term concern.

Malabsorption/maldigestion

Malabsorption presents as a diagnostic problem, not a specific disease. It is a state where there is inadequate digestion and/or inadequate absorption across the intestinal mucosa, related to digestive factors (e.g. pancreatic enzymes, bile) and/or absorptive factors (e.g. mucosal changes). The more common causes involve enzymes (cystic fibrosis [CF]) and mucosal surface area (coeliac disease). The presenting complaints may include failure to thrive, loose and frequent bowel motions, abdominal distension, short stature (e.g. coeliac disease), anaemia (folate, vitamin B_{12} or iron malabsorption), or chest infection (CF).

Aetiology

The common causes in the developed world include:

1. Cystic fibrosis (CF).
2. Coeliac disease.
3. Post-gastroenteritis syndrome.
4. Giardiasis.
5. Bacterial overgrowth (usually associated with congenital gut anomalies or prior gastrointestinal surgery).

In contrast, in the developing world the most common cause of malabsorption is the combination of mucosal injury from repeated or persistent infections, plus poor hygiene and poor nutrition.

Other causes in the developed world include:

1. Inflammatory bowel disease (predominantly Crohn's disease [CD]).
2. Syndromic causes of pancreatic insufficiency:
   - Shwachman's syndrome (autosomal recessive). The abnormal gene is located on *7q11*. Features include short stature, skeletal anomalies, recurrent infections, bone marrow dysfunction, including pancytopenia and cyclic neutropenia.
   - Johanson-Blizzard syndrome. The abnormal gene is located on *15q15–q21.1*. Features include pancreatic insufficiency due to fatty replacement, gastrointestinal anomalies (e.g. imperforate anus), deafness, unusual whorls of tissue in scalp, absent nasal cartilage, hypothyroidism. Diabetes may also occur.
3. Short bowel syndrome (SBS): residual small bowel length less than 100 cm (e.g. post-necrotising enterocolitis).
4. Chronic liver disease (CLD) with cholestasis.
5. Others: immunodeficiency syndromes, intestinal lymphangiectasia, abetalipoproteinaemia.

Infants usually have congenital disorders of specific nutrient digestion or absorption/transport. These include disorders involving:

1. Aminoacids: e.g. enterokinase deficiency.
2. Fats: e.g. chylomicron retention disease, intestinal lymphangiectasia; abetalipoproteinaemia.
3. Carbohydrates: congenital intestinal enterocyte brush border enzyme deficiencies or transport defects (e.g. glucose-galactose transporter deficiency, sucrase-isomaltase deficiency, lactase deficiency, microvillus inclusion disease).
4. Electrolytes, vitamins, trace elements: e.g. congenital chloride diarrhoea, acrodermatitis enteropathica (zinc deficiency), selective B_{12} deficiency.

Mechanisms of malabsorption

Candidates should refresh their knowledge of the physiology of digestive and absorptive processes. These are normally divided into phases: intraluminal digestion, mucosal absorption, venous transport phase and lymphatic transport phase. Most nutrient absorption occurs in the proximal small bowel, although vitamin B_{12} and bile acids are absorbed in the terminal ileum. Malabsorbed bile acids irritate the colonic mucosa, having a detergent action which can lead to colitis and diarrhoea, especially in conditions like CD and SBS with disorders of the terminal small bowel.

Hepatobiliary and pancreatic secretions mix with nutrients in the duodenum and jejunum to digest fat. Long-chain fatty acids are absorbed and repackaged into chylomicrons, transported sequentially via lymphatics, the venous circulation, and finally the liver. Medium- and short-chain fatty acids are absorbed and transported directly to the liver via mesenteric venous blood flow.

Malabsorbed carbohydrates' osmotic properties lead to intraluminal fluid accumulation and diarrhoea, plus fermentation by ileocolonic bacteria to simple sugars, organic acids and gases (methane, carbon dioxide, and hydrogen—the basis for the hydrogen breath test). Generalised malabsorption usually does not cause azotorrhoea (excessive loss of nitrogen in the stool). Hypoproteinaemia in malnourished children with malabsorption is due to deficient dietary intake and excessive intestinal protein loss (protein losing enteropathy [PLE]).

Digestive factors

1. Insufficient pancreatic enzymes (e.g. CF, Shwachman's syndrome).
2. Lack of functioning bile salts:
   - Insufficient supply (e.g. CLD, ileal resection, coeliac disease).
   - Deconjugation (e.g. bacterial overgrowth).
3. Inadequate brush border enzymes (e.g. lactose intolerance).

Absorptive factors

1. Disordered mucosal villus function:
   - Congenital defects in villus structure: e.g. microvillus inclusion disease, tufting disease.
   - Reduced mucosal surface area: e.g. SBS, cytotoxic drug-induced epithelial injury, malnutrition.
   - Inflammatory disorders of villus: e.g. postinfectious diarrhoea (e.g. *Shigella*, *Escherichia coli*, *Campylobacter jejuni*, *Giardia lamblia*), coeliac disease (gluten sensitive enteropathy), allergic enteropathies (e.g. to cow's milk protein (CMP), soy, egg, or gluten), acute infectious enteropathy, immunodeficiency syndromes, autoimmune enteritis.
2. Defective intracellular lipid transport: e.g. abetalipoproteinaemia.
3. Inadequate lymphatic circulation of chylomicrons: e.g. lymphangiectasia (primary, or secondary to CD), mycobacterial gut infection, radiation enteritis, forms of congenital heart disease with chronically elevated right-sided heart pressure (impeded flow from lymphatics [thoracic duct] into systemic venous circulation).
4. Abnormal water and electrolyte transport (e.g. giardiasis).

Coeliac disease

This is an enteropathy in which intestinal inflammation is due to ingestion of gliadin and associated prolamins (proteins with a high content of proline and glutamine), which are present in wheat (gluten), barley (hordeins) and rye (secalins), in genetically predisposed patients. There is a strong association between coeliac disease and human leucocyte antigen (HLA) class II genes. DQ2 and DQ8 molecules present peptides derived from gliadin to intestinal T-lymphocytes (some after deamination by tissue transglutaminase [TTG]). Activated Th1 T-cells produce pro-inflammatory cytokines that cause (probably) the gut lesions of coeliac disease.

The gold standard in diagnosing this condition remains small bowel biopsy, with characteristic villous atrophy, crypt hyperplasia and increased intraepithelial lymphocytes. Although serology may be useful, it has yet to replace biopsy. Most cases with positive TTG antibodies and endomysial antibodies (EMA) have coeliac disease, and are HLA DQ2- or DQ8-positive.

History

Weight

Birth weight, progress of weight, timing of when weight gain started to diminish, current weight, rate of weight loss.

Chronology of symptoms

Age at onset of symptoms: for example, congenital villus dysfunction presents with intractable diarrhoea as neonate; coeliac disease may present between 3 and 9 months with severe diarrhoea, or later (9 months to late childhood) with moderate diarrhoea; inflammatory bowel disease is very rare before 8 years); it may present after a bout of known enteritis (e.g. *Shigella*).

Feeding

Dietary milestones, initial feeding, age at introduction of cow's milk (CMP intolerance), age at introduction of first solids, age at introduction of first cereals and the type of cereal (gluten-containing [wheat, rye, barley] in coeliac disease), age at introduction of first fruits (sucrase-isomaltase deficiency), appetite, poor feeding with irritability (iron deficiency associated with coeliac disease), parent-devised dietary restriction (attempting to avoid diarrhoea), iatrogenic dietary manipulation (decreased caloric intake and chronic non-specific diarrhoea).

Stools

Appearance, volume, fluidity, offensiveness, difficulty flushing stools (steatorrhoea or excess gas in stool), frequency, associated blood (CD).

Symptoms of specific nutritional deficiencies

Pallor (anaemia), night blindness (vitamin A), ataxia (vitamin E), bruising (vitamin K), rashes (zinc, various vitamins). See short case on nutritional assessment for a comprehensive list of possibilities.

Specific diagnostic clues

Chest infections (CF), susceptibility to infections (immunodeficiency states or neutropenic episodes of Shwachman's syndrome), arthralgia or rashes (e.g. erythema nodosum, erythema multiforme in CD), delay in pubertal development (CD), travel to giardia-endemic or exotic areas (giardiasis or other infestation), day-care (giardiasis).

Family history

CF, coeliac disease or other autoimmune disorders (e.g. type 1 diabetes, thyroid disorders, juvenile arthritis, autoimmune liver disease), disaccharidase deficiency, CD, infestations.

Social history

Beware of psychosocial causes of failure to thrive in the differential diagnosis.

Past medical history

Necrotising enterocolitis (NEC) as neonate, past bowel resections or other surgery.

Investigations thus far

The type and timing of investigations, the specialists involved, current thoughts on the diagnosis, planned future investigations.

Management

Current treatment approach (if any), plans for further treatment.

Examination

See short case on nutritional assessment and suggested examinations for IBD and CLD long cases. Start with growth parameters—weight, height and head circumference, then perform a nutritional assessment, and look for underlying IBD, CLD, and any suggestions of CF or immune deficiency. Carefully check for any abdominal distension, particularly with muscle wasting, as this can occur with an enteropathy. Perform a careful perianal examination. It is not necessary to perform a rectal examination, but this should be mentioned for completeness.

Investigations

Stool

1. Pus cells (colonic disease, e.g. CD).
2. Eosinophils (CMP intolerance).
3. Occult blood (IBD).
4. Cysts or trophozoites (e.g. *Giardia lamblia*).
5. Fat globules (CF or Shwachman's syndrome—maldigestion [luminal] rather than malabsorption. (*Note:* lubricants or ointments can produce false-positive results.)
6. Fatty acid crystals (coeliac disease—malabsorption [mucosal]).
7. Reducing substances (carbohydrate maldigestion or malabsorption).
8. Faecal alpha-1-antitrypsin excretion test (FA1AT). This screens for PLE. Elevated FA1AT result suggests a mucosal disorder, as inflamed mucosa allow transudation of serum proteins. This is common in CD and occurs in coeliac disease, but *not* in CF or CLD where there is an intraluminal maldigestive defect, which does not involve any mucosal damage.
9. Culture for pathogens (*Cryptosporidium, Yersinia*).
10. Three-day faecal fat assessment (more accurate than a qualitative stool stain).
11. Bile acids (in SBS with 40–80% ileal resection).
12. Colonic hydroxy fatty acids (in SBS with 80–100% ileal resection).
13. Ostomy output: electrolytes, osmolality (children with stomas).

Blood

1. Full blood count and film (anaemia, neutropenia [Shwachman's], lymphopenia [lymphangiectasia], acanthocytosis [abetalipoproteinaemia]).
2. Erythrocyte sedimentation rate, ESR (chronic infection, IBD).
3. Liver function tests (albumin, total protein, transaminases) (CLD, CD with PLE).

4. Vitamins: folate (serum and red cell), vitamin B_{12} (ileal disease), vitamins A, 25-OH D and E, and prothrombin time for vitamin K (fat malabsorption).
5. Minerals: calcium, magnesium, phosphate, iron, ferritin, zinc, copper, selenium.
6. Electrolytes, urea and creatinine (hydration, associated renal disease).
7. Fetal haemoglobin, HbF (Shwachman's).
8. Pancreatic isoamylase (Shwachman's).
9. IgA and coeliac disease serology (anti-tissue transglutaminase [TTG] IgA antibodies, EMA, anti-gliadin antibodies (IgG and IgA). In addition, testing for HLA DQ2 or DQ8 can be done, though this is not routine: 99% of patients with coeliac disease are positive for one of these.
10. IBD serology screening tests. None are routine but are included for completeness. Perinuclear anticytoplasmic antibodies (pANCAs) to neutrophil proteins may be elevated in UC. Anti-*Saccharomyces cerevisiae* (ASCA) antibodies may be present in CD (more sensitive and specific with elevated pANCA). Antibodies to *E. coli* (outer membrane porin C [anti-OMPC] antibodies) may correlate with diagnosis of IBD.
11. Immunoglobulins (severe combined immunodeficiency syndrome and other primary immune defects).
12. Human immunodeficiency virus (HIV) serology in high-risk groups.

Imaging

1. Bone age (delay in skeletal development; abnormal in Shwachman's syndrome with metaphyseal dysostosis; film will also show rickets).
2. Bowel contrast studies (anatomical lesions, CD).
3. Motility studies (nuclear medicine gastric emptying scan, upper gastrointestinal barium contrast study).
4. Liver scan (causes of CLD).
5. CT scan of liver and pancreas.
6. Radiolabelled Tc albumin lymphatic scan (lymphangiectasia).

Small bowel biopsy

This is the gold standard to diagnose villus injury. It is the standard test to diagnose coeliac disease, *Giardia lamblia*, intestinal lymphangiectasia, abetalipoproteinaemia (shows epithelial lipid). Severe villus atrophy occurs with coeliac disease and congenital microvillus inclusion disease. Less severe degrees of atrophy occur with giardiasis, immunodeficiency, allergic enteropathies and malnutrition. Biopsy can also determine mucosal enzyme deficiencies (e.g. disaccharidases).

Sweat test

The standard test to detect CF.

Others

Other potentially useful investigations include the following:

1. Breath hydrogen test (carbohydrate malabsorption, bacterial overgrowth).
2. Serum carotene and the 1 hour xylose test: indirect tests of absorptive function.
3. Pancreatic function tests: endoscopic retrograde cholangiopancreatography/ duodenal intubation for pancreatic enzyme analysis (CF including negative sweat test, Shwachman's, Johanson-Blizzard).
4. Urinary catecholamines and serotonin (carcinoid, neuroblastoma: causes of secretory diarrhoea).
5. Liver biopsy.

Note that all these investigations, except for pancreatic function tests and liver biopsy, can be performed as outpatient procedures. It is uncommon to need to admit a child to hospital for investigation of malabsorption, although a child with failure to thrive may require a period of hospitalisation for nutritional debilitation to resolve.

Short cases

Gastrointestinal system

This is a reasonably common short case, and is expected to be performed well. The introduction 'Examine the gastrointestinal system' is more detailed than 'Examine the abdomen', as it comprises not only abdominal but also nutritional assessment (which is a short case in itself), as well as a search for peripheral stigmata of various disease states. The most systematic method of approach, as in so many other cases, commences with inspection, followed by examining the hands, face, abdomen, lower limbs and then other systems depending on the findings.

The relevant findings sought are outlined in Figure 8.3. A more detailed listing of possible examination findings is given in Table 8.1.

Start by introducing yourself to the patient and parent. Have the child adequately undressed for examination. Note the child's parameters and visually assess the nutritional status. Request the percentile charts, as these are always helpful and often give a good indication of the underlying diagnosis before you examine the child. A good example of this is coeliac disease, where the weight percentile chart characteristically shows a falling-off of previously adequate weight gain, at the age that gluten-containing foods were introduced to the diet. The height chart can indicate disease chronicity and can suggest certain diagnoses that often present as short stature, such as Shwachman's syndrome or Crohn's disease. The head circumference is decreased in the congenital TORCH infections, which can present with poor growth and hepatomegaly.

Now, take 20 seconds or so to visually scan for those features outlined in the figure. After this, the child can be systematically examined, commencing with the hands, noting any clubbing, leuconychia or other peripheral stigmata of chronic liver disease. Move on to the head and neck, examining in particular the eyes and mouth. When examining the eyes, mention the relevance of examining the retinae, but defer actually doing it until you have completed the rest of your examination, as it is too time-consuming at this stage. This is followed by a thorough abdominal examination.

Next, inspect the lower limbs for erythema nodosum (inflammatory bowel disease, chronic active hepatitis) and feel for ankle oedema (chronic liver disease). The findings noted to this point will determine whether further assessment of other systems, such as the following, is needed.

Neurological assessment

A neurological examination is appropriate in the following circumstances:

1. Any jaundice or other suggestion of liver disease in a child over 5 years (e.g. vitamin E deficiency causing cerebellar ataxia and/or peripheral neuropathy, Wilson's disease causing ataxia, dysarthria, dystonia).
2. Any malabsorption or pigmentary retinopathy (e.g. abetalipoproteinaemia with vitamin E deficiency).

Figure 8.3 Gastrointestinal system

1. Introduce self

2. General inspection
Position patient: lying, fully undressed,
  after initial inspection standing
Parameters
- Weight
- Height
- Head circumference
- Percentiles
Nutritional status
- Muscle bulk
- Subcutaneous fat
Sick or well
Pallor
Jaundice
Bruising, petechiae
Peripheral stigmata of CLD
Oedema
Tachypnoea
Involuntary movements
Access devices

3. Demonstrate fat and protein stores
Subcutaneous fat
- Mid-arm, axillae, subscapular,
  suprailiac
Muscle bulk
- Biceps, triceps, quadriceps, glutei

4. Upper limbs
Nails
Palms
Xanthomata
Asterixis
Wrists
Other joints

5. Head and neck
Face
Eyes
- Lids
- Conjunctivae
- Sclera
- Iris
- Cornea
- Lens
- Retina
Mouth

6. Abdomen—anterior aspect
Inspection
- Distension
- Scars
- Access devices
- Injection sites
- Stoma
- Herniae
- Abdominal wall veins
- Striae
Palpation, percussion, auscultation
- Abdominal tenderness
- Hepatomegaly
- Hepatic bruit (hepatoma)
- Splenomegaly (portal hypertension)
- Enlarged kidneys (polycystic
  disease)
- Ascites
- Abdominal mass
- Inguinal herniae

7. Abdomen—posterior aspect
Inspection
- Purpura on buttocks (HSP)
- Xanthomata on buttocks (CLD)
- Gluteal wasting (malnutrition)
- Perianal fissures, fistulae (IBD)
- Imperforate anus (congenital)

8. Lower limbs
Inspect
- Bowing (vitamin D deficiency)
- Erythema nodosum (IBD, chronic
  active hepatitis)
- Joint swelling (IBD)
Palpate
- Ankle
  oedema
  (CLD, PLE)

9. Other
Urinalysis
Stool analysis
Temperature
Depending on
  findings
- Neurological
  system
- Respiratory
  system
- Cardio-
  vascular
  system

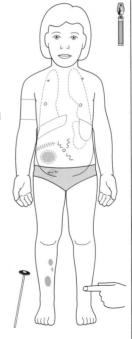

CLD = chronic liver disease; HSP = Henoch-Schönlein purpura; IBD = inflammatory bowel disease;
PLE = protein-losing enteropathy.

3. Dysmorphism in an infant (marked hypotonia in Zellweger syndrome).
4. Microcephaly (congenital TORCH infections, with developmental delay).

In older children, assess the gait and then formally test the lower limbs. In infants, a gross motor developmental approach, followed by lower limb assessment, is more appropriate.

Respiratory assessment

If there is any evidence of liver disease, respiratory distress or diabetes (think of CF), a full respiratory assessment is needed, including asking the child to cough and requesting inspection of a sputum specimen.

Cardiac assessment

If there is any evidence of jaundice or hepatomegaly in an infant (pulmonary arterial stenosis in Alagille syndrome, or in congenital rubella) or any suggestion of cystic fibrosis (for evidence of cor pulmonale), then a full praecordial assessment is warranted.

At the completion of clinical examination, request inspection of any urine or stool specimens available, as well as the urinalysis, stool analysis and temperature chart.

Table 8.1 Additional information: details of possible findings on gastrointestinal examination

General inspection

Pallor (GIT blood loss, CLD, nutritional deficiencies in iron, folate, various vitamins)

Jaundice (CLD, vitamin B_{12} deficiency with ileal resection or disease)

Bruising (CLD, thrombocytopenia in hypersplenism, HSP)

Petechiae (hypersplenism in portal hypertension)

Peripheral stigmata of CLD: spider naevi, scratch marks (pruritis with cholestasis), xanthomata (cholestasis)

Oedema (CLD, PLE)

Tachypnoea, cyanosis, cough, barrel chest (CF)

Irritability (iron deficiency, coeliac disease)

Mental state (hepatic encephalopathy)

Dysarthria (Wilson's disease)

Involuntary movements: athetoid, choreic, tremor, dystonia, or myoclonus (all can occur in Wilson's disease)

Access devices (venous ports used in CF for administering antibiotics; intravenous access for total parenteral nutrition, or hyperalimentation)

Nasogastric tube

Dysmorphic features
- Arteriohepatic dysplasia (Alagille syndrome)
- Zellweger syndrome (infants)
- Various other syndromes

Joint swelling (associated with IBD)

Evidence of rickets (bow legs, prominent wrists and ankles, rib rosary) (vitamin D deficiency)

Abdominal distension, scars, access devices, stoma

Skin
- Various rashes related to nutritional deficiencies
- Dermatitis herpetiformis (coeliac disease)
- Erythema nodosum (IBD, chronic active hepatitis)

Upper limbs

Nails
- Clubbing (CLD, IBD, CF)
- Leuconychia (CLD)
- Koilonychia (iron deficiency)
- Cyanosis (CF)

Palms
- Crease pallor (anaemias)
- Erythema (CLD)
- Crease pigmentation (Addison's)

Xanthomata (between fingers and on extensor surfaces)

Continued

Table 8.1 *(Continued)*

Dark brown spots on nails, hands (Peutz-Jeghers syndrome)

Asterixis (liver failure, CO_2 retention in CF)

Wrists: palpable epiphyseal enlargement (vitamin D deficiency)

Joints: swelling (arthritis with IBD)

Head and neck
Facial characteristics
- Cushingoid facies (steroid-treated IBD or chronic active hepatitis)
- Doll face 'cherub' (glycogen storage diseases types 1 and 3)

Eyes
- Pigmentation around eyes (2–3 mm brown-black spots in Peutz-Jeghers syndrome)
- Lids: xanthelasma (hyperlipidaemia)
- Conjunctivae: pallor (anaemias, associated with nutritional deficiencies, GIT blood loss (CLD, Wilson's disease), xerosis (vitamin A deficiency)
- Sclera: jaundice (note depth thereof)
- Iris: iritis (IBD)
- Cornea: xerosis, clouding, opacification (vitamin A deficiency), Kayser-Fleischer rings (brown/green pigmentation in limbic region, reported in several conditions including Wilson's disease)
- Lens: cataracts (congenital TORCH infections, steroid-treated IBD or chronic active hepatitis, Wilson's)
- Retina: retinal pigmentation (abetalipoproteinaemia, Alagille syndrome), chorioretinitis (TORCH), retinopathy of prematurity (ex-premature with NEC)

Mouth
- Breath: hepatic fetor (liver failure)
- Lips: angular cheilosis (iron deficiency): pigmentation (Peutz-Jeghers syndrome)
- Buccal mucosa: areas of brown-black pigmentation (Peutz-Jeghers syndrome, Addison's disease)

Abdomen—anterior aspect
Distension
- Weak abdominal muscles (protein calorie malnutrition [PCM], coeliac disease)
- Ascites (CLD, PLE, PCM)

Operative scars (Kasai, colectomy, liver transplant)

Access devices (e.g. venous port for antibiotics in CF)

Injection sites (insulin in CF with diabetes, venous port site in currently treated CF)

Stoma (colostomy, ileostomy, gastrostomy)

Prominent abdominal wall veins (portal hypertension)

Striae (Cushing's syndrome in steroid treated IBD, chronic active hepatitis)

Urine, stool, temperature chart
Request inspection of
- Urine: dark (cholestasis)
- Stool: acholic (cholestasis); blood (portal hypertension)

Urinalysis
- Bilirubin (hepatobiliary disease)
- Urobilinogen (increased hepatic dysfunction)

Temperature chart (infectious hepatitis, chronic active hepatitis)

Neurological system
Infants
Alertness (decreased in Zellweger, TORCH)

Hypotonic posture (Zellweger)

Choreoathetoid movements (kernicterus)

Gross motor assessment (hypotonic with Zellweger, hypertonic with TORCH)

Primitive reflexes: pathological persistence (TORCH, bilirubin encephalopathy)

Hearing: deafness (congenital rubella, bilirubin encephalopathy, Zellweger's)

Older children (over 5 years)
Gait examination
- Cerebellar ataxia (vitamin E deficiency)
- Peripheral neuropathy (vitamin E deficiency)
- Involuntary movements (Wilson's)
- Antalgic gait (arthritis with IBD)

Romberg's sign (vitamin E deficiency)

Hold arms horizontally: wing beating tremor (Wilson's disease)

Diminished reflexes (vitamin E deficiency)

Diminished sensation (vitamin E deficiency)

Continued

Table 8.1 *(Continued)*	
Respiratory examination Full respiratory examination, including getting child to cough and inspecting any sputum (CF)	**Cardiac examination** Full praecordial assessment (Alagille syndrome, congenital rubella, CF)

CF = cystic fibrosis; CLD = chronic liver disease; GIT = gastrointestinal tract; HSP = Henoch-Schönlein purpura; NEC = necrotising entercolitis; PLE = protein losing enteropathy; TORCH = toxoplasmosis, other (e.g. HIV, syphilis), rubella, cytomegalovirus, herpes (both simplex and varicella).

The abdomen

This is a common short case, but is often failed due to several simple errors. 'Examine the abdomen' is not the same as 'Examine the gastrointestinal system', but is often interpreted as such. The other common misconception is that the abdomen can be examined with the examiner standing up: this is inappropriate, as the hand and forearm should be at the same level as the abdomen, which can be achieved only by kneeling at the bedside or sitting on a chair. The other point worth noting is that after inspection, when initially palpating, you should look not at the abdomen or examining hand but at the face of the child, as that is the only way to assess if there is any abdominal tenderness.

First have the child fully undressed. Initial inspection can be performed with the child standing, as this is the best position from which to gain an overall impression of the child's height and nutritional status, and also to assess abdominal distension. Then lay the child flat on the bed, with one pillow under the head, and, after completing an initial visual scan, sit on a chair or kneel next the bed so that the examining hand is at the same level as the abdomen for palpation.

Begin with general palpation, commencing in one or other iliac fossa and proceeding clockwise. Watch the child's face throughout, to detect any abdominal tenderness. Then palpate for the liver, noting its size, consistency, surface, edge and vertical downward movement with inspiration. Percuss in the midclavicular line, from resonant to dull, first from above, then from below, and measure the span with a ruler or tape measure (in centimetres). Palpate for the spleen next, starting in the right iliac fossa so as not to miss massive splenomegaly. Note the movement towards the umbilicus with inspiration, and feel for the splenic notch; percuss and measure the span in centimetres.

Next, ballotte for the kidneys, noting their size and percuss for resonance above them. Percuss for ascites; if resonant to percussion to the flanks, there is no need to test for shifting dullness. If not, then check for the latter by rolling the patient away from you, waiting 20 seconds for any fluid to settle, and percuss again. Note any change in the site where the percussion note became dull. Measure this distance. Also check for a fluid thrill if there is evidence of any shifting dullness. An assistant (e.g. an examiner) is required to test for a fluid thrill.

Next, examine the inguinal regions for herniae or lymphadenopathy. Examine the genitalia: note the Tanner pubertal staging and the size of the external genitalia and, in a boy, the size, shape and consistency of the testes. If there is any mass here, then transilluminate it. After completion of palpation and percussion, auscultate over the liver, spleen, renal arteries and bowel. Finally, check the abdominal reflexes.

Figure 8.4 The abdomen

1. Introduce self

2. General inspection
Position patient: lying down (after initial
    inspection standing)
Rapid visual scan (take no more than
    20 seconds)
Parameters
- Weight
- Height
- Head circumference

Sick or well
Pallor (chronic haemolytic anaemia,
    CRF, leukaemia)
Bruising (CLD, haematological
    malignancies)
Jaundice (CLD, chronic haemolysis)
Sallow complexion (CRF)
Nutritional status
Oedema (CLD, nephrotic syndrome,
    protein-losing enteropathy)
Dysmorphic features (various)
Facial characteristics
- Rodent facies (thalassaemia)
- Cushingoid facies (adrenal
    tumour, treated nephrotic
    syndrome)
- Doll face 'cherub' (glycogen
    storage diseases types 1 and 3)

Hemihypertrophy (Wilms' tumour,
    hepatoblastoma)

3. Abdomen—anterior aspect
Inspection
- Distension
- Scars
- Access devices
- Injection sites
- Stoma
- Herniae
- Abdominal wall veins
- Striae
- Genitalia

Palpation, percussion, auscultation
- Abdominal tenderness
- Hepatomegaly
- Hepatic pulsation (tricuspid
    incompetence)
- Hepatic bruit (hepatoma,
    haemangioma)
- Splenomegaly
- Splenic rub (splenic infarct)
- Enlarged kidneys
- Renal bruit (renal artery stenosis)

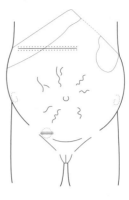

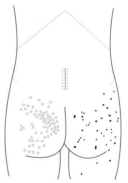

- Ascites
- Abdominal mass
- Inguinal lymphadenopathy
    (leukaemia, lymphoma)
- Empty scrotum (undescended
    testes)
- Enlarged testis (seminoma,
    teratoma)
- Enlarged scrotum (hydrocoele)

4. Abdomen—posterior aspect
Inspection
- Buttocks
- Midline anomalies
- Needle marks
- Anus

Palpation, percussion, auscultation
- Pelvic tenderness on springing
    (ALL)
- Spinal tenderness (ALL, bone
    tumours)
- Renal bruit (renal artery stenosis)
- Absent anal wink (spina bifida)

Continued

Figure 8.4 *(Continued)*

5. Other Urine inspection (dark in obstructive jaundice, haematuria in renal diseases) Urinalysis (UTI, CRF)	Stool inspection (acholic in obstructive jaundice, melaena from bleeding oesophageal varices) Stool analysis (CF, coeliac disease, IBD, giardiasis)

ALL = acute lymphoblastic leukaemia; CF = cystic fibrosis; CLD = chronic liver disease; CRF = chronic renal failure; UTI = urinary tract infection.

This completes the anterior abdominal examination. The posterior abdominal examination is also important, as many signs here may explain findings noted anteriorly (e.g. spina bifida associated with enlarged bladder or kidneys; bone marrow biopsy sites over the iliac crests, accompanying hepatosplenomegaly).

Roll the child over to inspect the posterior abdominal wall. Spring the pelvis and percuss the lumbar spine for any tenderness, and also auscultate over the kidneys for any bruits.

Next, roll the child on one side and, after asking the examiners for permission, inspect the perianal region, test for the anal wink, and mention performing a per rectal examination (you will not be expected to do this in the examination setting).

Always request the urinalysis, stool analysis and temperature chart at the completion of your examination.

Common findings in the examination setting include hepatosplenomegaly, ascites and enlarged kidneys.

In view of the large number of possibilities in this case, they are best enumerated in list form. Figure 8.4 shows several of the findings sought. For further details on the many possible signs on inspection, see Table 8.2.

The abdominal findings will determine the remainder of the general physical examination.

- If the only finding is minimal tenderness, proceed to a gastrointestinal or renal examination, depending on the site of tenderness.
- If the finding is hepatosplenomegaly, proceed to a gastrointestinal and haematological assessment.
- If the finding is enlarged kidneys, proceed with a renal examination, after requesting the blood pressure and urinalysis.
- If the finding is lymphadenopathy and splenomegaly, examine the haematological system.
- If ascites is the finding, proceed as outlined in the short case approach to the child with oedema.
- If ambiguous genitalia is the finding, request the blood pressure, look for hyperpigmentation and then proceed as in the short-case approach to ambiguous genitalia in Chapter 7.

Common findings on abdominal examination and their causes are outlined in the following sections.

Hepatomegaly

The following two lists give different classifications of hepatomegaly. The first is a mnemonic, SHIRT, which the author has found useful. The second describes the more common findings found in three different age groups: infant, preschool (less than 5 years) and school age (5 years and over), further subdivided into jaundiced or not jaundiced. This second classification is more practical than comprehensive.

Causes of hepatomegaly (mnemonic *SHIRT*)

S *Structural*

Extrahepatic biliary atresia (EHBA), choledochal cyst, intrahepatic biliary hypoplasia, polycystic disease, congenital hepatic fibrosis.

Storage/metabolic

1. Defective lipid metabolism—Gaucher's disease, Niemann-Pick disease, hyper-lipoproteinaemias, cholesteryl ester storage disease, carnitine deficiency, mucolipidoses.
2. Defective carbohydrate metabolism—diabetes mellitus, glycogen storage diseases (types 1, 3, 4, 6), hereditary fructose intolerance (HFI), galac-tosaemia, Cushing's syndrome, mucopolysaccharidoses.
3. Defective amino acid/protein metabolism—tyrosinaemia (type 1), urea cycle enzyme disorders.
4. Defective mineral metabolism—Wilson's disease.
5. Defective electrolyte transport—cystic fibrosis (CF).
6. Defective nutrition—protein calorie malnutrition (PCM), total parenteral nutrition (TPN).
7. Deficiency of protease—alpha-1-antitrypsin deficiency.

H *Haematological*

Thalassaemia, sickle cell disease (chronic haemolysis and transfusion haemosid-erosis), acute leukaemia, chronic myeloid leukaemia.

Heart

Congestive cardiac failure (CCF), constrictive pericarditis, obstructed inferior vena cava (IVC).

I *Infection*

1. Viral infections—congenital rubella, cytomegalovirus infection, coxsackie virus, echovirus, hepatitis (A, B, C, D and E) viruses, infectious mononucleosis.
2. Bacterial infections—neonatal septicaemia, *E. coli* urinary tract infections, tuberculosis, congenital syphilis.
3. Parasitic infections—hydatid disease, malaria, schistosomiasis, toxoplasmosis, visceral larva migrans.

Inflammatory

Chronic active hepatitis, chronic persistent hepatitis, IBD associated liver disease.

Infiltrative

Histiocytosis X, sarcoidosis.

R *Reticuloendothelial*

Non-Hodgkin's lymphoma, Hodgkin's disease.

Rheumatological

Systemic onset juvenile idiopathic arthritis, SLE.

T *Tumour/hamartoma*
1. Primary hepatic neoplasms—hepatoblastoma, hepatocellular carcinoma (hepatoma).
2. Secondary deposits—neuroblastoma, Wilms' tumour, gonadal tumours.
3. Vascular malformation/benign neoplasm—infantile haemangioendothelioma, cavernous haemangioma.

Trauma
Hepatic haematoma.

Causes of hepatomegaly (practical classification)

Note that some diseases occur in both the 'jaundiced' and 'not jaundiced' lists. These are not misprints, but reflect the wide spectrum of clinical findings in these conditions.

Infants
Jaundiced
1. EHBA (most common).
2. Alpha-1-antitrypsin deficiency.
3. Arteriohepatic dysplasia (Alagille syndrome).
4. Metabolic—HFI, galactosaemia, tyrosinosis, cystic fibrosis.
5. Choledochal cyst.
6. Infection—echovirus 11, TORCH, *E. coli* urinary tract infection.
7. Hypopituitarism.

Not jaundiced
1. Tumours. ⎫
2. Choledochal cyst. ⎬ Most common
3. Haemangioma. ⎭
4. Glycogen storage diseases types 1, 3 and 6.
5. Lipid storage disease.
6. Congenital hepatic fibrosis.
7. CCF.
8. Metabolic—as above.

Preschool (less than 5 years)
Jaundiced
1. Metabolic—alpha-1-antitrypsin deficiency, HFI, CF.
2. Chronic active hepatitis.
3. Choledochal cyst.

Not jaundiced
1. Infection—hepatitis (A, B, C, E), infectious mononucleosis, cytomegalovirus, toxoplasmosis.
2. Metabolic—HFI, glycogen storage diseases, cholesteryl ester storage disease.
3. Structural—choledochal cyst, tumours, congenital hepatic fibrosis.

School age (5 years and over)
Jaundiced
As above, plus Wilson's disease and chronic active hepatitis.

Not jaundiced
As above, plus Wilson's disease and chronic active hepatitis.

Splenomegaly

A mnemonic (**CHIMPS**) is helpful to remember the causes of splenomegaly.

C *Cardiac*

Subacute bacterial endocarditis (SBE).

Connective tissue disease

Systemic onset juvenile chronic arthritis, systemic lupus erythematosus.

H *Haematological*

Chronic haemolytic anaemias—hereditary spherocytosis, glucose-6-phosphate dehydrogenase (G6PD) deficiency, thalassaemia.

I *Infection*

1. Viral infection—infectious mononucleosis, cytomegalovirus.
2. Bacterial infection—SBE, typhoid, septicaemia.
3. Protozoal infection—malaria, toxoplasmosis.

Injury

Haematoma.

M *Malignancy*

Leukaemia, lymphoma.

P *Portal hypertension*

1. Extrahepatic—post-neonatal umbilical vessel catheterisation or sepsis.
2. Hepatic—the various causes of cirrhosis, congenital hepatic fibrosis.
3. Suprahepatic—Budd-Chiari syndrome.

S *Storage diseases*

Gaucher's, Niemann-Pick.

Splenic cyst or hamartoma

Hepatosplenomegaly

The causes of hepatosplenomegaly can be seen by perusing the previous two sections for diseases on both lists. In general terms, the causes are as follows:

1. Congenital hepatic fibrosis.
2. Haematological—thalassaemia.
3. Infection—infectious mononucleosis, TORCH.
4. Malignancy—leukaemia, lymphoma.
5. Storage diseases—Gaucher's (long term), Niemann-Pick, mucopolysaccharidoses.

Renal enlargement

Unilateral flank mass

1. Tumour
   - Renal—Wilms' tumour, renal cell carcinoma, congenital mesoblastic nephroma.
   - Non-renal—neuroblastoma, adrenal cell carcinoma.

2. Hydronephrosis.
3. Hypertrophied solitary kidney.
4. Renal cyst.
5. Renal vein thrombosis.

Bilateral flank masses

1. Polycystic kidney disease (infantile—autosomal recessive, adult type—autosomal dominant).
2. Hydronephrosis—posterior urethral valves, vesico-ureteral reflux, neurogenic bladder.
3. Tumour—Wilms', leukaemia, lymphoma, tuberous sclerosis.
4. Metabolic—glycogen storage disease type 1 (A and B), tyrosinaemia type 1.

Ascites

1. Hepatic—cirrhosis and portal hypertension.
2. Renal—nephrotic syndrome.
3. Gastrointestinal—protein-losing enteropathy (e.g. coeliac disease, inflammatory bowel disease), nutritional (PCM, beri-beri), intestinal lymphangiectasia.
4. Cardiovascular—right ventricular failure, constrictive pericarditis, IVC obstruction, hepatic vein obstruction (Budd-Chiari syndrome).
5. Lymphatic—acquired chylous ascites (thoracic duct obstruction by enlarged lymph nodes or neoplasms).
6. Infection—chronic tuberculous peritonitis.

Table 8.2 Additional information: details of possible findings on inspection of abdomen

Inspection	Pubertal status (precocity)
Anterior aspect of abdomen	External genitalia (ambiguous)
Distension, best assessed standing (ascites, coeliac disease, PCM, organomegaly)	Enlarged testis (seminoma, teratoma)
	Posterior aspect of abdomen
Operative scars (e.g. Kasai, renal transplant, peritoneal dialysis, exomphalos repair)	Purpura on buttocks (HSP)
	Xanthomata on buttocks (cholestasis)
Access devices (e.g. Tenckhoff catheter, subcutaneous venous port)	Buttock asymmetry (sacral tumour)
	Gluteal wasting (malnutrition)
Injection sites (e.g. insulin, desferrioxamine)	Midline anomalies related to spinal dysraphism
Stoma (colostomy, ileostomy, ileal conduit, gastrostomy)	• Lipoma
	• Midline hair tuft
Herniae (umbilical, paraumbilical, inguinal, incisional)	• Myelomeningocoele
	Midline scars (repaired spina bifida, resection spinal tumour)
Prominent abdominal wall veins (portal hypertension)	Needle marks over iliac crests (bone marrow biopsy site)
Striae (Cushing's)	Perianal fissures, fistulae (IBD)
Visible peristalsis (pyloric stenosis)	Patulous anus (spina bifida)
Inguinal lymphadenopathy (leukaemia, lymphoma)	Imperforate anus (congenital)
	Faecal soiling (habitual constipation)

HSP = Henoch-Schönlein purpura; IBD = inflammatory bowel disease; PCM = protein calorie malnutrition.

Jaundice

The approach to this case depends on the child's age. In view of this, two separate diagrams of suggested approaches are included, one for the age group below 2–3 years, and one for those older. There is, of course, some overlap, but the author certainly found this division helpful.

The infant

Start by introducing yourself to the parent. Note the infant's growth parameters and any obvious dysmorphic features. Alagille syndrome (arteriohepatic dysplasia) can be associated with a prominent forehead, a small pointed chin and hypertelorism. Zellweger syndrome, a peroxisomopathy, is associated with hypotonia, especially of the neck, a high forehead and huge anterior fontanelle, which may have metopic extension, and hypertelorism. Infants with a congenital TORCH infection may be small, microcephalic and neurologically abnormal, and infants with hypothyroidism can have coarse facial features and be relatively inactive. Note if the child looks well. Children with biliary atresia usually look very well despite the serious nature of their disease. Children with congenital TORCH or urinary tract infections or galactosaemia can look very sick. Listen to the infant's cry, as it may be quite hoarse in hypothyroidism. Also note the infant's posturing, which may be hypotonic (with 'frog leg' positioning of the lower limbs in Zellweger syndrome) or hypertonic (with signs of upper motor unit involvement in the TORCH group). Inspect carefully for any stigmata of chronic liver disease.

The systematic general examination of the infant commences with the hands, followed by the head and neck, the abdomen, a neurological assessment, cardiac and chest examinations and, finally, interpretation of the urinalysis, stool analysis and temperature chart. This approach is outlined in Figure 8.5. Note that the sequence outlined also includes assessing for complications of (unconjugated) hyperbilirubinaemia itself (that is, kernicterus) or for bilirubin encephalopathy, and also examines for complications of cholestasis (if that is the underlying mechanism suspected), namely deficiencies in the fat soluble vitamins A, D, E and K. All but vitamin E deficiency can manifest themselves clinically in this age group.

In the examination of the abdomen, the presence or absence of hepatomegaly is particularly important. The most common four causes of an obstructive jaundice with hepatomegaly in an infant are as follows.

1. Extrahepatic biliary atresia (EHBA).
2. Alpha-1-antitrypsin deficiency.
3. Alagille syndrome.
4. Ex-premature graduate of neonatal intensive care (multiple mechanisms).

The other possibilities at this age include the following.

1. Metabolic—galactosaemia, tyrosinaemia, hereditary fructose intolerance (HFI), cystic fibrosis (CF).
2. Structural—choledochal cyst.
3. Infective—echovirus 11, TORCH.

Several clues can help differentiate between these. If a child is older than a few months and has no large surgical scars, it is unlikely that EHBA is the problem. Conversely, if the child has a large Kasai scar, then do not mention a metabolic disease as the most likely diagnosis! If the infant looks unwell, then infectious or metabolic causes are more likely. If the infant is only several weeks or a few months old, looks well and has acholic stools, then EHBA or choledochal cyst are the most likely diagnoses.

Figure 8.5 Jaundice in infants

1. Introduce self

2. General inspection
Position patient: lying, fully undressed
Parameters
- Weight
- Height
- Head circumference

Sick or well
Activity
Dysmorphic features
Posture
Peripheral stigmata of CLD
Abdominal scars
Cry

3. Hands
Leuconychia (CLD)
Clubbing (CLD)
Palmar erythema (CLD)
Xanthomata (between fingers and on extensor surfaces)

4. Head and neck
Head
Face
Eyes
- Lids
- Conjunctivae
- Sclera
- Cornea
- Lens
- Retina

Mouth
Neck

5. Abdomen
Inspect for
- Distension: ascites (CLD)
- Scars: Kasai procedures (EHBA)
- Caput medusae (CLD)
- Umbilical hernia (hypothyroidism)
- Delayed separation of umbilical cord in neonate (hypothyroidism)

Palpate and percuss
- Hepatomegaly
- Splenomegaly
- Ascites

- Auscultate liver (vascular malformation)
- Genitalia (small with hypopituitarism)

Nappy (if nappy not available, request it)
- Dark urine (cholestasis)
- Acholic stool (cholestasis)

6. Neurological
Alertness
Posture
Involuntary movements
Gross motor assessment
Primitive reflexes
Hearing

7. Cardiac
Examine praecordium for congenital heart disease

8. Chest
Auscultate for any evidence of cystic fibrosis

9. Other
Urinalysis
Temperature chart

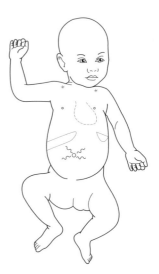

CLD = chronic liver disease; EHBA = extra hepatic biliary atresia.

Associated splenomegaly can occur in chronic hepatic disease and in infective processes such as TORCH. Massive splenomegaly should lead to suspicion of a lysosomal storage disorder.

Ascites and jaundice occur with chronic liver disease, but can also coexist in spontaneous perforation of the bile duct, which stains the umbilicus and scrotum yellow-green.

The neurological examination is directed towards detecting underlying aetiologies, such as TORCH infection or Zellweger syndrome, as well as the complications mentioned above. Evidence should also be sought of malformations which cause hypopituitarism (e.g. septo-optic dysplasia).

In the cardiological assessment, there are several possible findings of relevance. In Alagille syndrome, there can be a congenital hypoplasia or stenosis of the pulmonary artery, and other cardiac anomalies. In congenital rubella, pulmonary artery stenosis, patent ductus arteriosus or septal defects can occur. Other less common associations linking jaundice and cardiovascular problems include the following.

1. Polysplenia/asplenia syndromes, in which biliary atresia indistinguishable from EHBA can occur in association with dextrocardia and congenital heart disease.
2. Arteriovenous malformation of the liver, which can lead to heart failure.
3. Congestive cardiac failure can cause hepatomegaly and jaundice.

In assessing urinalysis, as well as bilirubin and urobilinogen, ask whether any reducing substances are present (if the child is taking lactose in the diet) for galactosaemia, and whether there is blood or nitrites suggestive of a urinary tract infection. _E. coli_ urinary tract infections, in particular, cause cholestasis and often occur in patients with galactosaemia.

The most important condition to identify early is EHBA, as its optimal treatment should be undertaken before 6 weeks of age. The examiners may therefore ask how you would investigate a child for whom this is the likely diagnosis. The following is a suggested approach.

1. Stool inspection—EHBA causes acholic stools.
2. Ultrasound of abdomen—EHBA is associated with a gall bladder less than 2.5 cm in diameter. Ultrasound can also identify choledochal cysts and exclude calculi.
3. Nuclear DISIDA scan—extrahepatic or intrahepatic biliary atresia and severe cholestasis can be indistinguishable. All are associated with lack of tracer in the gastrointestinal tract. For this test the patient should be primed with choleretic therapy with phenobarbitone and cholestyramine.

Exclude all other causes of cholestasis, as all can cause acholic stools. Investigations should include the following:
a. Blood
- TORCH screen.
- Organic acids (Zellweger).
- Amino acids (tyrosinaemia).
- Alpha-1-antitrypsin (AT) assay and phenotype (AT deficiency).
- Thyroid function tests, including TSH assay (hypothyroidism).
- Glucose (hypopituitarism).
- Red blood cell (galactose-1-phosphate uridyl transferase) assay (galactosaemia).
- CF DNA mutation testing (CF).
b. Urine
- Reducing substances (galactosaemia).
- Metabolic screen (Zellweger, tyrosinaemia).
- Culture (urinary tract infection).

   c. Sweat: iontophoresis (CF).

   d. Radiology: chest X-ray to identify butterfly vertebrae (Alagille).

   e. Cardiac assessment: to exclude pulmonary artery stenosis (Alagille).

If all the above are normal, proceed as follows.

4. Liver biopsy (percutaneous)—EHBA shows extrahepatic biliary obstruction, and bile duct proliferation (discriminate EHBA from other diagnoses in 80% of cases).
5. Percutaneous transhepatic cholangiography (PTC), usually done with biopsy.
6. Operative cholangiogram—the 'gold standard' for diagnosing EHBA.
7. Wedge liver biopsy (if above inconclusive).

Table 8.3 gives details of the possible findings on examination of an infant with jaundice.

The older child

The examination of the older child is more like that of an adult. Again, commence by introducing yourself to child and parent. Listen to the child's voice for any evidence of dysarthria, which can occur in Wilson's disease (but is very rare in children under 10 years of age). Note the child's growth parameters and whether the child looks sick or well. Look for dysmorphic features (Alagille syndrome) and any involuntary movements (Wilson's disease). Visually scan the patient for any evidence of the peripheral stigmata of chronic liver disease. Also, assess whether there is any joint swelling, particularly in an adolescent patient (inflammatory bowel disease or chronic active hepatitis).

Systematic examination commences with the hands, followed by the head and neck, abdomen, heart and chest, neurological assessment and then interpretation of the urinalysis, stool analysis and temperature chart. This is outlined in Figure 8.6.

As with the infant, the sequence also detects complications of cholestasis, and in children over 4 years signs of vitamin E deficiency can become manifest as cerebellar ataxia and peripheral neuropathy.

The diseases in this age group are somewhat different from those outlined in the section on the jaundiced infant. The main groups of disease that cause hepatomegaly and jaundice are as follows.

1. **Infective**
   a. Hepatitis A, B, C.
   b. Infectious mononucleosis.
   c. Toxoplasmosis.
   d. Cytomegalovirus.
2. **Metabolic**
   a. Alpha-1-antitrypsin deficiency.
   b. Hereditary fructose intolerance (HFI).
   c. Cystic fibrosis.
   d. Wilson's disease (if child is older than 5 years).
3. **Structural**
   Choledochal cyst.
4. **Autoimmune**
   Chronic active hepatitis.

Note that cystic fibrosis is the most common cause of liver disease in the 0–5 age group in Australia. There are few reports to date of Wilson's disease occurring in a child under 5 years, so it is not wise to mention it early in the differential diagnosis of a 3-year-old with jaundice. Important points regarding Wilson's disease are given below.

Table 8.3 Additional information: details of possible findings on jaundice examination (infant)

Inspection
Dysmorphic features
- Arteriohepatic dysplasia (Alagille syndrome)
- Zellweger syndrome (cerebro-hepato-renal syndrome)

Posture (hypotonic in Zellweger)
Peripheral stigmata of CLD: bruising, bleeding, spider naevi
Scratch marks (pruritis with cholestasis)
Abdominal scars (Kasai)
Hoarse cry (hypothyroidism)

Head and neck
Head
Facial changes of syndromes
- High forehead, hypertelorism, large fontanelle (Zellweger)
- Prominent forehead, hypertelorism, small pointed chin (Alagille)
- Down syndrome

Coarse facial features (hypothyroid)
Increased head circumference (extramedullary haematopoiesis in chronic haemolysis)
Microcephaly (TORCH)
Craniotabes (vitamin D deficiency)
Very large anterior fontanelle (Zellweger)
Large posterior fontanelle (hypothyroidism)
Eyes: nystagmus (septo-optic dysplasia with hypopituitarism)
Lids: xanthelasma
Conjunctivae
- Pallor (haemolytic anaemia)
- Xerosis (vitamin A deficiency)

Sclerae: depth of jaundice
Cornea: xerosis, clouding, opacification (vitamin A deficiency)
Lens: cataract (galactosaemia, TORCH)
Retina
- Chorioretinitis (TORCH)
- Retinal pigmentation (Zellweger)

- Optic atrophy (septo-optic dysplasia)

Midline defects (e.g. clefts): hypopituitarism
Tongue: enlarged, protruding (hypothyroidism)
Neck: goitre (hypothyroidism)

Neurological
Alertness (decreased in Zellweger, hypothyroidism, TORCH)
Posture: hypotonic (Zellweger)
Choreoathetoid movements (bilirubin encephalopathy, indicating unconjugated hyperbilirubinaemia)
Gross motor assessment
- Hypotonic (Zellweger)
- Hypertonic (TORCH)

Primitive reflexes: pathological persistence (TORCH, bilirubin encephalopathy)
Hearing: deafness (congenital rubella, bilirubin encephalopathy, Zellweger)

Cardiac
Palpate apex to exclude dextrocardia (polysplenia and asplenia syndromes)
Auscultate praecordium for:
- Pulmonary artery stenosis (Alagille, congenital rubella)
- Patent ductus or septal defects (Zellweger, congenital rubella)

Other
Urinalysis
- Bilirubin (hepatobiliary disease; its absence implies unconjugated hyperbilirubinaemia)
- Urobilinogen (increased in haemolysis and hepatic dysfunction)
- Blood (UTI)
- Nitrites (UTI)
- Reducing substances (galactosaemia)

Temperature chart (infection, e.g. UTI)

CLD = chronic liver disease; TORCH = toxoplasmosis, other (e.g. HIV, syphilis), rubella, cytomegalovirus, herpes (both simplex and varicella); UTI = urinary tract infection.

1. Neurological problems are extremely rare in children (although they are listed here for completeness).
2. If there is neurological disease, Kayser–Fleischer rings are usually present.
3. Cystic fibrosis often presents when screening an asymptomatic sibling of a child with Wilson's disease.
4. It may present as a psychiatric problem or with deteriorating school performance.
5. It can present early in childhood, around 5 years, as a haemolytic anaemia, which can be associated with jaundice.
6. It is crucial not to miss the diagnosis, as it is one of the few curable causes of cirrhosis.

In the child over 10 years, chronic active hepatitis and Wilson's disease are more likely to be seen in the examination setting. If chronic active hepatitis seems likely, then it is worthwhile mentioning, and examining for, associations of the autoimmune variety: namely thyroiditis (feel for goitre), glomerulonephritis (request the blood pressure and urinalysis) and erythema nodosum (make a point of carefully inspecting the legs). In this age group, it is also worth assessing for evidence of inflammatory bowel disease, which can be complicated by liver disease, and may be associated with arthritis and erythema nodosum, as well as uveitis.

Investigations

The examiners may ask what investigations you would perform. Obviously this depends on the findings in the particular child you see, but in general it is better to assess the severity of the problem before a long differential discussion about the cause, as this is what would apply in practice. Therefore, first mention basic investigations.

Liver function tests (LFTs)
1. Serum bilirubin (direct and indirect): total indicates severity of jaundice; fractional determination (conjugated or unconjugated) valuable in diagnosis.
2. Serum enzymes:
   a. transaminases—AST (SGOT) and ALT (SPOT)—indices of hepatocellular dysfunction;
   b. alkaline phosphatase (SAP)—indicates biliary tract disease;
   c. gamma–glutamyl transpeptidase (GGT)—confers specificity to an elevated SAP, as normal GGT activity occurs in children with bone disease.
3. Serum proteins: albumin—index of liver capacity for protein synthesis.

Clotting studies
Prothrombin time (PT) is not a sensitive indicator of hepatic disease but has prognostic value (if response to vitamin K given parenterally, good prognostic value).

Assessment for deficiency of fat soluble vitamins
1. Serum retinol level (vitamin A).
2. Serum calcium, phosphate, SAP (vitamin D).
3. Serum vitamin E level.
4. Vitamin K assessed by PT as above.

After these have been discussed, mention appropriate investigations to clarify the diagnosis.

The single most important disease that must not be missed is Wilson's disease, as it is curable. Further important diagnoses include hereditary fructose intolerance and choledochal cyst, for similar reasons.

Figure 8.6 Jaundice in older children

1. Introduce self

2. General inspection
Position patient: lying down, fully
    undressed
Parameters
- Weight
- Height
- Head circumference
- Sick or well
Dysmorphic features
Dysarthria
Involuntary movements
Peripheral stigmata of CLD
Abdominal scars
Joint swelling

3. Hands
Leuconychia (CLD)
Clubbing (CLD)
Palmar erythema (CLD)
Xanthomata (between fingers and on
    extensor surfaces)
Asterixis (liver failure)
Wrists: epiphyseal widening (vitamin D
    deficiency)

4. Head and neck
Head
Face
Eyes
- Lids
- Conjunctivae
- Sclera
- Iris
- Cornea
- Lens
- Retina
Mouth
Neck

5. Abdomen
Inspect
- Distension: ascites (CLD)
- Scars: liver transplant, Kasai
- Caput medusae (CLD)
Palpate and percuss
- Hepatomegaly
- Splenomegaly
- Ascites
- Inguinal lymphadenopathy
    (infectious mononucleosis)
Auscultate liver (haemangioma,
    hepatoma)
Inspect perianal region (IBD)

Mention rectal examination for
    haemorrhoids (portal hypertension)

6. Chest
Sternal deformity (vitamin D deficiency)
Rib rosary (vitamin D deficiency)
Auscultate praecordium for pulmonary
    artery stenosis (Alagille syndrome)
Auscultate chest for any evidence of CF

7. Gait and lower limbs
Inspection
Bowing (vitamin D deficiency)
Erythema nodosum (IBD, chronic active
    hepatitis)
Joint swelling (IBD)
Gait examination (in children over
    4 years)

8. Other
Inspection
- Urine
- Stool
Urinalysis
Temperature chart

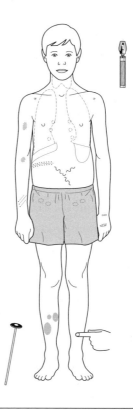

CF = cystic fibrosis; CLD = chronic liver disease; IBD = inflammatory bowel disease.

Table 8.4 Diagnostic investigations in the older child with jaundice

Disease	Investigations
Wilson's disease	Reduced serum copper (usually) and caeruloplasmin Elevated urinary copper excretion Markedly elevated liver copper content on liver biopsy (most reliable)
Chronic active hepatitis 1. HBsAg negative	Markedly elevated serum gammaglobulin (over 90% cases) Positive for antinuclear antibody (75%) High-titre smooth muscle antibody Positive direct Coomb's test (75%)
2. HBsAg positive	Mildly elevated serum gammaglobulin Negative for antinuclear antibody (95%) Low-titre smooth muscle antibody Negative direct Coomb's test Positive (often) HBsAb
3. HCAb positive alpha-1-antitrypsin deficiency	Pi phenotyping: PiM allele; phenotype MM (normal level alpha-1-antitrypsin) PiZ allele; phenotype ZZ (5%–15% of normal level of alpha-1-antitrypsin) PiMZ allele; phenotype MZ (60% of normal level of alpha-1-antitrypsin)
Hereditary fructose intolerance	Fructose-1-phosphate aldolase assay on liver or jejunal biopsy specimen
Sclerosing cholangitis in inflammatory bowel disease	Visualised on percutaneous transhepatic cholangiography (PTC) or endoscopic retrograde cholangiography (ERCP)

Table 8.4 gives an incomplete list of some of the more important possible investigations. Table 8.5 details the possible findings on examination of an older child for jaundice.

Nutritional assessment

The simplest approach to this case comprises three successive components:

1. Assessment of growth parameters.
2. Assessment of fat and protein stores.
3. Assessment of other nutrients, systematically.

First, introduce yourself to the child and the parent. Ensure the child is fully undressed, then stand back and inspect the child carefully. Visually scan for subcutaneous tissue and muscle bulk. Comment on the child's height and weight, request the percentile charts and interpret these. If only one measurement is given, request previous measurements to observe their progression. Work out the weight age and height age; compare these and comment. Next, if the child is underweight, work out the weight for height, to quantitate the difference in kilograms between this value and the child's actual weight.

Table 8.5 Additional information: details of possible findings on jaundice examination (older child).

Inspection
Dysmorphic features (Alagille syndrome)
Dysarthria (Wilson's disease)
Involuntary movements: athetoid, choreic, tremor, dystonia or myoclonus (all can occur in Wilson's disease)
Peripheral stigmata of CLD: bruising, bleeding, spider naevi
Scratch marks (pruritis with cholestasis)
Abdominal scars (liver transplant, Kasai)
Joint swelling (IBD)

Head and neck
Head
Facial features of Alagille syndrome
Coarse facial features (hypothyroid)
Frontal and parietal bossing (thalassaemia)
Craniotabes (vitamin D deficiency)
Eyes
Lids: xanthelasma
Conjunctivae
• Pallor (haemolytic anaemia) (can occur in Wilson's disease)
• Xerosis (vitamin A deficiency)
Sclerae: depth of jaundice
Cornea
• Xerosis, clouding, opacification (vitamin A deficiency)
• Kayser-Fleischer rings (Wilson's disease)
Lens: cataracts (steroid treated IBD)
Mouth
Poor state of dentition (vitamin D deficiency)
Palatal petechiae (infectious mononucleosis)
Tonsillar exudate (infectious mononucleosis)
Neck

Cervical lymphadenopathy (infectious mononucleosis)
Goitre (hypothyroidism)

Gait and lower limbs
Most of this section is only applicable to a child over 4 years of age, as vitamin E deficiency and Wilson's disease do not exhibit neurological effects until later in childhood.
Gait examination
• Cerebellar ataxia (vitamin E deficiency)
• Peripheral neuropathy (vitamin E deficiency)
• Involuntary movements (Wilson's disease)
• Antalgic gait (arthritis with IBD)
Romberg's sign (vitamin E deficiency)
Hold arms horizontally: wing beating tremor (Wilson's disease)
Knee and ankle reflexes
• Diminished (vitamin E deficiency)
• Delayed return (hypothyroidism)
Sensation: diminished (vitamin E deficiency)

Other
Request inspection of:
• Urine: dark (cholestasis)
• Stool: acholic (cholestasis); blood (portal hypertension)
Urinalysis
• Bilirubin (hepatobiliary disease; its absence implies unconjugated hyperbilirubinaemia)
• Urobilinogen (increased in haemolysis, and hepatic dysfunction)
• Blood (UTI)
• Nitrites (UTI)
Temperature chart (hepatitis, UTI, chronic active hepatitis)

CLD = chronic liver disease; IBD = inflammatory bowel disease: UTI = urinary tract infection.

On interpretation of percentiles, the common finding is poor weight gain, but height can also be significantly decreased by chronic disease, protein calorie malnutrition (PCM), zinc deficiency and rickets. Head circumference can be decreased in PCM, but increased in vitamin D deficiency rickets.

After interpreting the percentile charts, demonstrate the amount of subcutaneous fat tissue by examining the skin fold thickness, between your thumb and index finger, at the mid-arm over biceps and triceps, the axillae, and the subscapular and suprailiac regions. Demonstrate muscle bulk at the arms, thighs and buttocks, muscle wasting

Figure 8.7 Nutritional assessment

1. Introduce self

2. General inspection
Position patient: fully undressed, standing, then lying down
Parameters
- Weight
- Height
- Head circumference
- Percentiles
- Weight age versus height age
- Weight for height (quantitate)

Sick or well
Nasogastric tube
Intravenous access
Posture
Skeletal deformity
Pot belly

3. Demonstrate fat and protein stores
Subcutaneous fat
- Mid-arm
- Axillae
- Subscapular
- Suprailiac

Muscle bulk
- Biceps
- Triceps
- Quadriceps
- Glutei

4. Skin
Pallor
Jaundice
Bruising
Dermatitis
Erythema nodosum

5. Head and neck
Head
Hair
Eyes: detailed examination
Mouth
Teeth
Tongue
Gums
Neck

6. Upper limbs
Palms, nails
Pulse
Wrists, forearms
Blood pressure

7. Chest wall
Rib rosary (vitamins C, D)
Sternal deformity (vitamins C, D)
Harrison's sulcus (vitamin D)

Sacral oedema (PCM, CLD)

8. Abdomen
Distension
Ascites (PCM, CLD)
Weak abdominal muscles (PCM, vitamin D)
Hepatomegaly (fatty infiltration with PCM, linoleic acid)
Hepatosplenomegaly (CLD, zinc)
Pubertal delay (zinc)

9. Gait
Full gait examination (vitamins B_1, B_6, B_{12}, E)
Examine back (vitamin D)

10. Lower limbs
Palpation
- Muscle bulk
- Ankle oedema
- Tenderness

Neurological examination

11. Cardiovascular system
Full praecordial examination looking for:
- Cardiomegaly (vitamin B_1, phosphate, selenium)
- Cardiac failure (vitamin B_1, phosphate, anaemias)

12. Other
Urinalysis
Low specific gravity (CRF)
High specific gravity (dehydration)
Glucose (diabetes)
Stool analysis
Malabsorption
Giardiasis
Temperature chart (hypothermia with PCM)

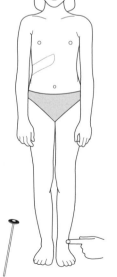
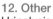

CLD = chronic liver disease; CRF = chronic renal failure; PCM = protein calorie malnutrition.

being best demonstrated over these areas, particularly the buttocks (glutei). In infants, poor muscle bulk can be reflected by hypotonia on picking the child up.

The next step is a systematic general examination directed at detection of various deficiencies. It commences at the hands, continues up to the head, and then essentially moves from head to toe. Figure 8.7 outlines the order of examination, and Table 8.6 at the end of this section gives additional information. Each deficiency sought is given in parentheses after the relevant physical sign.

Check the skin thoroughly before examining the patient. There are numerous dermatological manifestations of many deficiencies. Some of the relevant deficiencies include marked flakiness (PCM), dryness (linoleic acid, vitamin A), bruising (vitamin C, K), pellagra (niacin) or hyperpigmented hyperkeratosis (zinc deficiency).

Examine the child's hands next. Look at the palms for crease pallor (anaemia associated with several deficiencies) or palmar erythema (chronic liver disease, CLD), and the nails for koilonychia (iron), brittleness (iron, protein), leuconychia (CLD) or clubbing (cystic fibrosis, CLD, Crohn's disease).

Feel the radial pulse for bradycardia (PCM, iodine) or tachycardia (vitamin B_1, dehydration). Check the wrists for palpable epiphyseal enlargement (vitamin D), forearms for tenderness (vitamin C) and joints for swelling (vitamin C). Take, or request, the blood pressure, supine and standing (sodium, dehydration), and offer to look for Trousseau's sign (cuff inflated to greater than systolic pressure for 3 minutes) at the end of the examination (calcium).

Next, examine the head and neck. Look for thinning of hair or areas of alopecia (linoleic acid, zinc), and for dyspigmentation of hair (PCM), and feel the hair for dryness (iodine) or excessive pluckability (PCM).

The eyes are the next area on which to focus, and many signs are possible here (see Table 8.6). In particular, look at the conjunctivae for pallor (iron, copper, B group vitamins, folate), or dryness and wrinkling (vitamin A), or Bitot's spots (silver plaques of desquamated epithelial cells and mucus) on the bulbar aspect (vitamin A). Look for scleral icterus (vitamin B_{12}, CLD), corneal dryness, wrinkling or clouding (vitamin A), or opacification (vitamin A, zinc). Quickly assess the external ocular movement (vitamin E), and check for photophobia (riboflavin, zinc). Offer fundoscopy for optic nerve inflammation (vitamin B_{12}) or atrophy (vitamin B_1); usually this will not be required.

Next, percuss over the facial nerve, for Chvostek's sign (calcium). Then, inspect the mouth for angular cheilosis (iron, riboflavin), gums for swelling or bleeding (vitamin C), teeth for caries (fluoride), enamel defects (vitamin D) or looseness (vitamin C), tongue for moistness (hydration) or glossitis (B group vitamins), and buccal mucosa for reddening, ulceration (B group vitamins) or petechiae (vitamin C). Examine the neck for goitre (iodine).

Examine the chest for sternal deformity (vitamin C, D), or any 'rib rosary' (vitamin C, D).

Next examine the abdomen for evidence of pot belly (weak abdominal musculature, coeliac disease), hepatomegaly (PCM, linoleic acid), hepatosplenomegaly (CLD) or ascites (PCM, CLD). Assess Tanner staging for pubertal delay (zinc).

Now, ask the child to walk, looking for evidence of cerebellar ataxia (vitamin E, zinc) or peripheral neuropathy (vitamins B_1, B_6, B_{12}). Check for Romberg's sign (vitamins E, B_{12}). While the child is up, check the back for scoliosis, lordosis or kyphosis (vitamins D, C), and look again for any evidence of bow legs or knock knees (vitamin D).

Proceed with a lower limb examination, feel for ankle oedema (PCM, CLD) and test muscle tone (decreased in PCM). Check muscle power for weakness (PCM, sodium, potassium). Tap out the knee and ankle jerks, which may be decreased (vitamins, B_1, B_6, B_{12}, E), increased (vitamin B_{12}) or have slowed return (iodine). Examine sensation for peripheral neuropathy (vitamins B_1, B_6, B_{12}, E) or posterior column dysfunction (vitamins B_{12}, E).

Examine the heart for cardiomegaly (vitamin B_1, phosphate, selenium) or congestive cardiac failure (vitamin B_1, phosphate, anaemia).

Finally, request the urinalysis for specific gravity (high with dehydration, low with chronic renal failure) and glucose (diabetes), and the stool analysis for evidence of malabsorption or giardiasis.

Table 8.6 Additional information: details of possible findings on nutritional assessment

Inspection
Activity, awareness (PCM)
Irritability (vitamin C, iron, coeliac)
Nasogastric tube
Intravenous access for total parenteral nutrition
Posture
- 'Frog leg' (vitamin C)
- Bow legs (vitamin D)
Prominent wrists, ankles (vitamin D)
Rib rosary (vitamin C, D)
Harrison's groove (vitamin D)
Pot belly (PCM, coeliac, vitamin D)

Skin
Pallor (vitamins A, B_1, B_2, B_6, B_{12}, C, E, folate, iron, copper)
Jaundice (CLD, vitamin B_{12})
Bruising (vitamins C, K)
Poor wound healing (vitamin C, PCM, zinc)
'Flaky paint' dermatitis (PCM)
Desquamation (linoleic acid, biotin)
Dry (vitamin A, linoleic acid)
Rough, scaly skin (pellagra) in sun-exposed areas (niacin)
Seborrheic dermatitis (vitamin B_2)
Eczematous scaling around mouth, elbows, knees, genitals, anus (zinc)
Waxy (vitamin B_1, in wet beri beri)
Dermatitis herpetiformis (coeliac)
Erythema nodosum (Crohn's disease, ulcerative colitis)

Upper limbs
Palms: crease pallor (anaemias), erythema (CLD)
Nails: leuconychia (CLD), koilonychia (iron), brittle (iron, PCM)
Pulse: bradycardia (iodine, PCM), tachycardia (vitamin B_{12}, hydration)
Wrists: palpable epiphyseal enlargement (vitamin D)

Forearms: tender (vitamin C)
Joints: swollen (vitamin C)
Blood pressure: hypotension (sodium, hydration)
Trousseau's sign (calcium)

Head and neck
Frontal and parietal prominence (vitamin D)
Increased head circumference (vitamins A, D)
Soft skull (craniotabes) (vitamin D)
Fontanelle
- Large (vitamin D)
- Bulging (vitamin A)
- Depressed (hydration)
- Sutures separated (vitamin A)
Hair
- Alopecia (zinc, linoleic acid)
- Dyspigmented (PCM)
- Thinning (PCM)
- Pluckable (PCM)
- Dry (iodine)
Eyes: sunken (hydration)
Lids
- Ptosis (vitamin B)
- Blepharitis (vitamin B_2, zinc)
Conjunctivae
- Pallor (anaemias)
- Xerosis (vitamin A)
- Conjunctivitis (vitamin B_2, C)
- Bitot spots (vitamin A)
Scleral icterus (vitamin B_2, CLD)
Cornea
- Xerosis (vitamin A)
- Cloudy (vitamin A)
- Keratomalacia (vitamin A)
- Opacification (vitamin A, zinc)
- Vascularisation (vitamin B_2)
Retina
- Optic neuritis (vitamin B_{12})
- Optic atrophy (vitamin B_1)

Continued

Table 8.6 *(Continued)*

Eye movements: ophthalmoplegia
(vitamin E)
Photophobia (vitamin B_2, zinc)
Facial nerve: percuss for Chvostek's sign
(calcium)
Mouth: angular cheilosis and stomatitis
(iron, vitamin B_2, niacin)
Teeth
- Caries (fluoride)
- Loose (vitamin C)
- Enamel defects (vitamin D)
Tongue
- Glossitis, reddening and ulceration
(vitamin B group)
- Moisture (hydration)
- Cyanosis (CHD, vitamin B)
Buccal mucosa
- Reddened and ulcerated (vitamin B
group)
- Petechiae (vitamin C)
Gums: swollen, bleeding (vitamin C)
Contour of lower face
- Prominent salivary glands (vitamin C)
- Pendulous cheeks (PCM)
Neck: goitre (iodine)

Gait and back
Full gait examination, looking for:

- Cerebellar ataxia (vitamin E, zinc)
- Peripheral neuropathy (vitamins B_1,
B_6, B_{12})
- Romberg's sign (vitamins E, B_{12})
Examine back for scoliosis, kyphosis and
lordosis (vitamin D)

Lower limbs
Palpate
- Muscle bulk (PCM)
- Ankle oedema (PCM, CLD)
- Long-bone tenderness (vitamin C,
phosphate)
- Calf tenderness (vitamin B_1, selenium)
Power: decreased (PCM, vitamin C,
sodium, potassium, phosphate)
Tone: decreased (PCM)
Reflexes
- Decreased (vitamins B_1, B_6, B_{12}, E)
- Increased (vitamin B_{12}: note that B_{12}
deficiency can cause either decreased
or increased reflexes)
- Slowed return (iodine)
Sensation
- Peripheral neuropathy (vitamins B_1,
B_6, B_{12}, E)
- Posterior column dysfunction
(vitamins B_{12}, E)

CHD = congenital heart disease; CLD = chronic liver disease; PCM = protein calorie malnutrition.

Failure to thrive

This is a very complicated short case and fortunately uncommon. The approach outlined is essentially a nutritional assessment modified to include relevant examination for chronic diseases of the main organ systems. To prevent unnecessary duplication, only aspects not mentioned in the nutritional short case are outlined in detail.

Commence with general inspection for obvious abnormalities, such as recognisable dysmorphic syndromes, central nervous system disease (e.g. cerebral palsy), neuromuscular disease (congenital myopathies, spinal muscular atrophy), tachypnoea (cardiac, respiratory, or renal—metabolic acidosis—in origin), cyanosis (congenital heart disease) and any findings related to nutritional status. Next, request the child's parameters. Failure to thrive as a term is used to describe failure of weight gain in particular, but—particularly if long standing—may include lack of linear growth as well. If the head circumference is significantly affected, this suggests an intrauterine onset.

The percentile charts should be examined. The pattern of the height, weight and head circumference curves relative to each other may well give a valuable indication of the underlying pathology.

1. If all percentiles are equally affected, the possibilities include intrauterine TORCH infections or chromosomal abnormalities.
2. If height is most affected, possibilities include endocrinopathies and skeletal dysplasias.
3. The common pattern for malnutrition is that the weight is most affected, the height less affected, and the head circumference relatively normal.

Demonstrate fat and protein stores, and then examine the skin fully, in particular for dermatitis herpetiformis (coeliac disease), erythema nodosum (inflammatory bowel disease) and pyoderma gangrenosum (inflammatory bowel disease). Note any ichthyosis (Shwachman's).

Look next at the hands, noting any clubbing (chronic lung disease, chronic liver disease, inflammatory bowel disease, congenital heart disease) and other nutrition-related signs. Examine the structure of the hands (dysmorphic syndromes), take the radial and femoral pulses (congenital heart disease, coarctation). Check the blood pressure (renal disease, coarctation).

Proceed to the head and neck. As well as nutrition-related signs, look for dysmorphic features, macrocephaly, scars and shunts. In the eyes, look for cataracts or chorioretinitis (TORCH), retinitis pigmentosa (abetalipoproteinaemia, Shwachman's syndrome), papilloedema (intracranial tumours, hydrocephalus), and check the extraocular movements (neurological disease). At the mouth, check for thrush (can occur in cell-mediated immunity defects), check the palate for a cleft, note the quality of sucking and test the gag reflex. If a bottle or breast is available, the method of feeding should be observed.

Now, move to examination of the chest. Look for sternal deformity (syndromes), hyperinflation, Harrison's sulcus, use of accessory muscles, intercostal recession (chronic lung disease), scars of cardiac or pulmonary surgery. Palpate tracheal position, apex beat, praecordium for thrills and heaves, percuss the chest and auscultate heart and lungs thoroughly to assess for chronic respiratory or cardiac disease.

Then, move on to the abdomen. Perform a full abdominal examination (see the short case on the abdomen). The findings sought include abdominal distension (ascites with chronic liver disease, coeliac disease, protein calorie malnutrition), prominent veins (chronic liver disease), scars of previous surgery (e.g. bowel resection with necrotising enterocolitis, Kasai procedure for biliary atresia), hepatosplenomegaly (chronic liver disease, TORCH, metabolic and haematological diseases), enlarged kidneys (polycystic kidneys, hydronephrosis), anal anomalies (syndromes), rectal prolapse (cystic fibrosis) and excoriated buttocks (carbohydrate intolerance).

Next, have the child stand up and walk, checking the gait for primary neurological disease, as well as for nutritional deficiencies. Examine the back for midline defects or skeletal abnormalities such as kyphoscoliosis (syndromes, cerebral palsy), and then return the child to the bed and examine the lower limbs, again predominantly to detect primary neurological disease, as well as nutritional parameters. Note that if the patient is an infant, a gross motor developmental assessment is more appropriate at this point, and this may be combined with checking the primitive reflexes.

Request the urinalysis for specific gravity (low with chronic renal failure, diabetes insipidus), glucose (diabetes), pH (renal tubular acidosis), protein (structural kidney disease, proximal tubular disease), blood (structural kidney disease, urinary tract infection), nitrites (urinary tract infection) and bilirubin (chronic liver disease). Also, request stool analysis, for evidence of steatorrhoea, fat crystals (coeliac disease) or globules (cystic fibrosis), low pH and reducing substances (carbohydrate intolerance), or giardia (cysts or vegetative forms). It is also worth mentioning inspection of any vomitus for bile (obstructive bowel lesions) or blood (portal hypertension) and the temperature chart for infection, as well as watching the mother feeding the child, noting their inter-action, the feeding technique and any maternal anxiety.

The examiners may ask how you would investigate the problem. If undernutrition seems possible, then a common approach would be to admit the child to hospital and document whether the child can gain weight with adequate calories, which confirms undernutrition. If the child does not gain weight despite adequate calories, then investigation for malabsorption, or for any chronic disease, would be appropriate (see the long case on malabsorption).

Poor feeding

This is a very similar case to failure to thrive, but the problem may be of shorter duration, such that poor somatic growth has yet to occur. The approach is essentially the same in content, with some additions, but the order is changed.

Commence with general inspection, as outlined in the previous section, and comment on parameters and percentiles. The resting respiratory rate is a guide to a cardiac or respiratory cause, and obviously abnormal posturing and movements may indicate a neurological cause (e.g. cerebral palsy, spinal muscular atrophy).

Next, watch the child feed. This will help to clarify the nature of the feeding problem—whether it is local or general and, if general, which system is affected.

Start the examination with the head, looking for local causes first, if no initial clues are apparent after inspection. If there are suggestions of specific problems, such as an infant with an alert face but paucity of movement, then 'go for the money', and 'chase' all the relevant clinical signs for the diagnosis that you suspect (in this example, demonstrate all the findings recognised in Werdnig-Hoffmann spinal muscular atrophy).

Note if there is any regurgitation of food through the nose, or any vomiting associated with feeding. Look for local structural problems, such as cleft palate. Check the gag reflex and note the quality of sucking. If the infant is breathless, check for nostril patency by holding a shiny metal object, such as one arm of a stethoscope, immediately below the nostrils, and inspect for condensation at the point underneath. The remainder of the head examination procedure suggested for failure to thrive is appropriate here.

The remainder of the general examination can also follow the failure-to-thrive pattern—that is, assessing the cardiorespiratory system, abdomen, and neurological system, as well as checking the blood pressure (renal disease), urinalysis and the temperature chart.

Weight loss — older child / adolescent

This is very similar in approach to failure to thrive, but there are numerous disorders that occur in older children that are not relevant to the infant or younger child in whom the term failure to thrive is used. The commonest cause of weight loss in adolescent girls in Australia and the United States is anorexia nervosa (AN). Other conditions that tend to affect older children need to be considered, including inflammatory bowel disease (IBD), thyrotoxicosis, Addison's disease, Wilson's disease and various malignancies. The usual lead-in will be 'This child is thin' or 'This child has lost weight over the past [specified time period]'.

The easiest way to think about the differential diagnoses for this case is going back to basic physiology: loss of weight can be due to any one or more of four groups:

1. Lack of caloric intake: voluntary (e.g. by desire in anorexia nervosa, to avoid nausea in Crohn's disease) or involuntary (e.g. protein calorie malnutrition [PCM]

in the third world, neglect, abuse, Münchausen's syndrome by proxy [a specific form of abuse], local structural craniofacial problems), or neuromuscular and neurodevelopmental disorders, making intake difficult.

2. Lack of calorie utilisation, from lack of food digestion (e.g. cystic fibrosis, Shwachman's syndrome) or food absorption (e.g. coeliac disease, severe Crohn's disease, short gut syndrome).

3. Excessive use of calories in metabolic processes. Any child with 'chronic [fill in the organ system here—anything] failure' can lose weight. Hence, numerous causes can be remembered easily: chronic renal failure (CRF), chronic liver failure (CLD), chronic respiratory failure (as in CF), congestive cardiac failure (various forms of congenital and acquired heart disease), chronic immune failure (immunodeficiencies such as HIV), chronic atopic dermatitis ('skin failure'), chronic adrenocortical failure (Addison's), chronic pancreatic endocrine failure (diabetes mellitus). Any child with cancer will lose weight. Any child with an active inflammatory process can lose weight (e.g. juvenile arthritis, IBD).

4. Excessive loss of calories/nutrients/water: various causes of diarrhoea (coeliac disease), various causes of polyuria (CRF, diabetes mellitus, diabetes insipidus), various causes of vomiting (anorexia nervosa patients with bulimic features, subacute bowel obstruction, intracranial pathology, malignancy).

Depending on the lead-in given, as alluded to above, malignancy may need to be considered. Leukaemia, intracranial tumours and solid tumours (lymphoma, neuroblastoma, Wilms') thus all come into the differential diagnosis. The approach given in Table 8.7 includes selected findings only; the list is by no means complete. While it is unlikely that a child with a malignancy would be a short-case subject in an examination format, it is still worth learning a comprehensive approach that will be useful in day-to-day practice.

For more detailed findings in the examinations for the various systems and their disorders, refer to the relevant sections (e.g. CF, IBD, CLD, CRF, oncology). Wherever a vitamin or trace element is noted in brackets, this refers to a deficiency of this, in the context of malnutrition.

Table 8.7 Weight loss in the older child: list of possible findings on examination

1. General inspection
Position patient: fully undressed, standing then lying down
Parameters
- Weight
- Height
- Head circumference
- Percentiles
- Weight age versus height age
- Weight for height (quantitate)
Sick or well
Cachectic (malignancy, AN, AIDS)
In pain (malignancy, IBD, JA)
Activity, awareness (PCM)
Irritability (hyperthyroidism, PCM, iron)
Depressed affect (AN)
Pigmentation (Addison's, beta thalassaemia major)

Nasogastric tube (AN)
'Raccoon eyes' (ecchymoses from neuroblastoma)
Intravenous access port (chemotherapy in oncology patients, TPN in IBD)
Chest AP diameter increased (asthma, CF)
Pot belly (PCM, coeliac)
Posture: bow legs (vitamin D)
Hemihypertrophy (hepatoblastoma, Beckwith [e.g. with adrenal carcinoma])

2. Demonstrate fat and protein stores
Subcutaneous fat
- Mid-arm
- Axillae
- Subscapular
- Suprailiac

Continued

Table 8.7 *(Continued)*

Muscle bulk
- Biceps
- Triceps
- Quadriceps
- Glutei

3. Skin

Pallor (deficiencies various vitamins, iron, CRF, ALL)

Acrocyanosis (AN)

Jaundice (CLD, vitamin B_{12})

Yellowish hue (from hypercarotenaemia in AN)

Bruising (CLD, ALL, neuroblastoma)

Petechiae: limited to SVC distribution (vomiting in AN)

Petechiae, purpura: generalised distribution (leukaemia)

Dry (atopic dermatitis, AN)

Dermatitis artefacta (e.g. cigarette burns, other self-injury in AN)

Scaling (AN)

Excoriated acne (self-injuring AN)

Hypertrichosis: lanugo-like, fine downy-like hair (AN)

Eczematous scaling around mouth, elbows, knees, genitals, anus (zinc)

Pigmented scars (Addison's)

Café-au-lait spots (NF-1 with associated tumours)

Axillary freckling (NF-1 with associated tumours)

Palpable non-tender subcutaneous nodules (neuroblastoma)

Dermatitis herpetiformis (coeliac)

Erythema nodosum (IBD)

Pyoderma gangrenosum (IBD)

Pretibial oedema (AN)

Necrobiosis lipoidica diabeticorum (red-brown plaques on shins, in IDDM)

4. Head and neck

Hair
- Loss of discrete areas (trichotillomania as self-injury in AN)
- Thinning (AN, PCM)
- Brittle, pluckable (AN, PCM)

Eyes: inspection (from above and from side, as well as in front)
- Exophthalmos (Graves', neuroblastoma, orbital tumour)
- Thyroid stare (hyperthyroidism)
- Blepharitis (zinc)
- Lid retraction (hyperthyroidism)
- Ptosis (intracranial tumour)
- Horner's syndrome: miosis, partial ptosis, anhydrosis (neuroblastoma)

- Heterochromia (associated malignancy)
- Aniridia (Wilms')
- Conjunctival pallor (anaemias)
- Scleral icterus (CLD)
- Cataract (diabetes, AN)
- Papilloedema (intracranial tumour)
- Extraocular movements: paresis of inferior oblique; muscles of convergence—medial, superior, inferior recti; lateral rectus
- Test for lid lag (hyperthyroidism)

Mouth: angular cheilosis and stomatitis (iron)

Tongue
- Glossitis, reddening and ulceration (vitamin B group)
- Cyanosis (CHD, CF)

Palate: scarring from self-induced vomiting (AN with bulimic features)

Buccal mucosa
- Reddened and ulcerated (vitamin B group)
- Petechiae (leukaemia, vitamin C)

Gums: gingivitis (ALL)

Teeth: erosion of enamel (AN who purge)

Contour of lower face: prominent salivary glands (AN with bulimia)

Neck
- Lymphadenopathy (lymphoma, ALL, CLL)
- Goitre (hyperthyroidism)

Full examination of cranial nerves, including motor cranial nerves (test first; for intracranial tumours)

5. Upper limbs

Tremor (hyperthyroidism)

Hands
- Russell's sign (calluses, scars or erosions over dorsal surface of hands, especially metacarpophalangeal joints with self-induced vomiting in AN)

Palms
- Pigmented creases (Addison's, beta thalassaemia major)
- Pallor (anaemias, CRF)
- Erythema (CLD)

Nails
- Clubbing (CF, IBD, CLD)
- Bitten (AN)
- Leuconychia (CLD)
- Koilonychia (iron)
- Brittle (AN, PCM)

Continued

Table 8.7 *(Continued)*

Fingers
- Fingertip prick marks (BSL testing in diabetes, CF)
- Hypertrophic pulmonary osteoarthropathy, HPOA (CF)

Pulse
- Bradycardia (AN, PCM)
- Tachycardia (thyrotoxicosis, phaeochromocytoma, vitamin B_{12})
- Irregular (atrial arrhythmia in AN)
- Flap (hypercarbia in CF, liver failure)

Wrists: tender, palpable epiphyseal enlargement (vitamin D)

Joints: swollen (juvenile arthritis, arthropathy with IBD, CF)

Epitrochlear node enlargement (lymphoma)

Blood pressure
- Hypotension: check for postural drop (Addison's, AN)
- Hypertension (CRF, phaeochromocytoma, other neuroendocrine tumour)

Full neurological examination of upper limbs, looking for:
- Cerebellar ataxia (posterior fossa tumour)
- Peripheral neuropathy (vitamin B_{12})
- Upper motor neurone signs (intracranial tumour, spinal tumour)

6. Chest
Full chest and cardiac examination. Findings can include:

Tachypnoea (CF, asthma, diabetic ketoacidosis, metabolic acidosis in AN)

Scars (previous cardiac surgery with CHD, lung transplant with CF, venous access port with CF, malignancy)

Chest deformity: pectus carinatum, increased AP diameter (asthma, CF)

Harrison's sulcus (CF)

Subcutaneous emphysema (with pneumomediastinum in AN)

Superior vena cava syndrome (malignancy)

Praecordium: palpate, auscultate (various forms of CHD)

Chest: ask to cough, palpate, percuss, auscultate (CF, secondary malignancy with effusion)

Sacral oedema (PCM, CLD)

7. Abdomen
Full abdominal examination. Findings can include:

Prominent veins (CLD with portal hypertension, malignancy)

Scars (gut surgery with IBD, hepatobiliary surgery, tumour removal)

Needle marks (diabetes mellitus, DFO in beta thalassaemia major)

Pigmented umbilicus, scars (Addison's)

Venous access port, below 'bikini line' (malignancy, CF)

Distension
- Ascites (malignancy,CLD)
- Weak abdominal muscles (PCM, coeliac)

Striae (corticosteroid treatment in IBD, asthma, CF)

Abdominal mass (Wilms', neuroblastoma, lymphoma, germ cell tumour)
- Full examination of all aspects of a mass: location (site), size (measure), if crosses midline, consistency, surface, tenderness, mobility, relations to adjacent structures, associated bruit, venous dilatation, enlarged draining lymph nodes, percussion note, associated ascites, extension into pelvis.

Hepatomegaly (hepatoblastoma, leukaemia, CCF, fatty liver: malabsorption)

Hepatic bruit (hepatoblastoma)

Hepatosplenomegaly (CLD, leukaemia)

Splenomegaly (portal hypertension in CF, CLD)

Renal mass (Wilms')

Genitalia/Tanner staging
- Pubertal delay (AN, Crohn's disease)
- Pubertal precocity (adrenal tumour, NF-1 with tumour)
- Testicular enlargement (ALL, testicular tumour)

Perianal disease (Crohn's disease)

Perianal or buttock mass (malignancy)

Rectal prolapse (CF)

8. Gait and back
Full gait examination, looking for:
- Cerebellar ataxia (posterior fossa tumour)
- Upper motor neurone signs (intracranial tumour, primary or secondary)
- Peripheral neuropathy (vitamin B_{12})
- Romberg's sign (vitamins E, B_{12})

Continued

Table 8.7 *(Continued)*

Examine back for:
- Tenderness (spinal tumour)
- Scoliosis (NF-1 with tumour; spinal tumour, neuroblastoma)
- Kyphosis and lordosis (vitamin D)

9. Lower limbs
Palpation
- Muscle bulk (AN, PCM)
- Ankle oedema (CHD, hypoproteinaemia in PCM)
- Tenderness (bone tumour, primary or secondary)

Full neurological examination of lower limbs, looking for:
- Cerebellar ataxia (posterior fossa tumour)

- Peripheral neuropathy (vitamin B_{12})
- Upper motor neurone signs (intracranial tumour, primary or secondary)

10. Other
Urinalysis
- Low specific gravity (CRF)
- High specific gravity (dehydration)
- Glucose (diabetes)

Stool analysis
- Malabsorption
- Giardiasis

Temperature chart
- Fever (ALL, AML)
- Hypothermia (PCM)

AIDS = acquired immune deficiency syndrome; ALL = acute lymphoblastic leukaemia; AML = acute myeloid leukaemia; AN = anorexia nervosa; AP = antero-posterior; BSL = blood sugar level; CF = cystic fibrosis; CHD = congenital heart disease CLD = chronic liver disease; CLL = chronic lymphocytic leukaemia; CRF = chronic renal failure; DFO = desferrioxamine; HPOA = hypertrophic pulmonary osteoarthropathy; IBD = inflammatory bowel disease; JA = juvenile arthritis; NF-1 = neurofibromatosis type 1; PCM = protein calorie malnutrition; SVC = superior vena cava; TPN = total parenteral nutrition.

Genetics and dysmorphology

Long cases

Down syndrome

Recent research has increased focus on Down syndrome (DS), as chromosome 21 has been sequenced fully, which should allow the relationship of genes, or groups of genes, to the neuropathogenesis of DS to be elucidated. Chromosome 21 has an estimated gene content of 329, including over 160 confirmed genes. These include 16 genes involved in mitochondrial energy production, 6 genes involved in folate or methyl group metabolism and 10 genes probably involved in brain development, neuronal loss and neuropathology as found in Alzheimer's disease. There are an increased number of associations noted with DS, in addition to Alzheimer's syndrome, including increased risk of coeliac disease and a greater awareness of co-morbid psychiatric and behavioural conditions, such as autism, depression and disruptive behaviour disorders. The median age of survival in DS has improved in recent years, as have many aspects of quality of life.

Background information

Definitions

A *syndrome* is a pattern of multiple structural defects, caused by multiple defects in one or more tissues, due to a single cause. In DS, the cause is three copies of chromosome 21 (trisomy 21) in 95% of cases, translocation between chromosomes 21 and 14 in 3%, and in the remaining 2% mosaicism, with two cell lines, one being trisomy 21 and the other being normal. It is the most common chromosomal anomaly, the prevalence being 1 in 1000 live births. The epidemiology has changed because of prenatal diagnosis and selected terminations.

DS is associated with a multiplicity of medical conditions, which are listed under 'History—Current state of health' below. Details and treatment for these conditions are outlined under 'Management'. Much of the management overlaps with several other sections in this book, to which cross-references are given.

History

Presenting complaint

Reason for current admission.

Diagnosis

When made (prenatal [increased nuchal fold thickness], birth, age in days), where, problems/symptoms at birth/diagnosis (e.g. cardiovascular [CVS] symptoms [cyanosis, tachypnoea, poor feeding], gastrointestinal tract [GIT] symptoms [vomiting, delay in meconium passage], haematological concerns [transient myeloproliferative disorder], vision and hearing aspects), who gave diagnosis, initial reaction to diagnosis, initial investigations done (karyotype, full blood examination, chest X-ray, electrocardiography, echocardiography, angiography, abdominal X-ray, ultrasound, brainstem auditory evoked response, ophthalmological assessment), genetic counselling given.

Initial treatment

1. Surgical (e.g. CVS—correction of atrioventricular canal; GIT—correction of duodenal atresia; staged reduction of omphalocoele).
2. Pharmacological (e.g. diuretics) and side effects thereof.

Past history

Indications for, and number of, previous hospital admissions. Pattern and timing of change in condition (e.g. CVS aspects—when cyanosis or heart failure developed, when and how it was controlled; GIT aspects—when operative procedures were undertaken, duration of hospitalisation, how long until feeding was established). Episodes of infection. Other complications of disease (e.g. development of hypothyroidism, coeliac disease, obstructive sleep apnoea [OSA], seizures, leukaemia).

Past treatment

- CVS: past surgery, complications thereof, plans for further operative procedures. Past interventional catheter procedures. Medications, past and present, side effects of these, monitoring levels, treatment plans for future. Antibiotic prophylaxis for dental procedures, maintenance of dental hygiene. Compliance with treatment. Any identification bracelet. Instructions for air travel and high altitude. Any recent investigations monitoring treatment. Any recent changes in treatment regimen, and indications for these.
- GIT: past surgery, complications thereof, plans for further operative procedures. Compliance with treatment (e.g. following diet for coeliac disease). Any recent investigations monitoring treatment. Any recent changes in treatment regimen, and indications for these.
- Hearing and vision: past ear, nose and throat surgical intervention, hearing aid placement, ophthalmologic intervention, glasses.
- OSA: past adenotonsillectomy, nasal mask continuous positive airway pressure (CPAP).
- Treatments for other conditions: hypothyroidism, atlantoaxial subluxation, seizures, leukaemia, arthritis, diabetes mellitus.

Current state of health

Note any of the following symptoms:

- CVS disease (fatigue, shortness of breath, cough, sweating, poor feeding, recurrent chest infections; symptoms suggesting arrhythmias such as syncope, alteration of consciousness, dizziness, palpitations, 'funny feeling' in the chest, chest pain).
- GIT disease (nausea, vomiting, change in bowel habit).

- Recurrent infection (how often, what sites [usually upper or lower respiratory tract], treatment required, any prophylactic antibiotics).
- Hearing impairment (compliance/problems with hearing aids, impacted cerumen, ventilation tubes for chronic otitis media).
- Visual impairment (development of refractive disorders, keratoconus, corneal opacities, cataracts).
- Weight concerns (obesity, non-compliance with diet, exercise, or sign of hypothyroidism)
- OSA symptoms (snoring, restless sleep, daytime somnolence).
- Skin problems (in children: seborrhoeic dermatitis, palmar/plantar hyperkeratosis, xerosis; in adolescents: folliculitis [especially back, buttocks, thighs, perigenital area], fungal infections [skin and nails], atopic dermatitis).
- Oral health (level of oral hygiene, dental caries, peridontal disease, bruxism [stereotyped orofacial movements with teeth grinding], intervention for malocclusion, non-compliance with dental recommendations).
- Respiratory problems (recurrent pneumonia due to silent aspiration).
- Orthopaedic issues (limping can be due to atlantoaxial subluxation, acetabular dysplasia with subluxing hips [not more common in DS, but may appear later], slipped femoral epiphysis, arthritis or leukaemia).
- Foot problems (hallux valgus, hammer toe deformities, plantar fasciitis, pedal arthritis).
- Joint problems (polyarticular onset juvenile arthritis-like arthropathy).
- Diabetes mellitus (increased drinking or eating, weight loss, lethargy).
- Hypothyroidism (dry skin, cold intolerance, lethargy).
- Haematological neoplasia (acute lymphoblastic leukaemia [ALL] or acute non-lymphoblastic leukaemia [ANLL] occur 10–15 times more frequently in DS, with usual symptoms of pallor, bruising, fever, hepatosplenomegaly and lymphadenopathy).
- Reproductive issues in adolescents (difficulties with menstrual hygiene, use of oral contraceptives, Depo-provera, presentation of premenstrual syndrome [PMS] with temper tantrums, autistic behaviour episodes, seizures, sex education, desire to reproduce).
- Neurological issues (seizures [more frequent than general population, but less than other causes of intellectual impairment], strokes [due to cyanotic CHD, or moyamoya disease]).

Current state of behaviour

Ask about possible co-morbid psychiatric/behavioural issues:

- Symptoms of ADHD (inattention, hyperactivity, impulsivity); any treatment for these.
- Symptoms of ASD (impaired social interaction, impaired communication, behaviour patterns including preferring own company, tendency to be loner, 'in their own world'), most problematic behaviours at present (e.g. rituals, anxiety, aggression, self-injury); any treatment for these.
- Other behavioural concerns: depression, conduct disorder, oppositional defiant disorder, aggressive behaviour; any treatment for these.
- Impact of these co-morbid issues (on family, educational facility [e.g. special school], therapists, carers).

Social history

1. DS impact on child: level of functioning in activities of daily living (ADLs), schooling (type of school, level of support from teachers, therapists, academic

performance, teachers' attitudes, peer attitudes, teasing, amount of school missed and whether schooling is appropriate).

2. DS impact on parents, e.g. financial situation, financial burden of disease so far, government allowances being received, marriage/partnership stability, restrictions on social life, plans for further children, genetic counselling, availability of prenatal diagnosis, contingency plans for child's future, guardianship and power of attorney issues.
3. DS impact on siblings, e.g. effect of family's financial burden, plans for siblings to act as guardians in future.
4. Social supports, e.g. social worker, contact with DS parent support groups, any available respite.
5. Coping: contingency plans (e.g. plan if child develops severe febrile illness); parents' degree of understanding regarding health supervision issues in DS.
6. Access to local doctor, paediatrician, neurodevelopmental clinic, various sub-specialty clinics attended (where, how often), other clinics attended, alternative practitioner (e.g. homeopathy) involvement.

Family history

Any other family members with DS or associated conditions.

Immunisations

Any delays, local doctor's attitudes, parents' understanding of importance of immunisation.

Examination

The examination of the child with DS in a long-case setting includes a full cardio-logical appraisal if the child has any CVS involvement, a documentation of the dysmorphic features of DS occurring in that child, plus an assessment for the de-velopment of any of numerous associated problems that may have arisen (e.g. thyroid disease, leukaemia). In addition, an assessment of function with respect to ADLs, a developmental assessment and an impression of behaviour based on direct interaction will give a complete picture, but time constraints may preclude these being assessed adequately. The approach given in Table 9.1 deals with the physical aspects of the child with DS that are able to be assessed objectively and within the time requirements. This approach can also be used in a short-case setting.

Management issues

The following directs you to most areas of management relevant in the long case.

Cardiac disease

Around 30–50% of children with DS have CVS disease, the most common being septal defects (particularly atrioventricular (AV) canal, then VSD, then ASD), patent ductus arteriosus, tetralogy of Fallot; left-side defects are uncommon. Cardiac disease may be entirely asymptomatic, so all neonates diagnosed with DS should have an echocardio-gram. The success rate for repair of septal defects is improving steadily: if not corrected, these conditions can lead to pulmonary hypertension, particularly if there is OSA, and shortened life span. Eisenmenger's syndrome (reversal of shunting, to cause right-to-left shunt), more common in DS than in the general population, is now rare. Children with DS under 2 years of age with cyanotic CHD have an increased risk of cerebrovascular accident (CVA); they may present with seizures or acute onset hemiplegia. Children

Table 9.1 The child with Down syndrome—physical examination

A. Measurements
Height
Head circumference
Request/plot weight
Assess percentile charts specific for
  Down syndrome
Calculate height velocity
Request/plot birth parameters
Request/plot parents' percentiles and
  ages at puberty

B. Systematic examination
The following is a selected listing of
possible physical findings in children with
Down syndrome. It does not include
behavioural aspects.

General inspection
Diagnostic facies
Tanner staging
Nutritional status
  • Obese (common after age 3; also,
    coexistent hypothyroidism)
  • Thin (commonly light for height in
    infancy; after age 3, unusual to be
    thin: consider coexistent malignancy,
    coeliac disease, hyperthyroidism,
    Crohn's disease, neglect)
Skeletal anomalies
  • Pectus excavatum
  • Scoliosis
Skin
  • Cutis marmorata (extremities)
  • Atopic eczema
  • Hyperkeratotic dry skin (especially
    palmoplantar)
  • Fungal infection (adolescents)
  • Pustular folliculitis (adolescents)
  • Vitiligo
  • Seborrhoeic dermatitis

Upper limbs
Manoeuvres: palms up (to detect simian
  crease, clinodactyly); check for
  hyperextensibility (hypotonia)
Structure of fingers
  • Brachydactyly (short fingers)
  • Fifth finger: hypoplasia mid-phalanx
    with clinodactyly
Nails
  • Clubbing (cyanotic congenital heart
    disease [CHD])
Palms
  • Simian creases

Blood pressure: elevated (occult renal
  disease)
Joints: hyperflexibility (usual), restriction of
  movement (arthropathy similar to
  juvenile arthritis)

Head
Size: small (measure and plot on Down
  syndrome specific growth charts)
Shape: brachycephaly, flat occiput; facial
  profile (flat)
Fontanelles: late closure

Hair
  • Midline hair whorl (parietal area)
  • Soft, sparse hair; alopecia
  • Excess skin back of neck (infant)
  • Webbed neck (occasional finding)
  • Low posterior hairline

Eyes
Inspection
  • Examine any glasses the child wears
    (myopia common): check vision with
    child wearing glasses
  • Epicanthal folds
  • Upward slant of palpebral fissures
  • Prominent eyes (coexistent
    hyperthyroidism)
  • Blocked tear duct (infant)
  • Ptosis
  • Squint
  • Nystagmus
Conjunctival pallor (iron deficiency,
  transient myeloproliferative disorder
  (infant), acute myeloid leukaemia
  [AML], acute lymphoblastic leukaemia
  [ALL])
Scleral jaundice (coexistent liver disease)
Iris: Brushfield's spots (white speckling of
  the peripheral iris)
Cornea
  • Large and cloudy (buphthalmos):
    glaucoma
  • Keratoconus
Visual fields: field defect (CVA from
  cyanotic CHD)
Eye movements
  • Nystagmus
Ophthalmoscopy: cataracts

Nose
Small, with flat nasal bridge

Continued

Table 9.1 *(Continued)*

Mouth and chin
Central cyanosis: various forms of CHD
Mouth: open (tendency to keep mouth
    open common)
Palate: short hard palate
Teeth: hypodontia, irregular placement,
    periodontal disease, dental caries
Tongue: prominent (small pharynx,
    normal-sized tongue), geographic
    tongue, fissured tongue
Tonsils: presence/size (can contribute to
    obstructive sleep apnoea [OSA]);
    absence (previous adenotonsillectomy
    for OSA)

Ears
Wearing hearing aid (hearing
    impairment in two-thirds of cases);
    check aid works, and child will
    wear it
Check hearing (for conductive,
    sensorineural or mixed loss)
Structure: small, overfolded upper helix,
    small/absent earlobes, low-set
Eardrums: ventilation tubes, chronic
    serous otitis media, permanent
    perforation, atelectatic eardrum,
    tympanic membrane scarring from
    previous infections or tubes, middle-
    ear cholesteatoma

Neck
Short, pterygium colli, scoliosis, excess
    skin back of neck (infant), low
    posterior hairline, goitre (coexistent
    thyroid disease).
Torticollis (spinal cord compression from
    atlanto-axial instability)

Chest
Inspection
• Scars: repairs of congenital heart
    defects (atrioventricular canal,
    ventricular septal defect, patent
    ductus arteriosus, atrial septal defect,
    tetralogy of Fallot), repair of tracheo-
    oesophageal fistula, insertion of
    access port (for chemotherapy for
    ALL, AML)
• Tanner staging in girls
• Sternal deformity: pectus excavatum
    or carinatum
Palpate and auscultate praecordium:

various forms of CHD, loud second
sound with obstructive sleep apnoea,
development of mitral valve or
tricuspid valve prolapse, or aortic
regurgitation

Abdomen
Inspection
• Scars: repairs of gastrointestinal tract
    anomalies (e.g. duodenal atresia,
    pyloric stenosis, Hirschsprung's
    disease, omphalocoele, imperforate
    anus), repairs of urinary tract
    anomalies (e.g. vesicoureteric reflux,
    posterior urethral valves, other
    obstructive uropathy), renal
    transplantation (e.g. dysplastic
    kidneys, glomerulosclerosis),
    operative interventions for other
    associated conditions (e.g. Crohn's
    disease)
• Prune-like appearance (prune belly
    syndrome)
• Tanner staging pubic hair (pubic hair
    tends to be straight)
Palpation
• Hepatomegaly (congestive cardiac
    failure [CCF])
• Splenomegaly (subacute bacterial
    endocarditis)
• Hepatosplenomegaly (ALL, AML)
• Enlarged kidneys (hydronephrosis)

Genitalia
Tanner stage genitalia: measure penis
    length and testes parameters,
    estimate testes volume
Penile anomalies: hypospadias (infant),
    corrected hypospadias
Testicular anomalies: cryptorchidism,
    enlarged (testicular cancer
    [seminoma], leukaemic deposits)

Gait, back and lower limbs
Inspection of lower limbs
• Clubbing of toes (various types of
    CHD)
• Gap between 1st and 2nd toes wide,
    with plantar crease between them
• Hallux valgus
• Hammer toes
• Fungal infection of nails (adolescents)
• Pes planovalgus

Continued

Table 9.1 *(Continued)*

Palpation: ankle oedema (CCF with CHD) Gait—standard examination (see short-case approach) to detect: • Quality of gait: often 'Chaplinesque' (externally rotated hips, flexed knees (in valgus), externally rotated tibiae) • Limp (hip dysplasia, dislocation, avascular necrosis, slipped femoral capital epiphysis) • Hemiplegic/circumducting gait (cerebrovascular accident [CVA] or cerebral abscess complicating cyanotic CHD) • Proximal weakness (e.g. developmental dysplasia of hip) Back • Look at the back to detect short neck or neck webbing • Bend over and touch toes to detect scoliosis	Lower limbs neurologically • Tone (usually decreased), power (usually normal) • Long tract signs (quadriparesis or quadriplegia—spinal cord compression from atlanto-axial instability); hyperreflexia (spinal cord compression from atlanto-axial instability, CVA or cerebral abscess complicating cyanotic CHD) Joints: hyperflexibility (usual), restriction of movement (arthropathy similar to juvenile arthritis) *Developmental assessment* See short case on developmental assessment. Most children with Down syndrome have developmental quotient (DQ) and later intelligence quotient (IQ) in the range 50–70.

with DS over 2 years of age with cyanotic congenital heart disease (CHD) have an increased incidence of brain abscess, the severity of which relates to the degree of hypoxia. They may present with fever, headache, seizures, or focal neurological signs. Around 50% of adolescents with DS syndrome and no previously known cardiac diagnosis develop mitral valve prolapse. This is an indication for antibiotic prophylaxis during dental and surgical procedures. Despite obesity and unfavourable lipid levels in DS, the incidence of hypertension and atheroma is low. See further discussion of cardiac disease issues in the long case on cardiology (chapter 6).

Hearing loss

Between 50% and 80% of children with DS have hearing problems. This increases to 90% in adults. The hearing loss may be conductive, sensorineural or mixed. The morphology of the head and neck predispose children with DS to hearing problems: the pinnae are small (harder to localise and concentrate sound), the canals are narrow, impacted cerumen is common (and can cause mild losses of 15 dB–25 dB), they may have conductive losses due to middle-ear fluid or structural abnormalities of the middle ear. Adolescents with DS have hearing losses in the high-frequency range, which are not seen in younger children.

Medical management for conductive loss includes treating otitis media and serous otitis media, surgical intervention with ventilation (pneumoeustacian) tubes, adenoidectomy and tonsillectomy (which also helps OSA). Some studies have questioned the effectiveness of ventilation tubes in DS, suggesting a lower cure rate, more sequelae (atelectatic eardrum, permanent perforation of eardrum, middle-ear cholesteatoma), more frequent episodes of otorrhoea, more antibiotic-resistant bacterial infection, and less hearing improvement after placement of tubes. Hearing aids are underutilised in DS, mainly due to compliance problems. Cochlear implantation may be required in severely hearing-impaired infants. Other management may involve speech therapy, signing and computer-based assisted communication devices.

Ophthalmologic disorders

Approximately 50% of children with DS have ocular impairments. These include strabismus, nystagmus, refractive errors, accommodation problems (resistant to correction by glasses), congenital (or later-forming) cataracts, blepharitis, hypoplasia of the iris, nasolacrimal duct obstruction with tearing, keratoconus, glaucoma. As well as standard visual screening, all children with DS should be assessed by a paediatric ophthalmologist by 6–12 months of age, and then yearly.

Behavioural and psychiatric issues

The most common behavioural issues include problems associated with ADHD-like behaviour and autism. See the discussion in the long cases in Chapter 5, Behavioural paediatrics, on each of these topics for relevant clinical aspects and their management. Depression is the other common psychiatric issue in DS, but tends to present beyond the paediatric age group. In those who appear depressed, thyroid function should be checked, as hypothyroidism can present in this way. Both the intellectual impairment and speech problems in DS complicate the prompt recognition of mental illness. Excluding sensory impairment in either vision or hearing, or both, should always occur before attributing new unusual behaviours to mental illness or Alzheimer's syndrome.

Obesity

The well-known high incidence of obesity (>120% of ideal body weight) in children with DS starts to develop in preschool years. Children with DS are less active, prefer indoor activities, and have a lower resting metabolic rate; living at home increases the propensity to obesity compared to a residential setting, and low rates of socialisation also increase the risk. By the time teenage years are reached, the average girl weighs 133% of ideal weight, and boys 124% of ideal weight. Obesity is notoriously difficult to prevent and manage in children with DS. Attempts at prevention should include decreased caloric intake, increased exercise, vitamin supplementation and weight-bearing activities (as bone density in the pelvis and spine is lower in children with DS compared to other children).

Dental problems

A high level of dental hygiene should be maintained. The immunological deficiency of DS results in periodontal disease in almost all children with DS, probably due to aberrations of mouth flora. Any carious teeth should be dealt with promptly with appropriate antibiotic cover. All DS children with congenital heart disease should be given a letter or card to show any dentist or doctor, explaining the need for antibiotic prophylaxis for any dental or similar procedure (e.g. tonsillectomy), including the recommended doses of antibiotics. Regular visits to the dentist and routine brushing can prevent periodontal disease. Orthodontic problems occur in almost all patients with DS, but compliance with orthodontic procedures and braces can be problematic.

Thyroid disease

The rate of congenital hypothyroidism in DS is around 1 in 140, versus 1 in 4000 for the general population. The recommendation is thyroid screening (for thyroxine and thyroid-stimulating hormone [TSH]) at birth, 6 months and then every year thereafter. The frequency of thyroid disease increases with age, such that it eventually affects 15% of people with DS. The symptoms and signs of hypothyroidism can be difficult to differentiate from those of DS itself. Children with DS who have a normal thyroxine level, but a TSH concentration above 10 mU/L, are considered to have compensated hypothyroidism and should be treated. Treatment with thyroxine in this group often results in increased growth velocity. For further discussion of the symptoms of hypo-thyroidism, see discussion in the short-case section on thyroid disease (Chapter 7).

Coeliac disease

The average time between the first symptoms of coeliac disease and definitive diagnosis approaches four years in patients with DS. The frequency of coeliac disease in DS is around 5–7%. It is sensible to screen all children with DS for coeliac disease: the Down Syndrome Medical Interest Group recommends this be done at 24 months of age, but there is yet to be consensus as to whether screening should be repeated later in life. See the short case on malabsorption for more details on screening tests (Chapter 8).

Obstructive sleep apnoea (OSA)

OSA is increasingly recognised in DS, and in children previously incorrectly labelled as having ADHD. OSA has also been a major contributor to pulmonary hypertension and the development of Eisenmenger's syndrome in children with DS and cyanotic CHD historically. See further discussion of clinical and management aspects in the long case on OSA in Chapter 15.

Haematological disorders (including leukaemia)

Transient myeloproliferative disorder is a form of self-limited leukaemia that is almost exclusive to neonates with DS, spontaneously regressing by 2–3 months. It occurs in 10% of infants with DS. These infants must be followed up carefully, as some of them later develop myelodysplastic syndrome or, more often, megakaryoblastic leukaemia aged 1–3. Both ALL and AML occur 10–20 times more frequently in children with DS compared to the general population. ALL and AML (most often acute megakaryoblas-tic leukaemia) occur with equal frequency (about 1 in 300 children with DS). In DS, AML usually occurs between ages 1 and 5 years (median 2 years). From 20% to 70% of patients with DS and AML present with myelodysplastic syndrome with thrombocy-topenia, followed by anaemia, developing over months. For further discussion of leukaemia, see the long case section on oncology (Chapter 14). The other haematolog-ical aberrations seen in DS are neonatal polycythaemia (occurs in two-thirds of babies with DS) and macrocytosis (also in two-thirds).

Seizures

Seizures occur in around 8% of patients with DS. There is a bimodal distribution of age of onset: 40% of seizures commence by 12 months of age, and 40% commence just outside of the paediatric age group, in the third decade of life. Children with DS tend to develop infantile spasms and generalised tonic clonic seizures with myoclonus; about half of those with infantile spasms will go into remission without relapse, and there can be some restoration of development. For further discussion on seizures, see the long-case section on seizures and epilepsy in Chapter 13, Neurology.

Atlanto-axial instability

Atlanto-axial instability refers to excessive mobility of the articulation of the atlas (C1) on the axis (C2). The standard method to detect this has been a lateral X-ray of the neck in neutral, flexion and extension. If there is an atlanto-dens space of more than 4.5–5.0 mm, this is considered subluxation, irrespective of presence or absence of symptoms. Around 13% of DS patients have an increased space but are asymptomatic; a further 2% become symptomatic. The symptoms and signs of spinal cord compression may include: altered gait (including limp), neck pain, torticollis, loss of bladder and bowel control, hyperreflexia, and quadriparesis or quadriplegia. Management of symptomatic patients involves immediate referral for stabilisation and surgical consultation. Follow-up of asymptomatic patients shows no progression to becoming symptomatic.

Diabetes mellitus

At least 1% of children with DS will develop diabetes. Screening is not indicated, but vigilant observation for any symptoms developing is appropriate.

Turner's syndrome

Turner's syndrome (TS) is due to haplodeficiency (see below) of some or all genes on the X chromosome. There may be complete absence of one X chromosome or structural anomalies of one X chromosome. The consequent phenotype is variable, relating to the underlying chromosomal pattern. The classic phenotype is 45 X, but the majority of (possibly all) patients with TS demonstrate mosaicism (see below), usually with a second, normal cell line (e.g. 45 X/46 XX or 45 X/46 XY). Other cell lines can include 47 XXX. There can also be structural anomalies of the X chromosome, including rings, deletions, translocations and isochromosomes (equal length chromosome arms, from transverse division of centromere rather than the normal longitudinal division). A Y chromosome is present in about 6% of patients with TS; an additional 3% have a marker chromosome (structurally abnormal chromosome unable to be identified by conventional cytogenetics) derived from the Y or another chromosome.

The physical signs of TS may be very subtle in childhood and adolescence. In the newborn, there may be characteristic features, such as lymphoedema of the hands and feet, nuchal folds, left-sided heart lesions, webbed neck and low hairline. In childhood, TS should be considered in any girls with declining growth velocity (falling below the 5th centile), even if there are no obvious dysmorphic features. In adolescence, TS may cause short stature, absence of breast development by 13 years of age, or amenorrhoea with elevated follicle-stimulating hormone (FSH) levels. TS can also present with the phenotypic expression of conditions that are X-linked recessive, such as haemophilia A, Duchenne's muscular dystrophy, or red–green colour blindness, which suggests X monosomy.

Definitions

A *syndrome* is a pattern of multiple structural defects, caused by multiple defects in one or more tissues, due to a single cause. *Mosaicism* means the presence of two or more chromosomally different cell lines both of which derive from the same zygote. *Haplodeficiency* means the presence in the cell of one set of genes instead of the usual two sets.

TS is associated with a multiplicity of medical conditions, and this leads to a large number of discussion areas in the long-case format. The relevant conditions are enumerated in the current state of health section of the history below, and in the management section. Much of the management overlaps with several sections in this book; the reader will be directed to these accordingly.

History

Presenting complaint

Reason for current admission.

Diagnosis

When made (antenatal [ultrasound: renal anomalies, coarctation, cystic hygroma, increased nuchal fold thickness], birth [lymphoedema of hands and feet, left-sided heart problems, webbed neck, congenital glaucoma], childhood [decreased growth velocity, nail dysplasia, high arched palate, strabismus], adolescence [pubertal delay, amenorrhoea, short stature]); where; problems at diagnosis (e.g. cardiovascular (CVS) symptoms/signs [cyanosis, tachypnoea, poor feeding, hypertension], gastrointestinal tract (GIT) symptomatology [diarrhoea, rectal bleeding]; vision and hearing aspects; loss of weight (coeliac disease, Graves' disease, inflammatory bowel disease [IBD]), weight gain (hypothyroidism from Hashimoto's disease), growth delay (TS per se, coeliac disease, hypothyroidism, scoliosis); who gave diagnosis; initial reaction to diagnosis; initial investigations done (karyotype, full blood examination, chest X-ray, electrocardiography, echocardiography, angiography, abdominal X-ray, ultrasound, brainstem auditory evoked response, ophthalmological assessment), genetic counselling given.

Initial treatment

1. Surgical (e.g. CVS—correction of coarctation, hypoplastic left-heart syndrome [HLHS]; urinary tract—correction of duplex system).
2. Medical (e.g. antihypertensives, growth hormone (GH), oestrogen, progesterone, calcium supplementation, vitamin D, thyroxine for hypothyroidism, gluten-free diet for coexistent coeliac disease).

Past history

Indications for, and number of, any previous hospital admissions. Chronological progression aspects of TS: CVS problems (e.g. when hypertension developed, when and how it was controlled), urinary tract problems (e.g. frequency of urinary tract infections [UTIs], when operative procedures undertaken); ear problems (e.g. recurrent otitis media episodes); eye problems (e.g. strabismus, amblyopia); other complications of disease (e.g. hypothyroidism, coeliac disease, IBD).

Past treatment

- **CVS.** Past surgery, complications thereof, plans for further operative procedures. Past interventional catheter procedures. Medications, past and present, side effects of these, monitoring levels, treatment plans for future. Antibiotic prophylaxis for dental procedures; maintenance of dental hygiene. Compliance with treatment. Any identification bracelet. Instructions for air travel and high altitude. Any recent investigations monitoring treatment. Any recent changes in treatment regimen, and indications for these. Frequency of echocardiography or cardiac MRI to screen for aortic root dilatation.
- **Growth.** When GH started (fall below 5th centile), supervised by whom (paediatric endocrinologist), dosage given (usual commencing dosage 0.05 mg/kg/day [0.1 IU/kg/day]), any combination therapy (e.g. with oxandrolone in girls aged 9–12); when oestrogen replacement therapy commenced (after 12), when cyclic menstruation achieved.
- **Hearing.** When impairment detected, level of loss, whether hearing aids prescribed, compliance with hearing aids.

Current state of health

Note any symptoms of the following:

- CVS disease (symptoms suggesting dilation of root of ascending aorta: chest or epigastric pains, or 'funny feeling' in chest or epigastrium (preceding aortic dissection and rupture); symptoms of hypertension (headache); other symptoms of CVS involvement (fatigue, shortness of breath, sweating, poor feeding [infants], syncope, alteration of consciousness, dizziness, palpitations).
- Loss of weight (Graves' disease, inflammatory bowel disease [IBD], coeliac disease, renal disease, malignancy [colon, germ cell tumours]).
- Gain in weight (obesity, noncompliance with diet, exercise, Hashimoto's thyroiditis causing hypothyroidism).
- Hypothyroidism (dry skin, cold intolerance, lethargy).
- Orthopaedic problems: limp (associated developmental dysplasia of hips, juvenile arthritis, IBD-associated arthritis), back pain (scoliosis, kyphosis, lordosis, juvenile arthritis, IBD-associated arthritis).
- GIT disease: diarrhoea (coeliac, IBD), nausea, abdominal pain, rectal bleeding (IBD).
- Urinary tract problems (infection, haematuria, proteinuria).
- Hearing impairment (recurrent otitis media, recent hearing testing).
- Visual problems (development of strabismus).
- Weight concerns (obesity, noncompliance with diet, exercise, Hashimoto's thyroiditis causing hypothyroidism).
- Reproductive issues in adolescents (education about advisability or otherwise of pregnancy [high maternal mortality], education about donor oocyte pregnancies, sex education, discussion of desire to reproduce).
- Psychosocial/behavioural issues: being bullied, unsatisfactory peer interactions, ADHD-like symptoms (inattention, hyperactivity, impulsivity), immature behaviour, anxiety, depression; any treatment for these.

Social history

- TS impact on child: level of functioning in activities of daily living (ADLs), schooling (type of school, level of support from teachers, therapists, academic performance, teachers' attitudes, peer attitudes, teasing, amount of school missed and whether it is appropriate).
- TS impact on parents: e.g. financial situation, financial burden of disease so far, government allowances received, marriage/partnership stability, restrictions on social life, plans for further children, genetic counselling, availability of prenatal diagnosis, contingency plans for child's future, guardianship and power of attorney issues.
- TS impact on siblings: e.g. effect of family's financial burden.
- Social supports: e.g. contact with TS parent support groups
- Coping: contingency plans (e.g. parents' degree of understanding regarding health supervision issues in TS).
- Access to local doctor, paediatrician, paediatric endocrinologist, neurodevelopmental clinic, various subspecialty clinics attended (where, how often), other clinics attended.

Family history

Any other family members with associated autoimmune conditions.

Immunisations

Any delays, local doctor's attitudes, parents' understanding of importance.

Examination

The examination of the child with TS in a long-case setting includes a full cardiological appraisal if the child has any CVS involvement, a documentation of the dysmorphic features of TS occurring in that child, plus an assessment for the development of any of numerous associated problems that may have arisen (e.g. thyroid disease, coeliac disease). The approach given below deals with the physical aspects of the child with TS that are able to be assessed objectively and within the time requirements. This approach can also be used in a short-case setting.

Growth parameters are assessed first: measurements and manoeuvres are given below.

Measurements

Measure height and the lower segment (LS), i.e. pubic symphysis to ground. Calculate the upper segment (US) by subtracting the LS from the total height. Work out the US:LS ratio. Normal values (in normal children) are 1.7 at birth, 1.3 at 3 years, 1.0 at 8 years, and 0.9 at 18 years. If the US:LS ratio is increased, it suggests short lower limbs (e.g. hypothyroidism). If the US:LS ratio is decreased, it suggests a short trunk (e.g. scoliosis) or a short neck.

Measure the child's arm span, and compare this to the total height. The normal child's values (arm span minus height) are: −3 cm from birth to 7 years, 0 cm from 8 to 12 years, +1 cm (girls) and +4 cm (boys) at 14 years. An apparently long arm span can be seen with a short neck, or trunk.

Measure the head circumference and weight.

Plot available measurements on Turner's syndrome (TS) specific percentile charts, and calculate the height velocity. Check birth parameters and plot these. Plot parents' percentiles and ages of puberty. After all these parameters have been evaluated, proceed with the manoeuvres below, or commence a systematic head-to-toe examination and slot in the manoeuvres along the way as relevant.

Manoeuvres

With each manoeuvre, stand opposite the child and demonstrate, so that she will mirror your movements. The skin should be evaluated concurrently with inspecting from front, back and side. Note any pigmented naevi, any scars (keloid common).

1. Inspect from in front

- Screen for carrying angle: have the child hold arms out straight, with palms forward. This angle can be increased in TS.
- Screen for short limbs: have the child touch the tips of the thumbs to the tips of the shoulders. If the thumbs do not reach the shoulders, there may be middle-segment (mesomelic) limb-shortening, found in TS and the associated Leri-Weill dyschondrostenosis (caused by abnormalities of the same SHOX gene—the haplodeficiency [loss of one allele] which contributes to the TS stature).
- Screen the hands. Have the child hold the palms up: look for short mid-phalanx of fifth finger, Madelung's deformity (congenital subluxation or dislocation of head of ulna with radial deviation of hand). Turn the hands over (palms down) and check the nails (e.g. hyperconvex).
- Screen for short metacarpals by having the child make a fist and look for shortened third, fourth or fifth metacarpal.

2. Inspect from the side

The child should be standing with arms by her side. Note whether there is micrognathia. Note the shape of the back, for lordosis or kyphosis. Note how far the upper limbs reach. If the limbs are short, the fingers may only reach the proximal thigh; if the trunk is short, the fingers may reach the knees.

3. Inspect from the back

Examine for scoliosis. Have the child bend forward and touch the toes, to determine whether any scoliosis is structural.

Completing the examination

Formal physical examination flows well if commenced at the hands, working up to the head, and then downward—essentially a head-to-toe pattern. Table 9.2 gives a selected listing of possible physical findings in children with Turner's syndrome. It does not include behavioural aspects (see below).

Specific complications and associations

The mnemonic **TURNER ULLRICH'S** helps recall most of these:

T **T**hyroiditis and other autoimmune disease (JA, coeliac disease)
U **U**ndermineralised bone
R **R**oot of aorta dilatation risks (bicuspid aortic valve, aortic stenosis, aortic coarctation, hypertension)
N **N**eck short, webbed, **N**ails hyperconvex, **N**ormal intelligence (but impairments in memory, maths, spatial perception, goal-setting, goal-attainment, attention span)
E **E**ndocrine deficiency (pubertal failure, short stature), **E**ye findings (epicanthic folds, strabismus, ptosis, congenital glaucoma), **E**ars (unusual shape, rotation)
R **R**eproductive technology assistance (egg donor programs)

U **U**lcerative colitis/Crohn's disease
L **L**eft-sided heart problems, **L**inear growth deficiency
L **L**ymphoedema, **L**ymphatic malformations (e.g. cystic hygroma)
R **R**enal anomalies (hydronephrosis)
I **I**nfertility
C **C**ancer risks (gonadoblastoma, neuroblastoma, colonic carcinoma)
H **H**earing loss, **H**ypertension, **H**epatic cirrhosis
S **S**keletal (DDH, Madelung's), **S**pine (scoliosis, kyphosis, lordosis)

Management issues

The following directs you to most areas of management relevant in the long case.

Cardiovascular disease

Up to 60% of TS patients have some form of cardiovascular disease/malformation. Cardiac disorders are the sole source of increased mortality in TS. Patients with TS are at increased risk of aortic root dilation and rupture. Cardiac findings in TS may include left-sided heart defects that can present in infancy, such as bicuspid aortic valve (BAV) (50%), coarctation of the aorta (30%), aortic stenosis (10% of those without BAV) or mitral valve stenosis (under 3%). Systemic hypertension is common in TS and is a risk factor for aortic dilatation (as are BAV, aortic stenosis, aortic regurgitation, and obesity).

Table 9.2 The child with Turner's syndrome: physical examination

A. Measurements

Height

Lower segment (LS)

Calculate upper segment (US) by subtracting LS from height

Calculate US:LS ratio

Arm span

Head circumference

Record weight

Assess percentile charts

Calculate height velocity

Record birth parameters

Record parents' percentiles and ages at puberty

B. Manoeuvres

- Arms out straight (to detect cubitus valgus over 15 degrees between extended supinated forearm to upper arm)
- Thumbs on shoulders, to detect short limbs: can detect middle segment shortening
- Palms up: to detect short mid-phalanx of fifth finger; Madelung's deformity (congenital subluxation or dislocation of head of ulna with radial deviation of hand).
- Make a fist (to detect short third, fourth, fifth metacarpal)
- Look at the back to detect short neck or neck webbing
- Low hairline
- Bend over and touch toes (to detect scoliosis)

C. Systematic examination

Sitting up is the preferred position for the commencement of the systematic examination. The following is a selected listing of possible physical findings in girls with Turner's syndrome.

General inspection

Diagnostic facies

Tanner staging

- Delayed

Nutritional status

- Obese (coexisting undertreated hypothyroidism)
- Poor (coexisting inflammatory bowel disease, cancer)

Skeletal anomalies

- Broad shieldlike chest with widely spaced hypoplastic, and/or inverted nipples
- Pectus excavatum
- Scoliosis
- Kyphosis

Skin

- Lymphatic vascular malformations: congenital lymphoedema, residual swelling over hands and feet, dorsal aspect
- Haemangiomata
- Pigmented naevi

Upper limbs

Structure

- Short mid-phalanx fifth finger
- Short third, fourth, fifth metacarpal
- Madelung's deformity

Nails

- Dysplastic
- Hyperconvex, deep set

Pulse

- Radiofemoral delay (coarctation of aorta)

Blood pressure: elevated (essential hypertension, coarctation of aorta, renal disease)

Joints: swelling, decreased range of movement (coexistent juvenile arthritis)

Eyes

Inspection

- Epicanthal folds
- Ptosis
- Squint

Sclerae

- Icterus (coexistent liver disease)
- Blue

Cataracts

Fundi

- Hypertensive retinopathy

Mouth and chin

Central cyanosis: partial anomalous pulmonary venous return (PAPVR), hypoplastic left heart (neonate)

Narrow maxilla/high arched palate

Teeth: caries (risk of SBE)

Micrognathia

Ears

Wearing hearing aid (hearing impairment common): check aid works, and child will wear it

Continued

Table 9.2 *(Continued)*

Check hearing (for conductive, sensorineural or mixed loss)
Structure: malformed, rotated
Eardrums: ventilation tubes, chronic serous otitis media, permanent perforation, atelectatic eardrum, tympanic membrane scarring from previous infection

Neck/hairline
Pterygium colli
Short
Scoliosis
Low hairline

Chest
Inspection
- Shield-like broad chest
- Sternal deformity: pectus excavatum or carinatum
- Scars: repairs of left-sided heart lesions (e.g. coarctation, aortic stenosis, aortic root dilatation)
- Tanner staging: delay
- Wide-spaced, hypoplastic, inverted nipples
Palpation
- Praecordium (e.g. for CHD)
Auscultation
- Praecordium (e.g. for CHD)

Abdomen
Inspection
- Scars: gonadectomy, surgery for coexistent inflammatory bowel

disease, removal of tumour (e.g. gonadoblastoma, neuroblastoma)
- Tanner staging pubic hair: delay
Palpation
- Hepatomegaly (e.g. CCF from CHD)
- Splenomegaly (e.g. SBE)
- Hepatosplenomegaly (e.g. coexistent neuroblastoma)
- Enlarged kidneys (e.g. hydronephrosis)

Genitalia
Tanner-stage genitalia
- Delayed stage

Gait, back and lower limbs
Inspection of lower limbs
- Feet: short metatarsals
- Oedema of dorsa of feet
- Clubbing of toes (various types of CHD)
Palpation: ankle oedema (CCF with CHD)
Joints: swelling, decreased range of movement (coexistent JA)
Gait—standard examination screening for:
- Limp (e.g. developmental dysplasia of hip [DDH], coexistent JA)
- Proximal weakness (e.g. DDH)
Back
- Scoliosis
- Kyphosis
- Lordosis
- Decreased range of movement (coexistent JA)

CCF = congestive cardiac failure; CHD = congenital heart defect; SBE = subacute bacterial endocarditis; VSD = ventricular septal defect.

Aortic root dilatation can occur in up to 9% of patients. Aortic dissection and rupture have been reported rarely: there is one report of a 4-year-old patient dying from aortic rupture. The symptoms for aortic dilation are chest or epigastric pains, often misinterpreted as being of pulmonary or gastrointestinal origin.

Some patients with aortic dilation have had no risk factors. All TS patients must be screened for aortic root dilation. MRI may be more useful than echocardiography in delineating aortic pathology: MRI can detect aortic coarctation or dilation missed by echocardiography. Abnormalities of the aortic valve may not be seen on a neonatal echocardiogram, so that repeated echocardiograms or MRIs every year are essential. If a TS patient later becomes pregnant (through oocyte donation) this significantly increases the risk of aortic dissection or rupture. Patients with TS should have echocardiograms at least every 5 years throughout life.

Up to 40% of TS patients have hypertension, usually idiopathic, but cardiac or renal causes must be excluded. Once identified, hypertension must be aggressively treated. Blood pressure should be measured at all routine follow-up visits.

Less commonly seen cardiovascular diagnoses include mitral valve prolapse (5–15%), partial anomalous pulmonary venous drainage (PAPVD) (5–10%), ventricular septal defect (VSD) (<5%) and atrial septal defect (ASD) (>5%).

Cardiac anomalies are more common with a 45 X karyotype, and more common in patients with lymphoedema. Prophylaxis for endocarditis is important, particularly as dental malocclusion occurs in Turner's syndrome, and may require dental procedures. Those requiring cardiac surgery may develop keloid, another predisposition in Turner's syndrome. Ankle oedema may occur due to lymphoedema rather than a cardiac cause.

Growth

From the age of 2 years, growth should be plotted on TS-specific growth charts. GH treatment should be started as soon as the child falls below the 5th centile on the normal female growth charts (or 95th centile on the TS specific growth charts). The earlier GH treatment is started, the longer the duration of treatment can be, until oestrogen is commenced, which then leads to growth plate closure. Between the ages of 9 and 12, oxandrolone has been given with GH to improve skeletal maturity, but the drawbacks are potential masculinising effects and potential risk of hepatotoxicity. GH increases rate of growth without increasing bone age. Increases in final height of 15 cm have been described if there were at least 6 years of GH therapy, and oestrogen was delayed. The advantages and disadvantages must be covered fully in discussion with the parents. When GH is commenced, it can lead to enlargement of naevi, and recurrence of lymphoedema. In Australia, the approved doses are 4.7–9.3 mg/metres squared/week (0.16–0.32 mg/kg/week).

Induction of puberty

More than 90% of girls with TS have gonadal failure; however, up to a third may undergo spontaneous puberty and around 3% will have spontaneous menses. Oestrogen therapy is essential for the physical, emotional and psychosexual changes of puberty, and should be commenced around 12 years of age, and no later than age 14, otherwise adequate uterine size may not be achieved. Pelvic ultrasound can be done before starting oestrogen to check uterine size. The recommended preparation is oestradiol valerate, commencing at 0.5–1 mg on alternate days, increasing the dosage 6–12 monthly until feminisation is complete, which usually takes 2–3 years. Bone density needs to be checked around the time of late puberty to ensure adequate bone mineralisation has occurred. A progestin such as medroxyprogesterone acetate can be added when vaginal spotting occurs, or after 2 years of treatment with oestrogen, to enable regular withdrawal bleeding to occur. During treatment height, weight, Tanner staging and blood pressure should be checked, and blood should be taken for serum FSH and oestradiol levels every 3–6 months.

Renal and urinary tract anomalies

Around 30–60% of patients with TS have congenital renal anomalies, particularly horseshoe kidney and double-collecting systems. Only a small minority develop any renal impairment: there are reports of hypertension, urinary tract infection, hydronephrosis, focal segmental glomerulonephrosis and membranoproliferative glomerulonephritis (MPGN). Follow-up ultrasound examinations of the renal tract are recommended every 5 years.

Hearing loss

This is common, with most girls with TS having recurrent otitis media, which can lead to scarring and conductive hearing loss, even in early childhood. This is related to the morphology of the head and neck in TS: the palate is high-arched and there is Eustachian tube dysfunction. Also, there is a progressive sensorineural loss characterised by a sensorineural dip at a frequency of 1–2 kHz and high-frequency loss, due to anomalies of the outer hair cells of the lower middle coil of the cochlea. This is more frequent in patients with 45 X or 45 X/46 Xi (Xq) karyotype. Some children will need hearing aids, but hearing loss is progressive, and eventually at least 25% of adults with TS will require hearing aids because of this sensorineural complication.

Ophthalmologic disorders

Approximately 16% of children with TS have ptosis. Other ocular findings include strabismus, amblyopia, blue sclerae and cataracts. In addition to standard visual screening, all children with TS should be assessed by a paediatric ophthalmologist yearly.

Obesity

There is an increased incidence of obesity (>120% of ideal body weight) in children with TS. Attempts at prevention should include decreased caloric intake, increased exercise, vitamin supplementation and weight-bearing activities (as bone density is lower in children with TS compared to other children).

Thyroid disease

The incidence of Hashimoto's thyroiditis (leading to hypothyroidism) is increased in TS after the age of 10 years; the incidence of hypothyroidism is around 10–30% in later childhood, rising to 50% in adults. Patients with structural defects of the X chromosome have increased susceptibility to autoimmune disorders, including Hashimoto's thyroiditis and Graves' disease, IBD, myasthenia gravis and MPGN. The recommendation is thyroid screening every year from the age of 10 years (for thyroxine and thyroid-stimulating hormone [TSH], and for anti-thyroid antibodies). The symptoms and signs of hypothyroidism can be subtle. Once identified, hypothyroidism should be treated promptly. For further information about the symptoms of hypothyroidism, see the discussion in the short-case section on thyroid disease in Chapter 7, Endocrinology.

Craniofacial/dental problems

A narrow maxilla/palate occurs in over 80% of cases. Dental crowding is frequent, as is micrognathia (occurs in 70%). A high level of dental hygiene should be maintained. All TS children with congenital heart disease should be given a letter or card to show any dentist or doctor, explaining the need for antibiotic prophylaxis for any dental or other surgical procedure including the recommended doses of antibiotics. Regular visits to the dentist and routine brushing are important. Orthodontic evaluation is recommended around 8–10 years of age.

Gastrointestinal disease: coeliac disease, IBD, hepatic effects

The frequency of coeliac disease in TS is around 5%. It is sensible to screen all children with TS for coeliac disease, from mid-childhood, regardless of presence or absence of symptoms, repeating the screening every 2 years. See the short case on malabsorption in Chapter 8, Gastroenterology, for more details on screening tests.

IBD (especially Crohn's disease) is around two to three times more common in TS than in the general population. Either IBD or coeliac disease can present with poor weight gain or a range of gastrointestinal symptoms, and should be considered in these scenarios.

Elevation of serum hepatic enzyme levels occurs in 40–80% of TS patients, and is associated with up to a five-fold increase in cirrhosis in adult life. The aetiology of this is uncertain.

Osteoporosis

Osteopenia occurs commonly in TS. Peak bone mass attainment is inhibited in adolescents with TS, even with treatment: GH and oestrogen replacement improves, but does not normalise, bone mineralisation. To attempt to optimise bone mineral density, oestrogen should be used with adequate exercise, calcium and vitamin D.

Psychosocial aspects

Adolescents with TS are at increased risk for a number of behavioural abnormalities, including anxiety, depression, social isolation and poor self-esteem. Many of these girls demonstrate social immaturity for their age, and they often need support in becoming independent and in interacting with others socially (particularly with males). Girls with TS may be the subjects of teasing and bullying at school: once identified, this situation must be dealt with promptly and decisively by teachers and parents. Meeting with other girls with TS and their families is very beneficial and offers valued support for these girls and their parents. Patients with TS are not at any increased risk of significant mental health problems.

Education

Children with TS are known to have problems with visual-spatial processing. This affects them in mathematics and in areas needing fine-motor coordination. Educational and vocational training need to take these specific difficulties into account, as these problems persist into adulthood, and throughout life.

Short case

The dysmorphic child

This case potentially covers more clinical ground than any other and requires a very structured routine, quite similar to that used for the short-stature examination, except that many children with conditions making them dysmorphic are of normal height, or may be tall (e.g. Sotos', Marfan's). To simplify the initial approach, predominantly one subgroup of dysmorphic children (those with skeletal dysplasias) has been chosen to illustrate the procedure for measurements and manoeuvres. The subsequent systematic head-to-toe approach gives one or two differential diagnoses for each of the selected signs listed: these are merely examples, not the most frequent or important findings. This approach looks at each anatomical structure in turn (e.g. eyebrow, eyelid, conjunctiva, sclera, iris, pupil, lens, retina) and asks whether it appears normal or abnormal. If any finding appears abnormal, it is noted and may need checking later against reference values (e.g. if you suspect hypertelorism, take the outer canthal, inner canthal and inter-pupillary measurements and then compare these to standard percentile charts). The three areas in the examination that provide the most clues in the diagnosis of a dysmorphic child are often assessments of the head, heart and hands.

Definitions

Patterns of morphological defects include: sequences, syndromes and associations. Most often the term syndrome is used in a broader sense than its true meaning. The definitions of relevant terms are as follows:

1. A *sequence* is a pattern of structural defects caused by a single problem in morphogenesis (e.g. early amnion rupture sequence, Pierre Robin's sequence due to hypoplasia of the mandible before 9 weeks' gestation)
2. A *syndrome* is a pattern of multiple structural defects, caused by multiple defects in one or more tissues, due to a single cause (e.g. Down syndrome).
3. An *association* is a pattern of structural defects that are statistically related, that is, a non-random occurrence in at least two people of multiple anomalies not due to a sequence or syndrome. The classic examples are:
   the **CHARGE** association

C	**C**olobomatous malformation of the eye (retinal coloboma the most common)
H	**H**eart anomalies (e.g. tetralogy of Fallot)
A	**A**tresia of the choanae (bony and/or membranous)
R	**R**etardation: both cognitive and somatic growth
G	**G**enital anomalies and/or hypoplasia (males)
E	**E**ar anomalies and/or deafness

   and the **VACTERL** association:

V	**V**ertebral anomalies
A	**A**nal atresia with/without fistula
C	**C**ardiac anomalies (e.g. VSD)
T	**T**racheo-
E	**E**sophageal fistula with oesophageal atresia
R	**R**enal anomalies (urethral atresia with hydronephrosis)
L	**L**imb anomalies (polydactyly, humeral hypoplasia, radial aplasia and proximally placed thumb)

Examination

The lead-in may be quite general, such as 'Have a look at this child'. The approach outlined here is a blueprint for one method that can work and has proved successful in the examination. While it is true that 'spot diagnosis' short cases are best avoided, it is worth having a reproducible approach, as so many unusual-looking children will be encountered by a paediatrician or a general practitioner during their working life.

Listen to the child's age in the lead-in. Introduce yourself to the child and parent. Ask the child which grade he/she is in at school and note whether the response seems age-appropriate (intellectual impairment is a feature of numerous syndromes). Do not overlook the child's sex when discussing differential diagnoses. It would be embarrassing to talk about Turner's syndrome when assessing a boy, or discussing X-linked conditions in assessing girls. Stand back and look for evidence of an obvious diagnosis (e.g. Down syndrome), any particularly unusual body habitus (e.g. Marfanoid in Marfan's, homocystinuria and multiple endocrine neoplasia type 2b (MEN 2b), eunuchoid in Klinefelter's), obvious disproportion (skeletal dysplasias, rickets), obvious asymmetry (e.g. Beckwith-Wiedemann), abnormal posturing (e.g. hemiplegia in homocystinuria complicated by a cerebrovascular accident due to thrombotic tendency). Visually assess the pubertal status (hypogonadism being a feature of many syndromes e.g. Down, Prader-Willi, Fanconi's pancytopenia, Noonan's). Note if the child has a hearing aid (deafness can occur in Treacher Collins, CHARGE, fetal rubella effects, Waardenburg's syndrome). Comment on your findings.

Explain what you are doing as you proceed. Ask for the height and offer to measure the patient yourself: stand the child against a wall, position the head and heels appropriately, record the height and measure the lower segment (LS), i.e. pubic symphysis to ground. Then calculate the upper segment (US) by subtracting the LS from the total height. Work out the US:LS ratio: normal values are 1.7 at birth, 1.3 at 3 years, 1.0 at 8 years, and 0.9 at 18 years.

If the child is short:

- If the US:LS ratio is increased, it suggests short lower limbs (e.g. skeletal dysplasias, hypothyroidism).
- If the US:LS ratio is decreased, it suggests a short trunk (e.g. vertebral irradiation, scoliosis) or a short neck (e.g. Klippel-Feil sequence).

Next, measure the child's arm span, and compare this to the total height. The normal arm span minus height values: −3 cm from birth to 7 years, 0 cm from 8–12 years, +1 cm (girls) and +4 cm (boys) at 14 years.

- A short arm span can occur with skeletal dysplasias, and an apparently long arm span with a short neck, trunk or legs.
- If the span minus height is less than normal (a value more negative, e.g. −6 cm) with a high US:LS, this indicates short limbs and a normal trunk.
- If the span minus height is greater than normal (a value more positive, e.g. +8 cm) with a low US:LS, this indicates a short trunk and normal limbs.
- If the span minus height is less than normal (a value more negative) with a low or normal US:LS ratio, this indicates short trunk and limbs.

If the child is tall:

- If the US:LS is decreased, it suggests the lower limbs are disproportionately long (e.g. Marfanoid habitus, eunuchoid habitus).
- If the US:LS is normal, this is more in keeping with pituitary gigantism.
- If the arm span minus height value is longer than normal, this may be due to Marfanoid or eunuchoid body habitus.

Further measurements

Measure the head circumference (HC). HC can be increased in syndromes with hydrocephalus (e.g. X-linked hydrocephalus) or macrocephaly (e.g. Sotos'). HC is decreased in the many syndromes with microcephaly (e.g. Seckel's). The course adopted by the tape measure being placed around the skull can accentuate the abnormal skull shapes in cases of craniosynostosis (e.g. Apert's, Crouzon's, Pfeiffer's, Saethre-Chotzen).

Request the weight. Obesity occurs in many syndromes (e.g. Down, Prader-Willi, Bardet-Biedl), while a slim habitus (aesthenia) can occur in others (e.g. Marfan's, Caurati-Engelmann). Request percentile charts and progressive measurements (if not given), and calculate the height velocity. Request birth parameters (for intrauterine and chromosomal causes: numerous chromosomal syndromes have intrauterine growth retardation as a component).

After all these parameters have been evaluated, either (a) proceed with the manoeuvres below, particularly if the child is very short, or has obvious skeletal anomalies or clearly disproportionate short stature, or (b) commence a systematic head-to-toe examination, and slot in the manoeuvres along the way should they appear relevant. The order adopted is unimportant; it is the demonstration of a comprehensive approach that is required.

Manoeuvres

Inspect from front

Note any gross structural anomalies of the upper or lower limbs, such as limb deficiency (e.g. in early amnion rupture sequence, Holt-Oram), or aplasias of any long bones (e.g. radial aplasia in VACTERL association or in thrombocytopenia absent radius syndrome), contractures (e.g. distal arthrogryposis syndrome) or pterygia of axilla, antecubital and popliteal areas (e.g. Escobar's multiple pterygium syndrome). Next, a set of manoeuvres can be performed that very rapidly screens for a number of syndromes: most of these are relevant for short children. With each manoeuvre, stand opposite the child and demonstrate, so that he or she will mirror your movements.

Screen for asymmetry (irrespective of whether tall or short): have the child put the palms together with the arms out straight, and stand with legs together. Asymmetry occurs in Russell-Silver syndrome. It may also occur as a result of hemihypertrophy in several syndromes: e.g. Beckwith-Wiedemann (B-W), Klippel-Trenauney-Weber (K-T-W), neurofibromatosis type 1 (NF-1), congenital hemihypertrophy (CH). This manoeuvre may also detect approximation of shoulders (absent clavicles in cleidocranial dysostosis).

Focus on the upper limbs first, then evaluate the lower limbs: look at the knees, for any bowing (e.g. in hypochondroplasia, metaphyseal dysplasia), look at the feet for talipes (e.g. osteogenesis imperfecta) and the toes for their number (e.g. polydactyly in Ellis-van Creveld) and structure (syndactyly, and/or broad malformed distal hallux in Apert's).

Screen for carrying angle: have the child hold the arms out straight, with palms forward. This angle can be increased in Turner's or Noonan's syndromes. Also, restriction of elbow extension may be detected (e.g. hypochondroplasia).

Screen for short limbs: have the child touch the tips of the thumbs to the tips of the shoulders. If the thumbs overshoot, there is proximal segment (rhizomelic) limb shortening. If the thumbs do not reach the shoulders, there might be either middle segment (mesomelic) or distal segment (acromelic) limb shortening, or alternatively the limbs may be bent (camptomelic). Thus this manoeuvre should detect proximal segment shortening (e.g. achondroplasia, hypochondroplasia), middle segment shortening (e.g. Langer mesomelic dysplasia, Leri-Weill dyschondrostenosis) or distal segment shortening (e.g. acromesomelic dysplasia)

Screen the hands: have the child hold the palms up. Look for simian crease (Down syndrome) and clinodactyly (Russell-Silver syndrome). Note the structure of the fingers (e.g. short and stubby with hypochondroplasia), their number (e.g. polydactyly in Ellis-van Creveld) and any syndactyly (e.g. Apert's syndrome). Turn the hands over (palms down), note the structure of the hand (e.g. trident deformity in achondroplasia) and check the nails (e.g. hypoplastic in Ellis-van Creveld, hyperconvex in Turner's).

Screen for short metacarpals: have the child make a fist, and look for shortened third, fourth or fifth metacarpal (e.g. Gorlin's syndrome), first metacarpal (proximally placed thumb: e.g. in diastrophic dysplasia) or all metacarpals (e.g. in Poland anomaly).

Screen for joint laxity (relevant if short or tall): check degree of wrist extension and whether the child can appose the thumb to the radius (e.g. hypermobility in pseudoachondroplastic spondoepiphyseal dysplasia, osteogenesis imperfecta or Marfan's). If the child is tall or of normal height, check for arachnodactyly by having the child wrap the fingers of one hand around the other wrist. Check if there is complete overlap of the distal phalanx of the fifth finger on the distal phalanx of the thumb (the 'wrist sign'). Then check if the thumb can project from beyond the ulnar border of the hand when the thumb is apposed to the palm when making a fist ('the thumb sign'). Arachnodactyly classically occurs in Marfan's syndrome.

Inspect from side

The child should be standing with the arms by his or her side. Note whether there is a prominent forehead (e.g. achondroplasia), flat occiput (Down), proptosis (e.g. syndromes with craniosynostosis, NF-1), micrognathia (e.g. Pierre Robin's sequence), prognathism (e.g. achondroplasia). Note how far the upper limbs reach; if the limbs are short, the fingers may only reach the proximal thigh; if the trunk is short, the fingers may reach knees. Note the shape of the back, for lordosis (e.g. achondroplasia), thoracolumbar kyphosis (e.g. achondroplasia), crouched posture (e.g. diastrophic dysplasia).

Inspect from back

Examine for scoliosis (and any kyphosis, which should have been noted already). Have the child bend forwards and touch the toes to determine whether any scoliosis is structural. Scoliosis can occur in dozens of syndromes, including many skeletal dysplasias, several trisomies and a number of popular examination syndromes (fragile X, Marfan's, NF-1, Noonan's, Prader-Willi).

Do explain what you are doing as you proceed, so that the examiners will be aware of the significance of the manoeuvres.

Skin

The skin should be evaluated concurrently with inspecting from the front, back and side. Note any altered pigmentation; café-au-lait spots may occur with NF-1 and Russell-Silver; hypopigmented areas can occur in tuberous sclerosis. Freckling occurs in xeroderma pigmentosum and **LEOPARD** (multiple lentigines) syndromes. (The acronym stands for **L**entigines, **E**CG changes, **O**cular hypertelorism, **P**ulmonary stenosis, **A**bnormal genitalia, **R**etardation of growth, **D**eafness.) Small brown to blue-black macules occur in Peutz-Jeghers syndrome. Whorls of pigmentation occur in incontinentia pigmenti. Note any vascular malformations (e.g. Sturge-Weber, Klippel-Trenauney-Weber), telangiectasia (e.g. ataxia-telangiectasia, Osler's haemorrhagic telangiectasia syndrome), or telangiectatic erythema in butterfly distribution over the malar area (e.g. Bloom's, Cockayne's). Ichthyotic skin can occur in **CHILD** syndrome (acronym for **C**ongenital **H**emidysplasia, **I**chthyosiform erythroderma, **L**imb **D**efects). Alopecia or sparse hair may be noted in CHILD and Cockayne's syndromes, as well as incontinentia pigmenti. The above are merely a small sample of the vast number of skin disorders within syndromal diagnoses.

Completing the examination

Formal physical examination flows well if commenced at the hands, working up to the head, and then downward—essentially a head-to-toe pattern. Table 9.3 lists a small number of sample findings sought at each point.

Finally, summarise your findings succinctly, and give a brief differential diagnosis, placing the most likely diagnosis first.

Table 9.3 Dysmorphic child: measurements, manoeuvres and systematic examination

A. Measurements
Height
Lower segment (LS)
Calculate upper segment (US) by subtracting LS from height
Calculate US:LS ratio
Arm span
Head circumference
Request weight
Assess percentile charts
Calculate height velocity
Request birth parameters
Request parents' percentiles and ages at puberty

B. Manoeuvres
- Hands and feet together, to detect asymmetry (e.g. Russell-Silver), hemihypertrophy (e.g. Beckwith's, McCune-Albright, Proteus) and unilateral growth arrest (e.g. homocystinuria with cerebrovascular accident). This also detects approximation of shoulders (absent clavicles in cleidocranial dysostosis), genu valgum (e.g. homocystinuria), genu recurvatum (e.g. Marfan's), and pes planus (e.g. Marfan's)
- Arms out straight, to detect cubitus valgus (e.g. Turner's, Noonan's); over 15 degrees in girls; over 10 degrees in boys
- Thumbs on shoulders, to detect short limbs: can detect if proximal, middle or distal segment shortening
- Palms up, to detect simian crease (e.g. Down, Seckel), clinodactyly (e.g. Russell-Silver, Down, Seckel's)
- Make a fist, to detect short fourth metararpal (e.g. pseudo-hypoparathyroidism, Turner's, fetal alcohol)
- Check extensibility for hyperextensibility (e.g. Marfan's) and for limitation of extension (e.g. homocystinuria)
- Look at the back to detect short neck (e.g. Klippel-Feil, Noonan's), or neck webbing (e.g. Turner's, Noonan's)
- Low hairline (e.g. Turner's, Noonan's, Klippel-Feil)
- Bend over and touch toes, to detect scoliosis (e.g. Noonan's, Klippel-Feil)

C. Systematic examination
Sitting up is the preferred position for the commencement of the systematic examination. The following is a selected listing of possible physical findings in children with dysmorphic features.

General inspection
Diagnostic facies
- Dysmorphic syndromes (e.g. Russell-Silver, Down, Turner's, Noonan's, FAS)
Disproportionate stature
- Skeletal dysplasias (e.g. achondroplasia)
- Connective tissue disorders (e.g. osteogenesis imperfecta)
Tanner staging
- Advanced (e.g. McCune-Albright)
- Delayed (e.g. Noonan's)
Nutritional status
- Obese (e.g. Prader-Willi, Bardet-Biedl, Alström's, Down)
- Poor (e.g. Marfan's, homocystinuria)
Skeletal anomalies
- Asymmetry (causes of hemihypertrophy: Beckwith-Wiedemann, NF-1)
- Pectus excavatum (e.g. Marfan's, Noonan's)
- Scoliosis (e.g. Noonan's, Klippel-Feil)
Skin
- Vascular malformations (e.g. Klippel-Trenauney-Weber, Sturge-Weber)
- Hypopigmented macules (e.g. tuberous sclerosis)
- Café-au-lait spots (e.g. NF-1, Fanconi's anaemia, Russell-Silver)

Upper limbs
Structure
- Clinodactyly fifth finger (e.g. Russell-Silver, Down, Shwachman's, Seckel's)
- Short fourth metacarpal (e.g. pseudohypoparathyroidism, Turner's, FAS)
- Trident hand (e.g. achondroplasia)
- Polydactyly (e.g. Bardet-Biedl)
- Contractures (e.g. distal arthrogryposis)

Continued

Table 9.3 *(Continued)*

Nails
- Short (e.g. cartilage hair hypoplasia)
- Hyperconvex (e.g. Turner's)
- Hypoplastic (e.g. FAS)

Palms
- Simian creases (e.g. Down)

Wrists
- Splaying (e.g. X-linked hypophosphataemic rickets)
- Contractures (e.g. 'classic arthrogryposis': amyoplasia congenita disruptive sequence)

Pulse
- Radiofemoral delay (e.g. coarctation of aorta with Turner's, NF-1)

Elbows
- Contractures (e.g. 'classic arthrogryposis')

Blood pressure: elevated (e.g. coarctation of aorta with NF-1, Turner's, renal artery stenosis with NF-1, phaeochromocytoma with NF-1)

Head

Size
- Small (e.g. TORCH, numerous syndromes)
- Large (e.g. Sotos', X-linked hydrocephalus)

Shape
- Triangular (e.g. Russell-Silver)
- Frontal bossing (e.g. achondroplasia)

Consistency: craniotabes (e.g. X-linked hypophosphataemic rickets)

Fontanelle
- Large (e.g. Russell-Silver, X-linked hypophosphataemic rickets)
- Bulging (e.g. X-linked hydrocephalus with raised ICP)

Hair
- Sparse (e.g. hypohidrotic ectodermal dysplasia, progeria)
- Greasy (e.g. precocious puberty with NF-1)

Eyes

Inspection
- Prominent (e.g. Crouzon's)
- Microphthalmos (e.g. CHARGE, fetal rubella effects)
- Hypertelorism (e.g. Noonan's, Williams)
- Epicanthal folds (e.g. Noonan's, Williams, Turner's, Down)
- Ptosis (e.g. Noonan's, pseudohypoparathyroidism)
- Squint (e.g. Williams, Prader-Willi, septo-optic dysplasia)
- Nystagmus (e.g. septo-optic dysplasia)

Conjunctivae: pallor (e.g. Fanconi's pancytopenia)

Sclerae
- Icterus (e.g. Alagille)
- Blue (e.g. osteogenesis imperfecta, Marfan's)

Iris
- Coloboma (e.g. aniridia–Wilms' tumour association, CHARGE, cat-eye syndrome)
- Brushfield's spots (e.g. Down, Zellweger's)
- Pale blue (e.g. fragile-X, Angelman's)
- Heterochromia (e.g. Waardenburg's, Klippel-Trenauney-Weber)
- Stellate (e.g. Williams)

Cornea
- Large and cloudy (buphthalmos): glaucoma (e.g. aniridia–Wilms' tumour association, fetal rubella effects, Marfan's, NF-1, Marshall's, Stickler's)
- Keratoconus (e.g. Noonan's, xeroderma pigmentosa)

Visual fields: field defect (e.g. brain tumour with NF-1)

Eye movements
- Nystagmus (e.g. septo-optic dysplasia sequence, aniridia–Wilms' tumour association, Chédiak-Higashi)
- Lateral rectus palsy (e.g. Möbius' sequence)

Cataracts (e.g. rubella, aniridia–Wilms' tumour association)

Lens dislocation: Marfan's (goes up), homocystinuria (goes down)

Fundi
- Papilloedema (e.g. hydrocephalus with raised ICP)
- Optic nerve hypoplasia (e.g. septo-optic dysplasia)
- Chorioretinitis (e.g. TORCH)

Nose

Midface hypoplasia (e.g. FAS)

Anosmia (e.g. Kallmann's)

Continued

Table 9.3 *(Continued)*

Mouth and chin
Central cyanosis: various forms of congenital heart disease (CHD)
Midline defects
- Cleft lip (repaired): cleft lip sequence
- Cleft palate (repaired): cleft lip sequence

Teeth
- Hypodontia (e.g. Aarskog, Down, incontinentia pigmenti, Williams)
- Irregularly placed (e.g. Down: Crouzon's, Morquio's)
- Late eruption (e.g. incontinentia pigmenti, progeria)

Tongue
- Enlarged (e.g. Beckwith-Wiedemann, Pompe's)
- Ptosed (e.g. Pierre Robin's sequence)
- Prominent (e.g. Down, small pharynx, normal-sized tongue)

Facial hair or acne (e.g. precocity with NF-1)
Micrognathia (e.g. Russell-Silver, Turner's, Seckel's)

Ears
Low set (e.g. Turner's, Seckel's, Noonan's, Treacher Collins)
Posteriorly rotated (e.g. Russell-Silver)
Malformed (e.g. CHARGE, Treacher Collins, Beckwith-Wiedemann)

Hairline
Low (e.g. Turner's, Noonan's)

Neck
Pterygium colli (e.g. Klippel-Feil, Turner's, Noonan's)
Short (e.g. Klippel-Feil, Turner's, Noonan's, Down, CHARGE)
Scoliosis (e.g. Klippel-Feil)

Chest
Inspection
- Scars: repair of tracheo-oesophageal fistula (e.g. VACTERL, CHARGE), repair of diaphragmatic hernia (e.g. Marfan's, DiGeorge's)
- Tanner staging in girls, for precocity (e.g. McCune-Albright) or delay (Turner's)

Nipples
- Wide-spaced (e.g. Turner's, fetal phenytoin effects, several trisomies)
- Hypoplastic (e.g. Poland's anomaly)

Chest wall
- Sternal deformity: pectus excavatum or carinatum (e.g. Marfan's, Noonan's, Turner's, Kozlowski's spondylo-metaphyseal dysplasia, homocystinuria)
- Small thoracic cage (e.g. several skeletal dysplasias, Jeune's thoracic dystrophy, progeria)

Palpation
- Praecordium (e.g. for CHD)

Auscultation
- Praecordium (e.g. for CHD)

Abdomen
Inspection
- Scars: repair of duodenal atresia (e.g. Down), repair of Hirschsprung's (e.g. Down, Waardenburg's), removal of tumour (e.g. Wilms' in aniridia–Wilms' tumour association, adrenal tumour in Beckwith-Wiedemann), repair of inguinal herniae (e.g. Marfan's), repair of omphalocoele (e.g. Beckwith-Wiedemann)
- Prune-like appearance (prune belly syndrome)
- Tanner staging pubic hair, for precocity (e.g. McCune-Albright) or delay (Kallmann's, Klinefelter's, Noonan's)

Palpation
- Hepatomegaly (e.g. Shwachman's, storage diseases)
- Splenomegaly (e.g. storage diseases)
- Hepatosplenomegaly (e.g. various storage diseases)
- Enlarged kidneys (e.g. polycystic kidneys, hydronephrosis)

Auscultation
- Hepatic bruit (e.g. haemangioma, hepatocellular carcinoma associated with Beckwith-Wiedemann)
- Renal artery stenosis (e.g. NF-1)

Posterior aspect
- Midline scar (e.g. spina bifida repair)

Genitalia
Tanner staging genitalia
- Measure penis length
- Measure testes parameters; estimate testes volume
- Advanced stage (e.g. NF-1)
- Delayed stage (e.g. Noonan's)

Continued

Table 9.3 *(Continued)*

Penile anomalies
- Micropenis (e.g. Prader-Willi)
- Hypospadias (e.g. Noonan's)

Testicular anomalies: cryptorchidism (e.g. Noonan's)

Gait, back and lower limbs
Inspection of lower limbs
- Lower limb bowing (e.g. X-linked hypophosphataemic rickets)
- Proximal, middle or distal shortening (e.g. bony dysplasias)
- Oedema of dorsa of feet (e.g. Turner's)
- Clubbing of toes (various types of CHD)

Palpation: ankle oedema (CCF with CHD)
Gait—standard examination screening for:

- Long-tract signs (e.g. X-linked hydrocephalus; brain tumour with NF-1)
- Ataxia (e.g. ataxia-telangiectasia)
- Proximal weakness (e.g. myopathies, developmental dysplasia of hip)

Back
- Scoliosis (e.g. various skeletal dysplasias, NF-1)
- Kyphosis (e.g. achondroplasia)
- Focal spinal shortening (e.g. various skeletal dysplasias)
- Midline scar (spina bifida)
- Spinal tenderness (X-linked hypophosphataemic rickets)

Lower limbs neurologically
- Long-tract signs (e.g. brain tumour with NF-1)

CCF = congestive cardiac failure; CHD = congenital heart disease; FAS = fetal alcohol syndrome; ICP = intracranial pressure; LS = lower segment; NF = neurofibromatosis; TORCH = intrauterine infections with toxoplasmosis, other (e.g. HIV, syphilis), rubella, cytomegalovirus, herpes (both simplex and varicella); US = upper segment; VSD = ventricular septal defect.

Haematology

Long cases

Haemophilia

Discussion issues may include the use of recombinant factor VIII (F-VIII) or factor IX (F-IX) prophylactic replacement (the rationale, benefits, barriers, the terminology of various subgroups of prophylaxis, including primary [determined by age or first bleed], secondary, short-term, full dose, partial), the timing of placing of central venous access devices (CVADs), the management of joint disease, newer factor therapy products, advice regarding the management of carriers (siblings) and the initial results of gene therapy.

Background information

Definitions

Haemophilia A is factor VIII (F-VIII) deficiency, and accounts for 80–85% of haemophilia. Haemophilia B is factor IX (F-IX) deficiency, which accounts for 15–20% of haemophilia. Clinically, it is not possible to distinguish between them. Both are X-linked recessive conditions.

The F-VIII gene is at the telomeric end of the long arm of the X chromosome at band Xq28. It is a large gene, 186 kilobases (kb) long. Most of F-VIII is synthesised in the liver endothelial cells and immediately is linked to von Willebrand's factor (vWF) on entering the circulation; this prevents enzymatic degradation of factor F-VIII until it is required for coagulation. Molecular defects described include gross rearrangements of the DNA sequence, single gene rearrangements, deletion of some of the gene, and DNA insertions.

The F-IX gene is on the X chromosome at band Xq27. The gene is 33 kb long. F-IX is synthesised in the liver and released into the circulation in inactive form. Molecular defects described include single gene rearrangements, large deletions, additions and missense mutations. Over 60% of cases have a positive family history; over 30% are spontaneous mutations. Diagnosis is based on prolonged activated partial thromboplastin time (aPTT), F-VIII or F-IX assay, and DNA analysis; the last of these allows prenatal and carrier diagnosis.

Disease manifestations

Severity and frequency of bleeding complications are a reflection of the residual activity of F-VIII or F-IX. Patients with severe haemophilia (approximately 70% of type A and

50% of type B cases) have less than 1% residual factor VIII or factor IX. These children are predisposed to having spontaneous bleeding into joints, muscles and deep organs, including central nervous system bleeds. Patients with 1–5% of F-VIII, or F-IX, rarely have spontaneous haemorrhages, but may have significant haemorrhage with mild or moderate trauma. Those with mild disease, with over 5% of F-VIII or F-IX, may have bleeding with trauma or surgery. Some carrier females, who have low levels of these factors, may present clinically with gynaecological or obstetric haemorrhage.

Age-related presentation

Birth to 4 weeks
1. Bleeding following circumcision (infants of known carriers should not be circumcised until testing for F-VIII / F-IX rules out haemophilia).
2. Bleeding from heel puncture or other blood taking.
3. Central nervous system haemorrhage.

4–6 months
1. Large haematomas following immunisation (intramuscular injections).
2. Palpable subcutaneous ecchymoses.

6–24 months
1. Gingival haemorrhages when teething.
2. Bleeding from oral mucosa (e.g. from small lacerations of frenulum or tongue).
3. Increased bruising with mobilisation.

3–4 years
Joint and muscle haemorrhage become problematic.

Complications

Haemarthrosis
1. Results in destructive arthritis, joint instability and ankylosis.
2. Commonest joints affected are knees, followed by elbows, ankles and shoulders.

Neurological problems

Intracranial haemorrhage
1. One of the more common causes of death.
2. Survivors may have severe neurological deficits: see later discussion on neurological sequelae.

Haemorrhage into vertebral canal
1. Rare; 75% are extramedullary and 25% intramedullary.
2. Presents with severe neck or back pain followed by ascending paralysis.

Peripheral nerve compression
1. External compression or traction from intramuscular bleeds.
2. Nerves affected and relevant muscles often affected: femoral (iliopsoas), ulnar and median (forearm flexors), sciatic (glutei).

Life-threatening haemorrhages

Retropharyngeal
1. Usually associated with pharyngitis.

2. Presents with dysphagia and drooling.
3. Can be diagnosed by lateral neck X–ray.

Retroperitoneal
1. Can have loss of a large volume of concealed blood.
2. May be spontaneous or from trauma.
3. Diagnosed by ultrasound or CT scan.

Intracranial
See above.

History

Ask about the following.

Presenting complaint
Reason for current admission.

Past history
1. Initial presenting symptoms, diagnosis (when, where, how), subsequent management, progress of disease, hospitalisation details.
2. Complications of disease (e.g. neurological deficits, joint disease) or its treatment (e.g. inhibitor formation, hepatitis C seropositivity, liver disease).
3. Previous elective surgery or dental procedures (their management and outcome).
4. Outpatient clinics attended (where, how often).
5. Past treatments used (e.g. F-VIII, desmopressin [DDAVP], prothrombin complex concentrate).
6. Age when parents started administering F-VIII.
7. Age of self-administration.
8. Age of venous access port placement.
9. Recent change in symptoms or management.

Current status
1. Average number of bleeds per year, common sites involved (e.g. knee, elbow), 'target joint' (most patients with significant joint disease will typically develop one joint that is more affected by recurrent bleeds), any common precipitants (e.g. sport), treatment required (type of concentrate), usual outcome, where usually managed (home or hospital), who gives infusions (patient or parent), prophylaxis regimen, details of venous access port use.
2. Ongoing symptoms of joint disease (e.g. pain, stiffness), neurological disease (e.g. weakness from peripheral nerve compression, hemiplegia from intracranial bleed), immunocompromise from HIV. (Fortunately all children with haemophilia in Australia are now eligible to receive recombinant factor VIII or factor IX that has not been associated with transmission of HIV or hepatitis C but this remains a major concern for older patients.)
3. Management of bleeds away from home (school, on holidays, overseas).

Social history
1. Disease impact on patient (e.g. avoidance of participation in sports such as rugby, football, self-image, social rejection with HIV seropositivity, schooling

(attendance, performance, teacher awareness of, and attitudes towards, disease and its treatment, peer interactions, reactions to HIV status).

2. Disease impact on parents (e.g. marriage stability, fears for future, financial considerations [medical treatment, awareness of benefits available], modification of holiday plans).

3. Disease impact on siblings (e.g. sibling rivalry, hostility, genetic implications for girls).

4. Social supports (e.g. social worker, extended family).

5. Coping, e.g. who attends with patient, confidence with management, degree of understanding of disease (haemophilia or, later, AIDS), expectations for future, understanding of prognosis.

6. Access to hospital, local doctor, paediatrician, haematologist, orthopaedic surgeon, rheumatologist.

Family history and genetic aspects

Other boys with haemophilia, more children planned, prenatal diagnosis (and subsequent management for positive result), carrier detection in girls (normal factor VIII/factor IX level does not exclude a female being a carrier of haemophilia).

Immunisation

Routine, associated bleeding, hepatitis B.

Examination

The salient findings to be sought in the haemophilia long case are as follows:

General inspection

1. Position patient standing, undressed to underpants.

2. Parameters: weight, height, head circumference (subdural bleed).

3. Visually scan skin for bruises (number, size, age), joints for swelling and posture for evidence of neurological sequelae (e.g. hemiparesis [intracranial bleed] or foot drop [lateral popliteal palsy]).

4. Unwell (e.g. severe bleed) or well.

5. Pallor (anaemia from large bleed, e.g. retroperitoneal).

6. Jaundice (hepatitis).

7. Vital signs: respiratory rate (e.g. pulse [anaemia], blood pressure [hypotension from bleeding], urinalysis [blood]).

8. Distress due to painful bleed.

Directed examination for disease extent and complications

1. Full skin examination, for distribution of bruises, including mucous membranes (mouth, tongue).

2. Full joint examination for evidence of arthropathy, focusing on the range of movement of affected joints, associated muscle wasting, any supportive devices (wheelchairs, splints, orthotic devices), gait.

3. Full neurological examination for any evidence of intracerebral or intravertebral haemorrhage, or peripheral nerve lesions (or, later, HIV encephalopathy). Best commenced with gait examination, followed by examination of the motor system.

4. Abdominal examination for liver and spleen size (liver disease), or tenderness (gastrointestinal or retroperitoneal bleed).

5. As HIV still prevalent, check for generalised lymphadenopathy, oral candidiasis, evidence of herpes infections (simplex or zoster), parotid swelling or opportunistic infection (e.g. chest, ears, nose, throat).

Available treatment modalities

Concentrates

Recombinant DNA–engineered F-VIII and F-IX are the treatments of choice. Previously concentrates were made by refining cryoprecipitates and removing some of the fibrinogen. Their multidonor source meant concentrates carried the greatest risk of transmission of various infections (e.g. HIV, hepatitis C virus). Ultra-pure preparations are now made using monoclonal antibodies. Recently, there has been an emerging concern that some factor products that may contain small amounts of human or animal protein could transmit novel viruses (e.g. West Nile virus) or prions (e.g. variant of Creutzfeldt-Jakob Disease [vCJD]). Human protein free preparations are now becoming available. The Australian government now supplies recombinant factor VIII (Recombinate–Baxter) and factor IX (Benefix) for all patients with haemophilia.

Antifibrinolytics

Epsilon-aminocaproic acid (EACA) and tranexamic acid are useful ancillary agents. These inhibit clot lysis by the fibrinolytic system. They are commenced in conjunction with factor replacement therapy or DDAVP and continued for up to 14 days. They are particularly important in the management of oral haemorrhage, as saliva contains fibrinolytic enzymes. They are useful for tooth extractions and for uterine, gastrointestinal and intraocular bleeding, but are not recommended in haemarthrosis or haematuria, as in both their use may be associated with excessive fibrin deposition, possibly causing joint or renal tract damage/obstruction respectively. Antifibrinolytics are not given with prothrombin concentrates due to the risk of potentiating thrombosis.

Desmopressin (1-deamino 8-D arginine vasopressin: DDAVP)

A synthetic analogue of vasopressin which raises F-VIII level by up to five times in normal subjects and seven times in some mild haemophiliacs, but has no effect in patients with severe disease. The mechanism is not fully understood. It can be given intravenously (0.3 mcg/kg in 50 mL saline over 20 minutes, peaks at 30–60 minutes) or by intranasal spray (150–300 mcg, peaks at 60–90 minutes). Tachyphylaxis may occur after several doses. Complications include facial flushing, hyponatraemia (particularly in infants—contraindicated in children under 2 years) and thrombosis (rare). Fluid restriction and urine output monitoring are important considerations. It is best for use in controlled situations such as elective minor surgery.

Corticosteroids

Prednisolone has been used for haematuria, sometimes in conjunction with factor replacement. Brief courses (1–4 weeks) of steroids have been used for joint bleeds.

Fresh frozen plasma (FFP)

This contains all the clotting factors. Its use is limited by volume; 20 mL/kg can be given over 6 hours, followed by 10 mL/kg every 6 hours for maintenance. Harvested from one donor, FFP can be used for coagulopathy secondary to liver failure.

Prothrombinex

Formerly used for F-IX deficiency, this concentrate contains factors II, IX and X. It has been superseded by MonoFIX, a purified factor IX heat-treated plasma–derived concentrate, and recombinant F-IX. It is still sometimes used in the management of patients with factor VIII inhibitors.

Cryoprecipitate

This is a protein precipitate of fresh frozen plasma, rich in factors VIII and XIII and fibrinogen. On average it contains 100 units of F-VIII per bag and is normally derived from a single donor. It is no longer recommended.

Management

Treatment of acute haemorrhage

1. Control of specific bleeding problems
Clotting factors
The dose of F-VIII or F-IX required to achieve haemostasis varies with the severity of the bleed. One unit of F-VIII or F-IX is the amount that is present in 1 mL of 'pooled' normal plasma. One unit per kg of F-VIII increases the activity of F-VIII by approximately 2%. The factor VIII half-life averages 8–12 hours. F-IX has a longer half-life of 12–18 hours, and one unit per kg of F-IX increases plasma levels by approximately 1%.

F-VIII replacement guide
1. Minimal bleeds: first aid, antifibrinolytics if indicated. The need for factor VIII replacement should be assessed recognising the occasional difficulties with intravenous cannulation, particularly in young children.
2. Moderate bleed (e.g. joint, muscle, small oral mucosal or tongue laceration or bleed, epistaxis, gastrointestinal, or genitourinary): 20–40 units/kg, given 12–24-hourly, usually for 3 days. Frequent repeated doses may be required if bleeding does not settle.
3. Severe bleed (life-threatening haemorrhage, e.g. major trauma, retropharyngeal, retroperitoneal, intracranial, large oral mucosal bleeds): 50–75 units/kg initially, followed by repeat doses of 25–40 units/kg every 12 hours until bleeding has ceased, or continuous infusion (especially intracranial bleeds, trauma).

Generally, haemarthroses and soft tissue bleeds require 1–3 infusions, whereas serious bleeds, such as areas with peripheral nerves at risk (e.g. psoas), retropharyngeal or retroperitoneal bleeding, may require prolonged treatment, including continuous infusions of factor VIII.

F-IX replacement guide
F-IX doses are 1.5–2 times the doses for F-VIII listed above.

2. Other treatments
Musculoskeletal bleeds also benefit from **R**est/immobilisation, **I**ce, **C**ompression and **E**levation of the affected part (mnemonic RICE).

In addition to antifibrinolytics (EACA, tranexamic acid) and replacement therapy in oral or nasal mucous membrane bleeding and dental extractions, children should remain nil by mouth if they have oral or tongue bleeds/lacerations.

Analgesia

Haemarthrosis can be very painful. Temporary immobilisation in a splint, with infusion of F–VIII and wise use of simple analgesics that are free of any aspirin (e.g. paracetamol, codeine) may be sufficient. Narcotic analgesia should be avoided. Joint aspiration, under F–VIII cover, may be needed to stop the pain (rarely in childhood).

Restoring normal function

Physiotherapy should be initiated as soon as pain has diminished. Immobilisation should ideally not exceed 24–48 hours, and then static followed by active exercises should be introduced. Depending on the chronicity of the joint problem, F–VIII cover may be required to prevent physiotherapy-induced haemorrhage. The use of ultrasound may help to restore function after a large soft-tissue bleed.

Prevention of iatrogenic problems

With medical procedures, apply pressure for 10 minutes after any injection (e.g. venepuncture or subcutaneous injection). Immunisations can be given without clotting factor concentrate cover, but a small-gauge needle and deep subcutaneous injections rather than intramuscular injections are recommended. The injection site should be compressed for 10 minutes after the injection. For lumbar puncture (LP), give enough clotting factor to raise level to 50%, 30 minutes before the LP.

Complications of medical treatment

Analgesic abuse

This tends to be more of a problem in the adult haemophiliac population, but is well recognised in adolescents. Avoidance of addictive drugs is extremely important; this area should be considered in any adolescent.

Infectious agents transmissable in factor concentrates

Hepatitis viruses A, B, C and G

Each of these can be transmitted in factor VIII or factor IX concentrates derived from donor plasma. The most common problems are with hepatitis B (HBV) and hepatitis C (HCV). Children are immunised against HBV at diagnosis.

With current techniques, plasma-derived clotting factor concentrates are very safe, but the risk of viral transmission is still a possibility and so the preference is to use recombinant F–VIII and F–IX concentrates.

Before 1990 around 70–90% of patients receiving concentrates were infected with the hepatitis C virus (HCV). Long-term sequelae include chronic active hepatitis (CAH), cirrhosis and hepatocellular carcinoma. Alpha-interferon treatment for hepatitis C (chronic hepatitis patients) may be given for 6 months to see if there is any improvement; its effectiveness is controversial. Laboratory assessment should include second generation ELISA antibody testing, HCV genotyping (genotype may relate to disease severity and interferon responsiveness), HCV RNA levels in the serum, as well as liver enzymes.

HIV

Patients treated prior to 1985, when blood screening for HIV was introduced, have had a high frequency of seropositivity for HIV type 1. In many countries where recombinant DNA engineered factor VIII and IX are readily available, patients affected are now largely beyond the paediatric age range, and will not be seen in an examination format.

HIV infection will relentlessly progress to clinical AIDS in an increasing number of HIV-positive patients. The cumulative rate of AIDS is lower in children than in adults: the younger the age at conversion, the lower the risk of AIDS.

Since the implementation of HIV-1 screening in 1986 and the development of viral inactivation measures new HIV-1 seroconversions have been almost completely eliminated. Screening does not guarantee virus-free concentrates, as anti-HIV tests may still be negative during the early phase of HIV infection.

Other infective agents

Heat treatment may destroy HIV and hepatitis B and C viruses, but parvovirus B19 and hepatitis A virus can survive heat. Solvent detergent techniques are needed to deal with parvovirus. Recently, there has been an emerging concern that some factor products that may contain small amounts of human or animal protein could transmit novel viruses (e.g. West Nile virus) or prions (e.g. variant Creutzfeldt-Jakob disease [vCJD]).

Chronic problems

Neurological sequelae

Intracranial haemorrhage is one of the more common causes of mortality and morbidity. Between one-third and one-half of affected children die, and of the survivors half have neurological sequelae, including convulsions, and motor and cognitive impairment. All patients with any neurological symptoms or signs need appropriate imaging (CT or MRI) to diagnose small intracerebral bleeds early. The sequelae may require use of anticonvulsants, physiotherapy, occupational therapy, speech therapy and prolonged rehabilitation.

Joint involvement and synovectomy

Haemophilic arthropathy proceeds through many stages, with a cycle of haemarthrosis from inflammatory changes with erosion of cartilage and bone to proliferative chronic synovitis (highly vascular tissue) and increased haemarthrosis. Hypertrophied synovium causes destruction of cartilage, narrowing of the joint space, bone resorption and cyst formation, resulting in anatomical joint instability and chronic pain. Disuse leads to osteoporosis. Abnormal epiphyseal growth will occur, followed by atrophy of local muscles and further joint instability. Finally the joint becomes immobile, with repeated bleeding, leading to fibrous and bony ankylosis of large joints or complete destruction of small joints.

Haemophilic arthropathy can be staged radiographically:

Stage 1 Soft-tissue swelling due to haemorrhage into joint
Stage 2 Overgrowth of epiphysis
Stage 3 Joint disorganised
Stage 4 Cartilage destroyed, joint space narrowed
Stage 5 Fibrous contracture, loss of joint space, loss of joint

Magnetic resonance imaging (MRI) gives the best assessment of synovial hypertrophy, and can give additional information particularly in stage 2, demonstrating erosion, cysts, and joint effusions.

Optimal treatment to prevent this cycle is prophylaxis (see below), which is associated with a significant reduction in the average number of haemarthroses per year and in the rate of joint deterioration. When children are started on prophylactic replacement therapy to keep plasma factor levels above 1%, this effectively changes severe disease to moderate disease, and if commenced in children between 1 and 3 years of age, joint destruction will not occur.

Prompt treatment of any breakthrough bleeding and intensive physiotherapy are also important. Brief courses of oral corticosteroids (1–4 weeks) may be given in cases of severe synovitis as well, to decrease the synovium, but their beneficial effect is temporary. Non-steroidal anti-inflammatory drugs can be used, although ibuprofen has been associated with increased bleeding in some patients. The new COX-2 inhibitors can be used and are not associated with increased risk of bleeding.

If a joint remains chronically enlarged despite optimum medical therapy, surgical intervention may be considered (e.g. synovectomy). The rationale for synovectomy is that removing synovium decreases bleeds, thus reducing ongoing joint damage. Arthroscopic synovectomy is performed more commonly than the open-joint procedure. An alternative is isotopic or chemical synovectomy (synoviorthesis), where the synovium is ablated by intra-articular injection of colloidal P32 chromic phosphate (or 90-Yytrium, or 186-Rhenium, 169-Erbium or radioactive gold) or chemical agents (oxiteracicline chlorhydrate, osmic acid, hyaluronic acid, rifampicin). Radioactive agents seem to have better results long term with more rapid rehabilitation. Short-term results are very good with either mode of treatment. Complications of synovectomy can include rebleeding, long periods of rehabilitation, long-term ankylosis and potential requirement for total joint replacement (arthroplasty). Arthroplasty has very good short-term effects; the most common joints on which it is performed are the knees, hips, shoulders and, less often, the elbows or ankles.

Specific discussion areas

Home treatment

This is the cornerstone of modern management. The two forms of treatment are prophylactic (regular injections to prevent bleeds) and symptomatic (when a bleed has just started). Prophylactic treatment is the optimal therapy for severe disease recommended by the World Health Organization (WHO), the World Federation of Hemophilia (WFH) and various national haemophilia foundations (in Australia, USA, Canada and many European countries). Central venous access devices (CVADs) or 'ports' are placed to enable institution of home treatment at an early age, which avoids repetitive and difficult venepuncture. Most parents have a pager or mobile phone so they can be contacted when a bleed occurs at school and administer treatment without delay.

Prophylaxis

This is the standard approach for most boys with severe haemophilia. There are a number of types of prophylaxis; the specific terminology used is as follows.

Primary prophylaxis

Primary prophylaxis is the ongoing regular infusion of F-VIII from early childhood, before significant joint bleeding is established, to prevent most bleeding episodes. This is usually started after the first significant joint bleed (often at around 12 months of age) and is typically given through a venous access port (see below). In neonates who have intracranial bleeding, prophylaxis is best started as soon as possible (i.e. without waiting until after a first major joint bleed), implanting a venous access port during the hospital admission for the presenting intracranial bleed (in one of the author's patients this included a [successful] burr hole at age 4 days for a subdural haematoma with midline shift, a 'blown' pupil and incipient coning). Recombinant F-VIII is given three times a week, at a dose of 25–40 units/kg. Prophylaxis has led to a marked decrease in the number of bleeds suffered by these children. The age at which prophylaxis is started is an independent predictor for the development of arthropathy; the earlier it is started, the less joint disease will occur, irrespective of the variables of dose and infusion intervals used at the start of treatment before the age of 3 years. The increased cost of prophylaxis may be offset by the decrease in later interventions such as synovectomy and the avoidance of significant arthritis in the adult years.

Primary prophylaxis can be determined either by age, starting long-term continuous (52 weeks a year) treatment before 2 years and before any clinically evident joint bleeds, or by first joint bleed, starting long-term continuous (52 weeks a year) treatment before the onset of joint damage.

The advantages of primary prophylaxis include: the prevention of (a) haemarthroses, (b) chronic joint disease and (c) pain; less school interruption (and higher academic achievement in mathematics and reading); increased participation in physical activities; and less frequent hospital visits.

The disadvantages include port requirement in younger children, increased number of injections, increased usage of products, possible earlier development of inhibitors, requirement for compliant patient and family, and cost. In 2006 in Australia, the cost of recombinant F-VIII is approximately $1.00/unit; F-VIII is provided in 250-unit bottles ($250), so the dose is rounded up to the nearest number of bottles (that is, dose divisible by 250).

Prophylaxis will not prevent all bleeds. It should be continued until the patient is 18 years of age, and may continue indefinitely. There are no long-term studies of patients who discontinue prophylaxis in adulthood.

Secondary prophylaxis

This refers to a specified period of regular infusions of F-VIII after joint bleeding has been established. It is used for particular events such as surgical procedures or strenuous activities. Secondary prophylaxis is less successful in arresting recurrent joint bleeds.

Full-dose prophylaxis

This refers to infusion of F-VIII at least 2–3 times a week, or F-IX at least 1–2 times weekly, for a minimum of 46 weeks per year.

Partial prophylaxis

This is defined as 3–45 weeks of prophylaxis per year. *Short-term prophylaxis* refers to short-term treatment to prevent bleeding. *On demand therapy* means treatment given when bleeding occurs.

Central venous access devices (CVADs or 'ports')

CVADs allow easier access, with minimal discomfort (use of EMLA local anaesthetic cream), improved home treatment, and parent and patient acceptance. Negative aspects include the need for hospitalisation for insertion (usually 3–5 days) and significant risk of infection, given that the port is accessed 150 times a year. There is no lower age limit for CVADs. One port can last longer than 5 years. If a port is infected, attempted sterilisation with antibiotics may succeed, but once the port has been infected two or three times it is unlikely to be able to be salvaged. The usual infective agent is *Staphylococcus epidermidis*, although gram-negative organisms are not uncommon. The other complication of CVADs is thrombosis, which can occur in around 50% of cases by 4 years.

Elective surgery and continuous infusion of replacement factors
Before any elective surgical procedures, all patients with haemophilia should be assessed for inhibitors (see below) and to establish the optimum intervals of factor infusion. This comprises evaluation of increase in F-VIII or F-IX level per unit of F-VIII or F-IX per kilogram and the biological half-life of the factor in that child. It must be ensured that there are sufficient quantities of F-VIII or F-IX available on the day of surgery and for the week after. In general, for all surgical procedures, a dose to bring the patient's level to 100% can be given at induction for the procedure.

The use of continuous infusions of F-VIII makes surgery safer and easier. A pre-operative dose of 50 units/kg is followed by an infusion at a rate of 3 units/kg per hour to maintain a constant plasma level of factor VIII. The half-life of F-VIII is 8–12 hours. F-VIII is stable for 24 hours after reconstitution (longer than the product information states) provided it is not diluted with other fluids. A syringe driver should be used for administration, as factor VIII adheres to plastic bags. The exact regimen for clotting factor concentrate infusion will depend on the nature and extent of surgery.

When a CVAD is placed (usually the first surgical procedure undergone by these children), most units give continuous F-VIII or F-IX for 3–5 days, then access the CVAD for the first time postoperatively at 7 days.

Inhibitors and immune tolerance therapy
Inhibitors are polyclonal IgG antibodies usually directed against functional epitopes of F-VIII or F-IX. These develop in 20–30% of patients with severe haemophilia A, although in only 1–4% of those with haemophilia B. Of those with haemophilia A, some 35–50% are termed 'low responders', where the antibody circulates at low levels and no major anamnestic response occurs. The remaining patients are 'high responders', and do show an anamnestic response to F-VIII infusion.

Low responders may benefit from infusions at a greater dose or from more frequent infusions. Patients with high-responding inhibitors typically will not respond to standard clotting factor concentrate. These patients may require 'bypassing' agents, such as activated factor VIIa (NovoVII) or FEIBA for the treatment of bleeding. The recommended dose of recombinant factor VIIa is 90–120 micrograms/kg given every 2 hours until bleeding stops (for an acute bleed), or for at least 24 hours for major surgery (including total hip and knee replacement). F-VIIa enhances the generation of thrombin on platelets activated by the initial thrombin formation, and the formation of a firm fibrin plug that is resistant to premature fibrolysis. F-VIIa is expensive; in 2006 in Australia it cost approximately $1.00/microgram.

Immune tolerance therapy (ITT), also called tolerisation, refers to eradicating inhibitors by manipulating the immune system through recurrent exposure to regular infusions of F-VIII or F-IX. There is controversy over the ideal dosing, interval and product choice. Many patients can be tolerised on a regimen of plasma-derived F-VIII, in a dose of about 40 units/kg three times a week. An international study is under way to compare high-dose 200 unit/kg/day infusions of F-VIII with 50 unit/kg, three times a week. The advantages of ITT include better control of bleeds and reduced use of expensive products. The disadvantages include increased use of F-VIII in some cases, and a success rate of up to 80%. Inhibitors to F-IX are less common; around one-third of patients achieve successful immune tolerance. In response to exposure to F-IX replacement, severe allergic reactions have been described, including anaphylaxis; also, nephrotic syndrome can develop. Hence ITT must be considered very carefully in these patients. Rituximab, a monoclonal antibody directed against CD-20 positive cells, is being evaluated for those who fail to respond to ITT. Occasionally, immune modulation with steroids, or cyclophosphamide (to inhibit antibodies), IV immunoglobulin, plasmapheresis or protein A adsorption (to remove antibodies) is needed.

Sport

It is a myth that avoidance of strenuous activity prevents bleeding: only about 7% of recreational or sporting accidents lead to bleeding in an otherwise well child. Affected boys should be encouraged to participate in age-appropriate sporting activities with their school friends, the only exceptions being those where there is a definite risk of head injury (e.g. martial arts, boxing, rugby). A good level of physical fitness may help to reduce the number of joint bleeds.

Immunisation

Routine immunisations should be given to haemophiliac children (unless immunologically compromised by HIV, in which case live viral vaccines should be avoided). The risk of bleeding is minimal if pressure is applied over the injection site for at least 10 minutes. Routine immunisation against hepatitis A and B is recommended.

Dental extractions

A combination of tranexamic acid (15–25 mg/kg, 8-hourly) and F-VIII replacement to 30–60%, given at least 4 hours and 1 hour, respectively, before a dental extraction, may be used, with the former continued for 5–10 days. Repeat doses of F-VIII are seldom used.

Genetic counselling

The molecular lesions causing haemophilia are heterogeneous, including gross abnormalities (deletions, insertions) and single nucleotide abnormalities (point mutations). About half the mutations in severe haemophilia A are an inversion of intron 22, which can be detected by standard genetic tests.

Diagnosis at a DNA level allows the abnormal gene to be identified and marked and its inheritance to be traced. Carrier detection and prenatal diagnosis require only the ability to recognise the abnormal gene. Most families of patients with haemophilia can have DNA analysis to elucidate the carrier status of females, prenatal diagnosis (on chorionic villus biopsy at 9 weeks) and linkage analysis to trace the origin of the abnormality.

Progress

Cures for both haemophilia A and B have occurred with orthotopic liver transplantation (performed for liver failure). Gene therapy has made progress. The goal is to package the functioning F-VIII or F-IX into a vector, which is then incorporated into a target cell. Five gene therapy trials have enrolled patients and three have reported data. The method of delivery and vector vary from trial to trial. One trial was halted as the retroviral vector was found in the semen of one patient, and in another trial, adeno-associated viral vector DNA was found in bodily fluids of two patients. Both haemophilia A and B are particularly amenable to gene therapy, as the genes do not need tissue specific expression.

Sickle cell disease

Sickle cell anaemia (SCA) affects around 1 in 600 African Americans. The two main pathophysiological processes are haemolytic anaemia and vaso-occlusion. These are secondary to deoxygenation of the haemoglobin S molecule, which aggregates into a polymer, which then causes a distortion of the red blood cell to a 'sickle' shape. Sickle cells block the microvasculature; the consequent deleterious effects of SCA can involve most organ systems. The rate of sickling is related to the concentration of deoxy-HbS: it takes only seconds and if the cell is rammed through the capillaries it becomes reoxygenated and the polymers of HbS depolymerise. The cell shape lags behind and repeated hypoxic stress will alter the cytoskeleton of the cell and cause an irreversibly sickled cell.

Although the condition is less common in Australia than in the USA, Canada or the UK, children suffering from it do tend to appear in the examination setting. Because of their relative infrequency, candidates (and consultants) may find management of these children challenging.

Background information

Basic defect

Sickle cell anaemia is due to a homozygosity for the genetic point mutation (a single nucleotide change, GAT to GTT), whereby glutamic acid is replaced by valine at position 6 on the beta chain of haemoglobin: the resulting haemoglobin is HbS. Deoxygenated HbS polymerises, is denatured and releases toxic oxidants, distorting (sickling) the red cell shape. HbS adversely affects the erythrocyte membrane, leading to greater adherence to endothelial cells and shortened red-cell survival. Sickled red cells have difficulty negotiating the capillary beds. They block vessels (intermittent vaso-occlusive episodes leading to ischaemia) and are destroyed prematurely (haemolysis). In the homozygous state (HbSS disease) there is no HbA, and over 90% HbS. In the heterozygous state, red blood cells contain 30–45% HbS.

The gene has a wide geographic distribution, including equatorial Africa, the USA, the Caribbean, Italy and Greece, the Near and Middle East, and India. The beta globin gene cluster is on chromosome 11. The beta S gene is flanked by distinct haplotypes that are associated with specific ethnic groups of particular geographic regions, which may determine disease severity. They are named after the places where their initial identification occurred. Haplotype CAR (Central Africa Republic) leads to more severe disease than the Benin haplotype, which in turn is more serious than the Senegal haplotype.

Suggestions of more aggressive treatment for more aggressive haplotypes have been made, considering potential curative therapy such as bone marrow transplant (BMT) or gene insertion.

Note that there is an inverse relationship between the level of HbF and clinical severity. Children with high HbF have mild disease.

Definitions

The term sickle cell anaemia refers only to homozygosity for the sickle cell gene. The term sickle cell disease (SCD) is a more general one that can also include sickle cell/haemoglobin C disease, sickle cell/beta thalassaemia and other sickling disorders.

There are two groups of sickle cell syndromes:

1. Sickle states, which are relatively benign (e.g. sickle cell trait, HbAS).
2. Sickle cell diseases (SCDs), which present a variety of problems. These include sickle cell anaemia (SCA), HbSS, sickle beta-0 thalassaemia (beta thalassaemia without production of any beta globin), sickle haemoglobin C disease (HbSC), sickle beta+ thalassaemia (beta thalassaemia with decreased [not absent] production of beta globin). Patients with sickle beta-0 thalassaemia, and sickle beta+

thalassaemia, have a clinical features more like SCD than thalassaemia, because the sickle beta globin predominates as a result of inadequate production of normal beta globin.

Diagnosis

Haemoglobin electrophoresis is the most common technique used in the diagnosis of haemoglobinopathies. Several screening tests are available but none can differentiate between sickle cell anaemia and other HbS conditions. Tests include the classic metabisulfite sickle cell 'prep' (reduced HbS causes red cells to assume a sickled configuration), and dithionite solubility tests (deoxygenated HbS precipitates in aqueous solutions). In the USA, all 50 states now screen all newborns for the presence of SCD: the most common method used is electrophoresis and high-performance liquid chromatography (HPLC).

Sickle cell trait

Clinically benign, the major significance is genetic counselling. Growth and development are normal. Haemoglobin and reticulocyte counts are normal, and red cells are normocytic and normochromic. Affected people may have acute splenic infarction if exposed to significant hypoxia (for example, exposure to altitudes above 3000 metres). Also, renal sickling with spontaneous haematuria can occur. Partners of heterozygotes need screening to exclude haemoglobinopathies, which may lead to a child being born with a sickle disease.

Sickle cell anaemia (SCA)—clinical course

The course of SCA is one of ongoing haemolysis episodically punctuated by 'crises', which are clinical events that may be acutely painful or even life-threatening. Any crisis may be precipitated by infection and fever especially, as well as by hypoxia, exposure to extreme cold, dehydration or acidosis. Types of crises are sequestration crisis (especially affects infants), aplastic crisis, vaso-occlusive (infarctive) crisis and, least commonly, haemolytic crisis.

Effects of alpha thalassaemia

HbSS patients with alpha thalassaemia have a larger number of painful events (in extremities/back/abdomen/head) but fewer acute anaemic events (this does not include splenic sequestration).

Major complications

Vaso-occlusion and haemolysis are the main pathological processes in SCD. The organs most commonly affected are spleen, brain, kidneys and lung. Accordingly the most lethal complications (and common ages affected) are splenic sequestration (under 5 years), overwhelming sepsis due to functional asplenia (under 3 years), stroke (median 5 years), and acute chest syndrome (usually 2–4 years).

SICKLE CELL is a mnemonic for vaso-occlusive complications:

S   **S**equestration (spleen and liver)
I   **I**nfection
C   **C**erebrovascular accidents (CVAs)
K   **K**idney disease
L   **L**ung disease
E   **E**ye disease

C   Crises (painful, infarctive)

E   Erection (priapism)

L   Limb effects (bone infarcts, marrow necrosis, osteomyelitis and aseptic necrosis)

L   Leg ulcers

Painful crises (or vaso-occlusive pain events [VOE]) and acute chest syndrome (ACS) are the most common sickle-cell related complications in HbSS, HbSC, and beta/sickle thalassaemia patients. The risks of these begin in the first year of life; both are vaso-occlusive events.

The most dangerous complications are splenic sequestration, sepsis and CVAs.

Splenic sequestration crisis

1.   This is the most severe crisis in those under 5 years of age. It occurs in 10–30% of children with HbSS, most commonly between 6 months and 3 years.

2.   It results from acute entrapment of a large volume of blood in the spleen—often a large fraction of the circulating blood volume.

3.   These children get rapid splenic enlargement (at least 2 cm increase in spleen size from base line) with an acute fall in haemoglobin of greater than 2 g/dL, with raised reticulocyte count. They present with sudden collapse, shock, profound anaemia, and abdominal fullness due to the massive splenomegaly. This often occurs during an acute infection.

4.   It is life-threatening: it can be fatal within 30 minutes. Shock is treated with plasma expanders and whole blood.

5.   If the child is older (e.g. over 2 years), consider splenectomy in susceptible patients. If under 2 years of age, a chronic transfusion program may be needed.

6.   There is a tendency for recurrence: up to 50% of children have a second episode usually within 2 years. Elective splenectomy is generally recommended in patients presenting with the first episode of splenic sequestration.

Infection: overwhelming sepsis

1.   This particularly affects children under 3 years of age, as a result of poor development of immune response to polysaccharide antigens, complicated by early loss of splenic function (this 'autosplenectomy' occurs in 60% by 2 years, and 90% by 5 years).

2.   Pathogens are most commonly *Streptococcus pneumoniae* (pneumococcus)—various serotypes, and occasionally *Haemophilus influenzae* type B. Other pathogens include meningococcus, other *Streptococci*, *Salmonella* and fastidious gram-negative organisms such as DF-2 (*Capnocytophaga canimorsus*) after a dog bite.

3.   Prevention is by immunisation against pneumococci, *Haemophilus,* and meningococcus. Prophylactic penicillin is recommended until the age of 5 years, as it decreases the incidence of pneumococcal bacteraemia by 84%. Many units continue penicillin prophylaxis throughout childhood.

4.   If children with HbSS or sickle beta-0 thalassaemia present febrile, after clinical assessment it is prudent to take blood for a full blood count, blood cultures, plus type and cross-match if pale, spleen is enlarged, or there are neurological or respiratory symptoms. Then treat with ceftriaxone or cefotaxime (or vancomycin if in an area with a high prevalence of resistant pneumococci). Other investigations for sepsis (e.g. other cultures, CXR) and coexisting complications depend on presentation.

5.   The case fatality rate is up to 30%.

Cerebral infarction (cerebrovascular accident, CVA)

1. Central nervous system involvement is seen in up to 8% of patients; median age is between 5 and 8 years.
2. CVA particularly affects internal carotid (ICA), anterior cerebral (ACA) and middle cerebral (MCA) arteries. Stroke involves arterial occlusion, although SCA's haemoglobin deoxygenation and polymerisation occur in the microcirculation and venous system. Hence the aetiology of CVAs in SCA is unclear; possibly HbSS membrane procoagulant. Permanent sequelae can result (e.g. hemiplegia).
3. Without treatment, CVA recurs in 50–90% within 3 years; can be progressive.
4. MRI and MR arteriography are useful in evaluating the extent of the infarction.
5. Haemorrhage into infarcted areas (from bleeding from delicate vessels from neovascularisation), or ruptured aneurysm (in the contralateral circulation from compensatory increased blood flow) with subarachnoid haemorrhage can occur as early as 4 years of age and cause further neurological deficits.
6. The recommended treatment after cerebral infarction is long-term transfusion therapy maintaining HbS levels below 30%; this lowers the risk of recurrence to 10%.
7. Some studies show that subsequent stroke can occur after cessation of transfusion therapy. Many would recommend continuing transfusion indefinitely.
8. Prevention: some units suggest chronic transfusion of at-risk children. They may be detected by transcranial doppler (TCD) studies that have shown that high blood flow velocity through the ICA (over 200 cm per minute) clearly increases probability of arterial occlusive stroke. TCD studies are used in the USA but were not available in the majority of Australian centres in 2006.

Kidney involvement

1. Hyposthenuria (the inability to concentrate urine) is due to chronic sickling in the region of the loop of Henle (sickle cell–induced microvascular ischaemia, with obliteration of the vasa recta of the kidney medulla).
2. This leads to an obligatory urine output of up to 2 litres/m^2/day in infants, to 4 litres/m^2/day in adults, and associated nocturia, and puts patients at risk of rapid dehydration.
3. Other renal sequelae include renal tubular acidosis, impaired potassium excretion, microscopic haematuria, proteinuria and nephrotic syndrome.
4. Eventually, in adulthood, hypertension, ineffective erythropoiesis, renal osteodystrophy and end-stage renal disease (ESRD) can supervene, requiring top-up transfusion, recombinant human erythopoietin or renal transplantation.

Lung disease: acute chest syndrome (ACS)

1. Acute pulmonary disease with new respiratory symptoms (fever, cough, sputum production, dyspnoea, hypoxia), and new infiltrates on CXR.
2. May be due to pulmonary infarction or infection: e.g. bacterial (*Haemophilus influenzae, Staphylococcus aureus, Klebsiella pneumoniae, Mycoplasma pneumoniae, Pneumococcus, Chlamydia pneumoniae, Legionella pneumophila*, TB, *Cryptococcus*) or viral (respiratory syncytial virus, parvovirus, adenovirus, influenza, cytomegalovirus), or both; it can be difficult to distinguish between them. Definite aetiology is not established in 65–70% of cases with pneumonia. ACS also can be caused by rib or sternal infarction.
3. Pulmonary fat embolism (PFE) is the second most common cause of ACS. Marrow infarcts during a vaso-occlusive crisis (VOC) can generate fat emboli, which cause a marked inflammatory response in the lung. Secretory phospho-

lipase A2 (sPLA2) is an inflammatory mediator which liberates free fatty acids and causes the acute lung injury with PFE. In children with VOC and elevated sPLA2, blood transfusion may prevent development of ACS. ACS also can be caused by rib or sternal infarction.

4. ACS is most common in the 2–4 year age group and declines with increasing age. HbF seems to protect those under 2 years. Incidence is related to genotype: more common in HbSS and HBS beta-0 thalassaemia than in HbSC or HbS beta+ thalassaemia. Lower haematocrit also reduces incidence.

5. Repeated episodes of ACS associated with developing, in adulthood, chronic restrictive lung disease, pulmonary hypertension, cor pulmonale, hypoxia, osteonecrosis at multiple sites, and myocardial infarction.

6. Treatment: avoid hypoxia; judicious intravenous rehydration, analgesia, prevention of atelectasis (with incentive spirometry if possible), antibiotics (for all with fever, and most without), transfusion with packed cells (to increase oxygen carrying capacity), exchange transfusion for clinical deterioration or hypoxia, or unresponsive to other therapies. Transfusion risks include viral disease transmission, acute hyperviscosity and alloimmunisation. In adults, hydroxyurea treatment leads to a significant reduction in ACS.

7. It is the single largest contributor to mortality in children under 2 years.

Eye involvement: retinopathy

Sickle retinopathy is due to retinal blood vessels being plugged by sickled red cells. Lesions may be non-proliferative (e.g. intraretinal haematoma) or proliferative, with tufts of new vessels extending along the retina or into the vitreous. These forms can be seen as early as 5 years of age. Photocoagulation may be used.

Crises: vaso-occlusive crises (VOC) (infarctive crises)

Vascular occlusion in SCA involves both microvascular occlusion (mostly in the bone marrow, causing acute painful episodes or 'crises') and macrovascular occlusion (vessels affected by this [obstructed and injured] are the vulnerable vascular beds in the brain, spleen, lung, eye and heart). Crises and acute chest syndrome (ACS) involve components of bone marrow ischaemia and necrosis, embolisation and inflammation. Over 90% of hospital admissions of adults with SCD are for treatment of painful crises.

Dactylitis (hand-foot syndrome)

1. Infants as young as three months may present with painful swollen hands and feet due to symmetric infarction of red marrow and associated periosteal inflammation involving metacarpals, metatarsals and phalanges. Patients may be misdiagnosed with rheumatological disorders.

2. Dactylitis may be the first sign of diagnosis. Initial X-rays show swelling only, but after a few days' periosteal elevation and areas of osteoporosis and sclerosis may be seen.

3. Rare after 3 years of age, as the haematopoietic tissue in hands and feet is later replaced by fatty tissue.

4. Treatment is pain relief and hydration.

Abdominal involvement

1. Infarction within the spleen, mesenteric lymph nodes or liver.

2. It may present with signs of acute abdomen, with generalised abdominal pain and distension with vomiting, and diminished bowel sounds. X-ray is consistent

with ileus. Management is conservative with IV fluids and nasogastric aspiration.

3. Hepatic sequestration crisis can occur, with sickled cells held up in the liver.

Erectile problems: priapism

1. Painful failure of penile detumescence. 'Stuttering' priapism often occurs: development of erections lasting 1–2 hours. Priapism lasting for over 3 hours is a medical emergency. It is caused by obstruction between corpora cavernosa and spongiosa, followed by sickling within the corpora cavernosa, particularly in adolescents.
2. If the child cannot urinate, this indicates involvement of the corpora spongiosa.
3. Priapism may resolve within a few hours or last more than 24 hours, with extreme pain.
4. Management is medical initially, with analgesia, IV hydration, oxygen, sedation, warmth and exchange transfusion. Non-acute cases can be treated by conjugated oestrogens or vasodilators.
5. If medical treatment is unsuccessful after 12 hours, surgical intervention is required (e.g. cavernosa aspiration and irrigation, the earlier performed, the better).
6. Priapism may cause a fibrotic corpora cavernosa, penile atrophy and impotence.

Limb (bone and joint) involvement

1. Painful episodes usually occur after the age of 3 years.
2. Pathology includes infarction of bone marrow, cortical bone and periarticular tissues.
3. It may present with limitation of movement and swelling.
4. Osteomyelitis may occur, particularly under 5 years of age, with *Salmonella* as the pathogen in over half the cases.
5. Differentiating between infarction and infection can be hard; bone scans may help.
6. Infarcts are the most common in long bones, spine, sternum and ribs.

Leg ulceration

This is secondary to chronic haemolysis and anaemia.

Chronic haemolysis and anaemia

Sequelae include poor growth, delayed puberty and pigmented gallstones.

Haemolytic crisis

This is not common and is associated with a rise in reticulocyte count (which differentiates this from aplasia) and bilirubin level.

Aplastic crisis

1. This is due to compromise of compensatory response (increased red cell production) to ongoing haemolysis.
2. In SCA, red cell survival is only 10 to 20 days. If infection develops, patients may have red cell aplasia for 10–14 days. Causes include parvovirus B19, pneumococci, streptococci, *Salmonella* species, EB virus.
3. Present with pallor, tachypnoea, tachycardia and weakness.
4. White cell and platelet counts are normal; reticulocytes are decreased or absent.
5. Management is with transfusion (packed cells or exchange).

History

Ask about the following.

Presenting complaint

Reason for current admission.

Past history

1. Age and mode of presentation (e.g. screening as newborn, dactylitis as infant, sequestration as toddler, painful crisis as schoolchild).
2. Progress of disease, hospitalisation details, complications experienced (e.g. aplasia, sepsis, stroke), outpatient clinics attended.
3. Past treatment used (e.g. intravenous rehydration, analgesia, bicarbonate).
4. Recent changes in symptoms or management.

Current status

Nature and number of crises per year (e.g. bone, abdominal or chest pain), usual precipitants (e.g. infection), treatment required (e.g. analgesia with narcotics, transfusions), usual outcome.

Ongoing symptoms of complications: directed questioning regarding chronic haemolysis and anaemia (e.g. pallor, lethargy, poor growth, jaundice), neurological deficits (e.g. developmental progress), medications (e.g. prophylactic penicillin for hyposplenism), and management of crises when away from home (e.g. on holidays, travel to remote areas).

Social history

1. Disease impact on patient: effects of hospitalisations, behaviour, school attendance, self-image (e.g. short stature, leg ulcers, delayed puberty), peer group anxieties, narcotic abuse in older children.
2. Disease impact on parents: e.g. financial considerations (medical treatment, awareness of benefits available), modification of holiday plans.
3. Disease impact on siblings: e.g. sibling rivalry, genetic implications (screening for occult disease).
4. Social supports, e.g. social worker, extended family.
5. Coping: e.g. level of understanding of disease by parent (awareness of risks of sepsis, ability to palpate spleen to detect sequestration) and patient (understanding of precautions to take with risks of hypoxia, high altitude, exposure to cold, and of the necessity for penicillin prophylaxis); any problems with analgesic abuse.
6. Access to local doctor, paediatrician and hospital.

Family history

Ethnic origin, consanguinity of parents, other affected members, infant deaths in family, plans for further children, genetic counselling.

Immunisation

Routine, pneumococcal vaccine, meningococcal vaccine, hepatitis B vaccine.

Examination

The following is an outline of the main features to be sought in the long case with sickle cell disease; this approach would also be adequate for a short-case examination.

General inspection

1. Position patient: standing, fully undressed, and then lying down.
2. Parameters: height, weight, head circumference, percentiles.
3. Tanner staging (delayed).
4. Racial origin (e.g. African).
5. Well or unwell (e.g. sepsis, painful crisis).
6. Skin: pallor (aplastic crisis, haemolytic crisis), jaundice, scratch marks (haemolysis).
7. Joint swelling: periarticular infarction.
8. Posture: e.g. hemiparesis (cerebral sickling), restricted movement (bony infarction).
9. Dysphasia (cerebral sickling).
10. Abdominal distension (sequestration crisis).
11. Vital signs: respiratory rate (e.g. pneumonia), pulse (anaemia), blood pressure (hypotension from bleeding), urinalysis (low specific gravity, blood, white cells).

Directed examination for complications

Upper limbs
1. Screen joints for swelling.
2. Palpate bones for tenderness.
3. Neurological assessment.

Head and neck
1. Check eyes for visual field defects (cerebral infarction), conjunctival pallor, scleral icterus, proliferative retinopathy.
2. Examine the motor cranial nerves, especially noting whether there is an upper or lower motor neurone lesion of the seventh nerve (for localisation of damage in hemiplegia).
3. Check mouth for hydration.

Chest
Full examination of praecordium and lung fields for evidence of cardiac murmur, cardiac failure, pulmonary infarction or infection.

Abdomen
Full examination, noting any distension, tenderness, organomegaly.

Lower limbs
1. Inspect for ulcers (ankles).
2. Screen joints for swelling.
3. Palpate bones for tenderness.
4. Assess neurologically, commencing with gait examination for evidence of hemiplegia (or limp with joint involvement).

Management

Common management issues are as follows:
1. Management of acute crises.
2. Complications of medical treatment.
3. Prevention of crises: hydroxyurea.
4. Chronic problems.
5. Specific discussion areas.

Management of acute crises

Treatment of crises

There is no specific treatment, only symptomatic. All children should be admitted to hospital when having a crisis. Antibiotics are used for suspected infection; the ambient ward temperature should be warm. In suspected infarction/sickling, double maintenance intravenous fluids are given (5% dextrose is used as it is isotonic and decreases propensity for sickling). If there is pulmonary involvement, oxygen therapy may be given. In severe sickling episodes, blood transfusions can be used to reduce the percentage of HbSS to around 40–50%, which may prevent further sickling.

In cases with cerebral sickling, exchange transfusion can be performed. Adequate analgesia must be given (e.g. paracetamol, aspirin, codeine). Narcotic analgesia (e.g. morphine infusion) may be needed but the risk of addiction must be considered (see below). Some units give bicarbonate during a crisis as prophylaxis against acidosis.

Prevention of crises

Knowing the common precipitants of crises allows guidelines to be drawn up. Thus, patients should avoid the following:

1. Dehydration, to which they are prone because of their fixed hyposthenuria. Encourage the patient to drink plenty of fluids, especially during viral illnesses or in hot weather. During any infection, dehydration is anticipated and early hydration is instituted.
2. Infection with encapsulated bacteria. Prophylactic penicillin may be given, as well as immunisation against *Pneumococcus*, *Haemophilus influenzae* type b and *Meningococcus*.
3. Vascular stasis. Tight clothing (e.g. fashion jeans, cycling pants) and tourniquets when in hospital must be avoided.
4. Cold temperatures, either environmental (e.g. getting caught in the rain, swimming in rivers, cold baths, washing the car or doing the laundry [adolescents]) or related to ice-cold food or drinks.

A sequestration crisis may not necessarily be prevented by the above measures, but parents can be taught to palpate for splenic enlargement and seek medical attention more rapidly.

Elective surgery

Exchange transfusion should be undertaken before elective surgery. The other points worth noting are the avoidance of tourniquets, avoidance of preoperative dehydration, and ensuring administration of oxygen with any general anaesthetic agent.

Complications of medical treatment

Analgesic abuse is a well-recognised complication in adolescents, so narcotic analgesia is best avoided except when absolutely necessary. Chronic transfusion programs, which are occasionally needed (see later), can be associated with haemosiderosis, as in thalassaemic patients, and consequently the large number of related complications (see the long case on thalassaemia in this chapter). Recent chronic transfusion regimens involve elective red blood cell apheresis (where the patient's red cells are removed at the same time as the patient has a red blood cell transfusion). This reduces the percentage of haemoglobin S and also reduces the need for iron chelation therapy. Other complications of transfusion therapy, such as transmission of HIV and hepatitis C, are infrequent.

Prevention of crises: hydroxyurea

Hydroxyurea can induce production of fetal haemoglobin (HbF) and is used occasionally in some patients with problematic crises. The exact mechanism of action of hydroxyurea is not known, but may involve increasing the percentage of haemoglobin F which protects against sickling (increased intracellular HbF dilutes HbS and inhibits polymerisation) or alternatively reducing the white blood cell count that may be involved in the sickling process. Also, hydroxyurea increases red blood cell hydration, and decreases the expression of red-cell adhesion molecules. In a selected group of severely affected adults, its use clearly resulted in a decrease in the prevalence of painful crises and in transfusion requirements. Many studies subsequently have shown it has equal, if not better, efficacy and safety in children as young as 2 years of age. Hydroxyurea can ameliorate SCA's course to resemble the milder sickle cell–HbC disease, and leads to a decrease in acute chest syndrome and lower rates of painful crises. Hydroxyurea may cause bone marrow suppression and patients need to be monitored carefully during the initiation of treatment and as the dose of hydroxyurea is increased. There is a concern that long-term exposure to hydroxyurea in young patients may cause secondary malignancies.

Chronic problems

Related to intravascular sickling

The most severe problems are neurological sequelae, commonly hemiplegia, which may require extensive rehabilitation, physiotherapy, and occupational and speech therapy. Hemiplegia may be recurrent, causing progressive damage, and warrant chronic transfusion therapy. In adults, chronic failure of various organs (e.g. liver, kidney) is not infrequent, but this tends not to occur in children.

Related to susceptibility to encapsulated organisms

Parents need to be instructed to seek medical help if the child develops a significant fever (e.g. above 38.5°C). At hospital these children should have blood cultures taken, and consideration should be given to admission, and to intravenous or oral antibiotics.

This problem is life-long but is more common in infants. However, adolescents in particular must be reminded that the risk remains, as compliance can be difficult in this age group.

Related to chronic haemolytic anaemia

Chronic ankle ulceration is common in adolescent and adult patients, and is due to inadequate healing (a result of anaemia) of minor traumatic lesions. Management may include complete bed rest (immobilisation), debridement with proteolytic enzymes (or crushed papaya as used in Jamaica), clean dressings, antibiotics, oral zinc sulphate or pinch skin grafting.

Pigmented gallstones can occur from as early as 3 years old. Stones are usually small and multiple, and can block the cystic and bile ducts, or be associated with acute or chronic cholecystitis. May require laparoscopic cholecystectomy. Many units prescribe folic acid to prevent superimposed folate deficiency.

Specific discussion areas

Education

Given that parents assimilate a limited amount of information regarding SCA at any one time, essential facts should be delivered and reinforced incrementally during the course of regular follow up. Parents need to be taught about contingency plans for dealing with any of the following: fever, sudden pallor, abdominal distension, jaundice, recurrent pain (musculoskeletal, chest, abdomen), neurological symptoms (CVAs), swelling of hands and feet, and respiratory distress. A medialert bracelet is advisable. Family should be taught home management of pain, and given guidelines when to contact their doctor. The importance of routine immunisation, plus immunisation against pneumococcus, meningococcus and influenza, cannot be overemphasised. Penicillin therapy and folic acid therapy should be stressed also. Discussion of the child's involvement in appropriate sporting activities is important, while the need for adequate hydration, avoidance of temperature extremes and good dental hygiene must be stressed.

Most patients with SCA know the names of their medications, and their regimens, by the age of around 10 years. Also, they should understand the basics of the pathophysiology.

Issues of adolescence
Problems include poor self-image (especially related to delays in both the adolescent growth spurt and sexual maturation), inability to predict onset, complications, difficulty planning an uncertain future, depression and the realisation of their own mortality. Drug addiction is another concern: adolescents should devise an appropriate pain management plan that explores non-addictive analgesics, but fear of addiction should not lead to denial of narcotics for severe pain.

Pregnancy
This should be discussed with all adolescent female patients. Pregnancy is associated with an increased risk of infarctive crises, urinary tract problems and neonatal morbidity. In terms of contraception, combined oral contraceptives are not recommended as they may increase the risk of vaso-occlusive episodes. Intrauterine devices are unwise: they may produce pelvic sepsis, infertility or menorrhagia. This leaves progesterone-only contraceptives or barrier methods as the most appropriate options.

Genetic counselling
Parents need to be aware of the 1 in 4 risk of recurrence, and not assume that the next three children will be normal. Siblings need to be screened at the time of diagnosis of the child with HbSS. Parents should be given the option of antenatal diagnosis by chorionic villus biopsy at 9 weeks, and if the fetus is an HbSS homozygote, termination may be undertaken if desired. Neonatal testing and resultant improved outcome can be discussed with the parents should they opt for more children irrespective of the risk of an affected infant.

Neonatal screening and prevention of early mortality
Neonatal screening for early detection of HbSS (and related haemoglobinopathies), coupled with comprehensive medical management (immunisations, prophylactic penicillin) has decreased the mortality from sickle haemoglobinopathies.

Retrospective studies have shown previous mortality rates of up to 30% in the first 5 years for patients with HbSS disease. The three greatest risks to the young patient are acute splenic sequestration, aplastic crisis and overwhelming sepsis.

Sepsis has been reported in up to 30% of patients and in some areas is associated with a mortality rate of almost 50%. Commence regular penicillin at 3 months, with immunisation against pneumococcus, *Haemophilus* and meningococcus at 18–24 months, and boosters at 3–5 years. Children with HbSC or S-beta thalassaemia are similarly at risk and require the same approach. The most important feature in preventing early mortality is parental education.

Indications for chronic transfusion

The most common indications are cerebral sickling (particularly recurrent) and unremitting painful crises. A transfusion program may also be needed throughout pregnancy.

Pain

Sickle cell pain is secondary to tissue damage. 'Severe painful crisis' infers treatment at a hospital with parenteral opioids for 4 hours or longer. There are three useful groups of medications with which candidates should be familiar: non-opioids (e.g. paracetamol, non-steroidal anti-inflammatory drugs [NSAIDs]), opioids (e.g. morphine, meperidine) and adjuvants (e.g. antiemetics, antihistamines, laxatives).

Newer approaches to management

Haematopoietic cell transplantation (HCT)

In 1999 the first unrelated cord blood cell transplant was used to cure a 12-year-old boy of SCA. He had some graft-versus-host disease, which responded to prednisolone, and was free of crises and no longer required any transfusions after the procedure. Umbilical cord blood (UCB)—the blood remaining in the placenta after the birth of a child—contains early and committed haematopoietic progenitor cells in sufficient numbers for transplantation. There have been many successful reports of UCB transplantation in SCD from a related donor, the 2-year disease-free survival rate being 90%. Outcomes after UCB transplantation from sibling donors are similar to those after bone marrow transplantation (BMTx): see below. Cryopreserved placental stem cell banks, which collect and store UCB for families who might benefit from UCB transplantation, are becoming established in many countries.

Bone marrow transplantation (BMTx) is the best-established curative procedure, and the most conventional application of HCT, but its risks can outweigh its advantages. These include the risk of infertility, graft-versus-host disease, worsening of sickle-related vascular disease, other complications of conditioning for transplantation (e.g. side-effects of any of busulphan, cyclophosphamide, cyclosporine, methotrexate, anti-thymocyte globulin [ATG] or prednisolone), and a short-term mortality of 10%. Given that the average life span of an SCA patient is 50 years, this must be carefully weighed against the risks of BMTx, also knowing that other treatment modalities are improving rapidly. After BMTx, event-free survival among children with SCA has been around 85%.

Indications for BMTx have included recurrent ACS, CVA and recurrent severe vaso-occlusive crises. Graft rejection occurs in 10–15%. Only 10% of children with HbSS fulfil criteria for BMTx, and only 20% of those have a suitable donor. The best results have been achieved following transplantation from HLA-identical sibling donors. BMTx is a consideration for a child on a long-term transfusion regimen, with HLA identical siblings. Contraindications have included seropositivity for HIV, lack of compliance with medical care, severe lung disease, severe renal impairment, severe neurological impairment, acute hepatitis or severe portal fibrosis or cirrhosis.

Gene therapy

This is likely to be an available treatment within the next decade, but progress has been slow so far due to inadequate gene transfer, and low gene expression. Research has accelerated after the identification of a locus control region (LCR), which is necessary for transcriptional activity of the globin cluster. Research is focusing on gene therapy to inactivate the Hb-S gene, or its messenger RNA, increase the expression of the Hb-F gene, or utilise genes that produce inhibitors of Hb-S polymerisation.

Experimental therapies

Alternative agents for inducing Hb-F production include recombinant human erythro-poietin (r-HuEPO), which can be used in combination with hydroxyurea, butyrate, short-chain fatty acids and arginine butyrate. Trials of these agents have been small and have given conflicting and disappointing results. Clotrimazole, an imidazole anti-mycotic, can decrease HbS polymerisation and prevent red blood cell dehydration by blocking cation-transport channels in erythrocyte membranes: it is being evaluated, but is less effective than hydroxyurea in decreasing cell density.

Thalassaemia: beta-thalassaemia major

The thalassaemias are the most common single gene disease in the world. They are disorders of haemoglobin synthesis, classified according to the globin chain which is ineffectively produced. Beta-thalassaemia major is particularly prevalent in countries around the Mediterranean Sea and the Middle and Far East, and, with population migration, it is found throughout the world. Many components of management are just as relevant in other types of thalassaemia, or thalassaemia-like disorders (e.g. homozygous haemoglobin Lepore, beta-thalassaemia haemoglobin Lepore double heterozygotes, or haemoglobin-E beta-thalassaemia).

Background information

Basic defect (beta-thalassaemia major)

1. Decreased synthesis of the beta globin chain of haemoglobin.
2. Normal synthesis of the alpha chain of haemoglobin, leading to accumulation of unstable aggregates within the red blood cell, resulting in ineffective erythro-poiesis and haemolysis. In patients with concomitant alpha-thalassaemia, the symptoms of haemolysis may be ameliorated.
3. Hypochromic microcytic anaemia (*note*: mean cell volume may be in the normal range for children, but abnormal for that child). Number of reticulocytes is less than expected for the degree of the anaemia. Diagnostic blood film features include target cells, anisocytosis, poikilocytosis, schistocytosis, basophilic stippling and erythroblastosis.

Genetics

1. Autosomal recessive; beta globin gene on the short arm of chromosome 11, in a region that contains the embryonic and fetal globin genes. The expression of these globin genes is controlled by the LCR (locus control region), a major regulatory region containing a series of hypersensitive sites that interact with a variety of transcription factors.
2. Frequency of gene in Greek Cypriots is 0.2; in Italians and Lebanese, 0.04.
3. By 2002, over 200 different molecular defects were known, mostly involving single nucleotide substitutions or oligonucleotide insertions/deletions, that inactivate the beta gene expression by various mechanisms. Some mutations silence the beta globin gene (from mRNA modification at the splicing or cleavage steps, or from RNA mutations causing abnormal translation of the gene to a globin chain product, mostly caused by premature termination codon) resulting in beta-0 thalas-saemia; others reduce beta globin output resulting in beta+ thalassaemia (either by DNA transcriptional mutations at the promoter site, or from mRNA modification at the splicing or cleavage steps). Depending on the residual beta globin production, beta+ thalassaemia may be silent, mild or severe. Beta-0 thalassaemia mutations are usually severe.

Diagnosis

1. Usually not clinically evident until the child is 6–12 months old.
2. Definitive diagnosis is by haemoglobin electrophoresis: HbA is absent or minimal, HbF is elevated, and HbA_2 may be raised.

Major complications

Excess erythropoiesis

1. Bony changes to face: maxillary overgrowth, protrusion of teeth, separation of orbits, frontal bossing, chronic sinusitis and impaired hearing.
2. Bones (general): cortical thinning and risk of fractures. Most adult patients get osteopenia and osteoporosis, with backache, scoliosis, fractures, other spinal deformities. Males who are diabetic and have pubertal delay are most at risk for osteoporosis. DEXA (dual X-ray absorptiometry) assesses for bone density.
3. Spinal cord compression (vertebral expansion).
4. Lymphadenopathy (especially mediastinal).
5. Hepatosplenomegaly.

Iron overload

This is transfusional or from increased iron absorption. A packed red blood cell unit of 250 mL has around 175 mg of iron.

Endocrine failure (in order of frequency)

1. Short stature: growth is usually normal until about 12 years, but no pubertal growth spurt occurs: two-thirds of these children are below the tenth height percentile at 21 years. Possible pituitary or hypothalamic defect. Growth hormone level may be normal or raised.
2. Delayed puberty: gonadotropin levels are normal until puberty, but then no increase occurs.
3. Oestrogen/testosterone deficiency.
4. Hypothyroidism.
5. Diabetes mellitus.
6. Hypoparathyroidism.

Cardiac involvement

1. Cardiomyopathy from myocardial iron deposition, hypertrophy, dilatation, degeneration of myocardial fibres; unbound iron generates toxic oxygen metabolites; higher risk for myocarditis; occasional pulmonary hypertension.
2. Pericarditis: first attack usually after 10 years of age.
3. Arrhythmias, both ventricular and atrial, can occur. The risk is much increased after 150–200 units of blood.
4. Congestive cardiac failure: once this develops, the mortality is 90% within 12–18 months. Cardiac function can be reversed by aggressive chelation. Treatment may include angiotensin-converting enzyme (ACE) inhibitors, digoxin, diuretics and low-salt diet, in addition to chelation therapy. If refractory to medical treatment, heart transplantation is an appropriate consideration.
5. Measurement of liver iron correlates best with total body iron and predicts the threshold for risk for cardiac disease and early death (levels over 15 mg/g dry weight). Ferritin over 2500 microgram/L can help predict cardiac disease.
6. Heart disease is the main cause of death in transfusion-induced iron-overload patients.

Hepatic involvement

1. Cirrhosis and hepatic fibrosis: risk for this is increased after 7 years of treatment.
2. Liver function tests may be abnormal, but it is rare to see symptoms of cirrhosis. If hepatic enzyme levels are increased 4–5-fold, then there is a possibility of hepatitis and liver biopsy may be needed.
3. Common cause of morbidity and early death; worsened by coexistent hepatitis C.
4. If hepatitis C (HCV) is suspected, liver biopsy is needed and HCV RNA polymerase chain reaction (PCR) should be checked. Image to exclude hepatocellular carcinoma. Treatment with alpha interferon and ribavirin can improve liver disease, but side effects can include haemolysis, which increases transfusion requirements.

Chronic haemolysis

Gallstones are present in 50–70% of patients by around 15 years of age. Consider cholecystectomy only if biliary colic or obstructive jaundice occurs. At the time of splenectomy, consider ultrasound of the gall bladder and cholecystectomy if calculi are present. Appendicectomy at this time may be appropriate, because these patients are at risk of *Yersinia* infection, which can mimic appendicitis and might lead to surgery at a time when an operation should be contraindicated.

Hypercoagulable state

The mechanism involves platelet function, elevated endothelial adhesion protein levels and activation of coagulation cascade by damaged red cells. Deep venous thrombosis, pulmonary embolism (mostly asymptomatic) and cerebral ischaemia have been described.

Infection

There is increased risk of infection, particularly *Yersinia*, in iron-overload patients; patients may be splenectomised.

History

Ask about the following.

Presenting complaint

Reason for current admission.

Past history

1. Ethnic origin.
2. Diagnosis (age, where, how).
3. Age at first transfusion and at commencement of desferrioxamine (DFO).
4. Number of transfusions per year.
5. Previous hospitalisations (other than routine transfusions), previous surgery (e.g. splenectomy), medications given (e.g. penicillin with splenectomy, vitamin C).

Specific complications

Current status of the following complications (mnemonic **THALASSAEMIA**):

T	**T**anner stage (pubertal delay)
H	**H**eart (cardiomyopathy), **H**aematopoiesis (extramedullary), **H**ypercoagulable
A	**A**naemia
L	**L**iver, **L**ong tracts (neurological involvement) and **L**eg ulcers

A   **A**ppearance (thalassaemic facies, pigmentation)
S   **S**ugar diabetes
S   **S**hort stature
A   **A**rrhythmias
E   **E**ye and **E**ndocrine
M   **M**etabolic (hypocalcaemia) and **M**alocclusion
I   **I**ron overload, **I**cterus, **I**nfection and **I**atrogenic (DFO side effects)
A   **A**denopathy and hepatosplenomegaly.

Family history

Consanguinity of parents, other affected members, neonatal deaths in family, plans for further children, genetic counselling.

Social history

1. Disease impact on patient: e.g. effects of hospitalisations, behaviour, school performance, amount of school missed, self-image, pubertal anxieties, peer group anxieties, stigma of 'bad blood', adolescent denial, poor compliance, anxiety, 'live for today' approach, concerns about developing relationships, wanting a family.
2. Disease impact on parents: e.g. marriage stability, financial considerations (family income, cost of DFO and pump), dealing with noncompliance and teenage rebellion.
3. Disease impact on siblings: e.g. sibling rivalry.
4. Social supports: e.g. extended family, Australian Thalassaemia Association and state thalassaemia societies, social worker, financial benefits obtained (e.g. Children's Disability Allowance).
5. Coping: e.g. compliance, degree of self-management, perception of disease and its rate of progression, future plans, career thoughts.

Examination

See the short case on thalassaemia in this chapter.

Standard management principles

Blood transfusion

1. Regular transfusions every 4–6 weeks.
2. Timing of first transfusion usually at haemoglobin <60 g/L.
3. Maintain haemoglobin above 100 g/L (range 100–150 g/L, e.g. pretransfusion Hb about 95 g/L, post-transfusion 140 g/L, with a mean of about 120 g/L). This level is enough to suppress endogenous erythropoiesis and compensatory marrow hyperplasia, while avoiding unnecessary iron overload.
4. Use packed cells, or filtered red blood cells, negative for hepatitis B, C and HIV (phenotyped filtered red cells).
5. Watch for reactions at the time of transfusions.
6. Pre-transfusion investigations: group and cross-match (genotype); full blood count (for haemoglobin level, reticulocyte count, and to assess for hypersplenism); initial viral serology for hepatitis B, C (± G: research units), cytomegalovirus (CMV), toxoplasmosis, Ebstein-Barr virus, HIV; assessment for alloantibodies. Red cell genotype determines all the important red cell groups, including Duffy and Kell. Antibody screening at the time of cross-match is to detect any irregular alloantibodies.

Whenever the child is seen (at monthly transfusion and at regular outpatient review), assessment of transfusion requirements is needed, looking at pre-transfusion haemoglobin and transfusion interval. If the child needs more frequent transfusions than previously, the considerations include the following.

1. Development of hypersplenism ($\pm$ decreased platelet and white cell counts).
2. Development of red cell antibodies.
3. Concurrent gastrointestinal blood loss.
4. Use of 'old' blood.

Chelation with desferrioxamine

1. Start when ferritin level is around 1000–2000 mcg/L (before 3–4 years) or at preschool age.
2. Must be given subcutaneously or intravenously, aiming for negative iron balance.
3. Dosage is 40 mg/kg subcutaneously over 8–10 hours, 6 days per week.
4. Side effects include local irritation and hypotension if given too quickly intravenously. More severe effects were originally described when doses in the range 100 to 200 mg/kg/day were used. These included problems with vision (cataracts, night blindness, reduction of visual fields, decreased visual acuity, and pigmentary retinopathy) and hearing (sensorineural deafness). Other side effects described have included bone abnormalities (pseudorickets, metaphyseal changes, flat vertebral bodies) and altered renal function. Curently, doses are usually less than 50 mg/kg/day, and these effects are not often seen.
5. Pre-chelation evaluation may include clinical photography, bone X-rays, ferritin level, full blood count, liver function tests, thyroid function tests, fasting blood glucose level, tests of the hypothalamic–pituitary axis, calcium, phosphate and magnesium, audiovisual assessment (audiometry and slit-lamp examination), baseline electrocardiogram.
6. Avoidance of red meat and cereals should be recommended.
7. Patients who are compliant with iron chelation therapy should have a life expectancy of more than 50 years.
8. DFO treatment is suspended if the patient has sepsis, as DFO promotes *Yersinia enterocolitica* gastroenteritis.
9. New oral chelator therapies are available and under investigation.

Splenectomy

1. Main indication is hypersplenism, usually evidenced by increased transfusion requirements. Another indication is a 'large spleen', causing discomfort.
2. Most authorities recommend the use of pneumococcal and meningococcal vaccines (given before splenectomy) and prophylactic penicillin.
3. Consideration should also be given to gall bladder ultrasound for calculi, with a view to the possible need for cholecystectomy, which can be performed at the same time as splenectomy. Appendicectomy can be performed at the same time.
4. If a patient with a splenectomy is febrile, blood cultures should be taken and treatment instituted with intravenous antibiotics in hospital or oral antibiotics at home.
5. Some units recommend splenectomy only if transfusion requirements exceed 180–200 mL/kg/year.

Previous 'standard' therapies

1. Vitamin C is no longer widely used, as large doses, without DFO, have been linked to development of cardiomyopathy.
2. Vitamin E is no longer used, as there is scant evidence for its efficacy.
3. Folate has a place in treating children before they require transfusion, but is unnecessary after this.

Immunisation

Routine (should include hepatitis B), plus pneumococcal vaccine (before splenectomy, and boosters every 5 years), meningococcal vaccine (splenectomised) and influenza vaccine.

Common management issues

Although the previous section is headed 'Standard management principles', much is not 'black and white', but 'grey'. This section touches on some of these areas.

When to start transfusions?

This is really a clinical decision. There is no specific haemoglobin level, but if the level is below 50 g/L, there needs to be a good reason not to transfuse. Careful assessment in the first 2 months after diagnosis is needed, and treatment with folate. If there is any failure to thrive, significant anaemia or (especially) cardiac compromise related to anaemia, then transfusion should probably be instituted.

Which transfusion regimen?

The aim of transfusion is to correct anaemia and achieve marrow suppression to decrease myeloproliferation. Usually a level of between 100 and 150 g/L is desirable, but this depends upon the individual patient. Some patients with a haemoglobin level of 110 g/L will have multiple nucleated red cells and will need to be transfused to over 120 g/L, whereas in other patients 110 g/L may suffice. If the patient presents quite late (e.g. at 3 or 4 years of age) with splenomegaly, on occasion splenectomy can be offered first, which may cause a rise in the haemoglobin and defer the need to start transfusion therapy. Most children require transfusion every 4 weeks.

When to chelate?

Essentially, chelation should start when the child is big enough for the parents to manage needles. Another indicator is a rising ferritin level. By 3–4 years of age, most patients have been transfused for 2 years. These children may have ferritin levels over 2000 mcg/L. Some haematologists commence chelation when the ferritin level reaches 1000 mcg/L.

How to chelate?

Some units chelate daily for the first 6 months, then allow one day off per week. Thus most patients have chelation therapy 6 days a week, by subcutaneous infusion. When the child is having regular transfusion therapy, some units add desferrioxamine to the blood being transfused, whereas other centres are adverse to this idea for reasons of potential lack of sterility.

Are there alternative chelators?

DFO is standard therapy. It has high molecular weight (MW), is poorly absorbed from the gut and so is given parenterally. The DFO molecule has six binding sites and wraps itself around the iron nucleus. An oral chelator, deferiprone (DFP), is an alternative for patients who cannot tolerate DFO because of adverse effects, or who are non-compliant with (the injectable) DFO. DFP has only two binding sites: three molecules are needed to bind one iron atom. It has low MW and is readily absorbed from the gut; however, it can penetrate other cells and interfere with iron-requiring enzyme systems. DFP is used predominantly in countries where the effects of haemosiderosis outweigh the risks of DFP. DFP side effects can include neutropenia and agranulocytosis (idiosyncratic, but reversible), arthropathy (affects mainly large joints; usually reversible), zinc deficiency, gut symptoms and fluctuations in liver function. Other iron chelators are being developed, including a long-acting form of DFO. A newer chelator agent, ICL 670, offers promise.

Potential of haematopoietic cell transplantation (HCT)

BMTx from an HLA identical sibling is the most conventional form of HCT that can cure beta-thalassaemia. There appear to be three clinically important variables in patients under 16 that are predictive of the success of BMTx. If there is (a) no significant liver enlargement, (b) no liver fibrosis and (c) adherence to the regular high-quality iron chelation, there is around 90% event-free survival. The rate decreases as the risk factors increase.

The enthusiasm for this mode of treatment varies between countries. Some countries prefer to wait for breakthroughs in genetic engineering or a HbF switch mechanism, whereas in Italy BMTx is quite popular but has a 10% mortality rate related to infection or acute graft-versus-host reaction. The donor must be fully compatible (usually a sibling who is normal or heterozygous). It is not justified to offer any mismatched or matched unrelated donor transplantation. This treatment modality should be discussed with the parents of any child with thalassaemia, so that they are aware of this option in the future.

Cord-blood–derived stem cell transplantation (CB-SCT) can also cure thalassaemia major. Umbilical cord blood (UCB), the blood remaining in the placenta after the birth of a child, contains early and committed haematopoietic progenitor cells in sufficient numbers for transplantation. There have been many successful reports of UCB transplantation in beta thalassaemia from a related donor, the 2-year disease-free survival rate being 79%. Outcomes after UCB transplantation from sibling donors are similar to those after bone marrow transplantation (BMTx).

Gene therapy

This will produce a definitive cure for beta thalassaemia major eventually, but currently there remain problems in the development of high-level gene expression, safe vectors, and gene regulation.

Fetal haemoglobin augmentation: hydroxyurea, erythropoietin

Hydroxyurea can induce production of fetal haemoglobin (HbF). Hydroxyurea has been reported to eliminate transfusion requirements in some children with severe beta thalassaemia with specific mutations. Some studies have used recombinant human erythropoietin (r-HuEPO) by itself or with hydroxyurea. It is a very cost-effective treatment and an ideal option for millions of people in developing countries who do not have access to safe transfusion and chelation.

Hepatitis C

For patients who are positive for hepatitis C (HCV), alpha interferon and ribavirin are the only treatments shown to have any positive effect. Alpha interferon is given subcutaneously three times weekly. Monitoring is needed for neutropenia, thrombocytopenia, hypothyroidism (anti-thyroid peroxidase level can predict this), depression and retinopathy. Response to treatment can be monitored by HCV titres. Some units recommend 6-monthly liver ultrasound studies, and even yearly liver biopsies, to look for hepatocellular carcinoma.

Prenatal diagnosis

There are over 200 different molecular defects known for beta-thalassaemia. Within given communities, there are a dozen or so common molecular defects. Specific oligonucleotide probes are available to assess fetal DNA for diagnosis.

Follow-up

For the preschool child, some units recommend monthly pre-transfusion outpatient clinic reviews. For older children, an outpatient review is warranted on a 6-monthly basis, monitoring in particular the child's growth. In terms of investigations, some units recommend the following.

1. Check of ferritin level (degree of iron overload) every 3–6 months. Once on DFO, if ferritin levels are 2000 mcg/L, this suggests noncompliance. Levels over 3000 mcg/L may warrant liver biopsy (for dry-weight iron content) and hospital admission for continuous intravenous DFO once or twice a month.

2. Blood tests every 6 months for calcium, magnesium, phosphate (hypoparathyroidism), liver function (hepatitis or hepatic fibrosis), thyroid function (hypothyroidism), urea, electrolytes and creatinine (renal dysfunction from DFO). If ALT is elevated repeat in one month: if still up, check for hepatitis A, B, C, G, or CMV or EBV. If ALT is elevated for 3 months, consider liver biopsy and hepatitis viral titres by RNA analysis. HIV serology should be checked as well.

3. Yearly assessments for desferrioxamine toxicity (audiometry and slit-lamp examination) and of growth and pubertal status (bone age, and, over the age of 14, tests of the hypothalamic pituitary axis). By the age of puberty, essentially all these patients attend endocrine outpatient clinics. The boys usually require supplementation with testosterone preparations, and the girls low-dose oestrogens and progestogens. Screening for the development of diabetes mellitus includes testing for glycosuria and performing glucose tolerance tests. Approximately 50% of patients will have an abnormal glucose tolerance test by 10 years of age.

4. Yearly cardiac assessment, with a gated blood pool scan in children over 10 years to assess left ventricular ejection fraction (at rest and during exercise) is the preferred cardiac investigation. Some units recommend annual ECG, Holter monitoring and cardiac stress testing.

5. Annual dental examination is useful. Dental procedure antibiotic prophylaxis in splenectomised patients is important. Reminding these patients to take their antibiotics is another important point in follow-up.

Other points regarding clinic follow-up include the discussion of any emotional or social problems.

Prognosis

A favourite question is: 'What do you tell the parents of a child newly diagnosed with thalassaemia major?' The answer should include telling the parents the following:

- The child is very likely to need transfusions.
- A wait-and-see approach regarding the need for, and frequency of, transfusions should be adopted.
- A cure by HCT, or genetic engineering, may be possible (after discussing the more standard treatment options).
- Current treatment modalities allow patients to reach young adulthood, by which time better treatments and probably a cure may be available.

Compliance

Teenage rebellion is often a problem and is very difficult to manage, but must be addressed in adolescents with chronic disease.

The issue of further children

Parents are often angry that they have not 'beaten the odds' if they already knew the 1 in 4 risk, and had wrongly assumed that the next three children would be normal. This raises the issue of further children and prenatal diagnosis.

HIV risk

HIV infection is rare in patients with thalassaemia. Since donor screening commenced in 1985, the risk has declined towards zero.

Summary

In discussing your management, as well as being familiar with the above-mentioned areas, it is worthwhile asking the examiners for results of relevant investigations, such as the ferritin level, liver function tests, most recent chest X-ray and ECG, and the latest eye and hearing checks, as this is what you would need to know in practice. Of course, appropriate interpretation of this information is expected, if it is requested.

Short cases

The haematological system

The usual introduction involves assessment for anaemia or bruising.

First, note the child's sex (haemophilia and glucose-6-phosphate dehydrogenase deficiency [G6PD] are X-linked), nationality (thalassaemia is more common in children of Asian or Mediterranean descent, and SCA is more common in African children), growth (short with some syndromes, SCA or chronic renal failure [CRF]), and any dysmorphic features (Fanconi's anaemia, Blackfan-Diamond red cell aplasia, thrombocytopenia absent radius [TAR]; see later).

Check, and comment on, the growth parameters. The head circumference may be increased with a subdural haematoma from non-accidental injury (NAI), which may present with unexplained bruising. Weight may be decreased in children with a nutritional deficiency as the basis of their anaemia. Note pubertal status (delay in SCA, thalassaemia).

Assess whether the child looks sick or well. Patients with acute lymphoblastic leukaemia (ALL), CRF, haemophilia complicated by HIV, or purpura due to meningo-coccaemia look unwell. Patients with SCA may be in pain if a recent crisis has occurred. Infants with NAI may be wary of any attempts to get close. Note any pallor (various causes of anaemia).

Note any abnormal posturing suggesting hemiplegia, which can complicate haemophilia or SCA. Visually scan the joints for swelling, which can occur in haemophilia, SCA, Henoch-Schönlein purpura (HSP), ALL, inflammatory bowel disease (IBD) such as Crohn's disease, or juvenile idiopathic arthritis (JIA): the latter two can present with anaemia. Also note any abdominal distension (due to hepato-splenomegaly) and needle marks on the abdomen (DFO therapy).

Examine the skin for petechiae, purpura and ecchymoses. If any of these are present, make a thorough assessment of their distribution (e.g. purpura on buttocks in HSP, fingertip-shaped bruises in NAI). In the case of purpuric areas, note whether they are raised and/or tender (vasculitic) or flat and/or non-tender (platelet deficiency or dysfunction). Note any jaundice or scratch marks (haemolysis), haemangiomas (which can cause a consumptive coagulopathy), cigarette burns. Also look for the cutaneous manifestations of systemic lupus erythematosus (SLE) and peripheral stigmata of chronic liver disease (CLD), which can be associated with a coagulopathy.

The remainder of the examination is best commenced at the hands, working up to the head, and then downwards.

Look at the nails for koilonychia (iron deficiency), leuconychia (CLD), clubbing (CLD, congenital heart disease [CHD]), splinter haemorrhages (subacute bacterial endocarditis [SBE]). Inspect the palms for crease pallor (suggests haemoglobin level below 70 g/L) or palmar erythema (CLD). Note the pulse rate (anaemia). Moving up the forearm, examine the epitrochlear nodes bilaterally. Then request, or take, the blood pressure for evidence of hypertension (as the result of CRF, haemolytic uraemic syndrome (HUS), or as the cause of microangiopathic haemolytic anaemia [MAHA]) or hypotension (acute blood loss, cardiomyopathy from iron overload), or increased pulse pressure (anaemia). Then examine the axillary nodes bilaterally.

Next, examine the head and neck, followed by the chest wall, spine, abdomen, gait, lower limbs and heart. This is outlined in Figure 10.1.

A mnemonic that may be useful for outlining the order of the examination, is the eleven Ss: sex, syndrome, size, structure (hands), scone (head), sternum, spine, spleen (abdomen), stand (gait and lower limbs), SBE (heart) and stool.

At the completion of the examination, request results of stool analysis for blood, urinalysis for blood, protein, fixed low specific gravity (CRF) or infection, and the temperature chart for infection.

An alternative approach is based on assessing the three cell lines first, by looking at skin and mucous membranes: (a) the red cell line for deficiency (signs of anaemia) or excess (plethora from polycythaemia), (b) the white cell line for deficiency or excess (gingivitis, infected skin lesions), or (c) platelet deficiency (signs of bruising). After this, examine the three main areas of interest:

1. First all the lymph nodes (lymphadenopathy with ALL, AML, lymphoma), and the abdomen (hepatosplenomegaly, or abdominal masses, from ALL or AML infil-trates, or extramedullary haematopoiesis).
2. Next the musculoskeletal examination (skeletal tenderness at sternum, clavicles, ribs, spine, pelvis, tibiae [leukaemic infiltrates, SCA]; joint tenderness, swelling or decreased range of movement [ALL, AML, SCA, IBD, HSP, JIA]).
3. Finally dysmorphic features.

Figure 10.1 The haematological system

1. Introduce self

2. General inspection
Position patient: standing, undressed;
   then lying down

3. Upper limbs
Structure
Joint swelling
Nails
Palms
Pulse
Epitrochlear nodes
Blood pressure
Axillary nodes

4. Head and neck
Face
Ears
Eyes (include fundoscopy)
Nose
Mouth
Tongue
Gums
Palate
Throat
Neck (lymph nodes)

5. Chest wall
Spider naevi (CLD)
Supraclavicular nodes
Skeletal tenderness:
- Sternum
- Clavicles
- Shoulders
- Spine (ALL, NAI)

6. Abdomen
Distension
Splenomegaly
Hepatomegaly
Enlarged kidneys
Genitalia
Inguinal lymph nodes
Pelvis (spring)
Buttocks

7. Lower limbs and gait
Inspect
Palpate
Gait
Neurological
Joints

8. Cardiovascular system
Full praecordial examination

9. Other
Urinalysis
Stool analysis
Temperature chart

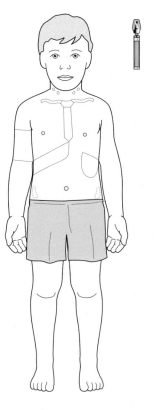

ALL = acute lymphoblastic leukaemia; CLD = chronic liver disease; NAI = non-accidental injury.

This approach thoroughly assesses one system at a time and is easy to remember. The only disadvantage is that it does not flow quite as smoothly as the 'Ss' approach.

A comprehensive listing of findings not listed above is given in Table 10.1. Which of the findings listed is relevant depends on the particular case involved.

After presenting your findings, you may be asked by the examiners which investigations you would perform. Depending on the presenting problem, a suggested plan is given below.

Table 10.1 Additional information: comprehensive listing of possible findings in the haematological examination

General inspection

Well or unwell (DIC, ALL, meningococcaemia)

Sex (haemophilia, G6PD deficiency in males)

Race

- Thalassaemia in Mediterraneans, Asians
- SCA in African-Americans, Jamaicans, Middle Eastern

Syndrome (Fanconi's, Blackfan-Diamond, TAR)

Thalassaemic 'chipmunk' facies

Parameters: height, weight, head circumference, percentiles

Pubertal status: delayed (thalassaemia, SCA)

Nutritional status

Posture: hemiplegia (haemophilia, SCA)

Skin

- Pallor
- Petechiae, purpura, ecchymoses (ALL, AML, aplastic anaemia, ITP)
- Pigmentation (thalassaemia)
- Jaundice, scratch marks (haemolysis, CLD)
- Cavernous haemangiomas (can cause Kasabach-Merritt syndrome; MAHA)
- Cigarette burns (NAI)
- SLE rashes
- CLD stigmata
- Subcutaneous nodules (ALL)
- Small angiomata (HHT)
- Eczema (Wiskott-Aldrich syndrome)
- Infected lesions (immune deficiency, ALL, AML)

Joint swelling (haemophilia, HSP, SCA, leukaemia, IBD, JIA)

Upper limbs

Structure of:

- Forearms (TAR)
- Thumbs (Fanconi's, Blackfan-Diamond)

Joint swelling (JIA)

Nails

- Koilonychia (iron deficiency)
- Leuconychia (CLD)
- Clubbing (CHD, CLD)

Palms

- Crease pallor (anaemia)
- Crease pigmentation (thalassaemia)
- Erythema (CLD)

Pulse: tachycardia

Epitrochlear nodes

Blood pressure

- Hypertension (CRF, HUS, or as cause of MAHA)
- Hypotension (acute blood loss, cardiomyopathy)
- Raised pulse pressure (anaemia)

Axillary nodes

Head and neck

Face (thalassaemic facies, syndromal, Cushingoid, SLE)

Ears

- Abnormal structure (Fanconi's)
- Discharge (Wiskott-Aldrich syndrome)

Eyes

- Squint (Fanconi's, sixth cranial nerve palsy with intracranial bleed)
- Ptosis (Fanconi's)
- Nystagmus (Fanconi's, intracranial bleeding)
- Conjunctival pallor
- Scleral icterus
- Subconjunctival haemorrhage
- Cataracts (DFO or corticosteroid therapy)

Fundoscopy

- Retinal haemorrhage (ALL, AML, NAI)
- Roth spots (SBE)
- Papilloedema (raised intracranial pressure with ALL, AML, NAI)
- Proliferative retinopathy (SCA)
- Retinopathy from DFO

Nose: evidence of epistaxis

Mouth: angular cheilosis (iron deficiency)

Tongue

- Pale atrophic (iron deficiency)
- Raw, beefy (B group vitamin deficiency)
- Red spots (HHT)

Gums

- Hypertrophy (ALL, AML)
- Inflammation (ALL, AML)

Palate: petechiae

Tonsils

- Hypertrophy (ALL, AML)
- Exudate (EB virus)

Continued

Table 10.1 *(Continued)*

Neck: enlarged cervical nodes (viral infections, lymphomas, ALL, AML)

Abdomen
Distension (due to hepatosplenomegaly)
Needle marks on abdomen (DFO treatment)
Splenomegaly
- Haemoglobinopathies
- Malignancy (ALL, AML)
- Infection (SBE)
- Osteopetrosis
- Storage diseases
- Congenital spherocytosis

Hepatomegaly: as above, plus hepatitis and Wilson's disease (decrease in clotting factors I, II and V)
Enlarged kidneys (ALL)
Adrenal mass (neuroblastoma)
Genitalia
- Tanner staging (delay with thalassaemia, SCA)
- Testes: enlarged (ALL, HSP: orchitis or bleeding)
- Penis: priapism (SCA, ALL, CML)

Inguinal nodes
Spring pelvis (bony tenderness)
Posterior iliac crests (bone marrow aspiration site)
Buttocks (HSP rash)
Perianal region: fissures, fistulae (IBD)

Lower limbs and gait
Inspection
- Joint swelling (see above)
- Ulcers (SCA)
- Erythema nodosum (IBD)

Palpate: tibial tenderness (ALL, NAI)
Stand: Rombergism (vitamin B_{12} deficiency)
Walk
- Antalgic gait (haemophilia with haemarthrosis, ALL, SCA)
- Ataxic gait (vitamin B_{12} deficiency)
- Hemiplegic (haemophilia with intracranial bleed, SCA with cerebral sickling)

Depending on above findings, further examination of:
- Joints
- Peripheral nervous system
- Central nervous system

Cardiovascular system
Full praecordial examination, looking for evidence of:
- SBE
- Cardiac surgery (fragmentation anaemia with artificial valves)
- Congenital heart disease (associated with bruising; syndromes)
- Cardiomyopathy (transfusion haemosiderosis with thalassaemia or SCA)
- Cardiac failure (anaemia)

Other
Urinalysis
- Blood (haemophilia, SCA, HUS)
- Haemoglobin (intravascular haemolysis)
- Urobilinogen (haemolysis)
- Protein (renal disease)
- Specific gravity (SCA, CRF)

Stool analysis: blood (HSP, IBD)
Temperature chart
Hess test can be offered in older child if relevant

Selected syndrome findings
Blackfan-Diamond red cell aplasia
- Turner syndrome-like phenotype
- Bone deformities
- Ocular abnormalities
- Abnormal ears
- Cleft lip
- Abnormal thumbs (bifid, double or triphalangeal thumbs)
- Talipes

Fanconi's anaemia
- Short stature
- Café-au-lait spots
- Pigmentation at groin, trunk and axilla
- Small head
- Squint, ptosis, nystagmus
- Abnormal ears
- Abnormal hands (aplastic, hypoplastic, or supernumery thumbs; syndactyly; decreased number of carpal bones; occasionally, absent radius)
- Small genitalia

Thrombocytopenia absent radius (TAR) syndrome
- Radius absent, but thumbs present

Continued

Table 10.1 *(Continued)*

Dyskeratosis congenita	*Wiskott-Aldrich syndrome*
• Male (usually)	• Eczema (severe)
• Nail ridging and atrophy	• Ear discharge, other infections
• Pigmentation (brown-grey) with	(middle ear, chest, skin)
telangiectasia and atrophy, at head,	• Immune deficiency, decreased IgM,
neck, shoulders, chest	infections (middle ear, chest, skin)
• Mucous membrane leukoplakia	• Thrombocytopenia, small platelets
• Sparse hair	
• Hyperkeratosis of palms and soles	

ALL = acute lymphoblastic leukaemia; AML = acute myeloid leukaemia; CHD = congenital heart disease; CLD = chronic liver disease; CRF = chronic renal failure; DIC = disseminated intravascular coagulation; G6PD = glucose-6-phosphate dehydrogenase deficiency; HHT = hereditary haemorrhagic telangiectasia; HSP = Henoch-Schönlein purpura; HUS = haemolytic uraemic syndrome; IBD = inflammatory bowel disease; JIA = juvenile idiopathic arthritis; MAHA = microangiopathic haemolytic anaemia; NAI = non-accidental injury; SBE = subacute bacterial endocarditis; SCA = sickle cell anaemia; SLE = systemic lupus erythematosus; TAR = thrombocytopenia absent radius.

Anaemia

The full blood examination and film is the most useful investigation. Classification based on the size and appearance of the red blood cells is well known and can be very useful. The three most commonly described morphologies are as follows.

1. Microcytic

The most common cause of this is iron deficiency. Other causes include thalassaemia minor and chronic inflammation.

2. Normocytic

This group can be subdivided into two groups, based on the reticulocyte count:

1. A low reticulocyte response occurs most commonly with transient erythroblastopenia of childhood. Other causes include aplastic crises and Blackfan-Diamond anaemia.
2. A high reticulocyte count occurs with bleeding or haemolysis. Haemolysis can be classified by extrinsic or intrinsic causes.

Extrinsic causes
1. Mechanical injury to red cells (e.g. small vessel disease in HUS or in disseminated intravascular coagulation [DIC], or larger vessel disease such as poorly epithelialised prosthetic cardiac valves).
2. Chronic renal or liver disease.
3. Haemolysis mediated by antibodies, including autoimmune haemolytic anaemia (e.g. warm antibody type in Epstein-Barr virus infections, cold antibody type in mycoplasma infections), and isoimmune haemolysis (e.g. incompatible transfusions).

Intrinsic causes
1. Membrane abnormalities (e.g. hereditary spherocytosis).
2. Enzyme abnormalities (e.g. G6PD).
3. Haemoglobin disorders (e.g. SCA).

3. Macrocytic

This can occur with folate or vitamin B_{12} deficiency.

Bleeding

This may be due to abnormalities of blood vessels, platelets or the coagulation system. The useful screening investigations include the following:

1. Full blood count and film, noting haemoglobin level (associated anaemia, e.g. in aplastic anaemia or ALL), white cell count (e.g. leucopenia in aplastic anaemia, blast forms in ALL), any thrombocytopenia, and also platelet size (large in Bernard-Soulier syndrome).
2. Prothrombin time, which assesses the extrinsic coagulation system.
3. Partial thromboplastin time, which assesses the intrinsic coagulation system.

In bleeding associated with vascular defects, the above tests will be normal.

Although mentioned in some texts, a bleeding time should not be done in children. It is painful, unable to be standardised and there are now better tests for von Willebrand's disease. These include:

1. Platelet aggregation studies with ristocetin (an antibiotic that causes vWF to bind to platelets and activate them). These studies reflect both plasma and platelet von Willebrand Factor (vWF);
2. vWF antigen (VIII-related antigen).
3. vWF activity (ristocetin cofactor).
4. vWF factor multimer analysis.

Thalassaemia

This case involves demonstrating the complications of extramedullary haematopoiesis, iron overload and desferrioxamine (DFO) therapy.

As mentioned in the long case, the mnemonic **THALASSAEMIA** helps list the important areas to examine:

T	**T**anner stage (pubertal delay)
H	**H**eart (cardiomyopathy), **H**aematopoiesis (extramedullary), **H**ypercoagulable
A	**A**naemia
L	**L**iver, **L**ong tracts (neurological involvement) and **L**eg ulcers
A	**A**ppearance (thalassaemic facies, pigmentation)
S	**S**ugar diabetes
S	**S**hort stature
A	**A**rrhythmias
E	**E**ye and **E**ndocrine
M	**M**etabolic (hypocalcaemia) and **M**alocclusion
I	**I**ron overload, **I**cterus, **I**nfection and **I**atrogenic (DFO side effects)
A	**A**denopathy and hepatosplenomegaly

Initial inspection should include assessment of growth parameters (usually short, head circumference often increased [due to skull bossing], pubertal status delayed), colour (pigmentation from melanin and iron deposition, pallor from anaemia, jaundice from haemolysis), whether the child has any respiratory distress (e.g. anaemia or cardiomyopathy causing congestive cardiac failure [CCF], or massive splenomegaly causing marked increase in intra-abdominal pressure), and description of any obvious

Figure 10.2 Thalassaemia

1. Introduce self

2. General inspection

Position patient: standing, adequately
  exposed; then lying down

Parameters
- Height
- Weight
- Percentiles

Tanner staging

Well or unwell

Colour
- Pigmentation
- Pallor
- Jaundice

Facial features
- Frontal bossing
- Parietal bossing
- Chipmunk facies
- Maxillary overgrowth
- Dental malocclusion
- Prominent malar eminence
- Broadened nasal bridge
- Mongoloid eye slant
- Epicanthal folds

Abdominal distension

3. Hands

Fingertip pricks
Palmar creases
Peripheral stigmata of CLD
Pulse

4. Head and neck

Eyes
- Conjunctival pallor
- Scleral icterus
- Cataracts (DFO)
- Retinopathy (DFO)

Teeth: dental malocclusion
Neck: goitre

5. Heart

Full praecordial examination: cardiomyopathy, CCF, haemic murmurs
Chest: pulmonary oedema

6. Abdomen

Distension
Splenectomy scar
Injection sites: DFO, insulin

Hepatosplenomegaly
Tanner staging

7. Lower limbs and gait

Leg ulcers
Ankle oedema
Bony tenderness
Gait examination: long tract signs
Delayed ankle jerk relaxation
Back examination: lordosis, tenderness

8. Other

Urinalysis for glucose
Chvostek's and Trousseau's signs
  (hypoparathyroidism)
Hearing (sensorineural deafness from
  DFO)

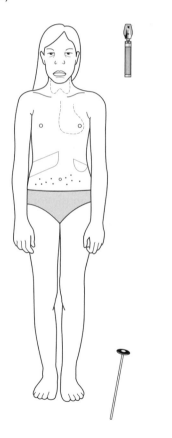

CCF = congestive cardiac failure; CLD = chronic liver disease; DFO = desferrioxamine.

bony abnormalities associated with the 'chipmunk facies' (see Figure 10.2). Note any obvious stigmata of CLD.

Commence general systematic examination by looking at the hands for fingertip prickmarks (blood sugar level testing), periungual pigmentation, palmar creases for pallor or pigmentation, and look carefully (if not done already) for any more subtle stigmata of CLD. Take the pulse (bradycardia with untreated hypothyroidism, irregularity with arrhythmias, pulsus alternans with CCF).

Examine the head, looking at the conjunctivae for anaemia and sclerae for icterus. Check for cataracts and retinopathy from DFO toxicity. Check the mouth for dental malocclusion secondary to maxillary hyperplasia, and the gum margins for hyperplasia (which may not be apparent in the well-transfused patient).

Feel the neck for goitre, secondary to iron deposition.

Examine the cardiovascular system fully, in particular for evidence of cardiomyopathy and pericarditis. Next examine the abdomen; inspect for distension (e.g. from organomegaly, or ascites with CLD), injection sites (from DFO and/or insulin), and splenectomy scar. Palpate for hepatosplenomegaly, percuss for ascites and assess Tanner staging.

Inspect the lower limbs for injection sites on the thighs (insulin), peripatellar fossa for increased pigmentation and ulcers on the lower leg. Palpate for ankle oedema (CCF, CLD) and bony tenderness (fracture, bony expansion). The gait should then be examined, followed by neurological assessment of the lower limbs on return to the bed, looking for evidence of long-tract signs secondary to vertebral bony expansion and cord compression. Also check the ankle jerks for delayed relaxation, from hypothyroidism. Following this, examine the back for lordosis and bony tenderness. Request the urinalysis for glucose.

If time permits, assess for hypocalcaemia secondary to hypoparathyroidism by testing for Trousseau's and Chvostek's signs, and check the hearing for sensorineural deafness due to DFO toxicity or bony expansion and compression of the eighth cranial nerve.

Neonatology

Short cases

The neonatal examination

A thorough perinatal examination is the most commonly performed systematic assessment in paediatric practice. All medical undergraduates, graduates and paediatric postgraduates should be able to perform a thorough 'baby check'. If there is ever a shortage of children with impressive signs around examination time, there is always a ready supply of neonates in level 2 nurseries, ideally suited to having a comprehensive baby check performed. The examination is standard irrespective of the gestation of the infant, although the interpretation of neuro-behavioural findings requires a thorough knowledge of the variations between different gestational ages. The gestational age can be assessed by the Ballard method; this is indicated where the gestational age is in doubt, but is fairly complicated and not covered in this section. The object of this section is to provide a framework for the perinatal examination that is easy to remember. Only a limited sample of possible findings is given here, as a comprehensive discussion could double this book's extent. Entire books can be, and have been, devoted to the examination of the newborn.

In hospital practice, ideally three checks are performed. An initial screening check is performed in the delivery room, assessing the baby's adaptation to the extrauterine environment. This includes assessing the Apgar scores at 1 and 5 minutes, noting any life-threatening conditions, obvious dysmorphic features (e.g. Down syndrome), gross congenital anomalies (e.g. neural tube defects), any birth injuries, and counting the umbilical cord vessels, making sure there are two arteries and one vein.

The second check should be the later comprehensive examination, within the first 24 hours of life. This is the check that must be done, irrespective of the introduction, in a neonate. The order of the examination is variable, depending on what the baby is doing at the time. Generally babies are quieter at the beginning of the examination, so always auscultate the heart first, before palpating anywhere else and disturbing the baby. The check may be approached in a somewhat opportunistic fashion: if the baby's eyes are open when first approached, check the eyes and red light reflexes (with the ophthalmoscope set at +10); if the baby yawns or cries with a wide open mouth, take your torch and check the pharynx. Do not palpate or move the baby until the cardiorespiratory auscultation is complete: crying does not interfere very much with the remainder of the check.

After listening to the heart, listen to the chest and then palpate the abdomen and the femoral arterial pulsations in particular. Then re-inspect, checking the baby from head to toe, but leave the less pleasant aspects until later (such as checking the mouth and palate with a spatula, checking the red reflex when the baby will not open his/her eyes, checking the hips). A detailed approach is given below.

A third check is required. This may be done in hospital on day 5, but is usually performed by the local doctor at 5–10 days of age. This examination should repeat the comprehensive examination, but with particular emphasis on the following:

- The cardiovascular system, particularly the heart and pulses for any evidence of cyanosis, murmurs, left-sided obstructive lesions or failure.
- The central nervous system, fontanelles and sutures.
- The skin for jaundice, evidence of dehydration (skin turgor) or rashes.
- The umbilical cord for any signs of infection (omphalitis).
- The abdomen, for any masses previously overlooked.
- Repeating the hip examination.

At this examination the urine and stool outputs are noted, and growth parameters are repeated as well, checking for adequate weight gain and feeding.

Inspect: growth, colour, respirations, posture, movements, cry

The initial thorough examination commences with inspection. Note the baby's weight, length, head circumference and nutritional status (muscle bulk, fat). Note the colour (peripheral cyanosis is common) and the respiratory rate (normal being 40–60 breaths per minute; periodic breathing is normal) and depth (retraction indicates some respiratory distress). Causes of tachypnoea include primary respiratory disorders (e.g. hyaline membrane disease, transient tachypnoea of the newborn, meconium aspiration, congenital pneumonia, pneumothorax), space occupying lesions (e.g. diaphragmatic hernia, congenital cystic lung lesions) or non-respiratory systems: cardiac (e.g. shunts, left-heart obstructive lesions, myocardial disease, arrhythmias), metabolic (e.g. hypoglycaemia), infective (e.g. septicaemia), haematological causes (e.g. anaemia, polycythaemia). Stridor may be noted with upper airway obstruction. It may be purely inspiratory if the obstruction is extrathoracic, and may involve expiration if intrathoracic. The causes are usually divided into site, intraluminal (e.g. meconium, mucus, blood or milk), intramural (e.g. subglottic oedema from overenthusiastic tracheal suctioning) or extramural (e.g. vascular ring). See the short case on stridor in Chapter 15, The respiratory system, for more details.

Posture, quality of movement and nature of cry are noted. The gestation of the infant must be considered with respect to posture. Normal full-term neonates usually lie with their hips abducted and slightly flexed, knees flexed, upper limbs adducted, flexion at the elbow and clenching of the fists (not tight) with fingers covering the thumb. Term babies with significant hypotonia may lie with their hips and thighs in the 'frog's legs position' (see case on floppy infant in Chapter 13, Neurology). Babies with serious intracranial pathology may lie with extended necks (opisthotonic posture), obligate flexion of thumbs or scissored lower limbs. Very premature infants (less than 30 weeks) normally have minimal flexor tone, like a rag doll; by 34 weeks, flexor tone appears in the lower limbs, and by 36 weeks in the upper limbs as well. A formal gestational assessment should be undertaken if the gestation is in doubt and the infant seems hypotonic, so as not to overinterpret normal findings of prematurity.

Normal movements may include alternating movements in all limbs, myoclonic jerks when asleep (sleep myoclonus) and jaw tremors when crying. Paucity of movement can occur in neuromuscular diseases (see the floppy infant case in Chapter 13). Involuntary movements can include tremulousness or 'jitters' (which can be stopped by gentle pressure) and seizures (may be subtle, tonic or more often focal, irrespective of the underlying pathology, and cannot be stopped by pressure, clearly differentiating them from jitters). Jitters can occur with hypoglycaemia, hypocalcaemia, sepsis and neonatal abstinence syndrome (NAS). Seizures can be due to neonatal encephalopathy (formally termed hypoxic ischaemic encephalopathy), intracranial haemorrhage, meningitis, metabolic causes (hypoglycaemia/hyponatraemia/hypocalcaemia/hypomagnesaemia; hypernatraemia/hyperammonaemia; kernicterus, various inborn errors, pyridoxine deficiency), developmental brain disorders, NAS, or can be idiopathic.

Asymmetric movement can occur secondary to cerebral malformations or intrauterine cerebrovascular accidents, or with birth injuries such as intracranial haemorrhage, or brachial plexus lesions such as Erb (C5,6) and Klumpke (C8,T1) palsies. Remember the myotomes of the upper limbs by the children's nursery rhythme 'five, six, pick up sticks [flex biceps], seven, eight, lay them straight [extension predominantly due to C7]'.

The cry is noted. A high-pitched cry goes with cerebral irritation, as in neonatal encephalopathy or meningitis. A hoarse cry can occur with upper airway obstruction and a cat cry occurs with the uncommon *cri du chat* syndrome (5p-syndrome).

Remember that you have to be opportunistic while a baby is settled. Do not examine the eyes or pharynx before other aspects of the examination that require a quiet baby. A suggested head-to-toe examination procedure is given below. The baby will determine in which order this occurs, however.

Systematic examination: head to toe

Head, neck and upper limbs

Initial inspection should detect any dysmorphic features. The head is examined for any traumatic injuries (abrasions, depressed fractures, haematomata or lacerations) and swellings (central [caput succedaneum] or to one [or both] side[s], stopping at suture lines [cephalhaematomata]). Fontanelles and sutures are palpated to assess size. They may be widened with increased intracranial pressure, as with hydrocephalus, or narrowed (or undetectable) and immobile with craniostynostosis.

The anterior fontanelle is highly variable in its shape and size. The head circumference (HC) must be measured, ideally with a paper (non-stretching) tape measure, around the head at the widest point: at term, the normal range is 32–37 cm. A useful rule of thumb is HC (cm) = height/2 + 10.

Next the eyes are checked (if the baby allows this at the time) including red light reflexes. Make sure that the eyes are examined. Even a baby who refuses to open the eyes at all (even on parental report) should have the corneas visualised (forcibly) to exclude glaucoma (which causes them to appear enlarged and very hazy). The nose is inspected. The metal condensation test can show bilateral nasal patency. A shiny pink lesion in the nostril can be a frontal lobe encephalocoele (not mucus, so do not try to suck it out: the author has seen an encephalocoele being assaulted with a suction catheter for several minutes in just such a case). The lips, gums, tongue, palate and oropharynx must be thoroughly assessed, including using a torch and spatula. A submucous cleft can easily be missed if direct inspection is not performed. The size of the tongue is also noted: macroglossia can be a clue to hypothyroidism or to Beckwith's syndrome.

The size and structure of the chin are noted. Micrognathia (mandibular hypoplasia) can occur separately or as part of Pierre Robin's sequence. At this point the suck can be checked by placing the little finger in the baby's mouth. The rooting reflex does not need to be tested. The ears are then checked for symmetry and positioning: deviations in each can occur with several syndromes.

The neck is then inspected for redundant skin posterolaterally, or 'web neck' (Noonan's and Turner's syndromes), checked for any masses (e.g. lymphatic malformation or 'cystic hygroma') or fistulae (e.g. branchial), asymmetry (transient as in persistent fetal posturing; permanent as in the maldeveloped cervical vertebrae of Klippel-Feil syndrome) and range of movement (torticollis from sternocleidomastoid fibrosis/tumour).

Check the hands, forearms and arms from a dysmorphic viewpoint (see the case on the dysmorphic child in Chapter 9, Genetics and dysmorphology).

Cardiorespiratory system

The conditions that must not be missed include coarctation (and other critical left-sided obstructive lesions such as hypoplastic left-heart syndrome, critical aortic stenosis and aortic interruption) and pulmonary hypertension, as evidenced by an active right ventricle (the presence of which, beyond day 3, may be associated with a significant systemic-to-pulmonary shunt, or an obstructed left-heart lesion, as above). A warm stethoscope helps to keep the infant quiet during auscultation. Localise the apex by auscultation. Note the heart rate (normal is 120–160 beats per minute). A murmur on day 1 can be due to a closing ductus arteriosus. This should disappear over the following days. Murmurs due to valvular lesions and vessel abnormalities (e.g. coarctation) will be present on day 1 also. Septal defects are unlikely to be heard on day 1 as there is minimal pressure differential between the left and right sides. As pressure changes occur (right ventricular pressure dropping, and left ventricular pressure increasing) the left side becomes dominant, and left-to-right shunts due to ventricular and atrial septal defects become audible after a few days. The second heart sound may be loud, and single or closely split, with pulmonary hypertension. After thorough auscultation, including all sites of possible radiation of any murmurs, listen to the chest. Finally, palpation of the femoral arteries and comparison with the brachial pulses is crucial to allow detection of the obstructed left-heart problems noted above.

Abdomen and genitalia

After inspection, gentle palpation for any masses or organomegaly is performed. The normal liver edge may be felt 1–2 cm below the costal margin in the midclavicular line, with the baby supine. The liver span at birth is around 2–2.5 cm. Kidneys may be easily palpable, especially the left one. Remove the nappy to check the groin, the genitalia and the anus. Any swelling in the groin is abnormal (e.g. indirect inguinal hernia).

In male babies, the scrotum is prominent, and should contain both testes (which should be of similar size). Hydrocoeles are common but often transient. Note the position of the urethral orifice (to detect epi- or hypospadias).

In female babies, the labia majora are prominent, and mucosal tags are frequent. There may be creamy vaginal discharge, replaced by day 3 with bleeding (pseudomenses). Labia should be spread to exclude imperforate hymen or other abnormalities (e.g. cysts of vaginal wall).

Ambiguous genitalia may represent virilised females (e.g. congenital adrenal hyperplasia [CAH], aromatase deficiency), inadequately virilised males (e.g. testicular defects, disorders of androgen production or action) or chromosomal defects. Take particular note of phallus size, the position of orifices, labioscrotal fusion, pigmentation (CAH) and whether any gonads are palpable. For more detail, see the short case on ambiguous genitalia in Chapter 7, Endocrinology. The baby's anus must be evaluated for patency and position.

Hip examination

The hip examination is most important—to detect developmental dysplasia of the hip (DDH, previously called congenital dislocation of the hip [CDH]). DDH can be difficult to detect on just one examination, even for very experienced clinicians, as the femoral head could be enlocated on that occasion. Thus, examination of the hip should be re-performed after the initial assessment. Asymmetric skin creases in the buttocks may occur with DDH, but are not a reliable sign of this. Similarly, unilateral DDH can be accompanied by a weaker femoral pulse to palpation on the affected side, but this is uncommon.

There are two standard manoeuvres:

1. **Ortolani's test** is to reduce a posteriorly dislocated femoral head. The middle finger is placed over the greater trochanter, with the hips and knees flexed to 90 degrees, the baby lying on a firm surface. With the knee in the palm, the thigh is gently abducted while the thigh is brought forward to enlocate the femoral head which should (may) produce a 'clunk' of relocation.
2. **Barlow's test** is to detect whether the femoral head can be dislocated. The pelvis is fixed with one hand (with the thumb over the pubic symphysis, and the other four digits behind the coccygeal area). The other hand firmly holds the thigh and adducts it gently downwards: in DDH the head dislocates over the posterior lip of the acetabulum, with an accompanying 'clunk'.

To remember which test is which, **O**rtolani's **O**pens **O**ut the lower limbs, **B**arlow's **B**umps **B**ack the femoral head. You need remember only one of these, the other being the opposite. Often, these manoeuvres will detect a 'click' or 'snap', which is ligamentous or muscular in origin and usually of no significance if the hip feels otherwise stable. If the clinical examination is equivocal, or normal but there is a history of breech presentation, a first-degree relative with DDH or significant oligohydramnios, hip ultrasound is indicated at 6 weeks.

Lower limbs

The lower limbs are checked for their length and shape. The feet are checked for postural and structural variations. Talipes calcaneovalgus is usually due to postural deformity secondary to intrauterine pressure. If full inversion can be achieved such that the sole is aligned vertically, the talipes is postural. Talipes equinovarus may be postural, or structural with muscle wasting. If full eversion is achieved, with the forefoot abducted and the little toe touched to the tibia (thus apposing the dorsum of the foot to the shin), the problem is probably postural.

Nervous system and spine

After having inspected for posture, symmetry and quality of movement, check the palmar grasp, pull the baby to sitting position, and note tone, degree of head control and head lag. Next, the baby can be positioned supine along the forearm, with the hand, palm upwards, supporting the neck and head and lifting the head gently. This support is transiently withdrawn by suddenly dorsiflexing the hand, eliciting the Moro (startle) reflex in a gentle fashion. The Moro reflex may demonstrate asymmetry of limb movement (e.g. with brachial plexus injury) or of facial expression (e.g. facial nerve palsy) or may be absent with significant intracranial pathology. If there are any concerns in any of the above areas, tap out the deep tendon reflexes.

The baby is then held in ventral suspension (normal being a convexity), and the spine is inspected carefully for abnormal curvature (e.g. scoliosis from vertebral anomalies), midline birthmarks, masses, pits or tufts of hair (e.g. diastematomyelia). Sacral or sacro-coccygeal pits and sinuses are common and of no clinical importance. The anus can be inspected at this time if previously omitted. The Galant (truncal incurvation) reflex can then be checked by stroking down one side of the spine from the neck to the coccyx; the spine should curve towards that side. The Galant reflex gives some indication of segmental integrity from T2 to S1.

Next, the stepping and walking reflexes can be tested. A supported baby will make walking movements when the feet are placed on a firm surface. The baby may then have the dorsum of each foot placed against the underside of a ledge, and will normally step up onto the ledge.

This completes the neurological assessment. Testing of deep tendon reflexes is not required.

Skin

Many benign, transient rashes may affect neonates and often worry new parents. The most common rash noted in the first days of life is erythema toxicum neonatorum, appearing on any part of the body except palms and soles as erythematous macules, usually with a central white or yellow papule. These 'pustules' are sterile, containing eosinophils. Milia are pinhead-sized white papules on the nose, forehead and cheeks containing keratogenous material. Miliaria is due to obstructed eccrine sweat glands, usually seen on the forehead, scalp and skin folds.

Several pigmented lesions are common, especially the Mongolian spot, a blue-grey area over the lumbosacral region seen in most Asian and black babies, which can be mistaken for a bruise initially. Multiple café-au-lait spots occur in neurofibromatosis and several other syndromal diagnoses. Hypopigmented macules occur in tuberous sclerosus.

Vascular birthmarks are common, and there are two distinct types:

1. **Vascular malformations**, which are always present at birth (e.g. trigeminal distribution 'port wine stain' in Sturge-Weber syndrome, with accompanying angiomatous malformation of the brain) and will grow in proportion to the rest of the body.
2. **Haemangiomata** (e.g. 'strawberry naevus'), which (usually) are not present at birth, and will grow out of proportion to the rest of the body for 24 weeks, then involute slowly, with 50% gone by 5 years. Haemangiomata are of concern in certain areas: e.g. near the eyes (can block vision, causing amblyopia), ears (can block ear canal causing 'auditory amblyopia') or 'beard' region (may indicate underlying laryngeal involvement), and may need to be treated with cortico-steroids or laser therapy. This is more likely an issue at the 6-week check.

To reiterate, unpleasant aspects of the baby check may be best left until last, but must not be forgotten. These include the inspection of the palate (using spatula and torch), checking the hips (some babies seem to hate this), the Moro reflex and checking the eyes if this was not possible earlier.

The 6-week check

The procedure for the examination of the infant at the 6-week check is essentially the same as for the perinatal examination. By 6 weeks, most term infants should be able to smile responsively (spontaneous smiling occurs later, from 6 weeks to 5 months), and some primitive reflexes have been fully incorporated (stepping and walking reflexes). The baby is now able to lift the head momentarily when prone (usually by 3 weeks) and can hold the head in line with the trunk when held in ventral suspension.

The key areas to re-examine include growth parameters, particularly weight gain (normal 150–200 g per week), head circumference (e.g. to exclude hydrocephalus), cardiovascular system (murmurs and femoral pulses) for defects that may not have been apparent at discharge from hospital (e.g. septal defects, coarctation), hip examination (you can never examine the hips too often, as DDH can still present late) and eye examination to exclude cataracts or causes of leucocoria (white eye) that may have been overlooked or more difficult to detect in the earlier examination and to check the ability to fix and follow to the midline (normally occurs by 5 weeks). If there is any jaundice, biliary atresia must be borne in mind, and direct and indirect bilirubin levels checked. Other, new problems may have arisen (e.g. nappy rashes, haemangiomata, umbilical granulomata). As with the neonatal examination, leaving the unpleasant parts until the end can be a good idea. The 6-week check is also a good time to discuss the importance of upcoming immunisation.

Nephrology

Long cases

Chronic renal failure

Several significant advances have occurred in the management of chronic renal failure (CRF) in the last decade, particularly in the area of renal transplantation (RTx) and immunosuppression. RTx, the treatment of choice for end-stage renal disease (ESRD), has become more routine, and now many children receive renal allografts before reaching ESRD. Pre-emptive RTx avoids the morbidity and mortality associated with dialysis. Many of the multiple long-term problems of CRF involving growth and neurocognitive development are improved with RTx. The rate of transition from chronic renal insufficiency to renal replacement therapy and RTx has accelerated in the last few years. There is now increased recognition of some conditions where pretransplantation native nephrectomy is considered, as these conditions can cause continued problems in the transplanted kidney.

There are a large number of newer immunosuppressive drugs being investigated including FTY20 (modulates T- and B-cell trafficking), everolimus (blocks proliferation of T- and B-cells), and atemtuzumab (antibody against CD52 antigen).

Children with CRF often appear in the long-case section of the clinical examination, most having ESRD, requiring renal replacement therapy to survive. The principles of management should be well understood, and the candidates should be fully conversant with treatment modalities such as continuous cycling peritoneal dialysis (CCPD), continuous ambulatory peritoneal dialysis (CAPD), haemodialysis, RTx and the commonly used immunosuppressive drugs and biologic agents.

Background information

Aetiology

1. Glomerulonephritis: 30%.
2. Malformation (structural) of kidney/urinary tract: 30%.
3. Hereditary nephropathies (e.g. nephronophthisis, cystinosis): 20%.
4. Others (e.g. haemolytic uraemic syndrome [HUS], nephrotoxins): 20%.

Causes can be divided into congenital and acquired. Congenital nephropathies and maldevelopments of the urinary tract tend to cause 'delayed' ESRD, by 5–15 years, with a protracted course of (perhaps subclinical) CRF, causing poor growth. Acquired conditions (rarer in infancy and early childhood) tend to progress faster, affected children having previously had normal growth before their illness. Congenital causes equate with groups 2 and 3 and acquired with groups 1 and 4.

At present the most common form of glomerular disease causing ESRD is focal and segmental glomerulosclerosis. In some patients with familial or sporadic forms of the disease, defects of proteins in the slit junction between podocyte foot processes are described. Other causes of ESRD are SLE, rapidly progressive glomerulonephritis, IgA nephropathy, Henoch-Schönlein purpura and mesangiocapillary glomerulonephritis.

Hereditary nephropathies are numerous (around 50 types: refer to the standard tomes).

There are two important points to remember:

1. *Structural* problems tend to cause salt- and water-losing forms of CRF.
2. *Glomerular* disease tends to cause anuria, salt retention and hypertension.

Glomerular filtration rate and clinical correlates

At a glomerular filtration rate (GFR) below normal, but above 25 mL/min/1.73 m², serum creatinine is usually up to 0.2 mmol/L (this depends on the size of the patient). This corresponds to the group of children with renal insufficiency who are monitored regularly (for their growth, development, blood pressure, serum creatinine, evidence of renal bone disease and calculated GFR) and may receive specific treatment for their specific diagnoses (e.g. cysteamine for cystinosis). They may also require antihypertensive agents, sodium supplements, bicarbonate supplements, calcitriol and phosphate binders. However, the majority of this group will progress to ESRD. Clinical problems are usually not evident until GFR falls below 25 mL/min/1.73 m².

At a GFR between 5–10 and 20–25 mL/min/1.73 m², the serum creatinine level is usually between 0.2 and 0.8 mmol/L. This corresponds to a group who require medical manipulation, but not dialysis or transplantation yet. In children in this group who are undiagnosed, symptoms develop (e.g. anorexia, fatigability) and finally bring the child to medical attention.

At a GFR below 5–10 mL/min/1.73 m², serum creatinine is usually above 0.8 mmol/L. This group requires dialysis or transplantation. If the GFR is below 5 mL/min/1.73 m², symptoms such as nausea, vomiting and oedema become severe, and, without treatment, pericarditis, bleeding diatheses and uraemic encephalopathy will supervene.

Aide-mémoire for GFR

An easy way to remember these groups is to think of two numbers—25 and 7. Thus:

* Above 25 (instead of 20–25): monitor.
* Between 7 and 25: medical manipulation.
* Below 7 (instead of 5–10): renal replacement.

Useful calculations

Calculation of GFR

The GFR can be approximated by an empirically derived formula, based on the relationship between muscle mass and serum creatinine: GFR equals 40 times height (in centimetres) divided by serum creatinine (in micromol/L). For example, the calculation for a child who is 120 cm tall and has a serum creatinine level of 400 micromol/L would be as follows:

$$GFR = 40 \times 120/400 = 12$$

Thus, that child's GFR would be 12 mL/min/1.73 m². Note that this formula is less useful in children under 2 years. For the formula for creatinine measured in mg/100 mL, the formula is 0.45 times height (in centimetres) divided by serum creatinine (in mg/100 mL). These formulae are not valid for patients with abnormal body proportions or markedly reduced muscle mass; in these cases GFR can be measured by DTPA clearance.

Assessment of rate of evolution of renal failure

The use of the reciprocal of creatinine to measure this has fallen out of favour. A graph was plotted of the reciprocal of the serum creatinine (on the vertical axis) against time (on the horizontal axis) for one year; at least five measurements over that time were needed, and the patient had to be stable (no development of hypertension, urinary tract infections, or such like) for it to be more accurate. This was thought to give the rate of decline of renal function, and the stage at which a given child will develop ESRD could be determined by extrapolating the graph to where it intersected the time axis.

History

Presenting complaint

Reason for current admission.

Current symptoms

Essentially, this is an extensive systems review.

1. General health (e.g. tiredness, coping at school, sports, poor growth, weakness, decreased exercise tolerance).
2. Urinary (e.g. polyuria, nocturia, anuria).
3. Gastrointestinal (e.g. anorexia, nausea, vomiting, abdominal pain, diarrhoea).
4. Neurological (e.g. headache, paraesthesiae, seizures, confusion).
5. Cardiovascular (e.g. hypertension, cardiac failure symptoms such as dyspnoea, oedema).
6. Skin (e.g. itching [from microscopic subcutaneous calcium deposits], bruising).
7. Skeletal (e.g. bone pain, muscle cramps).

Past history

Initial diagnosis (when, where, presenting symptoms, initial investigations, aetiology), number of hospitalisations, sequence of development of complications and their management.

Family history

Other members of immediate family affected (e.g. siblings), renal problems (e.g. nephronophthisis, polycystic kidney disease, cystinosis), deafness (e.g. Alport's syndrome).

Current management

Current diet, medications, dialysis routine, management problems, present treatment in hospital, usual treatment at home, sequence of prior treatment changes, use of growth hormone, erythropoietin, drug side effects (e.g. steroid effects), diet, compliance, degree of self-management (e.g. with CAPD), future treatment plans (e.g. living related donor transplant), usual follow-up (by whom, where, how often, routine investigations done), use of identification bracelet.

Social history

- Disease impact on child: e.g. amount of school missed, limitations on lifestyle, body image, self-esteem, peer reactions.
- Impact on family: e.g. financial considerations such as the cost of frequent hospitalisations, drugs (especially post-transplant if not eligible for [in Australia] a health care card—a problem for those over 16 years of age), special feeds (low-phosphate, high-calorie, low-protein, designed for renal patients; in Australia, Kindergen is now on the Pharmaceutical Benefits Scheme [PBS] and is useful for infants, but other feeds like Suplena and Nephro have to be bought from the hospital and can be expensive), pumps and disposables (many children are on nasogastric or feeds via gastrostomy overnight), surgery (renal transplant), treatment for other affected children, time lost from parents' work, transport, private health insurance.
- Parents as potential kidney donors.
- Impact on siblings: e.g. sibling as kidney donor, sibling rivalry.
- Benefits received, social supports (e.g. social worker, extended family, Kidney Health Australia [previously Australian Kidney Foundation], dialysis and renal transplant associations).
- Discussion on transition from paediatric to adult renal services. (In Australia, dialysis machines and disposables are provided by the government.)

Understanding of disease

Both the child's and the parents' understanding. Ask about the degree of previous education (e.g. in hospital, by local paediatrician), contingency plans (e.g. who to contact first when child unwell).

Examination

See the short case on renal examination in this chapter. Some of the findings mentioned there will, of course, not be relevant to the particular case you see, but the overall framework should be helpful.

Management

The candidate should avoid getting 'bogged down' in the acute management of electrolyte problems and should discuss issues such as bone disease, growth including use of rhGH, development and psychosocial issues (especially schooling in chronic patients, transition). Particularly discuss schooling, as children on dialysis often miss key parts of their education (especially maths) and have major problems at school later, often with some acting-out behaviour.

In patients with lesser degrees of CRF, discuss slowing of progression, such as controlling hypertension, excluding urinary tract infections, obstruction, use of angiotensin-converting enzyme (ACE) inhibitors and/or angiotensin receptors blockers (ARBs) in patients with proteinuria.

The candidate should recognise that CRF and ESRD are not synonymous.

The management of CRF can be divided into nine main areas, comprising the following.

1. Serum potassium: this is very important but the candidate should not go directly to this unless the child is already on dialysis. It is usually not the most important problem in CRF.
2. Salt and water balance (including hypertension).

3. Acid–base status.
4. Bone disease.
5. Nutrition and growth.
6. Anaemia.
7. Renal replacement therapy.
8. Social/school.
9. Uraemic complications (includes monitoring for development of neuropathy, encephalopathy; measuring serum urea and creatinine).

The examiners expect the candidate to be familiar with the standard management of all these areas.

Control of serum potassium

Hyperkalaemia

The potassium (K^+) level should be kept in the normal range. This is usually not difficult, as renal excretion of potassium remains fairly satisfactory in CRF. If the level rises above 5.0 mmol/L, dietary potassium restriction and administration of sodium polystyrene sulphonate may be adequate temporarily. However, if there is an acute rise in the potassium level (e.g. with intercurrent bacterial infection or haemolysis) above 7.0 mmol/L, this is poorly tolerated, and more acute intervention is needed.

The treatment of acute hyperkalaemia (serum potassium level above 7.0 mmol/L) should be known by all candidates. Note that dosages deliberately have been omitted, as it is unwise to try to quote doses in the examination unless you are absolutely conversant with the particular drug used. It is always safer to say that you would look up the dosage, based on weight or surface area.

Treatment of acute hyperkalaemia

1. Salbutamol, given nebulised (same doses as in asthma) or intravenously, works quickly and lasts a couple of hours. This is the easiest treatment to give in a paediatric service.
2. Calcium gluconate 10%, or calcium chloride 10% (cardioprotective) intravenously over 2–5 minutes, with electrocardiographic monitoring. This modifies myocardial cells' action potential, and protects for around 30 minutes.
3. Sodium bicarbonate intravenously over 30 minutes. Alkalosis shifts K^+ into cells.
4. An intravenous infusion of 50% dextrose with soluble insulin over 30 minutes. This shifts K^+ into cells.
5. Sodium polystyrene sulphonate orally in 70% sorbitol (or in water), or rectally in 1% methylcellulose suspension (or 20% sorbitol). This binds K^+ with ion exchange resin.
6. Acute dialysis.

The above measures are temporary only. If chronic hyperkalaemia cannot be managed with dietary restriction and oral sodium polystyrene sulphonate, definitive treatment (dialysis and eventually transplant) is needed.

Control of salt and fluid balance

Be careful, here, not to mix up CRF with ESRD. Most children with ESRD, regardless of cause, require restriction.

In CRF (but not ESRD) there are two main groups to consider: those who require fluid restriction, a low-salt diet, diuretics and dialysis for fluid overload; and those who waste salt and water well into the disease process, requiring a high fluid intake (often waking for fluids at night), require salt supplementation and intravenous hydration if vomiting with intercurrent illnesses. The former group commonly have a glomerular cause for their CRF and the latter group a structural cause, with tubular dysfunction and decreased concentrating ability. Consideration of the history (e.g. salt craving), examination (blood pressure, weight, oedema) and urinary sodium excretion help determine into which group the child falls.

Salt and fluid restriction

This is required for the majority of patients with ESRD and for some with advanced CRF. However, note that all patients with ESRD are thirsty (because hyperosmolality makes anyone thirsty, even if there is increased intravascular volume), and that all ESRD patients drink too much, leading to problems with oedema, hypertension and increased weight. Candidates should recognise this problem, but know that in practice it is unwise to confront the patient, as it is unhelpful (although some children will admit to drinking too much). The diet should have no added salt but not be so restrictive that the child stops eating.

High salt and fluid intake

Some children, particularly those in whom CRF is caused by congenital renal disease, have high output problems and require high fluid intake and salt supplementation. The amount given is guided by parameters such as urinary sodium excretion and weight. This is not a common problem in ESRD, as most children retain sodium and water, although a few continue to have a large urine output.

Hypertension

It is wise to have a logical plan for the introduction of antihypertensive agents. Fluid overload is the cause of the hypertension in CRF, so that when a child is finally on dialysis, antihypertensive agents (optimally) should not be needed, as dialysis should be able to manage fluid overload. If a patient is oedematous (i.e. fluid-overloaded), blood pressure cannot be controlled.

In children being medically managed, before needing dialysis, salt restriction and antihypertensive drugs can be used. The drugs widely used in CRF include diuretics, calcium channel blockers, ACE inhibitors, angiotensin receptor blockers (ARBs, e.g. irbesartan), beta blockers (e.g. atenolol, metoprolol) and prazosin (alpha$_1$ post-synaptic blocker). Different nephrologists have different preferences for the order in which various drugs are tried. One suggested general plan is as follows:

1. No-added-salt diet.
2. Diuretics (e.g. frusemide). They lose effectiveness once 70% of renal function is lost.
3. Calcium channel blockers (e.g. nifedipine, diltiazem).
4. ACE inhibitors (e.g. lisinopril, an easy-to-use tablet that can be dissolved and dose titrated for small children) or ARBs (e.g. irbesartan). Later they may reduce renal function; beware hyperkalaemia, which limits their use in advanced CRF or ESRD.

Acute hypertensive crisis

The following may be useful:

1. **For the conscious patient:**
   a. Clonidine (central sympatholytic action; given orally).
   b. Nifedipine (calcium channel blocker, given orally).
   c. Minoxidil (vasodilator, given orally).
   d. ACE inhibitors (given orally).

2. **For hypertensive encephalopathy (all given intravenously):**
   a. Clonidine (central action).
   b. Labetolol (alpha and beta blocker).
   c. Nitroprusside (vasodilator).
   d. Diazoxide (vasodilator).
   e. Hydralazine (vasodilator).

Differentiate between CRF and ESRD. Hypertension in ESRD is fluid overload until proved otherwise, and in compliant patients it is manageable with dialysis to remove fluid. Antihypertensive administration makes fluid removal on haemodialysis more difficult because of vasodilation.

CRF may require diuretics (e.g. glomerulonephritides), but reflux nephropathy is usually better controlled with nifedipine, or with ACE inhibitors (again, remember to beware of hyperkalaemia here). Amlodipine is an easy drug to use for longer-term control of blood pressure as a 5 mg tablet can be dissolved in water and then the required dose given. Breaking a nifedipine tablet turns it into a shorter-acting agent so it is difficult to titrate the dose in small children.

Remember that control of hypertension decreases the rate of decline of renal function. Be sure you know the side effects of any drug you mention.

Acid-base balance

Acidosis in CRF is caused by an inability to excrete acids (approximately 2–3 mEq/kg of H^+ ions produced from metabolism, daily) and an inability to retain bicarbonate. In advanced CRF and ESRD, metabolic acidosis is mainly related to problems with ammonium ion production and titrable acidity. Despite this, alkaline bone salts acting as buffers keep the plasma bicarbonate level stable at levels of between 14 and 18 mEq/L.

Acute severe acidosis is preferably treated by dialysis, as the patients are often fluid-overloaded and hypertensive, such that intravenous sodium bicarbonate administration would not be optimal.

For chronic acidosis, management includes administration of alkali (2–3 mEq/kg/day), which can be given as sodium bicarbonate tablets or liquid (1 mL of 8.4% sodium bicarbonate solution is equivalent to 1 mmol).

If acidosis is intractable, treat with dialysis.

Patients with ESRD on dialysis will not need bicarbonate supplements, as dialysis alone corrects acidosis.

Bone disease (renal osteodystrophy, i.e. renal rickets plus hyperparathyroidism)

Bone disease can be detected histologically within 6 months of the onset of ESRD, in almost all patients. It is due to a combination of lack of $1,25(OH)_2$ vitamin D_3 (calcitriol), secondary hyperparathyroidism and acidosis leading to use of alkaline bone salts as buffers. Secondary hyperparathyroidism is invariably present once there is a 50% reduction in GFR. Histological descriptions include a spectrum from high-turnover disease (osteitis fibrosa) to low-turnover disease (osteomalacia and adynamic lesion of bone), but there are no clear clinical correlates.

Clinical features tend to be fairly nonspecific, and may include muscle weakness, bone pain, bone deformity, and growth retardation. Bone deformities can lead to slipped epiphyses, bow legs or knock knees. Dental anomalies may occur, including defective enamel and malformed teeth, especially in those with congenital renal disease. Soft-tissue calcification can occur if serum phosphorus levels are too high. This can involve ischaemic necrosis of skin, muscle or subcutaneous tissues (termed 'calci-phylaxis'), and occasionally visceral calcification (e.g. pulmonary involvement causing restrictive lung disease).

A major objective of managing bone disease is preventing pain and deformity. Assessment includes measurement of serum calcium, serum phosphate, serum alkaline phosphatase, parathyroid hormone (PTH) levels, and taking bone X-rays. Serum alkaline phosphatase is used to monitor the success of treatment. Radiologically, the findings of renal osteodystrophy include widened growth plates, with fraying and cupping of metaphyses (renal rickets), plus subperiosteal bone resorption and osteo-penia (secondary hyperparathyroidism). The rachitic components are best seen at the ends of rapidly growing bones (e.g. proximal tibia, distal femur) and the hyperparathy-roid components on the radial aspects of the second and third digits. Delay in skeletal maturation also occurs. The overall plan of management is as follows.

Control of serum phosphate

This is important, as hyperphosphataemia can lead to a rapid decline in renal function. It is best to correct the hyperphosphataemia before trying to increase the serum calcium level. Calcium carbonate can be used as a phosphate binder, but needs to be given with food to be effective. Phosphate binders can be increased in dosage until the calcium level is also returning towards normal.

Calcium supplementation

The preparation of choice is calcium carbonate, which acts as a phosphate binder as well (as mentioned above). Note that when used as a calcium supplement, it is better given between meals. The serum calcium is not restored to normal until after the hyperphosphataemia is under control, because of the risk of metastatic calcification if hyperphosphataemia persists.

Vitamin D supplementation

This is usually given as $1,25(OH)_2 D_3$ (calcitriol). Serum PTH is used to monitor treat-ment, aiming for PTH to be 2–3 times normal. Higher levels indicate healing and the risk of overshooting with resultant hypercalcaemia. Lower levels of PTH are associated with adynamic bone disease, with reduced bone turnover. The main problem with management is non-compliance.

X-ray bones annually

Once a year (a) check bone age and (b) X-ray hips, knees and ankles (weight-bearing joints are usually the most severely affected).

Complications of uraemia: major issues

Growth

There are many factors that can adversely affect growth in CRF.

1. Deficient caloric intake: a most important factor in infants and young children.
2. Salt wasting: another important factor in infants and young children.
3. Disease onset (e.g. CRF from infancy [congenital renal diseases] leads to attained height of −3 Height Standard Deviation Score (SDS) at 3 years of age. Probably one-third of reduction in height occurs in the first 3 months of life, as most children with CRF have normal birth weights and lengths.
4. Disease type (e.g. cystinosis, or nephrotic syndrome requiring high-dose corti-costeroids, may lead to particularly poor growth).

5. Abnormalities in insulin-like growth factor-1 (IGF-1) and IGF-binding proteins (IGFBPs, especially IGFBP-3).
6. Growth hormone resistance, secondary to point 3 above.
7. Poor protein synthesis and low protein turnover.
8. Renal osteodystrophy.
9. Glucose intolerance (on steroids).
10. Acidosis.
11. Polyuria (decrease in extracellular volume).
12. Infection.

As noted above, growth problems are worse if the disease causing CRF dates from (before) birth. These children may have several problems, especially sodium wasting, leading to significant undernutrition in the first two years of life. Growth problems are also significant around puberty.

Each case may have several factors operating. Optimum nutrition, monitoring of bone disease, correction of acidosis and anaemia, avoidance of high-dose steroids and provision of adequate salt (especially in young children) may improve growth. Poor growth can have a devastating effect on the child's self-image and cause severe problems (e.g. being teased at high school). It may be the major issue in some cases.

Recombinant human growth hormone (rhGH)

A major breakthrough was the finding that supraphysiological doses of recombinant human growth hormone (rhGH) are very effective in increasing height velocity: e.g. in one study, from a baseline median of 4.1 cm/year to 9.2 cm/year after 12 months, and to 6.6 cm/year after two years of treatment. (The reduced GH-stimulating effect in the second year is also seen in children with idiopathic GH deficiency.) RhGH is used in children with CRF and a GFR below 30 mL/min/1.73 m^2, whose height is below the 25th centile for age, or whose height velocity is below the 25th centile for bone age. The maximum dose is 28 units/m^2 per week. If growth velocity fails to increase to at least the 50th centile for bone age, rhGH may be discontinued. Prepubertal patients respond particularly well to rhGH.

Mechanism: CRF causes decreased renal clearance of IGFBP-3, which binds 95% of IGFs. IGFBP-3 increases and binds to IGF-1, decreasing available, free, active IGF-1, hence causing uraemic GH resistance and growth impairment. RhGH is safe and effective in CRF, in patients with ESRD on dialysis (although slightly less effective) and in growth-retarded paediatric allograft recipients. RhGH should be continued until epiphyseal closure or renal transplantation occurs. Potential complications of rhGH therapy include hypercalciuria, aseptic necrosis of the femoral head, pseudotumour cerebri and suggestions of possible (although no evidence for this) induction of malignancy. The last of these, if correct, could be a consideration for those who have received cytotoxics, or have ESRD from Wilms' tumour.

Nutrition

The diet in CRF is a difficult therapy problem and depends on the stage of CRF. If CRF is advanced and dialysis is imminent, protein restriction may be used to keep urea at acceptable levels. Protein intake is no longer reduced to slow the progression to ESRD, as it has now been shown that it does not work in children, and there is a risk of reduced growth. Also, ACE inhibitors are effective and better tolerated than the previously recommended diet. Optimum nutrition is needed for these children with nutritional and growth failure, who are anorectic too.

A further problem is the intake of milk in infants. Milk has a high phosphate content and hyperphosphataemia is deleterious to renal function, so milk intake should be limited. Infant formulae can be used with added calories (e.g. polyjoule) and salt, or special formulae designed for renal patients (with high calories, and with low-phosphate and high-salt content).

Different units have different philosophies on diet. Candidates should learn (and understand) the regimen used by their training hospital and be able to discuss this.

Children with CRF have an inadequate intake of energy. Energy supplementation aims to raise this intake to the recommended daily allowance (RDA) calculated at mean weight for age. This can be achieved by adding glucose polymer to feeds, oral or flavoured supplements, but avoiding standard energy supplements (e.g. Ensure, Osmolyte) as these have high protein and phosphate content unsuitable for CRF. For infants, standard infant formulas can be supplemented with Polyjoule and Calogen (a long-chain fatty acid preparation).

In some children, volume constraints will limit the amount of nutritional supplementation that can be given. For younger children with structural disease, nutrition can be optimised by supplemental feeding (e.g. overnight by gastrostomy, or nasogastric feeding), as volume overload is not a problem. Should fluid restriction be necessary, high-calorie supplements (e.g. Suplena, Nutrison Energy Plus or Nepro) can be used for overnight feeds. If overnight feeds are not tolerated because of coexistent gastro-oesophageal reflux, fundoplication may be needed.

The general principle is to encourage a normal, balanced diet, in order to maximise growth potential, while correcting electrolyte and acid-base imbalances by medications where needed. Nutritional supplementation by itself does not lead to catch-up growth, but does allow stabilisation of growth rates.

Recombinant human erythropoietin (r-HuEPO)

Probably the greatest advance in nephrology in two decades, r-HuEPO has been added rapidly to the therapeutic arsenal. Erythropoietin increases the terminal differentiation of erythroid progenitor cells, increases cellular haemoglobin synthesis, and increases reticulocyte release from bone marrow. Several symptoms previously attributed to uraemia are definitely improved by r-HuEPO, including fatigue, poor exercise tolerance, anorexia, pruritis, uraemic bleeding, sleep disturbance, cold intolerance and cognitive dysfunction (typical problems being difficulties staying on task, concentrating, poor short-term memory, and suboptimal performance at school). The benefits of r-HuEPO are improved overall well-being, increased energy levels, increased exercise tolerance, improved school attendance, increased physical activity and improved overall cognitive functioning. Other improvements have included regression of ventricular hypertrophy and normalisation of impaired brain-stem auditory evoked responses.

The avoidance of transfusions, with their attendant risks of sensitisation and transmission of infective agents, and the amelioration of anaemia are the main advantages of using r-HuEPO. Disadvantages include the cost and the potential side effects of r-HuEPO: hypertension, hyperkalaemia (remember the first symptom of hyperkalaemia is death), iron deficiency and vascular access thrombosis.

R-HuEPO can be given intravenously (IV) or subcutaneously (SC). Previously it was given intraperitoneally (IP), but this increased the risk of peritonitis. It may be given SC, twice a week, if the haemoglobin level is below 10. This is continued until the Hb level is around 11–12, at which stage once a week is enough. The child's B_{12}, folate and iron status should be checked also. The preparation used now is darbepoetin, which can be given SC or IV, but needs to be given only weekly or less frequently. The original erythropoetin (Eprex) has been withdrawn for SC use.

Suboptimal responses occur with several conditions: iron deficiency, aluminium intoxication, hyperparathyroidism, inflammation and infection. If there is such a response, check the ferritin, iron and total iron-binding capacity (TIBC) and transferrin saturation (iron/TIBC). If there is iron deficiency (iron saturation of <20% is the most useful indicator), replacement oral iron is given. If the oral preparation is insufficient to replete iron stores, IV iron sucrose (this is the only IV preparation available now) may be warranted; this is a common problem in haemodialysis patients. Also, check parathyroid hormone levels, to exclude hyperparathyroidism.

Dialysis

Dialysis is only waiting for a transplant. Occasionally parents are not aware of this, so make a point of assessing their understanding of this point.

Dialysis is commenced when the complications of CRF can no longer be managed by medical therapy. It is usually started when the GFR is below 5–10 mL/min/1.73 m^2. Indications include inability to control the main management headings (electrolytes, hypertension, oedema, acidosis, bone disease) and uraemic symptoms not corrected by treatment with r-HuEPO. Other considerations include availability of donors. Some children can have a transplant as their initial renal replacement therapy, known as a 'preemptive transplantation' (PET): see below. Overall, it is an individual clinical decision for each child. It is better if the child is still fairly stable and reasonably well, when first started on dialysis, rather then waiting until he or she becomes very sick.

A child may be excluded from the transplant program if there are congenital malformations with very poor functional prognosis. Infants under 6 months may be excluded for technical reasons. It is a joint decision made by the doctor, child and parents.

The modality of dialysis varies—haemodialysis, continuous ambulatory peritoneal dialysis (CAPD) or continuous cycler-assisted peritoneal dialysis (CCPD). Most children in the long-case setting will be on home-based peritoneal dialysis (although more and more are on inpatient haemodialysis). CAPD uses gravity to instill prefilled bags of dialysate into the peritoneal cavity three or four times a day. It has the advantages of not causing any pain and providing continuous dialysis. CAPD is a simple portable procedure and is relatively cheap. Disadvantages include no days off, the requirement for repeated connections and disconnections, and the attendant risk of peritonitis (usually from *Staphylococcus aureus* or *Staphylococcus epidermidis*).

CCPD involves use of an automated cycler for overnight instillation and drainage of dialysate fluid. CCPD has the advantages of only one connection and disconnection between the cycler and the peritoneal catheter per day, hence less risk of infection, and decreased time demands on the family. It does interfere with the child's social life, especially for teenagers.

Children are admitted to hospital, have a peritoneal (e.g. Tenckhoff) catheter inserted and are trained (along with their parents) in the management of CCPD and CAPD, usually for 3 weeks. All get cyclers, but they need to know CAPD for holidays or machine breakdowns. The volume of dialysis fluid instilled into the peritoneal cavity on each occasion is usually between 40 and 60 mL/kg (this partly depends on the child's tolerance). In CAPD, bags are changed three or four times a day. Bag sizes are 500 mL, 1000 mL, 1500 mL and 2000 mL. In CCPD, there are a variable number of bags overnight, 5–8 cycles, and fluid dwells in the abdomen during the day.

Solution strengths (different glucose concentrations) available are: 1.5%, 2.5% and 4.25%. Which one is used depends on the amount of fluid one wishes to remove. Of all dialysis modalities, CAPD is associated with the best growth, best control of anaemia and best patient tolerance. When started on dialysis, the child is usually put on the transplant program.

Common complications of CCPD or CAPD include peritonitis, exit–site and catheter-tunnel infections and catheter blockage. To counter peritonitis, which occurs in about 1 in 8 patient months, or three times every 2 years, the standard IP antibiotics are cephalothin and gentamicin. Antibiotics are added once daily to fluid that dwells in the abdomen all day. Insertion of catheters can be covered with antibiotics. If the child develops abdominal pain and the fluid becomes cloudy, treatment with intravenous and intraperitoneal flucloxacillin and gentamicin is effective. Catheter life varies, averaging about 9 months.

Haemodialysis (HD) takes 4–5 hours, three times a week. It is usually undertaken in a tertiary renal centre, and access is via central venous double lumen catheter designed for HD. These are percutaneously inserted for acute HD and short term, or inserted like Hickman catheters for longer term. Infection and obstruction are the main catheter problems. Fistulae and vein grafts may be required in some long-term HD patients. A school teacher and a play therapist are required in that case.

Renal transplantation (RTx)

RTx is the treatment of choice for ESRD. It is particularly beneficial in terms of growth. Living related donor (LRD) grafts are preferable to cadaveric donor (CD) grafts, as they give a better rate of patient survival at 5 years (95% for LRD, versus 80% for CD) and of graft survival at 5 years (80% for LRD, versus 60% for CD: less difference with newer immunosuppressives like tacrolimus). The allograft half-life (time for half of the transplanted kidneys from a particular cohort to be lost) for a LRD graft is more than 25 years, versus 16 years for a CD graft. Adult kidneys can be used, even in children under 5 years of age. The use of LRD has increased steadily; now around 60% of RTx in children have used LRD allografts. Over 80% of LRD allografts come from a parent.

Preemptive transplantation (PET) is where children have a transplant as their initial renal replacement therapy, if there is a living related donor. PET is performed before reaching ESRD and dialysis, and has become increasingly popular, with around 30% of transplants being PETs in the USA. PET recipients have improved patient and allograft survival.

Pretransplantation native nephrectomy may need consideration if the diseases causing the renal failure are likely to cause ongoing problems in the transplanted kidney. In Australia today, it is rare that paediatric renal units need to consider native nephrectomy before transplant. If necessary, one or both native kidneys can be removed at transplant. The most common reason for this to be done is to make room for a transplant. For completeness, the conditions which very rarely may require pretransplantation are listed here:

1. Very significant polyuria (e.g. obstructive uropathies, dysplastic kidneys). Polyuria can persist in the native kidney, causing dehydration and exacerbating nephrotoxic effects of post-RTx immunosuppressive regimens.
2. Significant electrolyte disturbances.
3. Persistent proteinuria (e.g. FSGS, SLE, MPGN, congenital nephrotic syndrome). Oedema, poor nutritional status, hyperlipidaemia and hypercoagulability all can increase risk of allograft thrombosis.
4. Hypertension (many glomerulonephritides). Pre-transplant native nephrectomy can lead to improved blood pressure control, less reliance on antihypertensives, and improved surgical and long-term graft survival.
5. Recurrent pyelonephritis (can occur particularly with bladder dysfunction, obstructive uropathy, reflux nephropathy).

Initial work-up for transplantation includes adding the name of the child to the cadaveric waiting list and sending blood, monthly, to the blood bank. The average waiting time for RTx in Australia is around 4 years: in New South Wales, children under 15 have a priority rating, which operates once they have been on dialysis of more than a year, so that children are waiting around 18 months for a cadaveric transplant. Blood grouping and tissue typing is done on all family members if an LRD is considered, this being increasingly the case. Donors must be ABO blood group compatible; otherwise pre-formed isohaemagglutinins interact with renal vascular endothelium, leading to loss of the graft. HLA matching clearly is beneficial in LRD transplants, although there is less evidence for its importance in cadaver donor grafts. HLA matching does improve the outcome of second or subsequent transplants.

Pre-transplant immunisation is very important. Varicella vaccination should be given before RTx if possible, while viral surveillance for serological evidence of any prior exposure to cytomegalovirus, herpes simplex virus, hepatitis B, hepatitis C, HIV and Ebstein-Barr virus allows consideration of prophylactic antiviral therapies.

Work-up also involves assessing the bladder for vesicoureteric reflux and outlet obstruction. Recipients must weigh at least 6 kg, which can be a problem. For example, in a very small 2-month-old infant with ESRD, transplant would be preferable to dialysis, so if there is a related donor available, the best plan would be to supplement the child's caloric intake (such as by nasogastric tube) and 'feed up' the child to 6 kg.

Immunosuppressive therapy

A major problem with transplantation is the need for long-term immunosuppressive therapy, with the associated risk of opportunistic infection and an increased risk of malignancy later in life. Corticosteroids are still used. The most standard treatment is now prednisone, mycophenolate mofetil (MMF) and cyclosporine A (CSA); tacrolimus is also used. In many centres, tacrolimus is preferred to CSA, as the data from RCTs show that it is more effective in preventing rejection. Standard therapy usually comprises basiliximab, tacrolimus, mycophenolate mofetil (MMF) and prednisolone.

There has been a rapid expansion in the number of newer immunosuppressants. The following agents may be used to prevent graft rejection. They are arranged as the ABC of immunosuppression for mnemonic purposes only. The main side effects are listed.

Antiproliferatives
1. *Azathioprine (AZA)* is a prodrug of 6-mercaptopurine, which inhibits growth of immune cells. It is being used less in RTx, replaced by MMF. Side effects are bone marrow suppression, susceptibility to viruses, pancreatitis, alopecia, malignancy, gastrointestinal upset.
2. *Mycophenolate mofetil (MMF)* is an antimetabolic agent that interferes with purine metabolism in B- and T-lymphocytes. It is metabolised to mycophenolic acid, which blocks conversion of inosine monophosphate (IMP) to guanosine IMP. It is more effective than AZA in preventing acute rejection in the first year post-transplant, and has similar toxicities to AZA.
3. *Sirolimus* is a product of *Streptomyces hygroscopicus*. It forms a complex with FK binding proteins in lymphocytes, which interrupts second messenger signalling, leading to blockage of cytokine-mediated proliferation of T- and B-cells. With the combination of sirolimus and CSA there is a synergistic effect that allows a lower dose of CSA to be given. Sirolimus is not nephrotoxic, and has no adverse effect on blood pressure. There is a competitive drug interaction with CSA and sirolimus, such that sirolimus should not be given within four hours of CSA.

*B*iologic agents

1. **Monoclonal antibodies**

    a. *OKT3* binds to the lymphocyte-CD3 complex. It is used as induction therapy, and can reverse acute rejection, but subsequent treatment is limited by the production of anti-OKT3 antibodies. Infusion-related side effects (due to foreign protein being given) are fever, chills, vomiting, diarrhoea and anaphylaxis. Other complications are pulmonary oedema, nephrotoxicity, neurological complications (headache, aseptic meningitis). Drug-related side effects are increased susceptibility to infection, anti-OKT3 sensitisation, and risk of malignancy. The infusion-related side effects are associated with the first few doses and can be decreased by pretreatment with high-dose steroids, antihistamines and antipyretics.

    b. *Basiliximab* is a chimeric human/murine antibody directed against the CD 25 antigen (the interleukin-2 [IL-2] receptor alpha chain on the surface of activated T-cells), which causes IL-2 receptor blockade. It is used instead of ATG (see below), together with CSA, mycophenolate and prednisone, for prevention of rejection. It has almost no side effects.

    c. *Daclizumab* is a humanised antibody directed against the alpha chain of the IL-2 receptor. Adding this to CSA, AZA and prednisone therapy reduces acute allograft rejection. It has almost no side effects.

2. **Polyclonal antibodies**

    Antilymphocyte globulin (equine) is a horse-derived antilymphocyte antibody, with efficacy levels similar to OKT3. A newer agent is a rabbit-derived *antithymocyte globulin (ATG)*. ATG causes prolonged lymphocyte suppression. Side effects are allergic reactions, serum sickness, neutropenia, thrombocytopenia and increased propensity to infections. As with OKT3, fever, chills, arthralgia and dyspnoea can occur, but are decreased with pre-treatment with high-dose steroids, antihistamines and antipyretics. Both these agents can be used in the treatment of rejection. ATG is also used to prevent rejection, especially in patients likely to suffer acute tubular necrosis (ATN) post-transplant, so that CSA or tacrolimus does not have to be started immediately (which would increase the risk of prolonged ATN).

*C*alcineurin inhibitors

1. **Cyclosporine A (CSA)** is a fungus-derived cyclic peptide that blocks T-cell response. It binds to cellular proteins (cyclophilins), blocks IL-2 production and inhibits T-cell proliferation and differentiation. Side effects are nephrotoxicity, hypertension, hyperkalaemia, anaemia, hypertrichosis, gingival hyperplasia, susceptibility to infection and increased risk of malignancy. The newer microemulsion form of CSA has improved, more consistent absorption. If used during induction, it can be given intravenously by continuous infusion or 8-hourly. CSA has more rapid metabolism in children than adults, such that children have higher doses. The dose of CSA is lower when used with sirolimus, as the two drugs have a synergistic immunosuppressive effect.

2. **Tacrolimus** is a fungus-derived macrolide, like cyclosporine. It inhibits T-cell–derived lymphokines, including IL-2, IL-3, IL-4 and gamma interferon, and clonal expansion of helper and cytotoxic T-cells. Tacrolimus is effective in inducing graft tolerance. Its side effects are similar to those of CSA, including nephrotoxicity, neurotoxicity, diabetes, infection, plus lymphoproliferative disease (more common than with CSA).

Management

The above agents can be divided into two groups:

- Induction therapy agents: biologic (OKT3, ATG, basiliximab, daclizumab).
- Maintenance therapy agents: steroids, calcineurin inhibitors (CSA, tacrolimus) and antiproliferative agents (AZA, MMF, sirolimus).

Prednisone, CSA, MMF and basiliximab are becoming the standard immunosuppressive agents. Quadruple regimens are preferred in many centres, especially in the USA. Candidates should be familiar with the side effects of the above treatments.

After transplantation, children usually remain in hospital for a fortnight or less, after which they are reviewed regularly (daily for the first month or so). Often patients will have one or more episodes of rejection, with clinical findings of tenderness over the graft and fever (although this sign is less useful in cyclosporine-treated patients), and laboratory findings of a rising serum creatinine level and leukocytosis. High-dose intravenous steroids or OKT3 are usually effective. Some units use cotrimoxazole prophylaxis against pneumocystis for 6 months. Most units now use valganciclovir, the prodrug of ganciclovir, as it is better absorbed and ganciclovir has been withdrawn from the market. It is used in many units for 3 months in all renal transplants except donor CMV-negative to recipient CMV-negative. Others use it for donor CMV-positive to recipient CMV-negative or when giving OKT3 or ATG, where there is an increased risk of CMV disease.

At each outpatient visit, check growth and blood pressure (hypertension can occur in up to 85% of transplant recipients), and look for signs of opportunistic infection and side effects of drugs (e.g. Cushing's syndrome from steroids, hirsutism from CSA, pallor from AZA). Check the skin and all lymph nodes (skin cancer and lymphomas can be seen in paediatric transplant recipients). Take blood to check renal function and for a full blood count (if on AZA). If the serum creatinine level is rising, think of the following possibilities: rejection, infection, obstructed blood supply to graft, or obstructed ureter or nephrotoxicity if taking CSA. It can be particularly difficult to decide between rejection and CSA toxicity. Blood glucose should be checked when taking tacrolimus.

Allograft loss

1. *Chronic rejection* (most common cause): incomplete understanding of mechanism; presumed combination of immunological and nonimmunological mechanisms, noncompliance, drug toxicity and recurrent disease; risk increased by multiple acute rejection episodes, late acute rejection. No effective therapies yet available.
2. *Acute rejection* (second most common cause). Complete rejection reversal can be achieved in around two-thirds of patients, but reversal is less likely with an increased number of rejections, increased age of recipient, and late (over 12 months post-RTx rejection) rejection episodes.
3. *Vascular thrombosis* (third most common cause). The risks are decreased by use of CSA or antilymphocyte antibody on day 0–1, and increased by peritoneal dialysis pre-RTx, cadaver donors under 5 years of age, recipients under 2 years of age or repeat RTx recipients.
4. *Recurrent disease*. See the list below. FSGS is a particular problem, and the most important, as most lose their grafts quickly. Children with FSGS are twice as likely as all other diagnostic groups (below) to have primary acute tubular necrosis (ATN) requiring dialysis post-RTx. If it does recur once, there is an 80% chance it will recur in any subsequent RTx.

Recurrence rates in transplants (histologic recurrence)
1. Membranoproliferative glomerulonephritis (MPGN) type II: 100%.
2. Membranoproliferative glomerulonephritis (MPGN) type I: 70%.
3. Henoch-Schönlein purpura (HSP): 55–85%.
4. IgA nephropathy: 25–45%.
5. Focal segmental glomerular sclerosis (FSGS): 25–30%. FSGS is the most important as most lose their grafts quickly.
6. Haemolytic uraemic syndrome (HUS): 12–25%.
7. Systemic lupus erythematosis (SLE): 5–40%.

Histologic recurrence does not correlate with clinical recurrence, the latter being much rarer. Recurrence can also occur in oxalosis, cystinosis (but no adverse effect on graft function) and congenital nephrotic syndrome.

Social problems

Although mentioned last, often these are the most important discussion points in the long case. Ensure that a full social history is taken, and that the social circumstances have at least been thought over before you confront the examiners, knowing all the side effects of OKT3 but not knowing if the family have their own transport or receive the Child Disability Allowance.

Schooling is a particular problem. ESRD patients go to school but do not seem to learn as much as other children (poor self-esteem, depression) and tend to miss school for no good reason. How well the family copes is extremely important.

Compliance with medications is a real problem. A significant proportion (around 25%) of grafts lost from rejection are associated with non-compliance.

Minor issues

Anaemia

This is mainly due to lack of erythropoietin. Other contributing factors include increased red blood cell destruction, blood loss (nose, gut, skin), decreased erythropoiesis by uraemic toxins, marrow suppression by drug treatment, poor intake of protein, iron and vitamins, and defective utilisation of iron. Anaemia can be alleviated by treatment with r-HuEPO (SC), aiming for a haemoglobin level of 110–120 g/L. A patient should probably be transfused when the haemoglobin drops below 60 g/L, to avoid the risk of cardiac decompensation.

Congestive cardiac failure

This is usually related to fluid overload. Management includes normalising blood pressure, maintaining haemoglobin above 90 g/L, salt restriction, cautious use of diuretics and dialysis. Cardiomyopathy is not uncommon and generally resolves post-transplant. It is related in part to nutrition.

Drugs

Many drugs require reduced dosage in CRF. It is impossible to remember them all, so it is safest to simply obtain a pharmacology book and look up any drug that is being considered. A brief list of commonly used drug groups that require decreased dosage in CRF is as follows:

- Aminoglycosides.
- Some cephalosporins.
- Some penicillins.

- Sulphonamides.
- Digoxin.
- Thiazide diuretics.
- Paracetamol.
- Phenobarbitone.

Other issues

Genetic counselling

In children with hereditary nephropathies, genetic counselling is a very important and necessary component of the overall management.

Monitoring

The examiners may ask what follow-up you would recommend for your long-case subject. The following is a brief checklist to consider.

1. Routine check of growth, blood pressure, oedema.
2. Electrolytes, bicarbonate, creatinine, urea, serum calcium, phosphate, serum alkaline phosphatase.
3. Haemoglobin, white cell count, platelet count.
4. Cholesterol, triglycerides, uric acid.
5. Bone X-rays—hips, knees, ankles, hands.
6. Chest X-ray.
7. Calculated GFR.
8. Follow-up by dietician, social worker, occupational therapist, especially for adolescent issues, and in younger children, development.

Nephrotic syndrome

Children with nephrotic syndrome often appear in the examination. Those chosen as long-case subjects are unlikely to have uncomplicated idiopathic nephrotic syndrome (INS), but may present with therapeutic dilemmas, difficult-to-control disease, or significant side effects from drug treatment.

Background information

Definition

Nephrotic syndrome (NS) is characterised by four components:

1. Proteinuria above 40 mg/m^2/hr (or 1 g/kg/24 hr) *or* urinary protein (mg/dL)/creatinine (mg/dL) ratio of 2.0 or more; alternative units—ratio more than 0.2 mg/micromol.
2. Hypoalbuminaemia (serum albumin less than 25 g/L).
3. Hypercholesterolaemia (serum cholesterol over 200 mg/dL [5.17 mmol/L]).
4. Oedema.

The primary abnormality is proteinuria. The other features are secondary to this. Other characteristic findings include:

- Hypocalcaemia (ionised fraction normal): below 9.0 mg/dL (2.25 mmol/L).
- Hyperkalaemia: over 5.0 mmol/L.
- Hyponatraemia: below 135 mmol/L.
- Hypercoagulability (decreased partial thromboplastin time [PTT]).

Aetiology

The most common cause of NS is INS. This was previously called minimal change nephrotic syndrome (MCNS), or minimal change disease (MCD). The name has been changed because it is now uncommon for children with NS to have renal biopsies. INS accounts for 80–90% of all forms of NS in childhood, with the remainder accounted for by other glomerulonephropathies and inherited renal diseases. INS is further subdivided into corticosteroid-sensitive INS (CSINS) and corticosteroid-resistant INS (CRINS).

Other important causes of NS are as follows:

1. Focal segmental glomerulosclerosis (FSGS). This is the most common progressive glomerular disease in children, and the second most common cause of ESRD (the most common cause being congenital renal anomalies). It can be idiopathic, or secondary to postinfectious glomerulonephritis, obstructive uropathy or systemic diseases (e.g. sickle cell disease [SCD], systemic lupus erythematosis [SLE]).
2. Mesangial proliferative glomerulonephritis (MesPGN). This can be due to chronic infection (bacterial or viral), SCD, SLE, renal transplant or bone marrow transplant.
3. Membranous glomerulonephritis. This can be idiopathic, or due to SCD, SLE, drugs (e.g. nonsteroidal anti-inflammatory drugs [NSAIDs], captopril), toxins (heavy metals) or infections (e.g. hepatitis B or C).
4. SLE. This can cause FSGS, MesPGN or membranous glomerulonephritis.

These are the only diagnoses likely to come into the differential diagnosis of NS. Textbooks often give the impression that each type of glomerulonephritis has one particular type of presentation. Note, however, that *any* clinical picture can be caused by *any* histologic picture, which can have *any* clinical outcome.

Idiopathic nephrotic syndrome (minimal change disease)

INS tends to affect younger children (2–5 years), and more often boys (until puberty, then the sex incidence is equal). It is thought to be due to a defective electrostatic glomerular barrier (the defect caused by a circulating lymphokine). An associated defect is a proliferation of a T-cell subclass. INS characteristically shows fusion of epithelial foot processes on electron microscopy (although this is characteristic of all proteinuric states if 'nephrotic'). It is associated with loss in the urine of low-molecular-weight anionic proteins (e.g. albumin), but some higher-molecular-weight proteins such as IgG are also lost.

Clinically, hypertension and haematuria occur in 10% of children with INS, but are transitory. Most children with INS respond to corticosteroids (CSINS). Up to 80% of children have a frequently relapsing course (see below). Children may have one or more episodes per year for many years, and sometimes into adult life.

Other glomerulonephropathies

The other glomerulonephropathies tend to present in older children (6–15 years) with variable sex ratio depending on the particular condition. Generally, in this group there tends to be a greater leakage through the glomerular filtration barrier, and higher-molecular-weight proteins may be lost. Clinically, haematuria is often present, and hypertension may also occur. If there is reduced renal function, then consideration of rarer causes of NS may be appropriate. Most of this group do not respond to steroids. In particular, FSGS is often the finding in a child who has CRINS.

Definitions used in INS

- **Remission:** urinary protein excretion less than 4 mg/m^2/hour, or no trace of protein on urine dipstick, or protein/creatinine ratio below 0.02 g/mmol for 3 consecutive days.
- **Relapse:** recurrence of proteinuria as defined in definition of INS, or 2+ or more on dipstick for 3 consecutive days.
- **Frequent relapsers:** children with two or more relapses within the first 6 months of initial response, or more than four relapses in 12 months.
- **Corticosteroid dependence:** two consecutive relapses while on prednisone or within 2 weeks of ceasing prednisone.
- **Corticosteroid resistance:** failed response after 8 weeks of 2 mg/kg/day prednisone.
- **Cyclosporine (CSA) dependent:** relapses when CSA is tapered or stopped; it refers to the group of steroid-dependent children who achieve remission with CSA.

Differentiating between INS and other glomerulonephropathies

In practice, in children with uncomplicated NS, initial differentiation is not crucial, as they are all given a trial of steroids. Ultimate prognosis seems to depend on steroid response rather than selectivity of proteinuria or biopsy findings.

Complications of NS

Infection

Children with NS have increased susceptibility to infection with encapsulated bacteria (e.g. *Pneumococcus, Haemophilus, E. coli*), including cellulitis, peritonitis and urinary tract infections. This is due to multiple factors, including urinary loss of immunoglobulin (IgG), loss of factor B of the alternate complement activation path, loss of transferrin, altered T-cell function, plus the burden of steroid therapy or other immunosuppressive drugs, and mechanical factors such as oedema and ascites. Peritonitis occurs in 2–6% of patients. The risk is further increased by decreased mesenteric blood flow and increased coagulability (see below), with decreased flow and sludging causing microinfarction.

Complications of treatment

Steroids often cause Cushingoid effects, but poor growth is the most serious complication. Medications used as steroid-sparers or in resistant NS (cyclosporine [CSA], cyclophosphamide [CPA], chlorambucil [CAB], cyclosporine [CSA], levamisole [LVS], angiotensin-converting enzyme [ACE] inhibitors, mizoribine and mycophenolate mofetil) have significant potential side effects, which are discussed later under 'Other agents'.

Oedema

Children with *rapid* onset of INS develop loss of oncotic pressure: fluid moves from the intravascular space to the interstitium, resulting in hypovolaemia. In these patients infusion of albumin with administration of a loop diuretic (e.g. frusemide) leads to increased excretion of salt and water loss. Children with *chronic* nephrotic syndrome, however, have increased or normal plasma volume. In these patients, diuretics alone can be given (e.g. frusemide, together with spironolactone). Angiotensin-converting enzyme (ACE) inhibitors (e.g. enalaprin) have been used in children with CRINS to reduce proteinuria, raise serum albumin and reduce oedema.

Thrombosis and embolism

NS can be associated with hypercoagulability, due to increase in plasma fibrinogen and clotting factors II,V,VII,VIII, IX, X, XIII (due to increased hepatic synthesis), decreased plasma antithrombin III (lost in urine), platelet abnormalities (thrombocytosis, increased aggregability), increased blood viscosity, decreased blood flow and hyperlipidaemia. This leads to increased risk of major vessel thrombosis, usually venous (risk around 2–5%). Most commonly this involves renal veins or sagittal sinuses, but can occur also in the deep vessels of the limbs and the pulmonary venous system. The likelihood is further increased by any coexisting illness leading to fluid loss, and by haemoconcentration, from vomiting or diarrhoea, from diuretic use, immobilisation and the presence of indwelling catheters.

Hyperlipidaemia and cardiovascular disease risk

Hyperlipidaemia is reversed quite quickly in CSINS, in 4–6 weeks, and is not usually a clinical concern. Concerns for cardiovascular sequelae include exposure to corticosteroids, hypertension, hypercoagulability and anaemia (erythropoietin-responsive anaemia has been reported in NS). In children with unremitting NS, persistent hyperlipidaemia raises concerns, reflecting adult NS experience of increased risk of coronary heart disease, and the rare reports of myocardial infarction in children with NS. In adults, HMG-CoA-reductase inhibitors are used successfully to limit hyperlipidaemia and its complications. These drugs have been used in children, but adequate safety and efficacy data have yet to emerge.

Growth disturbance

This is noted particularly in congenital nephrotic syndrome, and is thought to be due to urinary loss of insulin-like growth factor (IGF) binding protein, decreasing the levels of IGF-I and IGF-II, and decreasing IGF-receptor mRNA. Use of recombinant human GH (rhGH) in treatment is as yet unproven. Growth disturbance can be compounded by use of corticosteroids.

Hypocalcaemia

This is due to loss of vitamin D-binding protein in the urine. It can lead to bone demineralisation in the long term.

Negative nitrogen balance

Loss of protein in urine, plus poor appetite, and nausea contribute to poor intake.

End stage renal disease (ESRD)

Only a small minority of children presenting with NS develop ESRD. The group most likely to do so have steroid-resistant FSGS. Around 8–10% of this group will ultimately develop ESRD. Rarely, children who were initially steroid-responsive become steroid-resistant and progress to ESRD.

History

Presenting complaint

Reason for current admission.

Current symptoms

1. General health (e.g. anorexia, weight gain, lethargy, poor height gain).
2. Oedema (e.g. periorbital or ankle swelling, ascites).

3. Urinary (e.g. haematuria, oliguria, concentrated urine).
4. Other (e.g. infections, abdominal pain, hypertension).

Past history

Initial diagnosis (when, where, presenting symptoms, initial investigations, established aetiology, initial treatment), number of episodes per year (usual precipitants, usual treatment), number of hospitalisations, sequence of complications, management.

Management

Current diet, medications, management problems, present treatment in hospital, usual management at home, home urine testing, sequence of prior drugs used, drug side effects (e.g. steroid effects), compliance, future treatment plans (e.g. introduction of cytotoxic drugs), usual follow-up (by whom, where, how often).

Social history

Disease impact on child (e.g. amount of school missed, body image), impact on family (e.g. financial considerations such as cost of frequent hospitalisations), social supports.

Understanding of disease

By child and by parents.

Examination

See the short cases on oedema and renal examination in this chapter.

Management

Investigations

Any child with NS should probably have the following tests.

Urine

Urinalysis, including looking for cellular casts, which do not tend to occur in INS but may well occur in other glomerulonephropathies (note that hyaline or waxy casts are common in INS).

Blood

1. Urea, creatinine and electrolytes (renal function is usually normal in INS; may be abnormal in other glomerulonephropathies).
2. Albumin and total protein levels (to evaluate severity).
3. Serum complement C3 and C4 (low with MesPGN, SLE; normal in INS).
4. Full blood examination. Haemoglobin level is normal in INS. If anaemia is present this suggests other diagnoses.
5. Hepatitis B and C serology (hepatitis B is associated with membranous nephritis; hepatitis C is associated with MesPGN).

Renal biopsy indications

Note that renal biopsy should be reserved for those with very atypical features. It is not a routine requirement. There is probably no indication for biopsy before commencing non-steroid agents if the child is completely responsive to prednisone (i.e. proteinuria absent for over 3 days). Indications include:

1. Onset: before six months of age.
2. Onset: macroscopic haematuria.
3. Persistent hypertension with microscopic haematuria.
4. Persistent abnormal serum complement level.
5. Elevated (or rising) serum creatinine level.
6. Steroid resistance.

Other tests

Another test that is often mentioned is the 24-hour urinary protein estimation. This is not very useful as it is almost impossible to perform accurately and does not add to the diagnosis (although it may be useful in non-INS forms of NS or in non-nephrotic proteinuric states). Demonstration of steroid responsiveness may require the simpler test of urinary protein:creatinine ratio (normal ratio less than 0.02 mg/micromol). Serum cholesterol and triglycerides are often requested, as is protein electrophoresis, but they do not aid diagnosis or management. Antinuclear antibody (screening for SLE) is not necessary in younger patients with uncomplicated NS.

Treatment

1. Corticosteroids

The mainstay of therapy remains steroids. Protocols vary between different units; it is wise to learn the regimen of your own teaching hospital. There is good data that, in the first episode of NS, when oral prednisone is given for 4 weeks and then on alternate days for 2 months or more (increase in benefit up to total course of prednisone of 7 months), fewer children relapse than those who are given 'standard therapy' of daily prednisone for 4 weeks (2 mg/kg/day or 60 mg/m^2/day) and then alternate daily for 4 weeks. This standard therapy leads to remission within an average of 2 weeks in those with INS. There is good evidence that increasing the total dose of prednisone during the first episode and increasing duration results in fewer children relapsing by 12–24 months. Around 50–70% of children relapse after 8 weeks of therapy, with the relative risk of relapse falling by 13% for each month that the initial duration of therapy is extended beyond 8 weeks. In subsequent episodes, prednisone can be used until remission occurs for more than 3 days, and then alternate daily prednisone, considering other agents when toxicity of steroids exceeds side effects of other agents. Most children will grow quite well on alternate day steroids until they go into puberty, when growth slows.

The other use of steroids is for steroid-resistant NS, usually due to FSGS, using IV methylprednisolone. This is given at a dose of 30 mg/kg, three times a week for 2 weeks, then tapering gradually over 80 weeks with concurrent prenisolone on alternate days. This regimen can provide a remission rate of 60–70%, but it is very toxic (side effects: hypertension, delayed growth, cataracts, infections) and has not been subjected to a randomised control trial.

2. Other agents: additional options including cytotoxic drugs

The main agents that can claim success in NS (mnemonic: CLAIM) are:

C **C**yclophosphamide (CPA: 2–3mg/kg/day for 8 weeks), **C**hlorambucil (0.2 mg/kg/day for 8–12 weeks), **C**yclosporine A (CSA: 2.5 mg/kg 12-hourly for 12 months)

L **L**evamisole (2.5 mg/kg alternate daily for 6–12 months)

A **A**ngiotensin-converting enzyme (ACE) inhibitors

I   **I**mmunisation with pneumococcal vaccine

M   **M**ycophenolate mofetil (25 mg/kg/day for up to one year)

- **CPA** has significant side effects, short term (e.g. bone marrow suppression, risk of viral infections such as varicella, measles) and long term (e.g. gonadal toxicity and risk of carcinogenesis).
- **CSA** can cause nephrotoxicity, hypertension, gingival hyperplasia, hirsutism.
- **CPA** given for 8 weeks and CPA given for more than 6 months are equally effective in maintaining remission while CSA is being given. However the effect of CSA is not sustained while that of CPA is.
- **Levamisole** causes enhanced cellular immune responses in certain conditions with depressed immune function. Levamisole may help to maintain remission in steroid-dependent INS, is well tolerated and has few side effects (neutropenia, rarely vasculitis, liver toxicity, convulsions) and these are all reversible on withdrawing the drug.
- **ACE inhibitors** reduce glomerular hyperfiltration. Adverse effects include hypotension, cough.
- **Immunisation** as per schedule for pneumococcal vaccination of immunocompromised children: heptavalent conjugated pneumococcal vaccine (7vPCV) in children under 5, polysaccharide pneumococcal vaccine (PPV23) in children 5 or older.
- **Mycophenolate mofetil** can be used for diffuse proliferative lupus nephritis. It is also used for steroid sensitive NS (although no RCTs).

Indications for commencing these agents include:

1. Failure to respond to steroids (depends on pathology—only CSA and ACE inhibitors have been shown to reduce proteinuria significantly in RCTs).
2. Unacceptable steroid side effects (e.g. reduced height gain).
3. Steroid-dependent NS (only if side effects are unacceptable).
4. Relapses with hypertension or thrombosis (only if frequent relapser or steroid dependent).

Poor compliance is not an indication, as monthly intravenous methylprednisolone can be given. One notable (relative) contraindication for use of CPA is lack of varicella antibodies. While a patient is taking these drugs, the full blood count must be checked regularly, to detect development of marrow suppression (e.g. neutropenia).

3. Antibiotics

Some units treat all episodes of remission with prophylactic daily penicillin, to avoid pneumococcal infection. Other units feel that penicillin increases the risk of infection with more serious organisms. *Haemophilus* can be a problem. Some units recommend broader cover than penicillin: e.g. a third-generation cephalosporin.

4. Immunisations

Live viral vaccines should be avoided in patients taking corticosteroids or immunosuppressive agents. Pneumococcal vaccine is recommended, as above, because of the increased risk of streptococcal infection.

5. Severe oedema

Children with INS with massive oedema (e.g. pleural effusions, ascites, scrotal or labial oedema) can receive intravenous concentrated (20%) albumin (1 g/kg infused over 4 hours) with intravenous frusemide (1 mg/kg) after the first hour of albumin. Note that albumin infusions can cause circulatory overload, hypertension and acute pulmonary oedema in patients with impaired renal function, or if INS is not the cause of the oedema. In the latter case, giving a diuretic may precipitate renal compromise. Albumin infusions should be used only when the child is very troubled by severe oedema symptomatically. They should not be used simply because albumin is very low, and should not be monitored by rise in albumin.

6. Hypertension
A minority of children with NS will have hypertension. Useful agents to treat this include nifedipine and beta blockers.

7. Diet
No added salt. No fluid restriction, except when very oedematous and diuretics are required. High biologic value protein.

8. In-hospital management
When these children are admitted, important observations include fluid balance chart, twice-daily weight, and 4-hourly temperature, pulse, respirations and blood pressure.

9. Activity
There is no need for bed rest or any restriction of activity.

10. Prognosis
The best prognostic indicator in NS is steroid sensitivity. Sixty to 80% of children with CSINS will relapse; 60% of them have five or more relapses. Most children ultimately 'lose' the nephrotic syndrome, towards adolescence (non-relapse rate 84% at 10 years). There are fewer relapsers if children are aged over 4 at presentation (remission occurs within 7–9 weeks of the start of corticosteroid treatment) and no microhaematuria. In children with steroid-resistant FSGS, most progress to ESRD and ultimately need renal transplantation. FSGS recurs in around 25% of renal allografts. For children with familial forms of NS, immunosuppressive treatment is ineffective, and transplantation is the definitive treatment, and the original disease does not recur in the graft. However, sometimes children develop an immunologically based nephrotic syndrome (e.g. development of antibody to nephrin in congenital nephrotic syndrome) in the transplanted kidney.

Short cases

Renal examination

A short-case approach to a renal examination is useful both in the long-case setting, for cases with chronic renal failure (CRF), and in the short-case setting for children with haematuria, proteinuria or other symptoms referable to the urinary tract.

Start by introducing yourself, and try to gain an impression of the patient's mental status (for encephalopathy, due to uraemia or aluminium toxicity, or depression, due to chronic illness).

Stand back and observe whether the child looks sick or well. Look at the growth parameters and percentile charts, and note the nutritional status (visually scan for

Figure 12.1 Renal examination

1. Introduce self
Assess mental state (encephalopathy)
Position patient: sitting up

2. General observations
Sick or well
Growth parameters
- Height (short with CRF)
- Weight (thin with CRF, obese with steroids)

Tanner staging (delay with CRF)
Nutrition
- Muscle bulk (poor in CRF)
- Subcutaneous fat (poor in CRF)

Skin
- Sallow (CRF)
- Pallor (CRF, HUS)
- Jaundice (hepatorenal syndrome)
- Bruising, petechiae (CRF)
- Scratch marks (CRF)

Valgus deformity of knees (CRF)
Hemihypertrophy (Wilms' tumour)
Tachypnoea (with acidosis in CRF)
Peritoneal dialysis catheter, bag
Arteriovenous fistula
Nasogastric tube
Gastrostomy

3. Upper limb
Pulse: tachycardia (dehydration, cardiac failure with CRF)
Hands/nails (vasculitis)
Nails: brown lines (CRF)
Palms: crease pallor (CRF, HUS)
Wrists
- Flaring; tender (CRF)
- Shunt (CRF)

Asterixis (CRF)
Blood pressure
Arms: proximal myopathy (CRF, steroids)

4. Head and neck
Face (e.g. hirsute)
Eyes (e.g. cataract)
Hearing (impaired)
Mouth (e.g. dry)
Neck (e.g. JVP)

5. Chest
Rib rosary
Praecordium
Lung fields

6. Abdomen
Inspect
- Intervention (e.g. CAPD)
- Scars
- Swelling
- Tanner stage

Palpate
- Musculature
- Tenderness
- Kidneys
- Lymph nodes
- Genitalia

Percuss bladder
Auscultate

7. Lower limbs and gait
Inspection
Palpation
Gait examination
Reflexes
Hips

8. Urinalysis
Blood
Protein
Specific gravity
Nitrites
pH
Glucose
  (various)

9. Temperature chart
Fever (e.g. infection, transplant rejection)

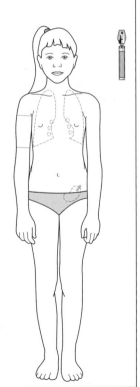

CAPD = continuous ambulatory peritoneal dialysis; CRF = chronic renal failure; HUS = haemolytic uraemic syndrome; JVP = jugular venous pressure.

muscle bulk and subcutaneous fat) and pubertal status (Tanner staging). Note any dysmorphic features (several malformation syndromes involve the genitourinary system). Look for any evidence of rickets (CRF) or hemihypertrophy (association with Wilms' tumour).

Look at the skin, for sallow complexion (CRF), pallor (anaemia of CRF or haemolytic uraemic syndrome [HUS]), and periorbital or peripheral oedema. Also note any jaundice (hepatorenal syndrome), bruising (CRF), uraemic 'frost' (CRF), or scratch marks (pruritis with CRF), although it is unlikely that patients that sick would participate in the examination. Note any hirsutism (steroids or cyclosporine [CSA]), or Cushingoid features (steroids for transplant or nephrotic syndrome). There may be other peripheral signs, such as nearby bags of peritoneal dialysis fluid (CRF), visible peritoneal dialysis catheter (CRF), arteriovenous fistula, subclavian or jugular venous catheter.

After initial inspection, a systematic examination can be performed, starting with the hands, followed by checking the blood pressure, and then examining in turn the head and neck, chest and abdomen, and finally the gait and lower limbs. This suggested order is outlined in Figure 12.1. Details of findings sought at each step are outlined in Table 12.1.

The urinalysis may be requested at any stage (e.g. before laying hands on the patient) but it must not be forgotten.

Table 12.1 Additional information: details of possible findings on renal examination

Head and neck
Face
- Malar flush (SLE)
- Hirsute (Cushing's, CSA)
- Periorbital oedema (nephrosis)
- Hearing aid (Alport's syndrome, aminoglycoside toxicity)

Eyes
- Aniridia (Wilms' tumour)
- Anaemia (CRF, HUS)
- Jaundice (hepatorenal syndrome)
- Band keratopathy (hypercalcaemia)
- Cataract (steroids)
- Uraemic retinopathy (CRF)
- Retinitis pigmentosa (nephronophthisis)

Hearing: impaired (e.g. aminoglycosides, Alport's syndrome)

Mouth
- Dry (hydration)
- Uraemic breath (CRF)

Neck
- Jugular venous pressure raised (cardiac failure with CRF); measure at 45 degrees
- Cervical adenopathy (e.g. CMV, lymphoma, if immunosuppressed)

Chest
Anterior aspect
Rib rosary (CRF)

Examine praecordium for:
- Cardiomegaly (fluid overload, CRF cardiomyopathy)
- Murmurs (anaemia)
- Pericarditis (CRF)
- Cardiac failure (fluid overload)

Posterior aspect
Sacral oedema (nephrosis)
Examine lung fields for pleural effusion (nephrosis) and pulmonary oedema (fluid overload)

Abdomen
Inspection
CAPD catheter
Other intervention, often related to congenital anomalies
- Ureterostomy
- Vesicostomy
- Ileal conduit
- Colostomy/ileostomy (e.g. related to imperforate anus)
- Nephrostomy or pyelostomy (e.g. related to sacral agenesis)

Scars (e.g. transplant [current or previous renal transplant has central abdominal scar in younger children, and scar in either iliac fossa for older children], CAPD)
Swelling (ascites due to CAPD fluid, or nephrosis)

Continued

Table 12.1 *(Continued)*

Prune belly appearance (triad syndrome)
Tanner staging (delay with CRF)

Palpation
Abdominal wall musculature (lacking in
  triad syndrome)
Tenderness (peritonitis)
Kidneys (e.g. enlarged with polycystic
  disease, hydronephrosis)
Transplanted kidney (also measure, note
  consistency, tenderness)
Lymph nodes (enlarged with CMV or
  lymphoma, from immunosuppression)
Genitalia
- Tanner stage of testes (delay with
  CRF)
- Cryptorchidism (e.g. triad syndrome)

Percussion
Bladder (for urine retention)

Auscultate
Renal arteries (renal artery stenosis)

Transplanted kidney (arterial stenosis)

Lower llmbs and gait
Inspection
- Muscle bulk (poor in CRF)
- Flaring at ankles (CRF bone disease)
Palpation: ankle oedema (nephrosis,
  cardiac failure)
Stand and reinspect: valgus deformity at
  knees (CRF bone disease)
Gait
- Foot slapping (peripheral neuropathy
  with CRF)
- Limp (slipped femoral epiphysis from
  CRF)
Squat: proximal weakness (CRF, steroids)
Return to bed:
- Reflexes (decreased with peripheral
  neuropathy of CRF)
- Hip movement (slipped femoral
  epiphysis from CRF)

CAPD = continuous ambulatory peritoneal dialysis; CMV = cytomegalovirus; CRF = chronic renal failure;
CSA = cyclosporine; HUS = haemolytic uraemic syndrome; SLE = systemic lupus erythematosus.

Hypertension

This is an infrequent case, and as such often 'stumps' the candidate. The lead-in can take
several forms: for example, 'This child has hypertension; examine her/examine her for
complications/examine her for the cause'. The approach given here includes both
causes and complications, and may need modification depending on the introduction.
It is essentially an extended cardiovascular examination. Likely cases would be renal
artery stenosis with bruits, NF-1, or infantile polycystic kidneys with large kidneys,
liver, portal hypertension and previous portosystemic shunts. Remember the vast
majority of children with chronic hypertension have a renal cause for their hypertension. The most common are reflux nephropathy (usually proteinuria) and renal
artery stenosis (usually bruits).

Begin by introducing yourself to the child and asking her or his name, age and
school grade, noting any irritability (hypertensive encephalopathy), dysphasia (intracerebral bleeding) or difficulty hearing your speech (deafness with Alport's syndrome,
or with congenital rubella). Any suggestion of developmental delay should be further
assessed (previous cerebrovascular accident or congenital rubella).

Commence general inspection with assessment of growth parameters. Children
with chronic renal failure (CRF), syndromal diagnoses (e.g. Turner's syndrome) or
other systemic disease such as neurofibromatosis type 1 (NF-1), or Cushing's
syndrome are often short. Children with congenital rubella (and associated renal
artery stenosis) and some with NF-1 may have small head circumferences, whereas
others with NF-1 may have large head circumferences. NF-1 is associated with renal

artery stenosis, phaeochromocytoma, coarctation of the aorta and neuroblastoma, all of which can cause hypertension. Weight is important in Cushing's syndrome. Truncal obesity with buffalo hump, loss of supraclavicular hollow and striae suggest this diagnosis.

While inspecting for growth parameters, note any asymmetry of limb size (hemi-hypertrophy with Wilms' tumour) or posture (hemiplegia from intracerebral bleed), and look for obvious scoliosis (NF-1).

Note any syndromal features (e.g. webbed neck in Turner's syndrome) and, in infants, the typical 'ex-premmie' appearance of the neonatal intensive-care graduate (umbilical arterial catheterisation leading to renal arterial thrombosis).

Look at the skin for pallor or sallow appearance (CRF), purpura (Henoch-Schönlein purpura, haemolytic uraemic syndrome, CRF), plethora (Cushing's syndrome), flushing and sweating (phaeochromocytoma), hirsutism (congenital adrenal hyperplasia, CAH, Cushing's syndrome), hyperpigmentation (CAH), café-au-lait spots or freckling (NF-1), depigmented macules (tuberous sclerosis with renal angiomyolipomata).

Note the facial characteristics. In particular, look for the moon face, hirsutism and acne of Cushing's syndrome, the heliotrope rash of dermatomyositis, the butterfly rash of SLE, the periorbital oedema of nephrotic syndrome and, in girls, the syndromal findings of Turner's syndrome (e.g. webbed neck, low hairline). Also note any asymmetry, either of facial movement—especially smiling (seventh cranial nerve palsy)—or facial structure (hemihypertrophy associated with Wilms' tumour).

After inspection, take the blood pressure (BP) reading yourself, in both arms. Make sure you use the right cuff size and the correct technique. The recommended cuff bladder width is 40% of the circumference of the mid-point of the upper limb, midway between the olecranon and the acromion. The cuff bladder must cover at least 80% of the circumference of the arm. The BP should be measured with the cubital fossa at the level of the heart, the arm being supported, with the stethoscope placed over the brachial arterial pulse, medial and proximal to the cubital fossa, inferior to the lower edge of the cuff. Note that current normative BP tables include height percentiles, age and gender, as BP depends on all these variables. A taller child will have a slightly higher BP than a shorter child of the same sex and age. Reference to the appropriate tables is essential. Note also that the fifth Korotkoff sound is used to define diastolic BP.

A rough rule of thumb is that an adult-sized cuff is appropriate in a normal-sized 6-year-old or older child. A thigh cuff can be used in large obese teenagers. Take particular note of the size (width) of the cuff supplied and, if it is too small, request a more appropriate cuff size. Question the values given if these were obtained with the same incorrectly sized cuff.

Note that most children and adolescents with BP levels at or above the 95th centile for their age and sex are overweight. Body size is the most important determinant of BP in childhood and adolescence. If the child has both diastolic and systolic BP above the 95th centile, there will be an underlying cause, usually renal disease. In children under 12 months of age, systolic BP is used to define hypertension.

Request the values for the lower limbs, or measure these yourself (make sure that you have practised this, as the exam is not the best place to start).

The remainder of the examination can commence at the hands, as in a standard cardiovascular examination, in particular feeling the radial and femoral pulses simultaneously, looking for coarctation, as evidenced by diminished strength of femoral pulsation. Then, work up to the neck, for jugular venous pressure and carotid pulses. The examination of vision, fundoscopy and hearing are best left until after abdominal examination, but scanning the face and head for signs such as conjunctival pallor is valid at this stage. After this, examine the heart, lungs and back. When examining the abdomen, it may be worth checking with the examiners that there is no contraindication to deep palpation, particularly if there is flushing or sweating, as palpation of a phaeochromocytoma can cause an acute hypertensive crisis. This need not be asked if the signs clearly suggest another diagnosis, such as renal disease (this is only a theoretical consideration as it is very unlikely that a patient with this tumour would be in the examination, but it is a point worth noting in practice). Next, check the vision and hearing, and then the gait.

The urinalysis is an essential part of the examination of the hypertensive child. It is valid to request the result of this before anything else, as it may direct the examination (and renal causes are by far the commonest) and will also prevent it being overlooked and the case consequently being failed.

The relevant findings sought at each point are listed in Table 12.2, and the suggested order of approach outlined in Figure 12.2.

Table 12.2   Additional information: details of procedure and possible findings in the hypertension short case

Introduction
Irritability (encephalopathy)
Dysphasia (CVA)
Hearing impairment (Alport's, congenital rubella, aminoglycoside toxicity)

General inspection
Parameters
- Height (short with CRF, Cushing's, NF-1, congenital rubella; with CAH, tall early, short later)
- Weight (obese with Cushing's)
- Head circumference
- Percentiles
Request urinalysis (protein, blood, casts, specific gravity)
Pubertal status
- Advanced (CAH)
- Delayed (Turner's)
Posture: hemiplegia (CVA)
Symmetry: hemihypertrophy (Wilms' tumour)
Scoliosis: NF-1, spina bifida
Skin
- Pallor (CRF, HUS)
- Purpura (HSP, HUS, CRF)
- Plethora (Cushing's)
- Flushing, sweating (phaeochromocytoma)
- Pigmentation (CAH)
- Café-au-lait spots (NF-1)
- Axillary freckling (NF-1)
- Depigmented macules (TS with renal involvement)
Facial characteristics
- Moon face (Cushing's)
- Acne, hirsutism (Cushing's, CAH)

- Butterfly rash (SLE)
- Periorbital oedema (nephrotic syndrome)
- Findings of Turner's syndrome (webbed neck, low hairline)
- Asymmetrical smile (seventh cranial nerve lesion)
- Hemihypertrophy (Wilms' tumour)
- 'Ex-premmie' appearance (UAC causing renal artery thrombosis)
Wears glasses (Alport's, medullary cystic disease, congenital rubella, NF-1)
Wears hearing aid (Alport's, congenital rubella, aminoglycoside toxicity)
Tachypnoea (pleural effusion with nephrotic syndrome, BPD in ex-premmies, LVF secondary to hypertension)

Head
This is best examined after chest and abdomen, unless obvious clues on inspection
Face: as under 'General inspection', above
Eyes
- Conjunctival pallor (CRF)
- Cataracts (Cushing's, congenital rubella)
- Leave testing vision and fundoscopy until later
Ears
- Low set or hypoplastic (congenital renal dysplasia)
- Hearing can be left until later
Facial nerve palsy due to hypertension

Continued

Table 12.2 *(Continued)*

Chest

Full praecordial examination for sequelae of hypertension
- Palpate for heaving apex, cardiomegaly
- Listen for: loud S2 (aortic); prominent S3 or S4; systolic murmur (coarctation)

Lung fields
- Percuss for hyperinflation (ex-premmie infants with BPD), pleural effusion (nephrotic syndrome)
- Listen for radiation of murmurs (coarctation), crackles (LVF).

Back

Inspection
- Midline scars (spina bifida)
- Sacral agenesis (renal anomalies)
- Buffalo hump (Cushing's)
- Scoliosis (NF-1): get child to bend forward to check this

Palpation
- Sacral oedema (renal disease, CCF)
- Spinal tenderness (Cushing's)
- Renal angle tenderness (nephritis)

Auscultation for renal arterial bruits (renal artery stenosis)

Abdomen

Inspect

Anteriorly
- Distension (ascites with renal disease)
- Dialysis catheter (CRF)
- Striae (Cushing's)
- Scar of renal transplant
- Tanner staging (CAH)

Posteriorly
- Midline scar (repaired myelomeningocoele)
- Sacral agenesis (associated renal anomalies)
- Buttock purpura (HSP)

Palpate

Kidneys
- Bilateral enlargement (polycystic disease, hydronephrosis)
- Unilateral enlargement (polycystic disease, Wilms' tumour, hydronephrosis, dysplastic kidneys, renal vein thrombosis, trauma)
- Tenderness (glomerulonephritis, pyelonephritis)

Suprarenal areas: mass (neuroblastoma)

Liver and spleen: enlarged (connective tissue diseases, congenital hepatic fibrosis associated with polycystic kidneys)

Bladder (after micturition): enlarged (posterior urethral valves, neurogenic bladder, obstructive uropathy)

Percuss

For ascites (nephrotic syndrome); over any masses to determine if retroperitoneal

Auscultate

Bruits (renal arterial in renal artery stenosis, abdominal coarctation)

Vision and hearing

Visual acuity decreased in Alport's, congenital rubella

Visual fields: hemianopia (intracranial bleed), constricted peripheral fields (medullary cystic disease)

Fundoscopy
- Papilloedema (raised ICP)
- Hypertensive retinopathy
- Perimacular degeneration (Alport's)
- Retinitis pigmentosa (medullary cystic disease [nephronophthisis])

Hearing
- Loss with Alport's, aminoglycoside toxicity
- Do Rinne and Weber's tests to confirm sensorineural loss

BPD = bronchopulmonary dysplasia; CAH = congenital adrenal hyperplasia; CCF = congestive cardiac failure; CVA = cerebrovascular accident; HSP = Henoch-Schönlein purpura; HUS = haemolytic uraemic syndrome; ICP = intracranial pressure; LVF = left ventricular failure; NF-1 = neurofibromatosis type 1; SLE = systemic lupus erythematosus; TS = tuberous sclerosis; UAC = umbilical artery catheterisation.

Figure 12.2 Hypertension

1. Introduce self

2. General inspection
Position patient: standing, fully
    undressed; then lying down
Well or unwell
Growth parameters
Request urinalysis
Tanner staging
Posture
Symmetry
Scoliosis
Skin
Facies

3. Blood pressure
Check the cuff size
Take the blood pressure in all four limbs

4. Upper limbs
Pulses
  • Tachycardia (CCF)
  • Absent (coarctation, Takayasu's
    arteritis)
  • Pulsus alternans (CCF)
Nails
  • Clubbing (SBE)
  • Splinter haemorrhages (SBE)
  • Brown lines (CRF)
Palms
  • Sweaty (phaeochromocytoma)
  • Pale creases (CRF)
  • Pigmented creases (CAH)
Wrists
  • Widened (renal osteodystrophy)

5. Neck
Jugular venous pressure (CCF)
Carotid pulse (may be absent with
    Takayasu's arteritis)
Carotid bruits (Takayasu)
Webbed neck (Turner's)
Buffalo hump (Cushing's)

6. Head
Face
Eyes
Ears
Facial nerve

7. Chest
Full praecordial examination, for
    sequelae of hypertension

8. Back
Inspect
Check for scoliosis

Palpate
Auscultate

9. Abdomen
Inspect
Palpate
  • Kidneys
  • Suprarenal area
  • Liver
  • Spleen
  • Bladder
Percuss for ascites
Auscultate for renal artery bruits,
    abdominal coarctation

10. Vision and hearing
Visual acuity
Visual fields
Fundoscopy
Hearing

11. Gait and lower limbs
Gait examination
Walk normally, on outsides of feet
    (Fog's test), run, hop
Lower limbs
  • Weak femorals (coarctation)
  • Examination
    for long tract
    signs due to
    intracranial
    bleed

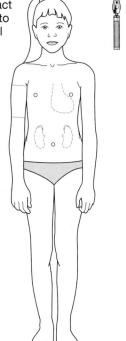

CAH = congenital adrenal hyperplasia; CCF = congestive cardiac failure; CRF = chronic renal failure;
SBE = subacute bacterial endocarditis.

Oedema

This short case is not infrequent and requires a rapid assessment of several major systems to determine the aetiology. Oedema can have the following causes:

1. Renal, e.g. nephrotic syndrome or chronic renal failure (CRF).
2. Liver, e.g. chronic liver disease (CLD).
3. Cardiac, e.g. congestive cardiac failure (CCF).
4. Bowel, e.g. protein-losing enteropathies, including inflammatory bowel disease (IBD) and cystic fibrosis (CF).
5. Nutrition, e.g. protein calorie malnutrition (PCM).
6. Local causes, e.g. lymphadenopathy causing leg oedema.

Each of these conditions deserves initial consideration.

This is one case where it is reasonable to request the urinalysis and blood pressure results before beginning to examine the patient, as these may well direct the candidate along a renal path (see the short case on renal examination in this chapter). If the urinalysis and blood pressure are unhelpful (i.e. normal), then a careful appraisal is necessary to detect other groups of causes.

A suggested way to approach this case is first to assess the extent of the oedema, and then to look for the cause.

Begin by asking the child to stand up (in underwear only) and inspect for periorbital oedema, findings of CRF (e.g. sallow complexion, pallor, skeletal changes of renal osteodystrophy), CLD (e.g. jaundice, spider naevi), CCF (e.g. raised jugular venous pressure), Cushingoid features of steroid-treated glomerulonephritis (especially idiopathic nephrotic syndrome [INS]), and nutrition and abdominal swelling from ascites. Also inspect from the side for ascites and kyphoscoliosis (osteodystrophy) and from the back for scoliosis (osteodystrophy) and buttock rash (Henoch-Schönlein purpura).

Next, demonstrate the distribution of the oedema. This can be done starting at the feet and working up (child lying down initially), or by starting at the head and working down (child standing up). The following abnormal signs should be sought:

1. Ankle oedema: press over the anterior tibiae for one minute (remember: one finger, one spot, one minute).
2. Ascites: shifting dullness, fluid thrill.
3. Sacral oedema: press over sacrum for one minute.
4. Pleural effusion: percuss the posterior chest wall.
5. Periorbital oedema: inspect.

Note that the time that you spend palpating for oedema can give you the opportunity to re-inspect the child and comment on whether there are any (previously overlooked) signs of CRF (e.g. transplant scar), CLD (clubbing, leuconychia, palmar erythema, caput medusae), bowel disease (e.g. clubbing, erythema nodosum, joint swelling with IBD).

After demonstrating the extent of the oedema, proceed to examine for the aetiology. A suggested order is as follows: hands, blood pressure (if not yet requested), face, chest, abdomen and urinalysis (again, if not already requested). Figure 12.3 outlines the findings sought at each stage of the examination procedure.

At the completion of the case, summarise succinctly, give a brief differential diagnosis and suggest which investigations you think appropriate.

Figure 12.3 Oedema

1. Introduce self

2. General observation
Position patient: standing
Periorbital oedema
Pale sallow complexion (CRF)
Jaundice (CLD)
Cushingoid (steroids for GN)
Nutritional status
Spider naevi (CLD)
Tachypnoea (CCF, CRF, pleural
    effusions)
Rickets (osteodystrophy)
Ascites: inspect from side as well
Kyphoscoliosis (osteodystrophy)
Buttock purpura (HSP)

3. Request
Blood pressure (CRF, various GNs)
Urinalysis (proteinuria with GNs)
Weight chart
Stool chart (IBD, other protein-losing
    enteropathies)

4. Demonstrate distribution of oedema
Ankle and leg oedema
Ascites
Sacral oedema
Pleural effusions
Periorbital oedema

5. Upper limb
Hands
- Clubbing (CLD, IBD, CF)
- Leuconychia (CLD)
- Pulse: rapid (CCF)
- Palmar crease pallor (CRF)
- Palmar erythema (CLD)
- Joint swelling (IBD)
- Wrist flaring (osteodystrophy)

Arms
- Spider naevi (CLD)
- Muscle bulk: poor (PCM, CRF, CLD)
- Subcutaneous fat: poor (as above)

6. Head and neck
Neck
JVP: elevated (CCF)
Face
Moon face, hirsute (steroids)
Malar flush (SLE causing GN)
Eyes
Scleral icterus (CLD)
Conjunctival pallor (CRF)

Mouth: uraemic foetor (CRF)
Tongue: glossitis (nutritional deficiency)

7. Chest
Palpate
- Rib rosary (osteodystrophy)
- Cardiomegaly (CCF, CRF)

Auscultate
- Flow murmur (CCF)
- Gallop rhythm (CCF)
- Crepitations (CCF)

8. Abdomen
Palpate
- Hepatomegaly (CCF, CLD)
- Splenomegaly (CLD)
- Nephromegaly (polycystic disease, hydronephrosis)
- Inguinal lymphadenopathy (if leg oedema only: local cause)
- Scrotal oedema

Demonstrate ascites
Inspect
- Buttock purpura (HSP)
- Perianal disease (IBD)

Stool analysis

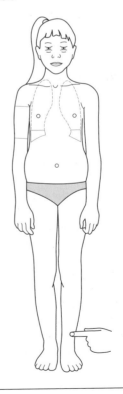

CCF = congestive cardial failure; CF = cystic fibrosis; CLD = chronic liver disease; CRF = chronic renal failure; GN = glomerulonephritides; HSP = Henoch-Schönlein purpura; IBD = inflammatory bowel disease; PCN = protein calorie malnutrition.

Neurology

Long cases

Cerebral palsy

Children with cerebral palsy (CP) often are used for both long- and short-case examinations. The following is a very brief listing of some of the major issues raised in the CP long case, plus a short case approach.

Background information

CP is a static encephalopathy—a non-progressive disorder of motion and/or posture, secondary to an insult in the developing brain. This excludes active degenerative progressive disorders. Despite its static nature, the peripheral manifestations may seem to progress and mimic progressive central nervous system pathology.

Classification

CP is classified according to the clinical type of neuromotor dysfunction:
1. Spastic (subgroups: monoplegic, diplegic, triplegic, quadriplegic).
2. Dyskinetic (extrapyramidal; subgroups may have athetosis, chorea, rigidity or dystonia).
3. Ataxic.
4. Atonic.
5. Mixed (subgroups including spastic-athetoid, ataxic-spastic).

Spastic diplegia is the most common subtype. Spasticity classically develops between 6 and 18 months. The most commonly affected muscles are the paraspinal muscles, hip flexors and adductors, hamstrings, gastrocnemius and soleus. Muscle spasticity and contractures can lead to bone and joint changes.

Causes

In around one-third of cases, the underlying aetiology is unknown. Known causes can be classified as follows:

1. **Prenatal problems**, e.g. cerebral malformations, intrauterine TORCH infection (toxoplasma, other [e.g. syphilis], rubella, CMV, herpes [simplex or varicella] or HIV infection), placental insufficiency, fetal coagulation and autoimmune disorders, cerebrovascular accidents or chromosomal anomalies.
2. **Perinatal problems**, e.g. prematurity, hypoxia (see below), hypoglycaemia, kernicterus.

3. **Postnatal problems**, e.g. trauma, cerebrovascular accident, intracranial infections.

Epidemiological studies show that in 90% of cases, the cause of CP could *not* be intrapartum hypoxia. In the remaining 10%, intrapartum signs consistent with hypoxic damage may have had maternal or intrapartum origins. Recommendations have been made that the term birth asphyxia should not be used, as it is inappropriate and inaccurate. Rather the terms antenatal hypoxia and intrapartum hypoxia, concerning correct timing of damaging hypoxia, should be used. Similarly the term hypoxic ischaemic encephalopathy is used loosely, in situations where hypoxia and ischaemia have not been proved; it should not be used in this manner.

Criteria have been developed defining acute intrapartum events sufficient to cause permanent neurological impairment:

1. Evidence of metabolic acidosis in the fetal umbilical arterial cord or early neonatal blood (pH less than 7.00; base deficit greater than, or equal to, 12 mmol/L).
2. Early onset of moderate to severe neonatal encephalopathy in infants of 34 weeks' gestation or more.
3. Spastic quadriplegic or dyskinetic types of CP.

For each child with CP, the above areas (classification, cause) should be defined, as well as functional severity, and prognosis. The long-case presentation should address the major problems (a) as the parent sees them and (b) as the various caregivers (e.g. doctors) see them; the interpretation may be quite different.

It is advisable to cover areas that were of interest to the examiners when they took the history and examined the child (ask 'What did the examiners ask about? What areas did they examine?').

History

Presenting complaint

Reason for current admission.

Current symptoms/functioning

1. Intellectual abilities (or present developmental status), current placement regarding education, domestic situation, employment.
2. Behaviour (e.g. hyperactivity), affect (e.g. depression).
3. Vision (e.g. cortical visual impairment, strabismus, myopia, hemianopia).
4. Speech, hearing and communication problems (e.g. expressive or receptive dysphasia, dysarthria, athetoid movements, use of aids such as communication boards and computers).
5. Activities of daily living (e.g. bathing, cleaning teeth, combing hair, dressing, writing and other hand usage, toileting, menses).
6. Feeding and nutrition (e.g. sucking and swallowing ability, tube feeds, gastrostomy, gastro-oesophageal reflux, aspiration, failure to thrive).
7. Seizures (e.g. type, duration, frequency, usual treatment including side effects, compliance and drug levels, last seizure).
8. Mobility (e.g. walking ability ['community', 'household' or 'non-functional' ambulator], gait pattern, wheelchair mobility), skeletal problems (e.g. kyphoscoliosis, lumbar lordosis, spondylolisthesis, hip subluxation and dislocation, pseudoacetabulum formation, contractures, unequal leg length), abnormal posturing.

9. Other problems: urinary incontinence, constipation, management of menses, chest infections, pressure sores.

Birth history

1. Maternal past history of miscarriages or infertility.
2. Pregnancy: hyperemesis, hypertensive disease of pregnancy, teratogenic medications, placental problems, clinical evidence of, or exposure to, infection (e.g. TORCH), quality of fetal movements, gestational age.
3. Delivery: presentation (e.g. breech, face), instrumental delivery, Apgar score, resuscitation required, birth weight, need for oxygen, nursery care.
4. Neonatal period: respiratory distress, feeding difficulties, seizures, hyperbilirubinaemia (phototherapy or exchange transfusion), intraventricular haemorrhage (IVH), periventricular leukomalacia (PVL), hydrocephalus, retinopathy of prematurity (ROP).

Developmental history

Age at which milestones achieved (including quality of attainment: e.g. bottom shuffling, bunny-hopping, gross motor development, early hand preference in fine motor development).

Family history

Any family history of CP.

Management

Recent management in hospital, usual treatment at home, daily routine, frequency of therapies, (e.g. physiotherapy, occupational therapy, speech therapy), usual doctors seen (e.g. local doctor, local paediatrician, subspecialists such as orthopaedic surgeon, neurologist), compliance with treatment, alternative therapies tried (e.g. acupressure, patterning).

Social history

Impact on parents and siblings, disruption to family routine, family financial considerations (e.g. private health insurance, visits to multiple specialists, cost of hospitalisations, surgical procedures, aids, home modifications, drugs, benefits received such as Child Disability Allowance), social supports (social worker, extended family, respite care, involvement of Spastic Centre, self-help groups), legal proceedings surrounding perinatal care.

Understanding of problems and prognosis

Parents' and siblings' understanding; degree of education regarding CP; question of resuscitation.

Important signs in examination of the child with CP

The procedure outlined below can be used for a long- or short-case examination. When presented in the long case, the examination of the child with CP should convey to the examiners an overall picture of the patient (e.g. 'a profoundly intellectually handicapped microcephalic girl with spastic quadriplegia') as the initial introduction.

In the short-case context, a wide number of introductions may be given; e.g. 'not walking', 'not developing as well as his siblings', 'has unusual movements', 'has a limp', 'wears out the tips of his shoes', 'has back arching', or more directed introductions such as 'This boy has cerebral palsy; please assess him for complications', or 'This girl was premature; please assess her for complications of prematurity'.

In the case of a child with hemiplegic CP, the lead-in may more likely be 'Please examine this boy's gait' or 'Please examine the peripheral nervous system'.

See the short case on hemiplegia in this chapter for a suggested examination procedure.

In each case, the initial 1 to 2 minutes spent standing back and inspecting should identify CP as the most likely problem and direct the examination accordingly.

General observations

1. Dysmorphic features (e.g. chromosomal anomalies).
2. Parameters: head circumference (often obvious microcephaly), weight (often failing to thrive), height (usually decreased), progressive percentile charts.
3. Posture (e.g. fisting, increased extensor tone, asymmetric tonic neck reflex (ATNR), hemiplegic, quadriplegic).
4. Movement: (a) involuntary (e.g. choreoathetoid movements, dystonic spasms, seizures); (b) voluntary (e.g. immature gait pattern with wide base, up on toes, arms out for balance; hemiplegic, diplegic gaits; note posturing of arms when walking).
5. Asymmetry (e.g. hemiatrophy: look at the size of the thumbnails and the great toenails for subtle clues of asymmetry).
6. Behaviour (e.g. lack of interaction with environment, crying).
7. Eye signs (e.g. squint, nystagmus).
8. Bulbar signs (e.g. dysarthria, drooling).
9. Interventions (e.g. nasogastric tube, gastrostomy tube, scars of orthopaedic procedures).
10. Clothing (e.g. nappies in child over 4 years old).
11. Peripheral aids (e.g. wheelchair, splints, orthoses).

Demonstration of signs of CP

1. If possible, perform a standard gait examination.
2. If the child cannot walk, but can crawl, look for abnormal crawling: (a) those with spastic diplegia or quadriplegia—buttock crawling and 'bunny-hopping' (jumping while on knees); (b) those with hemiplegia—asymmetrical crawl.
3. Gross motor '180-degree manoeuvre', incorporating primitive reflexes:
   a. Lying supine (assess position adopted, e.g. ATNR).
   b. Pull to sit by hands (to assess head lag and grasp).
   c. Sitting (assess sitting ability, then lateral propping).
   d. Hold up vertically, under axillae (to detect increased extensor tone, scissoring, automatic walking).
   e. Tilt sideways (to assess head righting).
   f. Ventral suspension (to detect excessive extensor tone).
   g. Parachute reflex (to detect asymmetry).
   h. Place prone (to detect back arching).
4. Inspect carefully for tendon release scars.
5. Palpate muscle bulk in each muscle group.
6. Tone: as above, plus assessment of upper and lower limbs, and evaluation of contractures (e.g. tight hip adductors, and tendoachilles).
7. Power: voluntary movement, functional power (grasp of toys, cloth cover test).

8. Reflexes: the head should be held in the midline (e.g. by an examiner) so that an ATNR does not give a false impression of unilateral hypertonia; note whether there is any crossed adductor reflex, spread of reflexes, clonus or upgoing plantar responses.

Complications of CP

1. Measure the head (for microcephaly, or macrocephaly due to hydrocephalus).
2. Check the vision, visual fields and extraocular movements (for myopia, squint).
3. Check the hearing (for sensorineural deafness).
4. Check the ears (for chronic serous otitis media).
5. Ask to check the gag reflex (bulbar dysfunction).
6. Look at the teeth (for dental caries).
7. Look at the back (for kyphoscoliosis).
8. Inspect and auscultate the chest (for chest infection).
9. Palpate the abdomen (for constipation).
10. Examine the hips (for dislocation).
11. Screen nutritional status (demonstrate fat and protein stores).
12. Perform a functional assessment for activities of daily living (e.g. offer cup, spoon, fork, knife, comb, toothbrush; ask the child to put on a piece of clothing).

Investigations

The examiners may ask which investigations you would think appropriate in the particular child you have seen. While this depends on the type of CP the child has, the following brief list may be helpful.

1. Brain imaging (MRI or CT scan) may show abnormalities in some patients with CP. It may show the basis of CP (e.g. gross malformations, hydrocephalus, intracranial calcification from congenital infection). It may suggest the timing of the aetiology (e.g. cortical dysplasias develop around 12–20 weeks' gestation; periventricular leukomalacia around 28–34 weeks' gestation; cortical and subcortical gliosis and atrophy in parasagittal watershed areas in term babies with intrapartum hypoxia) or show unexpected degenerative disorders (e.g. one of the leukodystrophies).
2. TORCH screen (including HIV), in infants, for intrauterine infection.
3. Urinary metabolic screen (various degenerative conditions).
4. Chromosomes (various anomalies).

Management

The management of CP is multifaceted and complex. It is beyond the scope of this section to give a comprehensive account of the various treatment modalities used. Rather, a list of the main treatment areas and issues is presented, as a framework around which to base further reading.

Role of the general paediatrician

The general paediatrician (the candidate) should coordinate and oversee the various caregivers involved in the management of the child with cerebral palsy. A multidisciplinary team is needed, including a social worker, occupational therapist, physiotherapist, speech therapist, orthopaedic surgeon and psychologist.

Information would routinely be requested when a child is transferred to the care of the local paediatrician looking after the child (which is how candidates should view themselves). As part of the management discussion, it is quite valid for the candidate to request information to clarify aspects of the past history, such as the neonatal notes, results of any investigations (e.g. imaging or metabolic studies) performed and summaries of previous hospital admissions.

General nursing care

Children with CP may require tube feeds, have trouble with gastro-oesophageal reflux requiring aggressive therapy, be very irritable, need attention to skin for pressure sores, tend to soil well into childhood (requiring attention to toileting) and may dribble. They can constitute a significant workload for the parent at home and for the nursing staff in hospital.

Physiotherapy, occupational therapy, splints/orthoses

These are important in maintaining range of movement and function of trunk and limbs, and preventing contractures. Physiotherapists (PTs) and occupational therapists (OTs) enable the child to perform the activities of daily living (ADLs) as well as his or her potential allows. They can evaluate whether there is a problem in the areas of dressing, washing, toileting, feeding, positioning, methods of carrying and lifting (which vary with the different types of CP), mobility aids and whether the furniture and bathroom fittings at home are appropriate. As much as possible, therapeutic manoeuvres can be built into everyday activities (e.g. handling/feeding/playing in younger children; in older children, simple activities such as lying prone watching television for those with hip flexion contractures).

Serial casting is useful for reversing ankle/foot equinus in younger children. Over 2–6 weeks, the calf muscle is stretched gradually, with the foot and ankle held in position by a below-the-knee plaster.

Orthoses (splints) act as exoskeletons, assist with position and function, and may prevent contractures developing. Soft orthoses may be made from high-density foam, neoprene or lycra (e.g. more for low tone, good for flexed knees). Hard orthoses include solid (fixed) ankle–foot orthoses (AFOs), hinged (articulated) AFOs (allow dorsiflexion); in-shoe orthoses (e.g. supramalleolar orthoses [SMOs]).

The selection of orthoses is aided by computerised gait evaluation in gait laboratories (see below). The ankle–foot orthosis (AFO) is the most commonly used orthosis. It may prevent ankle deformity and improve gait pattern.

Splinting is of great value in the prevention of contractures. Muscles kept in a normal position for the majority of the day will grow normally. Night splinting is beneficial.

Three-dimensional (3-D) gait analysis: computerised gait laboratories

Examination of gait in CP patients in gait analysis laboratories can detect primary movement problems, differentiating them from secondary or coping manoeuvres. Assessment of the complex gait deviations, which occur in three planes of motion, can direct an interdisciplinary team's clinical decisions as to the best course of treatment. This may be orthopaedic surgical intervention, or treatment that may be of more direct benefit than surgery, including orthotics, botulinum toxin A (BTX-A) therapy (see below) or PT.

Optical/reflective markers are placed at specific anatomical landmarks/limb segments, and as the child walks the 3-D location is detected by multiple infrared cameras. Gait analysis usually includes clinical lower limb examination, videotaped walking, measurement of limb segment motion (kinematics), and measurement of forces and moments causing that motion (kinetics). This includes 3-D joint motion at ankle, hip and knee; joint mobility; joint angular velocities; joint powers; gait parameters such as step, stride length and cadence; synchronised dynamic electromyography (EMG); ground reaction forces and foot pressure analysis. Children walk on a force plate to assess the amount of power generated. The energy cost of walking is also assessed: oxygen consumption, respiratory function and heart rate can be measured with a portable telemetric system. Most units have specific referral criteria, which may include being ambulatory (with or without aids) for at least 10 steps, being at least 4 years old, cooperative, and at least 100 cm tall.

Management of spasticity

Botulinum toxin A (BTX-A)

BTX-A is a neurotoxin produced by *Clostridium botulinum*, given by intramuscular (IM) injection, and taken up by endocytosis at cholinergic nerve terminals at the motor endplate, preventing release of acetylcholine from these terminals, which leads to a prolonged, reversible relaxation of skeletal muscle. BTX-A is useful for correcting gait abnormalities and for reducing the need for orthopaedic surgery. There are seven serotypes (A–G) of botulinum toxin; types A, B and F have been used clinically. BTX-A causes local paralysis in the injected muscle with an onset within 1–3 days of the IM injection. Duration of action is 3–6 months, by which time motor nerves generate new neuromuscular junctions by terminal sprouting, and there is then a clinical return of spasticity (from 12–16 weeks in most patients). Injections then may be repeated.

BTX-A reduces hypertonicity. Indication for use is dynamic contracture in the absence of a fixed deformity. Muscles typically targeted include gastrocnemius-soleus complex, tibialis posterior (to relieve equinovarus), hamstrings (to relieve crouch gait), adductors (improves positioning and perineal access for hygiene), rectus femoris (to relieve flexed stiff knee gait) and iliopsoas (to relieve dynamic deformity of hip flexion during gait). Decreased spasticity in iliopsoas and adductors may modify natural history of subluxation or dislocation of the hip. BTX-A may be used in the upper limbs as well as the lower. It may decrease muscle spasm after soft-tissue releases.

BTX-A is well tolerated, but there are several potential side effects. BTX-A can diffuse intra-axonally and across fascial planes, causing distant side effects. Side effects can be gait-related, including deterioration in walking, local weakness and falls. Other side effects have included aspiration pneumonia (impaired pharyngeal function from systemic spread of small amounts of BTX-A), local pain, muscle atrophy, global weakness and incontinence of urine and faeces. Drug interactions include non-depolarising muscle relaxants and aminoglycosides causing potentiation of neuromuscular blockade. Other disadvantages include cost and need for repeated injections. The neuromuscular junctions that are blocked are the same as those that cause meaningful movement. BTX-A may reveal underlying weakness or cause weakness by 'overcorrection', and 6 weeks later there will be a return of strength/function, but without the presenting problem. There have been very rare reports of intermittent tetraparesis after treatment. It may be used for relief of rigidity, but the effects in the extrapyramidal forms of CP are not so dramatic.

The majority of patients using BTX-A for treating spasticity demonstrate objective improvement in tone and function. Kinematic parameters of gait are improved in lower limb spasticity. Integrated multilevel BTX-A has a similar effect to a medical rhizotomy.

Intrathecal baclofen (IT-BLF)

This can cause decrease in tone in children with severe spasticity. Its greatest benefit is in the reduction of lower limb tone. It can be given by an implantable drug-delivery pump system for continuous infusion. However significant complications can arise, including central side effects such as apnoea, respiratory depression, bradycardia, hypotension and sedation, or various mechanical complications including pump or side-port failure, catheter kinks, extrusions or dislodgement, cerebrospinal fluid fistula, local infection and meningitis. Also, there have been reports of rapidly progressive scoliosis. IT-BLF has potential value, but more experience is needed to quantify the risk:benefit ratio.

Selective dorsal rhizotomy (SDR)

This has been widely used to treat spasticity in children with diplegic CP, but never shown to improve functional outcome conclusively. SDR involves intraoperative stimulation of lumbar nerve rootlets, monitored with EMG: the nerves that cause increased tone are cut. SDR decreases spasticity, but does not affect selective motor control, weakness, poor balance or fixed deformities. There are reports that SDR combined with PT and OT leads to greater functional motor improvement, compared to PT and OT alone.

Other treatments

Oral baclofen and oral diazepam have each been used for spasticity and a limited response can be seen. There have been some positive reports that physical training in CP increases aerobic power and isokinetic muscle strength, and that movement and swimming programs improve baseline vital capacity and water-orientation skills. It is likely that more research will be conducted in these areas. Other new therapeutic options in the management of spasticity include repetitive magnetic stimulation and the use of the anticonvulsant drug gabapentin.

Orthopaedic procedures

Single event multilevel surgery (SEMLS)

Multilevel orthopaedic surgical procedures for gait are performed at tertiary centres. The plan is based on comprehensive 3-D gait analysis. There are two surgeons and two operative teams. Generally 6–16 soft-tissue/bony procedures are undertaken, with postoperative epidural anaesthesia for up to 5 days and a total hospital stay of 7 days. Subsequently, there is community rehabilitation and review at 3, 6, 9 and 12 months in the 3-D gait laboratory. SEMLS allows correction and prevention of deformities, and has positive benefits as regards cosmesis. Procedures performed may include hip adductor tenotomies (help prevent hip subluxation and allow easier attention to perineal hygiene), hamstring releases (relieve knee contractures), lengthening of the tendoachilles (correcting equinus deformity), and surgery to correct valgus deformity of the foot.

Surgical procedures for spastic hip displacement

The natural history of hip displacement in CP is enlocation at birth, but with displacement occurring at 4–8% per annum. Displacement is easily missed on clinical examination, but easily detected and monitored by X-ray. There are preventative procedures (soft tissue), reconstructive procedures (osteotomies) and salvage procedures. These may be performed in the setting of SEMLS. The procedures available are as follows:

* **Preventative (soft-tissue surgery):** adductor longus release, gracilis release, adductor brevis release, iliopsoas lengthening, obturator neurectomy (anterior branch only).

- **Reconstructive (redirectional osteotomies):** femoral varus derotation osteotomy, pelvic osteotomy, combined femoral and pelvic osteotomy with or without open reduction.
- **Salvage:** excision of proximal femur, valgus osteotomy, interpositional arthroplasty, replacement arthroplasty, arthrodesis.

These procedures lead to significant improvements in function, including improved walking speed.

Other orthopaedic procedures

Upper limb surgery may be offered to correct a flexion–pronation deformity of the wrist, to achieve a better functional position; however, usually only cosmetic improvement is achieved, with little gain functionally, largely because of associated cortical sensory loss. Some children will require surgery for scoliosis (e.g. placing of Luque rods).

Gastrointestinal (GIT) problems and nutrition

Up to two-thirds of children with CP have disorders of GIT motility. Significant GIT symptoms include constipation (delayed colonic transit, especially of proximal colon), swallowing disorders (especially dysfunction of the oral and/or pharyngeal phase of swallowing), vomiting and/or regurgitation (delay in gastric emptying, abnormal oesophageal motility, gastro-oesophageal reflux [GOR]), abdominal pain (due to GOR-associated oesophagitis or constipation) and respiratory symptoms due to chronic pulmonary aspiration, secondary to GOR. GIT symptoms are not related to specific types of CP.

Children with CP often fail to thrive, due to GOR and/or impairment of swallowing. These children may require assessment and therapy by a speech therapist, nasogastric tube feeding or placement of a gastrostomy.

Speech therapy

The management of dysarthria, dysphasia and drooling requires assessment and treatment by an experienced speech pathologist.

Social implications

This is a major discussion point. Behaviour disorders in the child (e.g. attention deficits, depression from realisation of disability) are common. The siblings may be neglected inadvertently. There may be several significant burdens on the parents: emotional, physical and financial (e.g. hospitalisations, electric wheelchairs, home aids, home modifications, computer and communication devices). Inordinate amounts of time may be spent on the activities of daily living (ADLs), including feeding the child, physiotherapy and occupational therapy, and administering medications, with the parent/carer not having time for anyone else. Marriages may break up from the strain of managing a chronic disabling disorder such as CP.

It is vital to give parents the opportunity to detail their problems, offering to organise a social worker to discuss these, and encouraging the use of respite care. Ask the mother how much time is spent on the child's needs each day. The examiners will know the answer, having asked this themselves to ascertain the candidate's understanding of the implications of care in CP.

Seizures

The management of seizures in CP follows the same general approach as that of other seizure disorders. See the long-case approach to recurrent seizures in this chapter.

Visual impairment

A large number of children with CP have a squint (50–60%). Decreased visual acuity is common in spastic quadriplegia, and visual field defects are common in hemiplegic CP. Referral to an ophthalmologist is necessary. Management may include spectacles for refractive errors. For squint, which may cause permanent amblyopia after the age of 6 years, patching the good eye may be required. Surgical rearrangements of extraocular muscle actions to achieve parallel eye axes may well be needed. Educational aids will also be very important.

If the best-corrected acuity is less than 3/60, the child will require use of braille and teaching by methods not involving sight. 'Blind' means acuity of less than 6/60, not correctable by glasses. In 'partially sighted' children (i.e. acuity between 6/24 and 6/60) large print and magnifying aids will be useful.

Hearing impairment

Management depends upon the degree of hearing loss. Mild loss, that is 25–45 decibel (dB) loss, does not necessarily require intervention. Moderate loss (45–65 dB) requires some treatment with otological intervention or fitting of a hearing aid. Severe loss (65–85 dB) always requires amplification to hear speech. Profound loss (over 85 dB) requires special education for the deaf, as there is insufficient hearing for any useful communication. Intervention by an ear, nose and throat specialist may be necessary for conductive causes amenable to surgical intervention (e.g. suction myringotomy and insertion of ventilation tubes, tympanoplasty). For provision of hearing aids and information regarding auditory training facilities, referral to a competent audiology centre, e.g. in a large teaching hospital, or the Australian Hearing Service, is appropriate.

Schooling

Many children with CP have some degree of intellectual impairment, as well as physical disabilities. Many children with CP require special educational assistance to maximise their potential. Most states, regions or areas have their own centres that are designed to assist in all aspects of the management of CP (e.g. The Spastic Centre in New South Wales).

Intervention programs—orthodox

Most orthodox-trained therapists aim to enhance the child's quality of life and to give the parents realistic expectations of outcome. This goal begins from the early intervention stage, encouraging parents to modify how they handle their child to allow the full use of the child's motor abilities, and giving advice and support at all levels of developmental experience, in the home, child care, kindergarten, preschool, school, university and/or work-force settings. The main practice in Australia is based on facilitation techniques, with training in motor functional activities following the developmental sequence from head control to walking. This aids posture and movement control, towards eventual independence, recognising that those who are going to walk will usually do so by 7 years of age.

Intervention programs—less orthodox/unorthodox

There is no evidence that any specific intervention significantly changes the course of the motor disorder in CP. There are no convincing studies that show that outcomes from any 'unorthodox' therapies have any advantage over the outcomes from orthodox therapies, as practised by paediatric rehabilitation units in tertiary/teaching centres of excellence. A number of interventions have been available for many years. The better known include: Bobath's neurodevelopmental technique, conductive education (CE), acupressure, chiropractic, naturopathy, faith healing and the (largely abandoned) approaches of Vojta, and of Doman and Delacato (patterning). The American Academy of Pediatrics issued a policy statement in November 1999 on the treatment of neurologically impaired children using patterning, noting that it was 'based on an outmoded and oversimplified theory...current information does not support the claims of proponents that this treatment is efficacious, and its use continues to be unwarranted'.

Unfortunately, none of these methods has been shown effective in any well-designed randomised double-blind controlled trials. Despite this, many parents will try 'alternative' therapies; proponents of some may exhibit messianic zeal regarding their favoured therapy. A sensible approach to adopt is not to criticise these parents for doing so, as long as the child is not harmed in any way. One should explain to the family that there is no proof that these methods work better than more conventional treatment. The inadvertent engendering of false hope should be discouraged.

Excessive salivation

Anticholinergic drugs have been used for excessive drooling with some success, but ongoing excessive salivation may lead to consideration of operative intervention. Three procedures have been tried:

1. Transplanting the salivary ducts to the back of the pharynx.
2. Excising one of the salivary glands.
3. Section of the chorda tympani nerve.

Unfortunately, none of these procedures has any lasting benefit.

Drugs

Anticonvulsants for children with seizures are the only drugs consistently of use.

Duchenne's muscular dystrophy (DMD)

DMD is the most common childhood form of muscular dystrophy. Boys with DMD are often subjects for the long-case examination. Genetic counselling and prenatal diagnosis are likely discussion areas in the management of the DMD long case.

Background information on genetics of DMD

DMD is an X-linked recessive disorder, due to mutations (often deletions) in the dystrophin gene on the X chromosome (Xp21.2). It has a frequency of 1 in 3500 male births. The DMD gene is around 2000 kilobases in size and codes for dystrophin, a large, rod-like 427-kD protein containing 3685 amino acids and located at the inner face of the muscle cell membrane. Dystrophin binds with a group of 'dystrophin-associated proteins' (e.g. sarcoglycans, dystroglycans, merosin) that span the muscle membrane, linking the muscle cytoskeleton and the extracellular matrix. Absence of dystrophin disrupts the link, making the muscle membrane susceptible to damage from shearing stresses. Hence, dystrophin-deficient muscle is very susceptible to muscle injury, and degeneration of muscle fibres is a feature of dystrophic muscle. Dystrophin is undetectable in the muscle of DMD patients. Note that mutations in the dystrophin gene that result in the production of abnormal dystrophin (abnormal size or abnormal quantity) result in the milder Becker's muscular dystrophy. The tissue distribution of dystrophin correlates with clinical features. It is found in skeletal, cardiac and smooth muscle (resulting in skeletal muscle weakness and cardiomyopathy), and within the central nervous system (resulting in a static encephalopathy and cognitive deficits). Various forms of dystrophin are expressed in neurons and glia in the brain, especially the cortex, hippocampus, cerebellum and retina.

Molecular tests for DMD

1. Dystrophin detection in muscle (immunocytochemistry, protein electrophoresis [Western blotting]).
2. Dystrophin gene mutation detection, analysing DNA from peripheral blood by polymerase chain reaction (PCR). In DMD, deletions can be detected in 60–70% of patients, of whom two-thirds have intragenic deletions (which usually remove one or more exons). The remaining patients have intragenic duplications, which can now be detected by new molecular genetic techniques, or point mutations, which can usually be detected only by sequencing the gene. The latter is not performed routinely due to the large size of the gene.
3. Linkage studies are used for those in whom mutations are not detected by the assays currently available. In addition, linkage analysis using intragenic markers is the most reliable way to determine carrier status in families where the genetic mutation is known. Genotype predictions are always less than 100%, as there is a risk that meiotic recombination will alter the relationship between the marker locus and the disease locus.
4. Prenatal diagnosis is available by chorionic villus biopsy or amniocentesis by direct testing for abnormalities in the dystrophin gene.

Recent advances

In the last five years, research into DMD has accelerated, with a number of different treatment strategies being proposed. The role of steroids has become clearer. There is evidence that low-dose steroids can be useful when boys are still walking, to improve motor function. They need close monitoring, adjusting dose and timing to avoid unwanted side effects, especially weight gain.

It has been established that *prednisone* is effective in achieving delay in disease progression, prolongation of ability to walk, maintenance of strength and function, delay in, or prevention of, development of scoliosis, preservation of respiratory function by attenuating fibrosis of the diaphragm. The precise mechanism by which prednisone exerts a therapeutic effect is unknown. Prednisone is immunosuppressive, and also has direct effects on muscle cells. It can modulate proteolysis and calcium handling, increase myogenesis and inhibit apoptosis. A dose of 0.75 mg/kg per day can increase muscle strength within 10 days of commencement, and this effect can be maintained for 18 months. An ideal schedule for this is yet to be confirmed: some units use 10 days on, 10 days off; some units use alternate daily doses; some use weekly high doses (5–10 mg/kg per week). Side effects include weight gain, hypertension, osteoporosis, hyperglycaemia, easy bruising and behavioural problems. Prednisolone is used in children over 5 years of age. Side effects can preclude its ongoing use.

Another steroid which is as effective as prednisolone in maintaining muscle strength and function is *deflazacort*, a methyloxazoline derivative of prednisone. Deflazacort (DFZ) also enhances cardiac and pulmonary function and attenuates the development of scoliosis, including when ambulation is lost. DFZ may cause less severe adverse side effects (e.g. less weight gain) than prednisone. DFZ is not yet available in Australia except as part of a clinical trial.

A number of therapeutic approaches are being developed for DMD, but most of these are still at the experimental stage in animal models. Gene therapy trials using new generation adenovirus carriers known as 'stealth' or 'gutted' vectors (containing no original viral genes) are being developed to overcome the obstacle of the immune system. Work proceeds on alternative strategies to replace the defective dystrophin gene in DMD patients. These include 'exon skipping', where cells can read defective genes so some dystrophin is made, and 'utrophin upregulation', which attempts to increase muscle cell production of 'utrophin', a protein related to dystrophin, which can substitute or compensate for it if made in sufficient amounts. Primitive stem cells in bone marrow have been shown to migrate into muscle and become new muscle cells. Gentamicin has been found to permit cells to ignore an abnormal stop codon in the dystrophin gene and to proceed and synthesise the protein in the 15% of DMD patients who have premature stop codons as their underlying mutation.

Pharmacological approaches to develop a drug that can maintain muscles and function for a finite time are being explored, as they may be developed more rapidly than gene therapy techniques. The degradation of muscle fibres in DMD is predominantly caused by the enzyme *calpain*, a protease, activated by calcium. Muscle fibres contain an inactive form of calpain at their contractile structures. Inhibitors of calpain, such as *leupeptin*, can stop muscle degradation in the mouse model of DMD. A study in Italy in boys treated with leupeptin showed significant decreases in CK levels using low-dose leupeptin for one year. Another protease-blocking medication being trialled is Bowman–Birk inhibitor concentrate (BBIC), which blocks the dystrophic process in the mouse model of DMD. Myostatin, or growth differentiation factor number 8 (GDF-8), is made as an inactive protein. When a propeptide is split off, the resulting active myostatin initiates a sequence of reactions, ultimately leading to interruption of the genetic regulation that would usually result in the biosynthesis of new muscle proteins. By inactivating myostatin, regeneration of muscles may occur: this is being trialled in the mouse model as well, using a monoclonal antibody. A boy born without myostatin (both myostatin genes on chromosome 2 inactivated by a mutation) has muscles twice the normal size and is physically very strong. This has stimulated much interest in the potential of blocking myostatin in DMD. Other agents being researched include salbutamol, creatine, anabolic steroids, and calcium channel blockers.

History

Ask about the following.

Presenting complaint
Reason for current admission.

Current problems
1. Functional abilities with activities of daily living (e.g. dressing, writing); aids required (e.g. splints, supportive prostheses, computer-assisted communication/learning).
2. Mobility (e.g. long leg braces, wheelchair use, school and home access).

3. Home modifications required (e.g. ramps, bathroom fittings).
4. Transport needs (e.g. van with hoist).
5. Scoliosis (e.g. progression, any planned surgery).
6. Joint contractures.
7. Respiratory problems (e.g. symptoms of respiratory failure at later stage).
8. Cardiac symptoms (e.g. arrhythmias, symptoms of cardiac failure).
9. Gastrointestinal problems (e.g. incontinence, vomiting).
10. School (e.g. any access problems, educational problems, any help needed or provided with toileting; attitudes of class teacher, headmaster, fellow students).

Past history

1. Initial diagnosis—when, where, presenting symptoms (e.g. late walking, tendency to fall, method of rising after fall, clumsiness, muscle cramps, learning delay, cognitive impairment, global or gross motor developmental delay).
2. How long between onset of symptoms and diagnosis.
3. What investigations were done to make the diagnosis.
4. Stages of deterioration (e.g. age at which the child lost the ability to climb stairs, stand from the floor or walk independently).
5. Number of hospitalisations.
6. Development of complications (e.g. scoliosis, cardiac failure) and their management.
7. Surgical procedures (e.g. release of contractures).

Current management

Present treatment in hospital, usual treatment at home (including physiotherapy, exercise, breathing exercises, medications taken), future treatment plans (e.g. surgical procedures), usual follow-up (by whom, where, how often), alternative therapies tried (e.g. acupuncture, naturopathy).

Social history

1. Impact on child (e.g. difficulties at school, poor job prospects, limitations on lifestyle, body image, self-esteem, peer reactions).
2. Impact on family (e.g. parental coping, difficulties between mother and father, genetic implications for further children; financial considerations, such as cost of wheelchairs, home modifications, transport, hospitalisations, private health insurance; physical burden of helping children in and out of wheelchairs, cars, bed, bath).
3. Benefits received.
4. Social supports (e.g. social worker, DMD Family Support Group provided by the Muscular Dystrophy Association, visits to school by occupational therapist and community liaison nurse from hospital muscle clinic to meet class and teachers).

Family history

Other known family members with DMD, other males with developmental delay or late walking.

Understanding of disease

By the child, by the family (e.g. parents, grandparents, siblings) and by teachers. Ask the degree of previous education (e.g. in hospital, by local paediatrician), contingency plans (e.g. what to do when child develops a respiratory infection).

At the completion of the history, think about what particular problems this family is experiencing at the moment, from the viewpoints of the child, the parents and the attending physicians. These three perspectives may be quite different.

Examination

General inspection

Describe the resting posture (undressed). If the child can still stand, describe the standing posture. Usually this includes findings of small interscapular muscle bulk, small proximal upper limb musculature, abnormal anterior axillary fold (atrophic sternal head of pectoralis major), lordosis, some internal rotation of the femurs (due to muscle imbalance), small thighs with preservation of vastus lateralis, but prominent calves (pseudohypertrophy) and equinus deformity of the feet. If in a wheelchair, describe the child's posture, and also comment on the chair itself (that is, whether it is appropriate or needs some adjustments). Note whether the respiratory rate is raised (for intercurrent respiratory infection or cardiac failure). Also note the child's demeanour, apparent mood, intelligence and ability to communicate.

Gait

Ask the child to walk normally. Focus on each component of the gait in turn, starting at the feet (foot drop due to weak tibialis anterior, inversion due to strong tibialis posterior and weak peroneals, heels off ground partly due to tightened tendoachilles, higher step to gait than normal). Next inspect the knees (weakened quadriceps leading to knee locking gait, where the knee is snapped back into extension quickly for stability) and then the hips (weakened hip flexors require rotation of upper body to enable leg to swing forward; weakened hip abductors, gluteus medius, cause tilting of pelvis down on unsupported side with each step during walking—Trendelenberg's gait; weakened hip extensors, gluteus maximus and hamstrings, lead to a forward pelvic tilt and marked lordosis to maintain centre of gravity). Overall, the gait also has a wide base and the appearance of waddling.

Proceed with the other components of a full gait examination, including asking the child to run, hop, jump, squat and rise, walk up stairs, step onto a stool or chair, and do a sit-up and a push-up.

Boys with DMD can walk well on their toes, but are unable to walk on their heels, and if they try they end up inverting the feet. On squatting, these children are slow to return to standing, need to extend the knee before the hip, and lean on their thighs to assist extension at the hip.

Of particular importance is the elicitation of Gower's sign. The boy is asked to lie supine on the floor and then to get up. This first leads to rolling over to be prone (he cannot sit up because of weak neck and spine flexion), then onto the knees, then on 'all fours', i.e. hands and feet, then 'climbing up' the legs to stand.

Muscle power

All the muscle groups should then be tested and graded according to the Medical Research Council scale, i.e. 3 = full range against gravity, 4 = full range against resistance, 5 = normal.

Begin by testing against gravity. If this is attained, then test with resistance, but if it is failed, test with gravity removed. An example is the examination of the hip movements. First, testing against gravity: hip flexion (lying supine), hip abduction and adduction (lying on side), hip extension (lying prone). If extension is possible, then assess the gluteus maximus specifically by testing with the knee bent (if the knee is extended, this tests hamstrings as well). If the patient is unable to move against gravity, test with gravity removed, testing hip abduction and adduction (lying supine), hip extension and flexion (lying on side).

After comprehensive assessment of muscle power, check for contractures, especially at the ankles, knees and hips, tone and reflexes (knee jerks often lost).

Remainder of examination

The rest of the examination should comprise a full neurological assessment. In any child with a neuromuscular problem, this should include examining for myotonia, fasciculations, thickened nerves and abnormal sensation (although these do not occur in DMD). Examine the back (noting the details of any scoliosis), and the cardiorespiratory system (for evidence of respiratory infection or cardiac failure). Also an impression of any degree of intellectual impairment is important.

Management

The management of a child with Duchenne's muscular dystrophy is very complex and has much relevance to managing other chronic conditions.

A team approach is appropriate in the management of DMD. A hospital-based team would usually comprise a neurologist, geneticist, orthopaedic surgeon, physiotherapist, occupational therapist, orthotist, clinical nurse coordinator and social worker. The local paediatrician's (i.e. the candidate's) role, in the case of a child under the care of a muscle clinic team, includes keeping in full contact with the team regarding changes in medical care, being available to coordinate overall medical care and dealing with any problems that arise between clinic visits, such as managing intercurrent infections. Perhaps the general practitioner or paediatrician should be the principal advisor/counsellor, although this is seldom the case: the candidate may have views on this issue.

The main management areas are described below.

Psychosocial

1. Education of parents and patient. Clarification of misinformation from other sources requires multiple informative sessions with the various disciplines involved in the comprehensive management of these patients. Regular feedback is needed to ensure no misunderstandings occur. Other family members (e.g. siblings, grandparents, aunts, uncles and cousins) are often very much involved emotionally and tend to be neglected.
2. Expectation of grief reaction to diagnosis and its implications. Preparatory explanation to parents of probable feelings such as guilt, anger, depression. Explanation regarding any misapprehensions or strange beliefs about the nature of the illness.
3. Ensuring sufficient social supports, both from professionals (such as social workers) and non-professionals (such as other affected patients, families of other patients and groups such as the Muscular Dystrophy Association (MDA) or the Society for Crippled Children). The MDA provides parents' groups and a useful handbook that deals with the home situation, recreational activities, education and vocational possibilities. There is an excellent site on the Internet (at <http://mdausa.org>).
4. Informing about financial assistance measures, such as any government benefits (which may assist directly with the child's care, transport costs, accommodation costs, and provision of aids). The illness places a very large financial burden for home modification (such as ramps, bathroom modification, lifting machines) on the family.

5. Discussion of treatment difficulties (such as non-compliance), seeking other opinions, and understanding and acceptance of alternative therapies sought by parents.

6. A major point is helping the family to determine how various people (especially the affected son) are to be informed. The paediatrician may not be the person who will help most, but does have responsibility to ensure that it is done adequately. The consequences of failure in this aspect of management may include: parents who will not discuss the disease with their son, siblings, teachers or each other; one parent (usually the father) withdraws from reality; help is refused (because parents believe the child is cured by divine intervention).

Therapies

Physiotherapy

1. Stretches for contractures (e.g. flexion contractures at knees, hips, elbows, wrists, fingers); to minimise contractures, daily passive range of motion exercises of all joints of upper and lower limbs.

2. Exercises for strength (against gravity or resistance). Once the muscles are very weakened, these have little effect.

3. Chest physiotherapy for respiratory problems; teaching effective coughing. The use of inspiratory and expiratory exercises against resistance has increased over the last decade ('motivational breathing exercises'/'incentive spirometry' are used to open alveoli). Other devices include the intrapulmonary percussionator, the In-Exsufflator.

Occupational therapy

1. A very important function is prescribing specifications for equipment (e.g. wheelchairs).

2. Home visits and visits to the school (meeting with teaching staff, and question and answer sessions with the affected boy's class). These visits are very valuable.

3. Advice regarding aids to activities of daily living (e.g. getting in and out of wheelchairs, bed, bath or cars).

4. Aiding posture: avoidance of certain positions (e.g. postural scoliosis, flexion), orthoses (e.g. arm supports).

5. Assessment and advice on installation of ramps for adequate mobility at home. Assess the need for lifting machines (dependent on strength of care giver at home), modifications to home (e.g. bathroom access).

Equipment

1. Wheelchairs: generally a manual type is used from around 9 years of age, and a powered type from 11 years. An appropriate vehicle is required for transport (e.g. between home and school). New-generation wheelchairs have been developed, including one which has gyroscopic electronic sensors, and the ability to switch between four wheels and two to go through sand, up and down stairs and over kerbs, as well as a lift to tackle high counters and allow eye level interaction with standing adults.

2. Inclined standing board, to stretch tendoachilles.

3. Prone board.

4. Standing desks, or lying on inclined prone board.

5. Swivel feeders (make forearms essentially weightless).

6. Hoists: mobile, fixed and fitted to car.

Orthopaedic surgery

1. Elongation of tendoachilles if still walking, although it appears that weakness is the main problem inhibiting walking, not contractures per se.

2. Tendoachilles tenotomies, tibialis posterior transfer (either or both of these if wheelchair bound).

3. Management of scoliosis. Scoliosis commonly develops around 13–15 years, usually in the thoracolumbar region, becoming most apparent when in a wheelchair or during the pubertal growth spurt. This adversely affects appearance, body image and posture. Bracing does not work. There are a number of accepted criteria for surgical treatment:
   - Before the primary curve becomes greater than 25%.
   - Progressive curve.
   - Substantial growth capacity remaining.
   - Patient physically (and emotionally) fit for surgery.
   - Vital capacity has not gone below 50% predicted.

   The surgery comprises insertion of metal rods (e.g. Harrington-Luque rods or Luque rods for segmental spinal stabilisation), which may be accompanied by facet joint arthrodesis using autogenous bone from spinous processes.

4. An important area is fitness for surgery. Adequate presurgical assessment of respiratory function is essential (if respiratory function parameters are over 50% of predicted values for the child's size, surgery is possible). Postoperatively, early mobilisation should be undertaken to prevent deterioration in function while confined to bed. The occupational therapist helps to accommodate activities of daily living to increase sitting height (increased shoulder and elbow height) and rigid spine.

5. In any surgical procedure, neuromuscular depolarising agents such as succinylcholine should be avoided.

Common medical problems

Restrictive lung disease (RLD)

1. RLD is secondary to weakness of diaphragm, chest wall and abdominal musculature.

2. Patients tend to have recurrent chest infections, which should be treated aggressively. They may also require inhaled treatment (nebuliser or pressurised metered dose inhaler with spacer) with bronchodilators, mucolytics or antibiotics.

3. They may develop cor pulmonale secondary to hypoxia, due to ventilatory difficulties and ventilation-perfusion inequalities associated with scoliosis.

4. Monitor with regular (6-monthly) pulmonary function tests (PFTs), including forced vital capacity (FVC) and maximal inspiratory and expiratory pressure, the former reflecting diaphragmatic strength, the latter reflecting strength of the chest wall and abdominal muscles, correlating with the ability to cough and clear secretions.

5. Symptomatic respiratory failure with hypoventilation, hypercapnoea (e.g. restless at night, somnolent by day, morning headaches, anorexia, general malaise). Symptoms can resolve with nocturnal ventilatory support, such as bimodal positive airway pressure (BiPAP), a mode of positive pressure ventilation. An important aspect is the requirement for a good face or lip seal on the mask or nasal/oral orthotic interface. This may lead, within a couple of years, to a decision about daytime support and then 24-hour ventilation. Decisions about whether or not to go into long-term 24-hour ventilation have to be made in consultation with the respiratory physician;

the parents and the teenage boy, with the decision based on patient and family preference. Education and early discussion of options are the keys. Volume ventilators may be used when vital capacity is below 40% of normal. These use a soft plastic nasal or face mask (for connection to the airway) with Velcro head and chin straps to hold them in position. The ventilator can fit on a ventilator tray on the bottom of a power wheelchair. Eventually a tracheostomy may be appropriate, as masks may cause skin irritation due to constant skin pressure. A Passy-Muir valve can allow air through the vocal cords and improve voicing. The respiratory support area is a major current issue in management of DMD.

6. Main determinant of operative risk.
7. Usual cause of death. Median age of death was 22 years in 2005.

Cardiac disease

Most patients have cardiomyopathy. Cardiomyopathy usually develops when the patient is confined to a wheelchair and hence inactive. Heart failure from loss of contractility is common. About 10% of patients develop symptoms related to cardiomyopathy and respond well to ACE inhibitors and antifailure therapy. Current research is assessing whether ACE inhibitors and beta blockers should be given prophylactically to patients with DMD to prevent cardiac deterioration.

Obesity

This occurs because of lack of mobility and is managed by dietary manipulation.

Constipation

This is common and patients often have spurious diarrhoea. Management with diet and aperients can obtain good results, with a rigid, well-supervised regimen.

Urinary problems

Incontinence is uncommon, but frequent enough to be a feature of DMD and not a coincidence. It is managed with anticholinergic agents (e.g. penthienate bromide).

Schooling, career prospects, lifestyle

1. Most children with DMD are integrated into a normal school, or may attend a special unit in a regular school. Special schools are less often required.
2. Dystrophin is expressed in the brain (role not known). Boys with DMD have a decrease in IQ of 1 standard deviation (around 15 IQ points) compared with unaffected siblings. Thus the mean IQ is around 85, and a higher percentage have intellectual impairment (around 20–30% have an IQ below 70). Encephalopathy is static, unlike muscle disease. A problem is underestimating the abilities of DMD patients (and disabled people generally).
3. Outlook for work is poor.
4. Some children, or young adults, can have what they feel is a fairly reasonable lifestyle, such as those pursuing courses of tertiary education, working in quadriplegic workshops or working with computers.
5. Sex education is a very valid area, which should not be ignored. Often these patients can be quite ignorant of sexual matters, and education, such as group sessions discussing sexuality in disabled people, can be very useful.
6. Special accommodation needs should be addressed, such as the need for wide doors, special fittings, availability of lifting hoists, as these may represent an enormous financial burden to the family.

Genetic counselling

1. Recent advances allow improved detection of carriers and prenatal diagnosis in families with a child known to have DMD (see earlier, 'Background information on genetics of DMD').
2. A female is defined an obligate carrier if she has an affected son and at least one other affected male relative in a pedigree that corresponds to X-linked-recessive inheritance.
3. Mothers of isolated DMD patients are possible carriers, as are non-obligate carrier females related to affected males. Analysis of pedigrees and DNA analysis may clarify carrier status.
4. One-third of DMD patients represent new mutations. Effective genetic counselling will increase this proportion.
5. Involvement of a geneticist is very appropriate.

Seizures and epilepsy

Seizures are among the many problems of many long-case patients. Candidates should be aware of the numerous new antiepileptic drugs (AEDs) introduced in the last decade, improvements in neuro-imaging, genetic research and identification of putative epilepsy genes (see below), and surgical treatments in intractable seizures. The points outlined here may apply to any child with recurrent seizures.

Background information

Definitions: a *seizure* is a paroxysmal clinical episode that results from an excessive hypersynchronous discharge of neurons; the term *epilepsy* is used when recurrent unprovoked seizures occur. Recurrent febrile convulsions do not signify epilepsy.

Candidates should be familiar with the classification of epileptic seizures according to seizure type (ILAE, International League Against Epilepsy classification). There are three groups.

1. Partial seizures, which involve part of one cerebral hemisphere. These can be further subdivided into 'simple', meaning that consciousness is not impaired, and 'complex', where awareness and responsiveness are altered.
2. Generalised seizures, which involve both cerebral hemispheres. There may or may not be associated convulsive motor manifestations.
3. Unclassified seizures, which do not fit into the above groups.

Candidates should have knowledge of the following epilepsy syndromes:

- Infantile spasms (West's syndrome).
- Lennox-Gastaut syndrome (LGS).
- Childhood absence epilepsy (CAE, previously called *petit mal*).
- Benign rolandic epilepsy (BRE), or benign focal epilepsy of childhood (BFEC), or benign epilepsy with centrotemporal spikes (BECTS).
- Juvenile myoclonic epilepsy (JME, also called impulsive *petit mal*).
- Partial epilepsy syndromes (e.g. mesial temporal lobe epilepsy [TLE], frontal lobe epilepsy [FLE]).

In the context of the exam, epilepsy is symptomatic of the underlying problem and represents one aspect of management problems. The candidate should have an approach to the management of epilepsy.

Genetics of epilepsy

Advances in understanding clinical and molecular genetics have proceeded rapidly. A genetic predisposition to epilepsy (excessive neuronal membrane excitation) can be related to ion channel dysfunction or disorders of synaptic transmission. Dysfunction of ion channels has been demonstrated in several monogenetic epilepsies. It has been suggested that classification of disorders by clinical features alone is inadequate, given this emerging knowledge of channelopathies. Genetic heterogeneity is apparent in several monogenetic epileptic channelopathies: benign neonatal-infantile convulsions can be caused by sodium or potassium channelopathies; familial generalised epilepsy with febrile seizures plus (GEFS+) can be due to a sodium channel or a GABA receptor channel disorder.

Amongst the idiopathic epilepsies, a range of genetic defects are recognised in the following:

- Voltage-gated ion channels: sodium (GEFS+, severe myoclonic epilepsy of childhood, benign neonatal-infantile convulsions), potassium (neonatal seizures), chloride (generalised epilepsies), calcium (absence epilepsy).
- Ligand-gated ion channels: GABA receptors (GEFS+, absence epilepsy, juvenile myoclonic epilepsy), ACh receptors (autosomal dominant [AD] nocturnal frontal lobe epilepsy).
- Non-ion channel genes: temporal lobe epilepsy with auditory features (LGI1).

Idiopathic epilepsies with simple inheritance (usually quite benign) are now well recognised but are relatively rare: AD syndromes of early infancy (benign familial neonatal, neonatal-infantile and infantile; three different ages of onset; three different genes), AD nocturnal frontal lobe epilepsy, AD partial epilepsy with auditory features and familial temporal lobe epilepsies. In contrast, most common epilepsies have quite complex inheritance: such as idiopathic generalised epilepsies and idiopathic focal epilepsies.

History

The history of any seizure disorder depends on the description of the event by an eyewitness, with some input from the child, particularly with simple partial seizures. One must remain alert to the differential diagnoses, which are broad but more commonly include syncope (e.g. breath-holding spells), behavioural, parasomnia and postures of spasticity in children with cerebral palsy.

For each type of seizure the child has, the following must be established. The classification of the seizure type (e.g. generalised tonic clonic seizures [GTCS], absence, atonic) is determined from the history, taking into account the points below.

1. Any prodromal symptoms (e.g. irritability, pallor). The setting in which the events occur (e.g. from sleep, during exercise, when ill, when sleep-deprived). Any precipitating factors: tiredness, lack of sleep, fever, infectious illness, change of dosage or type of anticonvulsant, intake of other substances (in adolescents), falls or blows to the head, sensory stimuli such as flashing lights, television, computer games, sounds, startling by sudden noises or touch.
2. Any aura (e.g. a specific psychic or sensory symptom, as distinct from a prodromal symptom). This includes running to the parent for comfort. This is applicable to children with partial seizures.
3. Initial cry or scream.
4. Initial localising signs (e.g. twitching of one hand).

5. Description of all the manifestations (motor and autonomic) of the seizure (e.g. eyes 'rolling back', altered awareness, cyanosis, jerking movements of limbs, urinary and/or faecal incontinence).

6. The duration of the seizures—the range (e.g. between 5 and 20 minutes) and the 'usual' time (e.g. 5 minutes). Any episodes of status epilepticus (duration >30 mins).

7. The frequency of the seizures—range (e.g. none for 6 weeks to 6 in a day) and the 'usual' (e.g. once every 3 weeks).

8. Time of occurrence of seizures (e.g. on waking, or on going to sleep).

9. The date and time of the last seizure.

10. Postictal events (e.g. sleeping, confusion, headache, vomiting, Todd's paralysis).

The past history of the seizures—in terms of number of hospital admissions, previous anticonvulsants used and why they were changed, any previous complications of seizures or their treatment, and whether febrile convulsions occurred at a younger age—should be covered thoroughly. Past history of possible aetiological factors such as prematurity, cerebral infection or head injury should be sought. Note any family history of seizure disorders or other neurological problems.

The details of any anticonvulsant therapy must be known, including the dose, efficacy, when levels were last taken, what they were, recent dosage changes, and any current side effects. Common symptoms raised by parents that are often blamed on medication include drowsiness, cognitive slowing and poor behaviour.

Obtain an outline of how the parents manage when the child is having a seizure, what contingency plans exist for a prolonged seizure, their criteria for seeking hospital treatment, any medications given by them acutely at home (e.g. rectal diazepam), how long it takes to get the child to hospital in an emergency, and what restrictions are placed on the child because of the seizures (e.g. swimming). Remember to evaluate the parents' understanding of seizures, e.g. in terms of prognosis, chances of remission and complications. Are the parents afraid of the child dying? Are there steps of over-protectiveness, including sleeping in the parents' bed, excessive social restrictions. An assessment of the child's schooling progress is important. Compliance with treatment must be discussed.

Finally, remember to take a full social history, including any benefits the child is receiving (e.g. Children's Disability Allowance), social supports (e.g. Epilepsy Association) and impact of the disease on the child, schooling, parents and siblings. An enquiry into social isolation or bullying at school can be revealing. If the patient is an adolescent, this involves a whole range of new issues, including compliance, effects on career prospects, driver's licence, and menstrual and reproductive issues. Mental health issues often come to the fore with the high rates of teenage depression and anxiety seen.

Examination

This is outlined in the short-case section on recurrent seizures in this chapter.

Investigations

The extent of investigation depends on the clinical picture. The following is an incomplete list of some of the more commonly used investigations.

Electroencephalogram (EEG)

An EEG is performed to look for focal slowing or epileptiform activity—that is, spike or sharp wave (localised or generalised). However epileptiform activity on the EEG does not equate with the diagnosis of epilepsy. An EEG provides collateral information. Interictal epileptiform discharges (IEDs) are found in association with epilepsy. Their yield can be increased by activation methods such as sleep, sleep deprivation, hyperventilation and photic stimulation. Children with epilepsy should have an EEG performed and this may be helpful in making the diagnosis, particularly which type of epilepsy is present (e.g. CAE). However, it should be noted that children with epilepsy may well have normal EEGs (in up to 50% of cases) and, conversely, non-epileptic children may show 'epileptiform activity' on their EEGs (3–5% of children).

Certain patterns are well recognised and expected to be known (e.g. BRE with centrotemporal spikes). Interictal EEG provides valuable information in these epileptic syndromes: BRE, CAE, JME, LGS, benign occipital epilepsy and partial epilepsies.

Video/EEG monitoring is often reserved for when there are diagnostic issues (Is this epilepsy?) or management issues (What is the epilepsy syndrome?). It may be particularly useful in assessing a child who has a confusing or unconvincing history of 'funny turns', or possibly several seizure types. It may aid in assessing conditions such as atonic seizures (e.g. documenting the period of lost muscle tone, and the risk of head injury). Replaying the videotape to the parents may help them to appreciate aspects of their child's attacks that had not been noted, and allow many questions to be answered, based on what is seen. Video/EEG is indicated in children with medication-resistant epilepsy. It can guide further investigation and management, such as a presurgical evaluation.

Biochemical evaluation

A blood glucose level taken at the time of the seizure may detect a treatable metabolic cause, particularly in younger children. Serum calcium and magnesium should also be checked in someone presenting for the first time with an unexplained generalised seizure. An ECG is valuable to help exclude risk of an arrhythmia, such as the prolonged QT syndrome as a cause of syncope-seizure.

Other tests that may be useful in certain patients include serum electrolytes and metabolic evaluation (urine for amino acids, organic acids, acylcarnitine, acylglycines and mucopolysaccharides).

Imaging: structural

Brain-imaging studies by either magnetic resonance imaging (MRI) or computerised tomographic (CT) scanning may be indicated in the following circumstances. The present gold standard is MRI. Additional techniques such as spectroscopy and higher strength MRI have a limited clinical role.

1. Focal seizures, except for BRE (rolandic seizures), which is diagnosed on clinical and EEG features that are characteristic enough to make MRI/CT scanning unnecessary. However, a scan should be done if atypical features are present.
2. Focal EEG findings (again, except for those of BRE).
3. Abnormal neurological signs (particularly focal signs).
4. Developmental delay.
5. Seizures that are difficult to control.

Imaging: functional

Functional neuro-imaging modalities have become more widely used over the last decade. These modalities can help to accurately localise seizure onset without invasive means. They include:

1. Positron emission tomography (PET) scanning, which assesses cerebral metabolism (mnemonic: PET checks METabolism), using fluorodeoxyglucose. PET shows decreased metabolic rate of the epileptogenic area during the interictal period.

2. Single photon emission computed tomography (SPECT) scanning, which evaluates cerebral perfusion, using hexamethyl-propyleneomine axime (HMPOA) or iodoamphetamine or technetium-labelled Ceretec. There is interictal hypoperfusion, but ictal intense hyperperfusion at onset, with depression of perfusion after seizure. (Mnemonic for SPECT: **S**eizure [area] **P**erfusion **E**valuated by **C**eretec with **T**echnetium.)

3. Functional MRI: remains investigational but regional localisation of primary language, motor and visual cortical areas is possible with this technique.

Common management issues

The number of potential issues is enormous. This section addresses a small number of selected areas that may be quite relevant in the type of patients seen in the examination.

Increasing frequency of seizures and intractable epilepsy

If the seizures seem to be worsening in duration or frequency, or are changing in nature (such as the appearance of a different type of seizure), the overall management needs reconsideration. There are several important areas to question.

Question the diagnosis

There are a number of conditions which can mimic epilepsy, such as syncope, breath-holding attacks and pseudoseizures. Structural causes that are as yet undiagnosed (e.g. brain tumour) can present with seizures. Neurodegenerative conditions may present with seizures.

Concentrate carefully on the history for any suggestion of developmental regression. Physical examination may detect features of neurodegenerative conditions (e.g. macrocephaly, macular degeneration) or structural causes (e.g. focal neurological signs).

Question the medication

The dose may be wrong, the drug may be wrong, or adverse drug interactions may be occurring. The dosage may be too low, usually related either to non-compliance or to 'outgrowing' the dosage given (weight increase). The drug may not be the most appropriate choice for the types of seizure the child has (see below), or a drug appropriately chosen for one seizure type may worsen, or even 'unmask', another type of seizure (e.g. carbamazepine can worsen absence seizures). Insufficient numbers of medications may have been trialled.

Question an intercurrent problem

Intercurrent problems can include electrolyte imbalances consequent on drug side effects (e.g. hyponatraemia as a complication of carbamazepine, via the syndrome of inappropriate antidiuretic hormone secretion) or intercurrent infections (e.g. urinary tract infection).

Are there unrecognised precipitating factors?

The patient may have become increasingly exposed to unrecognised precipitants such as drugs, television, computer or video games.

Is this form of epilepsy commonly a treatment problem?
Certain types of epilepsy are notoriously difficult to control; examples are Lennox-Gastaut syndrome and infantile spasms.

Advice to parents (and school teachers)

Management during a seizure
Lay the child on the side. Do not put things in the child's mouth. Move away any nearby objects to avoid the child hurting himself or herself. Have a time plan: for example, if a seizure lasts longer than 5 minutes, call an ambulance.

Everyday childhood/adolescent activities: safety considerations
1. No swimming alone.
2. No bathing alone for younger children.
3. Showers rather than baths for older children (with the bathroom door open and someone nearby).
4. No climbing ladders or similar pursuits with a risk of falls.
5. No skateboard or bicycle riding on busy roads.
6. Use of helmets when riding on less busy roads.
7. Use of helmets for drop attacks (as in atonic seizures).

Avoid overprotection
Allow participation in normal sports and school activities. There is no contraindication to body-contact sports. Some neurologists prefer to encourage participation in non-contact sports such as tennis and athletics.

Driver's licence
The rules vary in different states and different countries. Commonly, the recommendation is that this is only allowed if the patient has had no seizures in the previous 2 years; however, guidelines are now more tailored to individual circumstances and type of epilepsy.

Avoid known precipitants
For example, in photosensitive epilepsy, avoid sitting close to the television in a dark room, and wear sunglasses outside, particularly in cars and buses, when sunlight dappling through trees combined with sitting in a moving vehicle can be a problem.

Rationale for treatment
Parents should have the reasons for recommending treatment explained to them, covering fully both the benefits and the possible side effects of whichever drug is chosen. Issues such as the morbidity and generally low mortality of epilepsy should be discussed.

Probable duration of treatment
All parents will want to know about this. A rough guide is that medication may generally be stopped when the child has been free of seizures for 2 years, depending on the syndrome. If the child had an abnormal physical examination or abnormal EEG, the treatment could be stopped later, e.g. at 3 to 4 years.

Remember that a number of factors are associated with an increased probability of seizure recurrence, once medications are stopped. The epilepsy syndrome itself is the best guideline. Other factors include abnormal neurological signs, mixed types of seizures, focal seizures (excluding BRE) and seizures that were originally difficult to control.

Genetic counselling

Parents often want to know whether there is a risk that their other children could develop the same condition. Accurate diagnosis is essential: if the problem is a known monogenetic problem, the risk can be predicted accurately, but for most clinically (not molecularly) diagnosed epilepsies, an estimate only is available. Overall, the risk to siblings of generalised epilepsies is around 10%, the risk to siblings of focal epilepsies is around 5%, and the risk to siblings of febrile seizures is around 8%. Most genetic epilepsies are benign.

Anticonvulsant medications

General aims

Monotherapy is the goal. One drug, given in the correct dosage for the child's body weight, with drug levels checked initially (if applicable) to confirm adequacy of dose when a steady state has been achieved (after five times the half-life of the drug). Many anticonvulsants need to be started at a low dosage and then gradually increased until the appropriate dose is reached over 1–2 weeks. In the case of lamotrigine, the process is usually over several months.

If one drug, given at the correct dosage and within the therapeutic range of serum levels, is unsuccessful in controlling the seizures, the next most appropriate agent can be started. Only after the first drug has reached steady state should it be slowly withdrawn.

Which drugs can have serum levels measured?

The candidate should know which drugs can have serum levels measured. Carbamazepine (CBZ), phenytoin (PHT) and phenobarbitone (PB) all have recommended 'optimal' ranges of serum drug levels, which may be useful in monitoring therapy. Valproate (VPA) is an exception: levels can be measured, but they do not correlate with efficacy or toxicity and so are unhelpful (except in suspected non-compliance, where a level of zero may confirm this suspicion). The same applies to the benzodiazepines (BDZs).

Which drug is preferable in which type of seizure?

Table 13.1 is an incomplete list of epilepsy syndromes and useful drugs in each.

What side effects are likely?

It is beyond the scope of this book to list all the side effects of the commonly used anticonvulsants. Behavioural and cognitive effects are among the most common side effects reported in children. Candidates should be familiar with the acute toxicities (e.g. drowsiness, nystagmus and ataxia with carbamazepine and phenytoin), acute idiosyncratic reactions (e.g. skin manifestations such as Stevens-Johnson syndrome), chronic toxicities (e.g. various effects on the haematological system, bones, connective tissue, cosmetic effects and teratogenic effects) and drug interactions, both between anticonvulsants (e.g. CBZ lowers PHT levels, VPA increases PB levels) and with other drugs (e.g. erythromycin increases CBZ levels).

Are any of the newer AEDs likely to be of use here?

Several new AEDs have been introduced over the last decade. Most drug research concentrated on the inhibitory neurotransmitter system, involving gamma-amino-butyric acid

Table 13.1 Epilepsy syndromes and examples of drugs used

Epilepsy syndromes	Drugs
Infantile spasms	VGB, prednisolone, ACTH, BDZs (e.g. nitrazepam), VPA
Lennox-Gastaut syndrome (childhood epileptic encephalopathy)	VPA, BDZs, LTG
Childhood absence epilepsy (CAE)	ESM, VPA
Benign rolandic epilepsy (BRE)	Sulthiame, VPA, CBZ
Juvenile myoclonic epilepsy (JME)	VPA
Symptomatic partial epilepsy	CBZ, VPA, LTG, clobazam

ACTH = adrenocorticotropic hormone; BDZs = benzodiazepines; CBZ = carbamazepine; ESM = ethosuximide; LTG = lamotrigine; VGB = vigabatrin; VPA = valproate.

(GABA). The importance of the excitatory system involving glutamate and the N-methyl-D-aspartate (NMDA) receptor is now recognised.

Vigabatrin (VBT)

An irreversible inhibitor of GABA transaminase, VBT increases the availability of GABA. Around 50% of patients have a 50% reduction in intractable partial seizures. It remains the drug of choice for infantile spasms, despite great concern involving the risk of some loss of peripheral visual fields, which can be irreversible despite cessation of the drug when detected. Side effects: sedation and fatigue, weight gain, agitation and hyperkinesis.

Lamotrigine (LTG)

This stabilises presynaptic neuronal membranes. It inhibits excitatory neurotransmitters (especially glutamate and aspartate) by blocking sodium channels. It is used as an add-on treatment for partial and generalised seizures. Around 25–33% of patients have a 50% reduction in intractable partial seizures.

It has a pharmacokinetic interaction with sodium valproate (VPA): elimination of LTG is prolonged if it is given with VPA, doubling the half-life. There is a pharmacodynamic interaction with VPA: LTG and VPA are a good combination, leading to greater efficacy than LTG with other agents, although there is a small chance of upper limb tremor, which stops on lowering the dose of either.

The most serious side effect is a skin rash, which can include Stevens-Johnson syndrome; this is increased by concomitant use of VPA. Care should be used with the combination of VPA and LTG: lower dosage and slower escalation rates are used. Other side effects of LTG: insomnia, double vision, blurred vision, dizziness, ataxia, drowsiness.

Topiramate (TPM)

This is an example of polypharmacy in one drug. A sulphamate-substituted mono-saccharide, it blocks seizure spread (similar to carbamazepine [CBZ] and phenytoin [PHT]), blocks glutamate receptors, increases GABA and weakly inhibits carbonic anhydrase. It has minimal interaction with other AEDs. It has no effect on CBZ, phenobarbitone (PB), PHT or VPA, but some of these AEDs (CBZ, PB, PHT) are enzyme inducers and can decrease serum concentration of TPM. TPM is used for simple partial, complex partial and secondarily generalised seizures. Side effects are drowsiness, cognitive dysfunction (in 10%) with word finding difficulties, dizziness, weight loss, renal stones, acute glaucoma. TPM needs to be introduced slowly, over 4–8 weeks.

Oxcarbazepine (OXC)

Indications are as for CBZ. There are fewer interactions with other drugs with OXC than with CBZ. Dose-related, idiosyncratic and chronic toxicity side effects are all less than for CBZ. Hyponatraemia has been described where OXC has replaced CBZ therapy, with Na level <135 mmol/L in 26.6%, Na <125 mmol/L in 2.6%; clinical symptoms of hyponatraemia have been described.

Levetiracetam (LEV)

This is unrelated to other AEDs chemically. The mechanism of action is unknown. It has been used in intractable symptomatic partial/generalised seizure disorders, including LGS. It is an adjunctive drug, never used alone initially. Side effects include blurred vision, sleepiness, dizziness, poor coordination. Behavioural symptoms have been reported in up to 37.6% of paediatric patients, including agitation, anxiety, apathy, depersonalisation, depression, emotional lability, hostility, hyperactivity, nervousness, neurosis and personality disorder.

Gabapentin (infrequently used)

Incorporates GABA into the cyclohexane ring; it is taken up into neurons. For intractable partial seizures, there is a 25% response rate. It has no specific interaction with other AEDs. Side effects are drowsiness, dizziness, diplopia, weight gain and behavioural change.

Tiagabine (TAB) (rarely used)

This blocks GABA uptake in glial cells and neurons, via a specific transport system (keeps GABA at receptor), and increases GABA in extracellular fluid and GABA-ergic mediated inhibitors in the brain. It is used for simple partial, complex partial and secondary generalised seizures. It has faster onset than VBT. Side effects are dizziness, tiredness and non-specific 'nervousness'.

What to try in intractable seizures?

In patients with intractable seizures all aetiologies should be considered, including metabolic (trial of pyridoxine). The ketogenic diet can be a valuable alternative, particularly in younger children. Any child with intractable focal epilepsy should be considered for surgery (see below).

Surgical treatment

Surgical treatment of epilepsy is now safe and effective for those with epilepsy that is medically refractory and surgically remediable, with an emphasis towards 'the sooner the better' in children. Most adult surgical work has been carried out involving the temporal lobe. In children, extratemporal cases are of similar frequency. About 1 in 7 patients with epilepsy are refractory to AEDs. Of these, 1 in 4 will be candidates for surgery. The commonest pathologies are focal gliosis, low-grade tumours and focal cortical dysplasia. Less frequent are conditions such as Sturge-Weber syndrome, tuberous sclerosis and hemimegalencephaly. Contraindications include any of the primary generalised epilepsies (PGEs), any neurodegenerative or neurometabolic disorder. Before surgery is even considered, an adequate trial of AEDs, including the newer AEDs if appropriate, is undertaken. If truly intractable, the localisation of the site of seizure initiation is detected using methods including clinical assessment, video-EEG monitoring, neuropsychology (to assess functional importance of site of onset: left-sided function includes verbal IQ and memory, right-sided function includes performance IQ and visual memory), CT, MRI, SPECT, PET, functional MRI and invasive monitoring. Electrical-stimulation mapping can be performed intra- or extraoperatively to identify eloquent cortex in relation to epileptogenic areas.

Examples of the types of surgery undertaken are as follows:

1. Seizures secondary to focal cerebral lesions: lesionectomy or partial lobectomy.
2. Seizures secondary to hemimegalencephaly or to Sturge-Weber syndrome or other large unilateral pathology: hemispherectomy.
3. Atonic seizures (drop attacks): corpus callosotomy.

Some centres offer vagal nerve stimulation to those intractable patients who are not candidates for surgery.

Overall mortality from focal resective surgery is very low. A higher mortality rate is seen with hemispherectomy, particularly if under 1 year of age. Morbidities, depending on the site of surgery, include hemiparesis (1–5%), visual field defects (1–5%), language dysfunction (1–3%) and global amnesia (1%).

In well-selected patients, seizure freedom can be seen in up to 80% of tumour cases and patients with other focal pathologies can be 50–70% seizure-free.

Management of the prolonged seizure

At home

In patients with neurological abnormalities (e.g. CP) and a history of unprovoked status epilepticus (particularly if at an isolated address), prolonged seizure can be treated with early administration of rectal diazepam, or buccal or nasal midazolam, while awaiting the ambulance.

In ambulance/at hospital

If the seizure has already gone on for longer than 5 minutes, an intravenous loading dose of phenobarbitone or phenytoin would be an appropriate next step.

A suggested 'ideal' time course for treating a seizure at presentation:

- Initial minute: intravenous diazepam or midazolam.
- 5 minutes: intravenous phenytoin infusion over 20 minutes.
- 10 minutes (still fitting): repeat intravenous diazepam or midazolam.
- 25 minutes (still fitting, phenytoin infusion complete): commence midazolam infusion, increasing dose every 10 minutes. The use of increasing midazolam doses requires the ability to ventilate the child if respiratory depression supervenes.

The underlying cause for the prolonged seizure must be thoroughly investigated. Investigations may include CT or MRI scanning, ± lumbar puncture. A common end point for a resistant prolonged seizure is for the child to be anaesthetised, while investigations continue, and treated (antibiotics, acyclovir, dexamethasone, plus continued anticonvulsants) to cover serious underlying pathology.

Management of the first non-febrile seizure

The chances of further seizures occurring after a single seizure, at 5 years of age, are as follows:

1. In neurodevelopmentally normal children, with a normal EEG: 25%.

2. In children with mild neurological problems: 70%.
3. In those with severe neurological problems (e.g. CP): 90%.

Different seizure types have different risks of recurrence. BRE, for example, is associated with a very high chance of recurrence (90% will have a second seizure). After a first epileptic seizure, EEG abnormalities are associated with an increased risk of seizure recurrence.

Psychosocial issues

The management of psychosocial issues is of particular importance in children with recurrent seizures. The key point in managing this area is clear communication and providing information to the family. The following points cover issues where education will resolve most of the difficulties.

Parents

The parents of an epileptic child often have concerns in the following areas:

1. Fear of brain damage.
2. Being uncomfortable with the label/stigma of 'epilepsy'.
3. False beliefs that the cause relates to themselves (e.g. 'stress' during pregnancy).
4. Equating an EEG with a treatment modality like electroconvulsive therapy.
5. Difficulty accepting the need for medication: ambivalence (forgetting to give medications); belief that the need for drugs equates with, or causes, 'retardation'; and suddenly stopping the medication when the supply is used up.

Children

Children with seizures not uncommonly have significant psychosocial problems. Their concerns include the following:

1. Fear of dying or being injured during a seizure.
2. Fear of loss of control, loss of friends, loss of continence.
3. Overprotection, inappropriate restrictions, 'vulnerable child' syndrome.

Other issues of concern to parents and doctors are actions that demonstrate significant underlying worries and conflicts in the child: denial, pseudoseizures, self-induced seizures.

Spina bifida

Over the last three decades, the frequency of new cases of myelomeningocoele and other neural tube defects (NTDs) has declined worldwide, one of the main reasons being widespread and improved prenatal diagnosis: careful, targeted ultrasound examination should identify at least 95% of all NTDs. Advances in the understanding of how NTDs occur and can be prevented have included the recognition that folic acid supplements before conception reduce both occurrence and recurrence risks of NTDs. Current recommendations include folic acid supplementation one month before conception and through at least the first 8–12 weeks of pregnancy. All women contemplating pregnancy should ingest a daily multivitamin containing 0.5 mg folic acid. If there is a family history of neural tube defect, one needs to advise that 5 mg is taken. It has been suggested that NTDs are not due to folate deficiency per se, but due to enzymatic abnormalities involving metabolic processes that depend on folate and its metabolites, tetrahydrofolate and 5-methyltetrahydrofolate, abnormalities that could be overcome with folate supplementation. The US Food and Drug Administration introduced fortification of staple foods with folic acid in 1998 to prevent NTDs. In Australia and New Zealand an application to fortify flour is in the pipeline.

Neural tube closure is believed to occur in five separate sites within the first 28 days of gestation: NTDs result from failure of closure at one site or failure of two sites to meet. Each site may be controlled by separate genes and influenced by differing external factors. Known environmental influences implicated in the development of NTDs include high first-trimester blood sugar levels (diabetic mother), elevated maternal temperature (from fevers or saunas), and AEDs, particularly sodium valproate and phenytoin.

Advances in prenatal diagnosis allow diagnosis of myelomeningocoele (MMC) as early as the first trimester. In specialised centres in the USA, in-utero repair of MMC has been performed at 19–25 weeks; this can theoretically reverse hindbrain herniation, decrease the need for postnatal ventriculo-peritoneal shunting due to hydrocephalus, and prevent late loss of function due to tethering.

A child with spina bifida gives a good example of an examination case with an enormous number of potential problems and management issues. In order to organise your assessment of the child, it is useful to structure history-taking and management issues as follows:

1. How does this child function in day-to-day life (i.e. a brief outline of the child's practical problems). This will make clear how the disability affects the child's life.
2. What medical problems are relevant in this child?

History

Current history

How does this child function?
1. **Mobility:** type, aids, therapy.
2. **Incontinence care:**
    a. What is the program for urinary incontinence (e.g. intermittent catheterisation, pads, pants, penile appliances, artificial sphincter)?
    b. What is the program for bowel care (e.g. regular toileting, laxatives, suppositories, enemas)?
3. **Education:** what type of schooling does the child have (e.g. regular school, special class, special school)? What particular problems are there with learning?
4. **Developmental problems:** related to age (e.g. awareness of disability, making friends, self-esteem, adolescent problems of identity, independence, sexuality, employment). How independent is this child in self-help skills such as bathing, dressing and feeding?

Specific medical problems
1. **Hydrocephalus:** does this child have a shunt? Any problems with the shunt?
2. **Urinary system:** infections, operations, any concerns on routine tests (reflux, kidney damage), any medications (antibiotics, anticholinergics)?
3. **Orthopaedic problems:** feet and hips (e.g. deformity, pressure areas, problems with splints, calipers, crutches or wheelchairs); back (e.g. scoliosis, kyphosis).
4. **Other medical complications:** (a) eyes (squint, amblyopia); (b) skin care: pressure ulcers; burns; latex allergy; (c) growth and development: precocious puberty; short stature; obesity; (d) problems with executive functioning, impaired ability to organise; (e) coordination problems.
5. **Issues of adolescence:** problems with motivation; transition to adult care.

Past history

This should include (a) pregnancy and birth history, (b) antenatal screening, (c) family history of neural tube defects, including anencephaly, (d) diagnosis, (e) initial management (counselling, understanding of the condition and expectations for the child), (f) early management, (g) complications (infections, hospitalisations, operations).

Social history

Ask about the impact on (a) the child (e.g. restricted opportunities, fewer friends, teasing, depression, poor motivation), (b) schooling and social integration (poor mobility limits opportunities, time in hospital, missing school, learning difficulties), (c) the family (extra time spent with child, effect on siblings, marriage and finances).

What assistance does the family receive?

1. Community supports: community nurse, community therapy, respite care, social worker, Spina Bifida Association, Crippled Children's Society.
2. Financial supports: Child Disability Allowance, Isolated Patients Transport and Accommodation Assistance Scheme, Provision of Aids for Disabled People (in Victoria this is now called the Victorian Aids and Equipment Program). After the age of 16, catheters are accessed via the Commonwealth CASS scheme.

Child's adaptation to disability

Ask what he/she thinks about himself or herself (self-esteem), friends, achievements, hopes for future.

Examination

See separate short case on spina bifida in this chapter.

Management

Entire books have been written on almost every aspect of spina bifida. This section gives a skeleton outline of the more common and important issues raised. Every child with spina bifida has a unique set of problems, the emphasis of each case being more individualised than the major texts would suggest. The problems tend to be more 'medical' in younger children, and more 'psychosocial' in older children and adolescents.

Major disabilities

Paralysis

Associated problems include immobility, dependence versus independence, joint contractures, anaesthetic skin risks, pressure necrosis of soft tissues.

Management involves a team approach:

1. Physiotherapy (e.g. ambulation training, wheelchair mobility).
2. Occupational therapy (e.g. functional training, activities of daily living).
3. Clinical motion analysis: Paediatric Gait Analysis Laboratory (see CP section).
4. Positioning orthoses (e.g. ankle–knee orthoses, hip-positioning brace).
5. Orthopaedic surgical procedures (e.g. tendon releases or transfers, surgery for dislocated hips).
6. Mobility aids (e.g. crutches, reciprocating gait orthoses, walkerette, parapodium, wheelchairs).
7. Education regarding risks to skin integrity (e.g. tight clothes, temperature of bath

water, sunburn, overtight tying of booties in babies or even hospital identification labels on ankles, ill-fitting orthoses, standing on hot sand at the beach). Aggressive management of pressure necrosis.

Sphincter disturbance

Associated problems include the social disability of incontinence and its medical implications (e.g. infection, renal impairment, hypertension).

Bladder and renal function

Bladder management depends on the type of dysfunction (e.g. dribbling urine, dribbling with increased abdominal pressure such as during crying or movement, urinary retention). Investigations may clarify this.

Anticholinergic agents may increase bladder storage capacity, and alpha-adrenergic drugs may increase bladder outlet resistance. The combination of these, plus intermittent catheterisation, can prevent residual urine retention and increase continence. Self-catheterisation is encouraged when the child is old enough. Many units' management involves starting all babies on intermittent catheterisation as soon as possible, usually within the first 2 weeks of life. It is very rare to see vesicostomies fashioned nowadays. Diversion methods such as ileal conduit are no longer favoured.

Those children who cannot store any urine can be managed by incontinence clothing (pads and pants). Boys can use a penile appliance from about 8 years of age. An artificial sphincter may be considered in this group, although this is very rarely done now because of high complication rates.

If catheterisation is difficult at all, then a Mitrofanoff procedure can be done (appendix used as a conduit to abdominal wall is fashioned and catheterisation is performed via this stoma). This is useful as children get older and need to be more independent, especially for those with tight adductors or fine motor difficulties who cannot catheterise themselves.

Urinary tract infections (UTIs) need a full course of antibiotics for the acute infection. Only give prophylactic antibiotics if frequent or severe urinary tract infections or vesico-ureteric reflux (VUR) occur. Urine specimens (MSUs) should be obtained regularly to check for infection, as well as when parents suspect urine infection (urine odour, child unwell). Surgery may be required for several urinary problems: augmentation cystoplasty if the bladder is small and hypertonic, bladder neck reconstruction or artificial external urinary sphincter. Surgery for VUR may be needed if recurrent urinary tract infections occur despite treatment, and if there is renal scarring or persistent hydronephrosis. Urolithiasis can occur secondary to immobilisation.

Renal review by nephrologist or urologist, with ultrasound or renal scan, and nuclear or radiographic cystogram are required yearly.

Chronic renal failure (CRF) can occur in about 5–10% of patients, and the medical management is along standard lines, including peritoneal dialysis and renal transplantation (RTx). It should be noted that, in peritoneal dialysis, an indwelling catheter in the peritoneal cavity with elevated risk of peritonitis is a consideration in patients with ventriculoperitoneal shunts who are prone to develop shunt infections. An ileal conduit is usually required for transplant as the neurogenic bladder is the cause of the renal failure.

Renal osteodystrophy in this population is of interest: children with spina bifida are at increased risk of fracturing their paraplegic lower limbs, even with normal renal function, so that with renal impairment, bone mineralisation is compromised further by metabolic acidosis, secondary hyperparathyroidism and impaired hydroxylation of vitamin D. This can be treated with dietary restriction of phosphate, administration of phosphate binders, and 1-OH-vitamin D. The correction of metabolic acidosis is particularly important, as spina bifida patients may have urinary conduits, bladder augmentation or urinary reservoirs, each of which can cause hyperchloraemic acidosis requiring alkali therapy. See Chapter 12, Nephrology, for more details on CRF, dialysis and RTx.

Bowel

Bowel management principles include managing constipation with a range of laxatives. Movicol (comprising macrogol, NaCl, KCl, sodium bicarbonate) has proved very useful in some children who have major problems with constipation and faecal impaction. A low-fibre rather than a high-fibre diet is recommended. Rectal emptying by suppositories or enemas may be necessary (when the child reaches the usual age of toilet training). In children with problematic faecal incontinence and constipation, some spina bifida teams recommend regular colonic enemas with hand–warm tap water or commercially prepared normal saline 0.9% solution given at home from once a day to twice a week. This approach has been reported in one series as permitting the use of nappies/diapers to decrease from 90% to 40% and allowing both faecal continence and high satisfaction with the procedure in two-thirds of patients.

Hydrocephalus

This is seen in 90% of all children with spina bifida, and is treated with a ventricular shunt. The caudal hindbrain anomaly of the Arnold–Chiari II malformation is present in almost all patients. Associated problems include an increased chance of intellectual impairment, and shunt complications such as infection, obstruction (underdrainage), low-pressure syndrome (overdrainage) or seizures. An average of two shunt changes are needed in the first 10 years.

Management includes appropriate schooling for intellectual impairment, and education regarding complications of shunts and their presentation. As well as all the usual immunisations, it is recommended that a child with a VP shunt receive pneumococcal vaccine as well.

Underdrainage can be due to blockage of the shunt tubing, the shunt breaking or parts becoming disconnected. Classic presentation includes headache (worse on waking, before rising in the morning), nausea, vomiting, dizziness, listlessness, lethargy, poor feeding, insidious deterioration in behaviour (e.g. irritable or disruptive) or intellectual functioning (worsening school performance), onset of, or worsening of, fitting. In addition, shunt malfunction can present as a change in motor performance (e.g. decreased muscle strength, loss of previously acquired motor skills, increase in spasticity in upper or lower limbs), alteration in gait, change in bladder or bowel habit, change in lower cranial nerve function, back pain, worsening scoliosis, worsening of lower limb orthopaedic deformities. Very rarely, the sole indicator of shunt malfunction is papilloedema, so it is worth checking the fundi every time a doctor is seen.

Over-drainage has a somewhat similar presentation: headache (worsened by getting up from lying down) dizziness, and fainting. If rapid, a subdural haemorrhage can result, with symptoms varying from headache to those of a stroke. If gradual, 'slit ventricle' syndrome can occur, and can cause high pressure to reappear, but with small ventricles on scanning). Various symptoms in a patient with a shunt may be attributed to the shunt unless a definite alternative diagnosis is apparent.

Infection of shunts is almost always due to bacteria getting into the cerebrospinal fluid (CSF) or shunt at the time of operation, hence it is most common within first 3 days of shunt placement. On occasion, infection can present as shunt blockage within weeks or months of operation. An infected shunt must be removed and replaced with a new clean shunt. Progress is being made in developing shunts that are resistant to bacterial infection.

In any child with a shunt, if there is any deterioration in neurological, orthopaedic or urological function, it should be assumed to be due to shunt dysfunction until proved otherwise. Generally a cranial CT scan is performed in the first instance to exclude blockage.

Other useful investigations with shunt problems may include cerebrospinal fluid analysis, plain X-rays (head, chest, abdomen) to demonstrate shunt position and to check for disconnection, cranial CT or MRI scan, radioisotope studies (e.g. computerised clearance study for clearance over 24 hours, or direct injection of isotope into the shunt to check shunt patency).

The Arnold-Chiari II malformation

This comprises downward displacement of the cerebellar tonsils and vermis through the foramen magnum, elongation and kinking of the medulla, caudal displacement of the cervical spinal cord and medulla, and obliteration of the cisterna magna. Descent of the hindbrain through the foramen magnum can cause compression of the brainstem and lead to dysfunction of the cerebellum, medullary respiratory centre and cranial nerves IX and X, and to hydrocephalus. It also incorporates other brain malformations (e.g. callosal dysgenesis, abnormalities of neuronal migration and brain sulcation) that may be associated with learning disabilities experienced by some children with spina bifida. It causes symptoms sufficient to require surgical treatment in about 15–35% of patients.

Symptoms can include: swallowing difficulties (due to lower cranial nerve or brain-stem dysfunction), choking on foods (especially liquids), nasal regurgitation or gastro-oesophageal reflux when drinking or vomiting, repeated aspiration pneumonia episodes, dysarthria, obstructive sleep apnoea, cyanosis, stridor (inspiratory), hoarse or high-pitched cry, weakness or spasticity of upper limbs, neck pain, headache, scoliosis, dizziness, clumsiness, poor coordination (the latter three being cerebellar symptoms).

Surgical treatment involves decompression of the medulla and upper cervical cord, then insertion of a dural patch graft (duraplasty) to increase the size of the dural sac. Cervical laminectomy is performed below the lowest level of the cerebellar tonsils. In response to surgical decompression, brainstem abnormalities improve in 50%, and upper limb weakness, cerebellar function and pain improve in 80% of cases.

The tethered cord

This is present in virtually all children with MMC, but only causes problems requiring surgical intervention in around one-third, who manifest symptoms or signs of tethering generally during growth spurts, as in adolescence. These include back or lower limb pain, worsening of motor function (decreased muscle strength or increased tone), change in sensory level, change in bladder or bowel habit, altered gait, progressive orthopaedic deformities of spine or lower limbs. Imaging includes MRI to confirm tethering and define the regional anatomy, and to identify any associated lesions (syringomyelia, lipomas) that could produce similar symptomatology or signs. Surgical untethering involves reopening the original repair wound, dissecting the scarred part of the cord from the dura and checking for any other areas of tethering (e.g. thickened filum terminale).

Syringomyelia

This is seen on MRI in around 80% of patients with MMC, but is symptomatic in only 2–5%. Usual presenting features are upper limb weakness, back pain, scoliosis and spasticity or motor loss in the lower limbs. Extension of syringomyelia can affect lower cranial nerves and brainstem function. Symptoms from syringomyelia can be due to associated hydrocephalus or shunt malfunction, and resolve when this underlying cause is corrected. A shunt from the syrinx to the peritoneal cavity can relieve the problem.

Other significant disabilities (the five Ss)

Spine: scoliosis and kyphosis

Associated problems of scoliosis: impairment of balance (changed centre of gravity); decreased total lung capacity, increased risk of infection, cor pulmonale; impairment of height; need for surgery (e.g. Harrington rods) and consequent prolonged hospitalisation.

Problems of kyphosis: increase risk of need for multiple shunt revisions. The natural history of sagittal plane kyphosis is progression at about 8 degrees per year, leading to intolerance of sitting and loss of independent use of the hands while sitting. Associated skin instability and breakdown can occur. Kyphosis has a serious negative impact on self-esteem. Some centres operate at age 2–5 years. Surgical correction techniques have included excision of apical vertebrae, stabilised with instrumentation, and multiple lordosing intervertebral osteotomies (decancellation kyphectomy).

Skin

With loss of sensation below the waist, pressure ulcers are among the main reasons for hospital admission. Any skin breakdown should be taken very seriously. Care in protecting the skin during simple activities of daily living can avoid prolonged hospitalisation. Burns can occur easily with normal activities (e.g. during a bath, resting against the hot tap). Anaesthetic areas of skin can also lead to missing significant pathology that would normally present with pain (e.g. significant infections or orthopaedic injuries that are not felt, and only noticed by swelling or redness). Poorly fitting calipers, crutches or wheelchairs can cause substantial skin breakdown before it is noticed. All of these areas become more of a problem with increasing independence and self-care. In treating pressure areas, avoid film dressings, as these, in combination with the excessive sweating often seen in these children, worsen skin breakdown. The majority of commercially available wound dressings are adequate for pressure ulcers.

Senses: vision (squint) and hearing

Squint is associated with hydrocephalus and can lead to amblyopia if missed. Referral to an ophthalmologist is necessary. Hearing should be assessed routinely.

Size

Small stature, short lower limbs, obese for height. Growth hormone levels are usually normal. Recombinant human growth hormone (rhGH) may be appropriate for some children with spina bifida and small stature, particularly if they have CRF.

Seizures

Epilepsy occurs in 15–20% of children with spina bifida and should be managed with careful consideration to possible pregnancy in female patients and to the issue of fit-free periods before applying for a driver's licence.

Other problems

Social issues

These can be the most important issues, particularly in older children. Problems include low self-esteem, ongoing dependence on parents, leading to living at home indefinitely, seeking partners who will 'care' for them (parent substitute), unrealistic expectations about marriage and employment prospects. One way to boost self-esteem is to encourage children to participate in decision-making (e.g. type of crutches, what kind of bracing, colour of wheelchair) and to include them in discussions about incontinence care and surgical interventions, if old enough. In terms of helping them to become more self-sufficient in society, their attention should be focused on the long-term picture, so that realistic educational and employment goals can be set.

Adolescence brings its own set of stresses. In these children, areas of concern include appearance and presentability. Problems such as pressure sores, obesity, leaking of urine, and progression of scoliosis become paramount. Other problems include denial of disability, difficulty establishing identity, independence, friendships with the opposite sex, and appropriate sexual functioning.

When patients reach adulthood, the attendance rate at multidisciplinary clinics drops by around 50%, lack of motivation being but one possible cause. Secondary effects may include neglect of skin care or of adequate catheterisation techniques. Apathy due to having the disorder per se, as well as secondary depression, are not uncommon in adults, and the use of antidepressants may be warranted. The local doctor is usually best placed to assess for these sorts of problems.

Sex education is an area of great importance. Because of years of incontinence, and catheterisation by helpers, modesty may not have been encouraged. This population is at risk of sexual abuse, and there is at least one paper that quotes 25% incidence (on self-report).

Some males can sustain an erection; however, ejaculation may be abnormal and many males will be infertile. Females, however, have normal fertility. Contraception must be discussed with any adolescent female patient. Group discussions regarding sexuality in disabled people may be very beneficial. Group outings may improve socialisation skills, and encourage appropriate friendships.

The adult patient with spina bifida has an increased risk (1 in 20) with each pregnancy of producing a child with spina bifida. Antenatal screening should be discussed.

The problems of caring for a child with spina bifida when the parent is also disabled are indeed considerable. Most young adults with spina bifida wish to have children of their own.

Latex allergy

Children with spina bifida have a predisposition to developing an allergy to latex, a substance derived from the sap of *Hevea brasiliensis*, the functional unit being the rubber particle—a spherical drop of polyisoprene. There is a clinical and immunochemical cross-reactivity between latex and avocado, banana, kiwi, papaya and chestnut.

Exposure to latex antigen can occur by skin, mucosal or parenteral routes. Latex gloves are dusted in cornflour powder, which is a potent carrier of latex antigen. Exposure to latex occurs with surgical procedures, rectal disimpaction and bladder catheterisation. Up to 50% of spina bifida patients may have latex-specific IgE. Children with a history of adverse reactions to latex should have serum RAST (radioallergosorbent test) or enzyme-linked immunosorbent assay to look for latex-specific IgE. The parents, carers and school, medical and allied health professionals involved with the child must be able to identify latex allergy reactions and respond appropriately if an allergic reaction does occur (e.g. availability of adrenaline if there has been a previous severe or anaphylactic reaction). The (obvious) treatment for the condition is avoidance of latex and the foods that cross-react with it. Operating in a latex free environment is the usual practice in many paediatric institutions.

Genetic issues

The parents of a child with a neural tube defect have an increased risk for neural tube defect in subsequent pregnancies of 1 in 20. Antenatal screening involves detailed ultrasound at 16 weeks (95% accurate in experienced hands) and amniocentesis to measure alpha fetoprotein and acetylcholinesterase, which are elevated with an open spina bifida lesion. The accuracy of ultrasound together with amniocentesis clearly should exceed 95%. If a fetus is affected, options available for expectant mothers to consider include termination or expectant management, in most countries; in specialised centres in the USA, a third option of in utero repair of the MMC at 19–25 weeks' gestation may be available.

Prognosis

Around 75% of children with spina bifida have IQs above 80. Among those with normal intelligence, 60% have some form of learning disability, particularly problems with mathematics, sequencing of information, problem solving and visual perception. Approximately 70% of surviving children walk well enough to function in the community. Social continence (free of urinary incontinence in social situations) is achieved in 85% of school-aged children. Of adult patients, 80% are independent in the community, 30% attend or finish tertiary education, but only one-third are gainfully employed.

Short cases

Developmental assessment

Entire books have been written describing the approach to evaluating a child's development. This section is not meant to be a detailed description, but merely a guide to the general areas that should be covered, and a suggested overall plan.

All candidates will be familiar with at least one type of developmental assessment system, and should continue using one with which they are comfortable (e.g. the Denver Developmental Screening Test).

Candidates often fear the lead-in, 'Would you please perform a developmental assessment', simply because there is an associated mythology of difficulty, which is unwarranted. Once you know the first 18 months of development 'backwards', including the times of appearance and incorporation of all the primitive reflexes, then you should be fairly well equipped to interpret your findings, as this tends to be the age range that is more popular as an examination subject.

The problem with this case is not one of interpretation but of inappropriate actions, such as distracting an infant with a noise-making stimulus when testing vision, or not undressing the patient when assessing gross-motor milestones. This section addresses those issues.

Begin by introducing yourself to the parent and patient. Inspect for the following:

1. Growth parameters: e.g. failure to thrive, associated with syndromal or chromosomal anomalies. Undernutrition or chronic illnesses can be associated with developmental delay, as may be small or large head size.
2. Evidence of any dysmorphic features (various syndromal diagnoses).
3. Appearance of the 'ex-premature' infant (beware the 'ex-premmie' whose age is not corrected for prematurity).
4. Obvious neurological abnormalities (including 'floppy infant' posturing, hemiplegic posturing, involuntary movements).

The next step depends on the age of the child. A child small enough to be comfortably sat on his or her mother's knee, should be positioned there for assessment of vision, hearing, language, personal–social interaction and fine-motor control.

It is unwise to remove a child from his or her mother to perform a gross-motor assessment first. Often, candidates seem too keen to do exactly that. It does not help rapport with child, mother or examiner. If a child is older, then he or she may prefer to be examined sitting on a chair.

Always test vision before hearing. Fixing and following, and an approximation of visual acuity (e.g. ability to pick up a 'hundred and thousand' for infants, ability to read in older children) are important. Testing of visual fields is not required. Testing each eye separately is desirable, but can be difficult to achieve without upsetting an infant.

Testing hearing, with the infant on the mother's lap, requires initial distraction with a non-noisemaking (i.e. purely visual) stimulus, directly in front of the child. This is then hidden, at which time the noise-maker (e.g. bell) is brought towards the ear from behind (out of range of visual fields) by an assistant (e.g. the chief examiner). On a signal given by yourself, the assistant makes a sound (e.g. rings the bell) at a certain distance from the ear (this varies for different ages), testing each ear in turn and noting whether the child's facial expression, or activity (in babies), changes, and if the head turns towards the stimulus, localising the sound (in older children). If the conditions are not optimal for testing hearing (e.g. fractious toddler), say so. If there is an equivocal result, it is reasonable to suggest a formal audiological assessment.

The fine-motor assessment can then be performed. If the child is severely visually impaired, this makes assessment very difficult, and explains the logic of always testing vision first. Ensure that you have appropriate objects in your case to test fine-motor functions, such as 'hundreds and thousands', raisins (testing pincer grip), 2.5 cm blocks (for stacking), different-sized beads and threads (threading a bead is a good test of co-ordination), a biro with a top (putting the top on a biro is another good test of coordination and fine-motor development), and a plastic knife, fork and spoon set.

Throughout the testing described above, assessment of personal–social interaction and language can be performed. Do not forget to comment on any vocalising the child does, or on interactions with you (e.g. smiling, waving, laughing) as these may give very valuable information, which can be overlooked if it is not actively considered as part of a developmental assessment.

Finally, perform a gross-motor assessment. In an infant, or severely impaired patient, this comprises the '180-degree examination', and in an older child, a gait examination.

The '180-degree examination' aptly describes the sequence of manoeuvres examined, as follows. Note that the gross-motor assessment should be performed on a firm surface, so if the examining couch is not firm, a sheet or blanket can be spread on the floor (the examiners must be aware that you realise the need for a firm surface).

First, with the child lying supine, note the posture (e.g. adopting abnormal asymmetric tonic neck reflex [ATNR] positioning) and movement (e.g. choreoathetoid movements with cerebral palsy [CP], paucity of movement with some neuromuscular diseases).

Next, draw the child into the sitting position, by traction on the arms, noting the degree of head control/lag (e.g. marked head lag with spinal muscular atrophy).

With the child in the sitting position, note the amount of head and trunk control, and ability to sit, supported and unsupported.

Next, hold the child up to check weight-bearing. This helps detect lower limb scissoring (as in CP), lower limb hypotonia and weakness (e.g. neuromuscular disorders causing the 'floppy infant' syndrome), and inappropriately 'advanced' weight bearing (in CP).

Then, hold the child in ventral suspension and describe the posture of the head, trunk and limbs. This position can demonstrate hypotonia well: if very severe, the infant describes a 'C' shape over the examiner's hand. The converse can occur with CP, where an exaggerated extensor posture may be adopted.

Finally, lay the child prone. Make sure that the hands are placed to either side of the infant's shoulders, with the palms apposed to the bed and elbows flexed, to optimise the ability to extend the upper limbs. Note the ability of the child to raise the head and trunk when placed prone.

The primitive reflexes may be checked separately after the 180-degree examination, or may be incorporated into the sequence (e.g. assessing the sucking, rooting, ATNR and neck-righting reflexes when supine, the grasp reflex when pulling the child to sit, the placing and stepping reflexes when held standing to check weight bearing, the Landau and Galant reflexes when held in ventral suspension), depending on personal preference. Whichever is chosen, leave the Moro and parachute reflexes until last, as they may upset the child.

If you are checking the primitive reflexes separately, the following is a suggested order, with the usual times of appearance and incorporation, or disappearance, of the reflexes. The elicitation of the lesser-known reflexes is detailed.

1. **Sucking** and **rooting** (birth to 4 months, when awake, and to 6 months when sleeping).
2. **Palmar grasp** (birth to 3 months).
3. **Placing, stepping** (both from birth to 6 weeks).
4. **Landau reflex**, a two-stage reflex. With the child supported prone (with your hand under the abdomen), the child should (normally) extend head, trunk and hips. This is the first, and more important stage. Next, flex the head and neck, and normally the response is flexion of trunk and hips, but this is less constant than the first stage (first stage from 4 months, plus second stage from 9 months; gone by 2 years).
5. **ATNR**. With the child supine, the head is rotated to one side. A 'fencing' posture develops, with extension of the ipsilateral upper and lower limb (i.e. the side towards which the head is turned) and flexion of the opposite side (2 months to 6 months). Persistence beyond 6 months is indicative of upper motor neurone problems, especially CP. Maintaining the ATNR posture throughout the time that the head is held turned, such that the child cannot 'break' from that position, is similarly significant.
6. **Neck-righting reflex.** Rotation of the trunk to conform with position of the head when the head is rotated to one side (6 months to 2 years).
7. **Moro reflex** (birth to 4 months). As with most primitive reflexes, persistence beyond the usual time of disappearance is pathological. Make a point of focusing not only on the limb movements, but also the facial response, for asymmetry (e.g. in hemiplegic CP).
8. **Parachute reflex.** With the infant held in the prone position, move him or her rapidly, face downwards, towards the floor. The normal reaction is to extend both upper limbs as if to break the fall (appears between 6 and 12 months, usually at 9 months, and persists; its absence beyond 12 months is abnormal). Asymmetry occurs with hemiplegia.

As the examination is proceeding, it is useful to comment on each finding as it is elicited, making sure that the examiners see that you know the significance of each sign found. Terms such as 'age-appropriate' may be useful when normal findings occur.

A succinct summary at the completion of the examination should attempt to give a developmental age to each of the areas assessed, and state whether any delay detected is global, or whether there is a scatter of abilities (e.g. gross- and fine-motor delay only in Werdnig-Hoffmann disease, visual and gross-motor impairment in an ex-premature baby, global delay in a child with congenital rubella or severe CP).

Eye examination

This is not an infrequent case. The number of possible pathologies is clearly enormous, but the candidate should be able to perform a comprehensive eye examination as outlined, and should be familiar with important paediatric eye conditions that can appear in examinations; a selected few are outlined below.

Background information: some important eye conditions

Lids

Ptosis (short for blepharoptosis)

The muscle involved in elevation of the lid is the levator palpebrae superioris, supplied by the third cranial nerve. Congenital causes of ptosis are the most common. Acquired causes include myopathies and third cranial nerve palsy (and Horner's syndrome causes a partial ptosis). Mechanical problems such as orbital cellulitis or haemangioma may also cause ptosis. Bilateral ptosis should prompt examination for a neuromuscular cause.

Iris

Aniridia

This is actually hypoplasia, not absence, of the iris; the root of the iris is present. Associated developmental anomalies of the eye include cataract, glaucoma and corneal opacification. There are at least two types of aniridia, one autosomal dominant, the other sporadic and associated with Wilms' tumour and genitourinary anomalies (deletion of chromosome 11).

Lens

Cataract

This opacity of the lens has a wide differential diagnosis, although in 50% of cases no cause is detected. Groups of causes include hereditary (e.g. autosomal dominant), chromosomal disorders (e.g. Down syndrome), other malformation syndromes (e.g. Noonan's syndrome), congenital TORCH infections, metabolic disorders (e.g. diabetes mellitus, galactosaemia), drugs (e.g. steroids). It is important to examine the child to detect these underlying problems.

Ectopia lentis

This displacement of the lens may be inherited as the sole anomaly, or may be associated with systemic conditions, such as Marfan's syndrome (where it usually displaces superiorly) and homocystinuria (where it mostly displaces inferiorly).

Retina

Colobomata

This defect, or lack of some portion, of tissue can involve any part of the eye. The most important types are chorioretinal and isolated optic nerve colobomata.

Optic nerve hypoplasia

This can be an isolated anomaly, or be associated with other eye anomalies (microphthalmos, aniridia) and neurological problems such as encephalocoele. It is associated with absence of the corpus callosum.

Retinopathy of prematurity (ROP)

This can only occur before the retina is vascularised. As the peripheral retina is the region that is vascularised last in the eye of the baby, it is the most commonly involved area. ROP affects around 80% of babies under 1 kg and almost 10% of these will have their vision threatened. Among those between 1 and 1.5 kg, 50% are affected with ROP, and 2% of these will have their vision threatened. The stage, location and extent of ROP are the standard three aspects that determine management.

There are five stages of ROP:

- **Stage 1:** flat white demarcation line between avascular and vascularised retina.
- **Stage 2:** ridge due to arteriovenous shunting (demarcation line raised into vitreous).
- **Stage 3:** extraretinal fibrovascular proliferation (new vessels elevated into vitreous).
- **Stage 4A:** partial retinal detachment, macula attached (visual prognosis still hopeful).
- **Stage 4B:** partial retinal detachment, macula detached (visual prognosis poor).
- **Stage 5:** complete retinal detachment.

'Plus' is added to each stage if there are dilated and tortuous vessels in the posterior retina. This indicates a worse prognosis and more progressive disease.

Three zones are described:

- **Zone I:** a circle centred on the optic nerve, the radius being double the distance from the optic nerve to fovea; disease here is the most dangerous.
- **Zone II:** edge of Zone I to oro serrata (nasal side), to anatomic equator (temporal side).
- **Zone III:** peripheral crescent on temporal side.

The extent is described relative to the circumferential distribution, in clock hours, with the entire eye comprising 12 clock hours, divided into single clock hours of 30 degrees.

If the disease is stage 3 in 5–8 adjacent clock hours with plus disease in Zone II, treatment with cryotherapy is warranted; this is the threshold level. The small (less than 1000 g) sick baby who goes from crisis to crisis is at greatest risk.

Squint (strabismus)

Certain terms should be known by the candidate:

- **Pseudostrabismus:** false appearance of squint (often due to epicanthal folds).
- **Orthophoria:** perfect condition of ocular balance.
- **Heterophoria:** latent tendency to squint (e.g. when tired).
- **Heterotropia:** permanent tendency to squint.
- **Non-paralytic squint:** not due to a problem with any extraocular muscles or cranial nerves supplying them.
- **Paralytic squint:** due to a problem with extraocular muscles or cranial nerves.
- **Esotropia:** convergent squint.
- **Exotropia:** divergent squint.

Squint can be divided into non-paralytic and paralytic types.

Non-paralytic
1. Convergent (i.e. esotropia). Types include infantile and accommodative. Accommodative squint typically presents around age 18 months to 2 years.
2. Divergent (i.e. exotropia). Types include intermittent and constant.

Paralytic
1. Third nerve palsy (frequently congenital; divergent squint, plus downward deviation of eye and ptosis).
2. Fourth nerve palsy (congenital or acquired from head trauma; accompanying head tilt towards opposite shoulder to eliminate a vertical deviation).
3. Sixth nerve palsy (frequently acquired from head trauma; convergent squint).

Procedure

The paediatric eye examination is best done with the child sitting on the side of the bed, in a chair or on the parent's lap, depending on the child's age. After introducing yourself, stand back and look at the overall appearance of the child, particularly for dysmorphic features (various malformation syndromes have eye involvement), facial features of the 'ex-premmie' (associated ROP) and growth parameters (e.g. may be small and microcephalic with intrauterine infection). Also note any head tilt (e.g. with fourth cranial nerve palsy). After brief comments on general appearance, direct your attention to the eyes.

Irrespective of the child's age, eye examination is always started by inspection for external abnormalities. Commence by looking from in front, from the side and from above to detect any proptosis. Next, focus successively on each of the anatomical structures of the eye to detect any abnormalities (i.e. look at the eyebrows, eyelids, cornea, iris, sclera and conjunctivae). This systematic approach should prevent important signs being overlooked. If the child wears glasses, examine these also.

After inspection, proceed with testing of visual acuity in each eye. Response to a face is the best way of trying to assess whether an infant can see or not. Note whether the infant can fix and follow by moving your face in front of him or her. After a face, the next best target is a large bright object (e.g. red ball of wool). See if the child is fixing and following. If he or she can see a large object, then proceed to test with smaller objects down to the pinhead size of a 'hundred and thousand' cake decoration. If there is no response to your face, use a torch to check response to a bright light. In older children, Sheridan Gardner Test Charts can be used (preschool age) or the Snellen Test Charts (school age). If these tests suggest a problem with acuity, then comment on the need for formal testing.

Testing of the visual fields can then be performed. Again the technique is age dependent. In infants, use a red ball of wool brought from behind the child's head: head turning indicates when it enters the visual field. In older children, a direct confrontation can be used, first with both eyes and then each eye separately. The classic 'red hat pin' technique can be used with adolescents.

Extraocular movements can then be tested (see the short case on motor cranial nerves in this chapter). It is probably easier to hold the child's head still with one hand, and have the child follow an interesting target (e.g. small bright puppet) held by the other hand, than to keep asking the child to stop moving the head. Both eyes can be tested together, and the child should be asked, at each position of gaze, to indicate any diplopia: 'say how many you see' or 'say if you see two'.

The evaluation of eye movements in the newborn infant can be difficult. One way to overcome this is to pick the baby up and move her or him in various directions, watching the eye movements produced because of the vestibular ocular reflex (when the child is rotated, eyes move in the opposite direction, and nystagmus occurs; when rotation is ceased, after-nystagmus occurs). Thus moving the child up and down, side to side, and backwards and forwards will permit evaluation of the main directions of eye movement.

At this stage, in older children, depending on the clinical findings so far, it may be appropriate to check for lid lag (if there is a suggestion of thyrotoxicosis) and fatigability on upward gaze (to screen for myasthenia gravis, particularly if there is bilateral ptosis or myopathic facies).

Near and far cover tests should be performed, with an interesting toy as the fixation target. If the child becomes upset when one eye is covered, this suggests poor vision in the uncovered eye (although this should have been detected when assessing visual acuity). Also, shine a torch into the eyes from a distance to detect a squint (although this will not detect microstrabismus).

Testing the pupillary light reflexes and fundoscopy are usually best left until the end, because of the cooperation required and time constraints. When assessing the pupils, note whether they are of normal size (or have been dilated for the examination) and if there is any asymmetry in size, and then check the light reflex (with a pen-torch; remember to place a hand between the eyes as a barrier to prevent any light reaching the opposite side to the one being tested; also watch for the Marcus Gunn phenomenon). Check the accommodation reflex.

Ophthalmoscopy is then performed. First, look for the red reflex. Then the anterior aspects of the eye should be examined, the cornea, the lens and finally retinoscopy. Remember one of the 'golden eye rules' is 'never give an opinion through an undilated pupil'. However, the examiners may expect an opinion (the pupils may already be dilated; if not, it may be appropriate to comment that dilating the pupils would be helpful).

Finally, for completeness, offer to test the corneal reflex (do not just go ahead and do it, as children tend to find this very distressing), palpate for evidence of raised intraocular pressure (glaucoma) and then auscultate over each closed eyelid with the bell of the stethoscope (with the child holding his or her breath while you auscultate, if possible) for bruits.

At the completion of the examination, the examiners may ask whether there is anything else you would like to assess. This will depend on the most obvious finding, as in the following examples:

1. **Finding: papilloedema.** The next steps could include a neurological examination for signs of raised intracranial pressure, measuring the blood pressure to detect hypertension and checking for asterixis from hypercapnia.
2. **Finding: retinopathy consistent with diabetes.** The next steps may include an endocrine assessment and urinalysis.
3. **Finding: nystagmus.** The next steps would include a full neurological examination: e.g. for cerebellar signs, if horizontal nystagmus.

Visual acuity

At birth, all normal children can see, but normal 'adult' acuity takes a few years to develop. Expected acuity is as follows:

1. At birth, normal visual acuity is approximately 3/60.
2. By 6 months, normal visual acuity is 6/30.
3. By 18 months, it is 6/9.
4. By 2 years, it is 6/6.

Stages of visual development (in relation to clinically applicable testing)

- Neonates turn their head towards a diffuse light source.
- By 6 weeks of age, babies follow a face or large, coloured (especially red) object (which should be silent, so that turning to sound is not misinterpreted). Also by this age the 'blink to menace' response is present.
- By 3 months, the eyes converge for finger-play.
- By 4 months, the infant follows objects through 180 degrees, turning the head.
- By 5 months, infants reach for a toy within their visual field and are able to regard a small raisin on a table.
- By 6 months, they move the eyes together in all directions. A squint at this stage is abnormal. This is the earliest age at which the Stycar graded balls test can be used to test the vision.
- By 9 months, they are able to pick up a raisin (raking grasp), look for fallen toys and play peek-a-boo.
- By 12 months, babies are able to pick up a raisin with neat pincer grasp. At this stage, it is possible to test with rolling balls as small as 3 mm at a distance of 3 m. Also the Stycar mounted balls test for ability to fixate and peripheral vision can be used. In the examination setting, a ball of red wool can be used for peripheral vision testing, bringing it from behind the child and watching the head turn towards the ball when it enters the child's visual field.

Between 1 and 2 years, the allure of rolling balls has diminished, and it is difficult to hold the child's attention, but if this is possible, the rolling and mounted ball tests remain useful. From 2 years, miniature toy-matching tests can be used. Remember that by the age of 2 years, acuity should be 6/6. For preschool children (3½ to 5½ years old), the Sheridan-Gardner test or the E test can be used. The former is a better test, as children are less likely to become confused because laterality is not involved. For school-aged children, the Snellen Test Charts can be used, or the E test if the child cannot recognise the Snellen Chart letters.

Motor cranial nerves

This is one of the most common neurological examinations requested. The introductions are variable (e.g. 'This child has had droopy eyelids since birth', or 'This boy has had facial weakness for several years'), but the specific instruction of 'Examine the motor cranial nerves' usually accompanies this type of lead-in. A smoothly performed motor cranial nerve examination can be comfortably achieved within 5 minutes. This is quite different from 'Cranial nerves', as the additional examination components of the vision, eyes, hearing and other sensory modalities are quite time consuming.

A suggested approach follows for children of preschool age or older. For younger children, improvisation involving the use of interesting-looking toys and play is necessary.

First, introduce yourself to the patient and parent. Shake hands with both (to detect myotonic dystrophy). Inspect the face carefully and scan the limbs, for any obvious signs such as ptosis, facial asymmetry or hemiplegic posturing.

Before checking the extraocular eye movements, the visual acuity needs to be quickly checked, to confirm that the child can see to follow an object (e.g. a finger puppet). Explain what you are doing as you proceed.

To test the extraocular movements, ask the child to follow your finger or other small object. Ask the child how many fingers (or objects) can be seen, in each of nine positions (right and left lateral gaze, up and down in central, right and left lateral positions, and straight ahead, i.e. central).

The findings sought include lack of movement, diplopia and nystagmus. If abnormalities are demonstrated, then each eye should be tested separately.

Third nerve lesions cause ptosis, a 'down and out' position of the involved eye, and paralysis of most eye movements, sparing only lateral rectus and superior oblique function. They also cause a dilated pupil and lack of direct pupillary light response, but pupil light reactions do not need to be tested in a motor examination. Fourth nerve lesions cause diplopia on looking down and in. Sixth nerve lesions cause lack of lateral movement, with diplopia most marked on looking towards the affected side.

Next examine the fifth nerve. You may ask the child the following, demonstrating each move as you proceed. 'Open your mouth': the jaw will deviate towards the weak side with a unilateral fifth nerve lesion, pushed by the normal pterygoid. 'Now keep it open; don't let me close it': this tests the pterygoids. 'Clench your teeth tight': feel the muscle bulk on each side. Then with your hand against the chin, 'Move your chin towards my hand', on each side. This tests each pterygoid in turn. Finally check the jaw jerk: 'Open your mouth a little; I'm just going to tap on your chin'. The jerk will be increased in pseudobulbar palsy.

The muscles of facial expression are then tested. 'Look up and raise your eyebrows': this tests the frontalis and is particularly useful in differentiating upper motor neurone lesions (upper facial muscles are preserved due to bilateral innervation) from lower motor neurone lesions, where the upper facial muscles are affected. 'Screw your eyes up tight': compare the two sides, noting any asymmetry between the degree the eyelashes are buried on either side. This may detect an obvious Bell's phenomenon, where there is rolling upward of the eyeball when attempting to shut the eyes forcefully, as eye closure may not be possible in lower motor neurone lesions. Then try to open each eye: 'Keep them shut; stop me opening them'. This tests the orbicularis oculi muscles. 'Now show me your teeth' allows assessment of any asymmetry of the nasolabial grooves. The mouth will be drawn towards the normal side if there is a unilateral lesion of either upper or lower motor neurone type. 'Puff out your cheeks; keep them like that': demonstrate this and then tap with your finger over each cheek to detect ease of air expulsion on the affected side.

The ninth, tenth and twelfth nerves are then tested. 'Open your mouth wide': look (with a torch) at the uvula for any deviation to either side. 'Now say aaah': watch movement of the soft palate. With unilateral lesions of the tenth nerve the uvula is drawn towards the normal side. Inspect the tongue for fasciculations (tongue not protruding). Then say 'Poke out your tongue' and note any deviation. With a unilateral lesion, the normal side pushes the tongue towards the affected (weaker) side. Also check that the tongue can be equally well protruded towards each side. (For some reason children love poking their tongues out at nervous examination candidates.) Get the child to speak (e.g. 'Which school do you go to?') to check for any evidence of hoarseness (unilateral recurrent laryngeal nerve lesion), and to cough to check for the 'bovine' cough of bilateral recurrent laryngeal nerve lesions: these are very rare in paediatric patients but are easy to test, for completeness.

The eleventh cranial nerve supplies the sternocleidomastoid and trapezius muscles. With your hand against the lateral aspect of the child's face say, 'Turn your head towards my hand', or if that is not understood, choose something for the child to inspect over his or her shoulder and say 'Look over there'. When this movement is performed, inspect and palpate the bulk of the sternomastoid, then repeat the process for the other side. Ask the child to 'shrug your shoulders' (demonstrate this), and then to repeat this against resistance (your hands). Note the bulk of the trapezius muscles.

At the completion of the examination, summarise your findings and give a differential diagnosis. The remainder of the examination should be directed towards confirming any suspected diagnosis, which may entail examination of the gait, lower limbs, upper limbs or neuromuscular assessment.

Neurological assessment of the upper limbs

This is a fairly common short case, and like most cases in neurology necessitates careful inspection before laying of hands on the patient. Perhaps because most candidates are quite comfortable with a standard neurological examination procedure, they may be eager to test power, tone and reflexes before careful inspection.

For adequate exposure, the child should be completely undressed down to the waist. Watching the child remove the pullover or shirt may provide valuable clues to the underlying problem.

Introduce yourself to the parent and child, and shake hands with the child (this may detect the inability to release your hand, which indicates myotonic dystrophy).

Inspection

Initial inspection is best done with the child standing, and then sitting in a chair or on the edge of the bed, directly facing the candidate.

Stand back and look at the child. Inspection should not be confined to the upper limbs; it should also include rapid scanning of the face, neck, lower limbs and skin, for clues to the underlying pathology (see Table 13.2 for details).

Next, focus on the upper limbs. Note their resting posture (e.g. hemiplegia). Look for: muscle wasting of arms, forearms or small muscles of the hands (marked wasting being more likely due to lower motor unit pathology); fasciculations (which indicate lower motor unit degeneration, such as anterior horn cell disease, when in the presence

---

Table 13.2 Additional information: possible useful signs on inspection

Head and neck Horner's syndrome (look for neck pathology) Myopathic facies (think of myopathies, myotonic dystrophy, myasthenia gravis) Facial nerve palsy (look for upper motor neurone signs, hemiplegia) Short neck (think of the Klippel-Feil anomaly; look for signs of spasticity, findings of syringomyelia) **Lower limbs** Posture Muscle wasting (e.g. peroneal atrophy of CMT) Involuntary movements Growth arrest Foot deformities (e.g. pes cavus)	**Skin** Stigmata of neurofibromatosis type 1 (NF-1) (e.g. café-au-lait patches, axillary freckling, neurofibromata) Stigmata of tuberous sclerosis (e.g. hypopigmented lesions) **Grading of power (National Health and Medical Research Council scale)** 0 Complete paralysis 1 Flicker of contraction 2 Movement possible if gravity removed 3 Movement possible against gravity, but not against resistance 4 Movement possible against gravity and some resistance 5 Normal power

CMT = Charcot-Marie-Tooth disease; NF-1 = neurofibramatosis, type 1.

of other signs of motor pathology); involuntary movements (e.g. chorea, tremor); contractures; scars (inspect thoroughly for these); growth arrest (compare size of thumb nail beds); trophic changes, neurocutaneous stigmata (e.g. neurofibromata). When looking at the hands, also note any 'classic' signs of brachial plexus lesions: 'true claw hand' due to a lower (Klumpke's) lesion (C8, T1); or the 'waiter's tip' position of an upper (Erb) lesion (C5, 6).

Also note any 'classic' signs of peripheral nerve lesions: wrist drop due to radial nerve palsy, 'monkey hand' due to median nerve palsy, and 'ulnar claw hand' due to ulnar nerve palsy.

After inspecting the upper limbs, quickly look at the neck for scars (e.g. removal of tumour) and the back, for scars of spinal surgery (e.g. spina bifida repair) or evidence of scoliosis (various neuromuscular causes such as anterior horn cell disorders, neuropathies, myopathies).

Have the child hold both upper limbs straight out in front, and ask her or him to close the eyes. Drifting of either arm may be due to loss of proprioception (posterior column disease), cerebellar hypotonia or weakness from pyramidal tract pathology.

Palpation

Feel the muscle bulk in each muscle compartment and, if possible, have the child contract the muscles while they are being palpated, for a more accurate assessment. Also note any muscle tenderness (e.g. dermatomyositis). Feel for any hypertrophied peripheral nerves, such as the ulnar nerve at the elbow (e.g. Charcot-Marie-Tooth disease).

Tone

Assess the tone at the wrists and elbows. When moving the joints, ensure that the rhythm and rate at which this is done is irregular and not predicted, and resisted, by the child. Passive pronation and supination of the forearms is probably the easiest way of assessing tone accurately. Note whether there is spasticity, rigidity or hypotonia.

Power

All candidates should be familiar with the grading of muscle power out of 5 (National Health and Medical Research Council Scale, see Table 13.2) and with the various motor root values and sensory dermatomes of the upper limb. While assessing power, note whether any weakness found is symmetrical or asymmetrical, is predominantly proximal or distal, involves a particular muscle group, motor nerve root, distribution of a particular peripheral nerve, or is in an 'upper motor neurone pattern', with weakness of abduction of the shoulder and extension of elbow and wrist.

Check the strength of the following:

1. Shoulder abduction (C5, 6): 'Hold your arms up like this [demonstrate abduction at shoulders with elbows flexed]. Stop me pushing them down.'
2. Shoulder adduction (C6, 7, 8): 'Hold your arms up like this again. Stop me lifting them up.'
3. Elbow flexion (C5, 6): 'Pull my hands towards you.'
4. Elbow extension (C7, 8): 'Push me away.'
5. Wrist flexion (C6, 7): 'Hold your hands like this [demonstrate full flexion at wrists]. Keep them like that; don't let me straighten them.'
6. Wrist extension (C6, 7): 'Hold your hands like this [demonstrate full extension at wrists]. Keep them like that; don't let me straighten them.'
7. Hand grip (C8, T1): 'Squeeze my finger as tight as you can. Don't let go.'

8. Finger abduction (C8, T1): 'Spread your fingers apart like this [demonstrate]. Stop me pushing them together.'

The following points may aid remembering motor root values:

1. The highest level is shoulder abduction (C4, 5).
2. Extensors (of elbow, wrist, fingers) are all supplied by C7.
3. Wrist flexion and extension have the same motor roots (C6, 7).
4. The lowest level is grip and the small muscles of hand (T1).

If there is a suggestion of a myopathic problem, at the end of assessing power ask the child to make a fist and then open the hand as quickly as possible, to assess for myotonia. If this is positive, go on to tap over the thenar eminence for percussion myotonia.

Reflexes

Check the reflexes. Remember to check with reinforcement, if there is no response on initial testing. Biceps and brachioradialis jerks both correspond to C5, 6. Triceps jerk corresponds to C7, 8 (so remember 5, 6, 7, 8).

Coordination

Check the finger–nose test: with the eyes open to assess for signs of cerebellar disease such as intention tremor, clumsy, jerking movements (dyssynergia) and overshooting the target (dysmetria); with eyes closed to assess for defective proprioception. In younger children, who cannot cooperate with the finger–nose test, putting a pen into a pen-top held out by the candidate may yield similar information. Also, threading a bead is a valuable test of coordination in young children. Check for dysdia-dochokinesis.

Sensation

Accurate testing of sensation is difficult in most children; it is also quite time consuming and is impractical in younger children. It may thus be appropriate in some cases to comment on the lack of reliability of testing in children and omit sensation. The following description is for older, cooperative children.

It may be wise to commence with testing for proprioception (posterior columns), as this is not time consuming and is fairly easy to do. Move the distal phalanx of the index finger (held from the sides) up and down, after demonstrating the procedure with the child's eyes open. Next test vibration (also posterior columns) using a 128 Hz tuning fork, with the child's eyes closed. Start distally (over the head of the ulna). Move proximally (over elbow) if there is lack of distal sensation. The best way to check is to ask the child to tell you when the 'buzzing' has stopped, and then to stop the fork vibrating. Then, proceed with checking light touch, in dermatomal distribution, with a wisp of cottonwool; this can be very difficult in younger children. Finally, check for pain sensation (spinothalamic tracts) using a new blunt pin. This is left until last, so as not to frighten the child. Ask the child to close the eyes and say whether the pin is sharp or dull. As with testing of light touch, test in dermatomal distribution.

The easiest way to remember the segmental cutaneous supply of the upper limb is as follows: numerically, start at the shoulder (C4) and proceed down the radial aspect of the limb (C5 arm, C6 forearm), reaching the tips of the fingers (C7) and then continuing up the ulnar aspect of the limb (C8 forearm, T1 elbow), until you reach the axilla (T2). It is useful to practise this 'counting' technique on your own upper limbs.

Function

Finally, if it seems relevant to the findings noted (e.g. spasticity, sensory deficits), it may be appropriate to perform a functional appraisal, although this is not part of the 'standard' neurological examination. (Note that this is really 'the icing on the cake', and omitting it would not be detrimental.) Ask the child to perform (or mime) some activities of daily living such as writing (if old enough), using a knife, fork, spoon, cup, comb and toothbrush, and undoing buttons or turning on a tap.

Summary

When summarising your findings, it may be useful to give a general description of the type of lesion (e.g. lower motor unit disorder) and then a more specific diagnosis (e.g. anterior horn cell disease), followed by a differential diagnosis of this.

It may be appropriate to request permission to examine other areas to confirm your impression of the most likely diagnosis. This may include, commonly, examination of motor cranial nerves and gait if a myopathy is suspected, or gait and lower limbs if a peripheral neuropathy is suspected, or further assessment of cerebellar function if a cerebellar lesion is likely.

If the suspected diagnosis is inheritable, also make a point of looking at the parents (e.g. in patients with Charcot-Marie-Tooth disease or myotonic dystrophy).

If the examiners ask which investigations would be useful, do not make the error of asking to see the electromyogram and nerve conduction studies, because if given actual copies of these, you must then be able to interpret them. It is more prudent to ask for the results of these studies (as interpreted by an expert).

Gait: a short-case approach

This is one of the most commonly encountered cases. A smooth and complete approach is mandatory. It can be the introduction to evaluating most pathological processes that affect the nervous system, and is an intricate component of many other cases outlined in this chapter on neurology (e.g. seizures, large head, scoliosis). But 'gait' does not necessarily mean a neurological diagnosis. A gait examination may also be the lead-in to a primary orthopaedic or rheumatological problem, or even more obscure problems such as haemophilia (presenting with a limp due to hip haemarthrosis or intrapsoas haemorrhage).

Begin by introducing yourself to the parent and patient. Stand back and rapidly scan for signs of neurological disorders, such as a large head, obvious eye signs (e.g. squint, ptosis or nystagmus), abnormal posturing (e.g. hemiplegic), abnormal movements (e.g. tremor, fasciculations), asymmetry (e.g. growth arrest with hemiplegia, rib asymmetry with scoliosis). Inspect the limbs very carefully. Note the muscle bulk (look systematically at buttocks, thighs and calves for any wasting), contractures, deformities of the feet (e.g. talipes, pes cavus). Look for skin signs such as neurocutaneous stigmata or scars of procedures (e.g. tendon releases, ventriculoperitoneal shunts). Then, with the child's lower limbs adequately exposed (watch how the child undresses), you may proceed with the following steps in this suggested order.

1. **Normal gait**. This is the initial screening procedure. Note any characteristic pattern of the gait: e.g. circumduction with hemiplegia, wide-based with cerebellar pathway dysfunction, waddling with proximal myopathies, antalgic gait (limp) with orthopaedic problems. If no obvious recognisable pattern is seen, then

look at each component of the gait in turn, focusing on pelvis, hips, knees and feet, or in the reverse order, and simply describe what you see.

2. **Heel–toe walking.** This tests for cerebellar pathway problems. If the child is over 2 years, and quite unable to walk steadily, this may be due to pathology in the cerebellar vermis, but it may also be due to weakness or sensory deficits. Do not overinterpret this sign by itself.

3. **Walking on toes.** This tests for strength of plantar flexion (S1). It is usually possible for children with cerebral palsy or Duchenne's muscular dystrophy to do this well, but children with lesions affecting S1 (e.g. low lumbar myelomeningo-coele, peripheral neuropathies, anterior horn cell disease) may find it impossible.

4. **Walking on heels.** This tests for strength of dorsiflexion (L5). It is often difficult in a large number of conditions (e.g. cerebral palsy, anterior horn cell disease, peripheral neuropathies, Duchenne's muscular dystrophy).

5. **Walking on outsides of feet.** This is the Fog test. It brings out signs of subtle hemiplegia, with the mildly hemiplegic child adopting either a frank hemiplegic posture, or demonstrating a notable asymmetry in arm and leg positioning. Walking on the insides of the feet, often called the 'reverse Fog', has similar significance. It is important not to overinterpret the sometimes bizarre bilateral postures children adopt when performing this part of the gait routine. It is the finding of asymmetry that is important.

6. **Running.** This also accentuates findings such as hemiplegia and proximal weakness (in the latter, a child may seem to be miming a run in slow motion).

7. **Standing on each foot.** By inspecting from behind, and noting the position of the pelvis, by iliac crest position, this allows detection of any proximal instability and positive Trendelenberg's sign.

8. **Hopping on each foot.** This assesses for unilateral weakness and for balance.

9. **Standing with feet together.** With eyes open, this tests for truncal (cerebellar) ataxia. With eyes closed, this checks for Romberg's sign (falling due to dorsal column pathology).

10. **Bending forward and touching toes.** This is to screen for scoliosis, which can occur with numerous neuromuscular disorders. The back should be inspected carefully for midline scars (e.g. myelomeningocoele repair), hairy patches or lipomas.

11. **Squatting and then rising** from the squatting position. Maintaining a squatting position tests more peripheral strength. This may be difficult in cases with peripheral neuropathy. Arising from the squatting position tests for proximal weakness.

12. **Lying on the floor and then rising** from this position. This is to elicit Gower's manoeuvre, which occurs with proximal weakness, and is classically associated with Duchenne's muscular dystrophy.

After the manoeuvres outlined above, probably the safest next step is to examine the lower limbs, as overinterpretation of certain signs may lead the candidate off on an inappropriate tangent (e.g. unsteadiness due to weakness could be misinterpreted as being ataxia due to a cerebellar problem, and may cause the candidate next to check for nystagmus and dysdiadochokinesis, rather than to methodically examine the lower limbs).

After the standard lower limb examination, you will probably have enough information to tell the examiners your thoughts about the probable pathology, and then to proceed to examine whatever else is relevant (this is most often the upper limbs).

Neurological assessment of the lower limbs

This is one of the most common neurological short cases. It is best started with examination of the gait (see the short case on gait), unless the examiners direct otherwise or the child is too young or too disabled to walk. The child's lower limbs should be adequately exposed, ideally undressed down to the underpants in younger children, but some older children can become embarrassed, and most adolescents prefer to maintain their modesty. The candidate should demonstrate to the examiners their sensitivity to the patient's modesty.

Note that examination of the back is essential in assessing the lower limbs.

Inspection

Initial inspection is done with the child standing (before full gait examination). More thorough inspection may be done when the child is on the bed, after the full range of gait manoeuvres.

Stand back and look at the child. Inspection should not be confined to the lower limbs. It should include rapid scanning of the face, neck, upper limbs and skin, for clues to underlying pathology (see the short case on the upper limbs for details). The back must be checked at some point, and this is most easily done when incorporated into the gait examination. Also note any peripheral signs, such as nearby crutches, splints, orthoses or wheelchair.

Focus on the lower limbs themselves. Note the resting posture (e.g. diplegia). Look for: muscle wasting of thighs, calves or feet (marked wasting being more likely due to lower motor unit pathology); fasciculations (which indicate lower motor unit degeneration, such as anterior horn cell disease, when in the presence of other signs of motor pathology); involuntary movements (e.g. myoclonus, chorea); contractures; scars (inspect thoroughly, including looking at posterior aspects of ankles and knees); growth arrest (compare size of great toe nail beds; may measure leg lengths); trophic changes; neurocutaneous stigmata (e.g. café-au-lait patches).

When looking at the feet, also note whether there is pes cavus, which reflects neuromuscular disease. This finding should prompt consideration of lower spinal lesions, spinocerebellar degenerations or peripheral neuropathies. Two 'classic' examination cases that may present like this are Charcot-Marie-Tooth (CMT) disease and Friedreich's ataxia.

Palpation

Feel the muscle bulk in each muscle compartment, and if possible, have the child contract the muscles while they are also being palpated, for a more accurate assessment. Also note any muscle tenderness (e.g. dermatomyositis). Feel for any hypertrophied peripheral nerves, such as the lateral popliteal at the knee (e.g. CMT disease).

Tone

Assess the tone at the knees and ankles. When moving the joints, ensure that the rhythm and rate at which this is done is irregular and not predicted, and resisted, by the child. Note whether tone is normal, increased (as in upper motor neurone or extrapyramidal lesions) or decreased (as in lower motor neurone or cerebellar lesions). Check for clonus at the knee and ankle. For the knee, place your hand on the lower quadriceps, and then push the patella down (towards the foot) briskly. For the ankle, position the limb with the knee bent and the hip externally rotated, then briskly dorsiflex the ankle. Sustained rhythmic contractions at either knee or ankle indicate upper motor neurone pathology. Note that up to 10 beats of ankle clonus may be present in the newborn, but this usually disappears by 2 months.

Power

All candidates should be familiar with the grading of muscle power out of 5 (see Table 13.2), and with the various motor root values and sensory dermatomes of the lower limb.

When assessing power, note whether any weakness found is symmetrical or asymmetrical, is predominantly proximal or distal, involves a particular muscle group, motor nerve root, or distribution of a particular peripheral nerve, or has an 'upper motor neurone' pattern (i.e. weakness of flexion at hip, knee and ankle).

Check the strength of the following:

1. Hip flexion (L1, 2, 3): 'Lift your leg straight up. Don't let me push it down' [by your hand placed above the knee].
2. Hip extension (L5, S1, 2): 'Keep your leg on the bed. Stop me lifting it up.'
3. Knee flexion (L5, S1): 'Bend your knee. Pull your foot in towards your bottom. Stop me straightening it.'
4. Knee extension (L3, 4): 'Straighten your leg. Stop me bending it.'
5. Ankle plantar flexion (S1): 'Push down. Push my hand away.'
6. Ankle dorsiflexion (L4, 5): 'Pull your foot back like this [demonstrate with wrist extension]. Stop me pushing it down.'

Reflexes

Check the reflexes. Remember to check with reinforcement (e.g. clenching teeth, or interlocking fingers in a 'monkey grip' and pulling apart hard just before the tendon hammer strikes the tendon) if there is no response on initial testing. Ankle jerk corresponds to S1, 2 and knee jerk corresponds to L3, 4 (so remember 1, 2, 3, 4).

Look for the crossed adductor reflex (adduction at the contralateral hip when the knee jerk is elicited) and other spread of reflexes (elicitable moving distally down the anterior aspect of the tibia) when checking the knee jerks. These indicate an upper motor neurone lesion in children older than 8 months. Check the plantar response. An extensor (Babinski's) response is normal under the age of 18 months, but after that time it reflects an upper motor neurone lesion.

Coordination

These manoeuvres are to detect cerebellar dysfunction. Check the heel–shin test: have the child slide his heel down his shin on each side, to check whether he can smoothly and accurately follow the line of the tibia. Next, check the toe–finger test (as with the finger–nose test): have the child lift his big toe to touch your finger, to detect intention tremor and past-pointing. Finally, test whether the child can tap the foot rapidly against your hand.

Sensation

Sensation is examined as for the upper limbs (see the short case on upper limbs). When testing proprioception, the big toe is used rather than the index finger. When testing vibration, the points for placing the tuning fork are the ankle (medial malleolus), the knee (tibial tuberosity or patella), and the pelvis (anterior superior iliac spine). Sensation for light touch and pain (pin prick) is tested in dermatomal distribution.

The easiest way to remember the segmental cutaneous supply of the lower limb is as follows. Numerically start at the groin (L1) and proceed down the anterior aspect of the limb: L2 supplies upper thigh, and L3 the knee. It becomes a little complicated below the knee: L4 supplies the medial aspect of the leg, L5 supplies the lateral aspect of the leg and continues down onto the medial aspect of the foot. (Mnemonic: L5 is the **l**owest **l**umbar, **l**ateral and **l**ong enough to reach the big toe). S1 supplies the sole. S2 supplies the central posterior aspect of the leg and thigh.

Summary

When summarising your findings, it may be useful to give a general description of the type of lesion (e.g. lower motor neurone disorder) and then a more specific diagnosis (e.g. peripheral neuropathy), followed by a differential diagnosis of this.

It may be appropriate to request permission to examine other areas to confirm your impression of the most likely diagnosis. This may include, commonly, examination of the upper limbs and motor cranial nerves, or further examination of cerebellar function. If the suspected diagnosis is inheritable, also make a point of looking at the parents (e.g. in patients with CMT, or myotonic dystrophy). See the case on the upper limbs for comments on investigations.

Cerebellar function

Occasionally the examiners may give a very directed lead-in such as, 'This boy has a problem with his coordination; would you assess his cerebellar function please?' If this is the introduction, then the following approach is useful.

First, make general observations, such as noting any nystagmus or tremor. Then ask the patient his name and age. With an older child, ask him to say 'sizzling sausage', which is more discerning in detecting cerebellar dysarthria. Next, examine the eyes for horizontal nystagmus (maximal if looking towards the side of the lesion). Have the child extend the upper limbs and note any drift or static tremor (due to hypotonia). Then check the finger–nose test for intention tremor and past-pointing. Test for dysdia-dochokinesis by having the child rapidly prorate and supinate the hand. In older children, it is also worth checking for 'rebound', where the child lifts his arms up very quickly from the side and then suddenly stops this movement. Cerebellar hypotonia may prevent the child from being able to stop the arms. Next, test for truncal ataxia by having the child sit up from lying down, with the arms folded. When the child is sitting up, test for pendular knee jerks (these only occur in severe cases).

Have the patient walk normally, then heel–toe. Also, have the child walk around a chair in both directions, as this will bring out staggering towards the affected side. Then, return the patient to the bed and examine the lower limbs for hypotonia, check the heel–shin test and the toe–finger test (the lower limb equivalent of the finger–nose test), and also have the child tap each foot rapidly against a firm surface (e.g. a clipboard).

This examination should take no more than 5 minutes, after which time a summary of the positive findings can be given and then the examination can be directed towards eliciting the cause. It may be worthwhile asking the examiners whether the child is taking anticonvulsants, if no obvious cause is discernible.

Large head

This is not an infrequent case, and is not difficult to perform quickly and comprehensively within the time constraints of a short case. The most important things to remember in this case are the following:

1. Always measure the head yourself, until a constant result around the largest diameter is obtained (usually three times is enough).
2. Always measure the parents' heads (in a similar fashion).
3. Always request the progressive percentiles of the child (the parents' percentile charts will not be available).
4. Always examine the back, to avoid missing spinal dysraphism.
5. Always examine the lower limbs before the upper limbs, as the lower limbs are first affected in hydrocephalus because the tracts supplying them run closer to the ventricles.
6. Always examine the eye movements, in particular the upward gaze (for Parinaud's syndrome) and lateral rectus function (for raised intracranial pressure compressing the sixth nerve).

Background Information

To interpret the abnormal, you must be able to remember the normal. There is a sex difference, and charts of head circumferences are readily available in all hospitals.

It is easy to remember the following average figures.

- 35 cm at birth.
- 47 cm (another 12 cm) at 12 months.
- 49 cm (another 2 cm) at 2 years.
- 50 cm at 3 years.
- 52 cm at 6 years.
- 53 cm at 10 years.
- 56 cm as adult.

In the actual examination, do not rely on remembering this, however. Always check the charts.

Correct interpretation of the percentile charts is mandatory. Measurements crossing percentile lines usually indicate significant pathology, except in the case of the benign condition, familial large head, where the 98th percentile line may be crossed (at, say, 12 months) and continue to deviate from the percentile curve, before it stabilises after 2 years of age.

The pattern of growth on the percentile chart can give an indication of the type of hydrocephalus a child has. An acquired hydrocephalus (e.g. from bacterial meningitis) will show normal growth until the time of the meningitis insult, and then will show deviation, whereas a congenital problem such as aqueduct stenosis will show much earlier deviation from the norm.

In simple terms, a large head can result from large bones, a large brain, large ventricles or a large bleed. This is outlined below with examples of each group.

Large bones—better referred to as 'bony disorders':
1. Achondroplasia.
2. Rickets.
3. Osteogenesis imperfecta (OI).
4. Chronic haemolytic anaemias.

Large brain (increased brain substance)

Generalised megalencephaly:

1. Sotos' syndrome (cerebral gigantism).
2. Neurocutaneous syndromes:
   a Neurofibromatosis type 1 (NF-1).
   b. Tuberous sclerosis (TS).
   c. Klippel-Trenauney-Weber syndrome (K-T-W).
   d. Sturge-Weber syndrome (S-W).
3. Inherited metabolic disorders:
   a Lipidoses (e.g. Tay-Sachs disease).
   b. Mucopolysaccharidoses (MPS).
   c. Leukodystrophies: e.g. Alexander's disease, Canavan's disease (also called 'spongy degeneration', actually a mitochondrial encephalomyelopathy).

Localised enlargement:

1. Cerebral tumours, e.g. glioma, ependymoma.
2. Cerebral abscess.

Large ventricles and/or subarachnoid spaces: due to excessive amounts of CSF, i.e. hydrocephalus.

1. Obstructive ('non-communicating' hydrocephalus): e.g. aqueduct stenosis, posterior fossa tumours.
2. Failure of CSF absorption ('communicating hydrocephalus'), e.g. meningeal adhesions after meningitis.
3. Overproduction of CSF (also 'communicating'), e.g. choroid plexus papilloma.

Large bleed: subdural haematoma (unilateral or bilateral), not infrequently due to nonaccidental injury (NAI).

The following approach should allow detection of any of the above groups. As the approach to the infant and older child is slightly different, both are discussed.

Examination

Infant

Start by introducing yourself to the parents and the child. Note the child's level of alertness, movement and any obvious features of syndromal diagnoses or neurocutaneous disorders. Look at the head for signs suggestive of hydrocephalus (e.g. 'sun-setting' of the eyes, and prominent scalp veins).

Measure the head circumference yourself, and then measure the head circumference of each parent. Request the percentile charts and comment on the findings. Inspect the shape of the head: this is best done with the child sitting up on the mother's lap. In this position, other important signs may be readily apparent, such as any titubation of head or trunk, or truncal ataxia from Dandy-Walker (D-W) syndrome. The shape of the head should be assessed from all angles, and is best described in terms of 'anteroposterior diameter' and 'biparietal diameter', and 'frontal bossing' and 'occipital prominence'. This is a good time to inspect the back for evidence of a repaired spina bifida lesion, in case it is forgotten later.

Palpate the head for suture separation, fontanelle patency (remembering that the posterior fontanelle normally closes by 4 months, and the anterior fontanelle closes by 18 months) and pressure, which must be checked in a sitting position, as a false impression of bulging may be obtained when the infant is prone or supine. Palpate carefully for shunts (there may be more than one, so be thorough) and, if present, trace shunt tubing, and inspect the chest and abdomen for scars indicating ventriculoatrial or ventriculo-peritoneal shunts. While palpating, interact with the child, watching eye movements and responsiveness.

Do not make the mistake of doing anything never done before, such as attempting percussion of the head, or transillumination (proper equipment for this is unlikely to be available).

Auscultate for evidence of an arteriovenous malformation involving the great vein of Galen. Listen over both temporal fossae, both eyeballs and both retroauricular regions.

Next, a full eye examination should be performed. When eye movements are being examined, do not forget that frontal bossing, if severe, can itself be a visual barrier, and may give a false impression of an upward-gaze palsy.

Examination of the back must not be forgotten, as children with spina bifida are frequent examination cases.

Following this, lower and upper limbs should be examined for motor and cerebellar signs. Testing sensation may be omitted in view of time restrictions, unless very relevant (e.g. sensory level in spina bifida).

Figure 13.1   Large head—infants

1. Introduce self
Interact with child, gain impression of
   development

2. General observations
Alertness
Dysmorphic features
Skeletal anomalies
Growth parameters
Movement
Skin

3. Head
Inspect
Measure
Percentiles
Shape
Look at back at this point
Palpate
Auscultate

4. Eyes
Inspect
- Visual acuity
- Visual fields
- External ocular movements
- Pupils
- Fundi

5. Back
Inspect
- Midline scar (spina bifida)
- Scoliosis (associated spina bifida, NF-1)

6. Lower limbs
Full examination of motor system
- Upper motor neurone signs (hydrocephalus, intracranial tumour)
- Lower motor neurone signs (spina bifida, leukodystrophies)
- Cerebellar signs (D-W)

7. Upper limbs
Full motor examination (as with lower limbs)

8. Developmental assessment
Gross motor
Fine motor
Hearing

9. Abdomen
Hepatosplenomegaly (MPS)

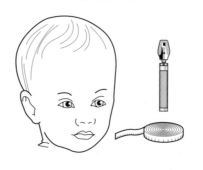

D-W = Dandy-Walker syndrome; MPS = mucopolysaccaridoses; NF-1 = neurofibromatosis, type 1.

A developmental assessment (gross motor, fine motor, personal–social and hearing) may then be performed. Abdominal examination may be performed if a storage disorder is suspected.

A suggested order of approach is outlined in Figure 13.1. A more comprehensive listing of possible findings, for reference, is given in Table 13.3.

Table 13.3 Additional information: possible physical findings in the child with a large head

General observations
Dysmorphic features (e.g. Sotos',
  mucopolysaccharidoses)
Skeletal anomalies (e.g. achondroplasia,
  OI)
Parameters
  • Height: tall (e.g. Sotos'); short
    (e.g. achondroplasia)
  • Weight: failing to thrive (e.g. Tay-
    Sachs, subdural from NAI, congenital
    toxoplasmosis)
Movement
  • Quality (e.g. hypotonia, poor head
    control in Tay-Sachs)
  • Symmetry (e.g. hemiplegia from
    subdural haematoma)
  • Upper limb versus lower limb
    (e.g. spina bifida)
Skin
  • Neurocutaneous stigmata (e.g. TS,
    NF-1, S-W, K-T-W)
  • Bruising (NAI)

Head
Initial inspection
  • Size, shape (see below)
  • Signs of hydrocephalus (scalp vein
    prominence, shiny skin, sun-setting
    eyes)
  • Eye signs, e.g. squint (see below)

Size
Measure head circumference: patient;
  parents
Request progressive percentiles

Shape
(Describe with infant supine initially; then
sit child up)
  • Frontal prominence (obstructive
    hydrocephalus)
  • Parietal prominence (subdural fluid,
    porencephalic cyst)
  • Occipital prominence (D-W)
  • Small posterior fossa (aqueduct
    stenosis)
(Look at the back at this point, for spina
bifida)

Palpate
(With child sitting up; interact with child
  and observe responsiveness, eye
  movements)
  • Craniotabes (rickets)
  • Split sutures (hydrocephalus)
  • Bulging fontanelle (hydrocephalus)
  • Absent fontanelle pulsation
    (hydrocephalus)
  • Shunts—trace shunt tubing, look for
    chest (VA) and abdomen (VP) scars

Auscultate
Bruit (AV malformation of great vein of
  Galen, causing increased CSF)

Eyes
Ptosis (third nerve palsy)
Nystagmus (brainstem tumour)
Squint (sixth, third nerve palsies)
Proptosis (NF-1 with orbital wall defect or
  optic nerve tumour)
Corneal clouding (MPS)
Visual acuity (impaired)
  • Retinal causes (e.g. optic atrophy,
    retinal haemorrhage)
  • Optic pathway causes (e.g.
    intracerebral glioma, optic nerve
    glioma—both can occur in NF-1)
Visual fields: field defect (e.g.
  porencephalic cyst, intracerebral
  tumour)
External ocular movements
  • Third nerve palsy (e.g. raised ICP)
  • Sixth nerve palsy (e.g. raised ICP)
  • Upward gaze palsy (e.g. pinealoma)
Pupils
  • Enlarged (third nerve palsy)
  • Unreactive to light (Parinaud's
    syndrome from dilated third ventricle)
Lens: cataracts (congenital
  toxoplasmosis)
Fundi
  • Papilloedema (raised ICP with closed
    fontanelle)
  • Optic atrophy (long-standing raised
    ICP)

Continued

Table 13.3 *(Continued)*

• Retinal haemorrhage (NAI) • Astrocytic hamartoma (TS) • Chorioretinitis (congenital toxoplasmosis) • Macular degeneration (lipidoses) **Developmental assessment** Gross motor: delayed (e.g.	hydrocephalus, inherited metabolic diseases) Fine motor: delayed (e.g. inherited metabolic diseases, neurocutaneous disorders) Hearing: impaired (e.g. post-meningitis, MPS)

AV = arteriovenous; CSF = cerebrospinal fluid; D-W = Dandy-Walker syndrome; ICP = intracranial pressure; K-T-W = Klippel-Trenauney-Weber syndrome; MPS = mucopolysaccharidoses; NF-1 = neurofibromatosis type 1; NAI = non-accidental injury; OI = osteogenesis imperfecta; S-W = Sturge-Weber syndrome; TS = tuberous sclerosis; VA = ventriculoatrial; VP = ventriculoperitoneal.

Older child

The approach to the older child is fairly similar to the examination of the infant. Again, begin with general observations and a full examination of the head and eyes, in a similar fashion to the examination for the infant. Then perform a full gait assessment, including looking for scoliosis, followed by examination of the lower and then the upper limbs. Next test the hearing, and then the abdomen.

Small head

A less common case than the large head, it requires a similar well-structured approach. There are several important points that must be remembered:

1. Always measure the head circumference of the patient, and of the parents and siblings, yourself (three times), and assess the percentile charts (including those of height and weight) before proceeding further.
2. Differentiate between true microcephaly (inferring microencephaly) and craniosynostosis.
3. Always include examination of vision and hearing in the assessment.

Background information

To interpret the abnormal, you must be able to remember the normal. Average head circumference measurements at various ages are given in the section on the large-head case. Correct interpretation of the head circumference percentile charts is mandatory. Measurements crossing percentile lines usually indicate significant pathology. The other growth parameters, height and weight, are very important, because they give valuable indications as to the underlying aetiology. Remember, percentile charts should be appropriate for the child's racial origin.

There are essentially three patterns of percentile findings:

1. Head circumference, height and weight all at the same percentile. Possibilities here include various syndromal diagnoses, endocrine causes such as hypopituitarism, and constitutional growth delay.
2. Head circumference small, but weight and height percentiles are even lower (i.e. relative sparing of the head). Possibilities here include various chronic illnesses, undernutrition and maternal neglect.
3. Head circumference small, height and weight at significantly higher percentiles

and may be within the normal range. Possibilities include all the causes of microencephaly (see below) and craniosynostosis.

It is the latter group that constitutes the bulk of discussion in this section, as this is the group most commonly represented in the short-case setting following the introduction: 'This child has a small head, would you please examine?'

In simple terms, a small head can result from 'small bones'—i.e. premature fusion of one or more sutures (craniosynostosis)—or from a small brain (microencephaly). These are discussed below.

Craniosynostosis

This is labelled according to which sutures are involved. If there is premature fusion of one or two sutures, there is no restriction of growth of the brain. However, if there is fusion of multiple sutures, this can prevent normal brain growth and lead to raised intracranial pressure and significant neurological impairments.

Table 13.4 gives a list of the sutures involved, the names given for premature closure of that suture, and the resultant head shape.

Microencephaly

Causes of microencephaly include primary defects in brain development, either of prenatal onset (e.g. chromosomal anomalies such as the trisomies; malformations such as holoprosencephaly, lissencephaly; malformation syndromes such as de Lange's syndrome; hereditary conditions such as autosomal recessive or autosomal dominant

Table 13.4 Sutures involved in craniosynostosis		
Suture	**Name for premature closure**	**Resultant head shape**
Sagittal	Scaphocephaly (also called dolichocephaly)	Elongated in the anteroposterior diameter, or boat-shaped, with decreased transverse diameter
Coronal	Brachycephaly	Widened in the transverse (biparietal) diameter, with high vault; decreased anteroposterior diameter
Single suture: unilateral coronal or lambdoid suture (or both), i.e. asymmetric craniosynostosis	Plagiocephaly	A 'skewed' shape
Metopic	Trigonocephaly	Midforehead ridging, with pointed, narrow appearance to forehead, and hypotelorism
Fusion of 4 or more sutures	Oxycephaly (also called turricephaly or acrocephaly)	A high, narrow, 'tower-shaped' skull; can cause significant neurological sequelae

microcephaly) or postnatal onset (e.g. malformation syndromes including Aicardi's, Angelman's, Fanconi's, Rubenstein-Taybi).

Secondary (acquired) abnormalities may similarly be of prenatal onset (e.g. intra-uterine TORCH infection, fetal alcohol syndrome [FAS], maternal phenylketonuria [PKU] or postnatal onset (e.g. perinatal asphyxia with resultant hypoxic encephalo-pathy, infections such as perinatally acquired herpes simplex encephalitis, or bacterial meningitis, head injury, undernutrition, inherited metabolic disease such as PKU, endocrine anomalies such as hypothyroidism and hypopituitarism). (Note: TORCH refers to **t**oxoplasmosis, **o**thers [includes syphilis, *Listeria monocytogenes* and HIV], **r**ubella, **c**ytomegalovirus and **h**erpes [both simplex and varicella-zoster].

Examination

Begin by introducing yourself to the parent and patient. Note the sizes of the parents' heads and whether they appear to have normal intelligence. Note the child's alertness. Scan for any dysmorphic features and note the presence of spectacles or hearing aids (e.g. intrauterine TORCH infection).

Look at the child's posture, as well as quality and symmetry of movement (volun-tary and involuntary). Also inspect the skin for neurocutaneous stigmata.

Measure the head circumference yourself, and then measure the head circumference of the parents. Request the height and weight of the child and the percentile charts. Comment on the findings. If the birth parameters are not given and a prenatal onset seems likely from the later percentile readings, request these. If prenatal onset is confirmed, this will direct the remainder of the examination towards disorders such as intrauterine infection and chromosomal anomalies.

Note the child's overall growth, in particular whether the child looks generally small (e.g. syndromal diagnoses, constitutional growth delay) or whether just the head is small (e.g. autosomal recessive microcephaly).

Request the percentile charts to confirm your impression. Note whether the head circumference lies at a lower, an equal or a higher percentile than the other parameters (weight and height). This is a very important step (see above).

Examine the head for any scars (e.g. surgical repair of craniosynostosis, closure of encephalocoele, decompressive craniotomy for severe head trauma) and visible ridging along suture lines (the metopic being seen most readily).

Next, focus on the shape of the head, assessing it from all angles. This is best done with the child sitting on the mother's lap. The shape of the head is best described in terms of 'anteroposterior diameter' and 'biparietal diameter'. Possible findings include the 'tower' skull of oxycephaly, or the sloping forehead and flat occiput of autosomal recessive microcephaly.

Palpate the head for ridging along suture lines and any deformities of skull contour (craniosynostosis) or bony defects (repaired encephalocoele).

Check the fontanelles. The posterior fontanelle closes by 4 months, and the anterior fontanelle by 18 months. A large anterior fontanelle occurs with the trisomies, congen-ital rubella and athyrotic hypothyroidism.

By this stage, it should be clear whether you are dealing with craniosynostosis or microencephaly. If it is the latter, then proceed as outlined below. If it is craniosyno-stosis, proceed as outlined later in this section.

Note any dysmorphic facial features (various syndromal diagnoses) as you proceed. Inspect the eyes for dysmorphic features. Perform a full eye examination (the relevant findings are given in the comprehensive list in Table 13.5). In particular, check the visual acuity (impairment from various pathologies, including TORCH or

Table 13.5 Comprehensive list of possible findings on examination for small head

General observations

Alertness

Dysmorphic features (e.g. de Lange's, Rubenstein-Taybi)

Wearing glasses (e.g. TORCH, CP, neurodegenerative disease)

Wearing hearing aid (e.g. TORCH, CP, Cockayne's syndrome, neuroaxonal dystrophy)

Skeletal anomalies (e.g. rhizomelia with RCDP)

Posture
- Hemiplegic (e.g. CP, Cockayne's)
- Quadriplegic (e.g. CP, neurodegenerative disorders)
- Decorticate (e.g. Krabbe's disease)

Voluntary movements
- Quality (e.g. poor head control with CP, neurodegenerative disorders)
- Symmetry (e.g. hemiplegia due to CP, Cockayne's, HIV-1)

Involuntary movements (beware CP or neurodegenerative disease)
- Choreoathetosis (e.g. CP, PKU, Pelizaeus-Merzbacher)
- Myoclonus (e.g. CP, PKU, infantile ceroid lipofuscinosis, Alpers', Aicardi's, incontinentia pigmenti)
- Tremor (e.g. PKU, HIV-1-related encephalopathy)

Skin
- Neurocutaneous stigmata (whorled splashes of brown pigmentation in incontinentia pigmenti)

Parameters

Head circumference: measure patient and parents

Request progressive percentiles

Height: short stature
- Same percentile as head (syndromal diagnoses, constitutional delay, endocrine disorders)
- Higher percentile than head (TORCH, Seckel's, Cockayne's, any severe encephalopathy in infancy)
- Lower percentile than head (causes of failure to thrive, chronic illness)

Disproportionate (RCDP)

Weight (failing to thrive): comparing weight and head percentiles, causes as outlined for height comparison above.

Head

Size (as above)

Shape (describe with child sitting up)
- Elongated AP diameter (sagittal synostosis)
- Wide with high vault (coronal synostosis)
- Asymmetric (e.g. unilateral lambdoid synostosis)
- Narrow forehead, midforehead ridge (metopic synostosis)
- Tower shaped (multiple synostosis)
- Sloping forehead (autosomal recessive microcephaly)

Palpate (with child sitting up; interact with child and observe responsiveness, eye movements)
- Ridging along sutures (craniosynostosis)
- Wide fontanelle (e.g. trisomies, congenital rubella)

Eyes

Dysmorphic features
- Microphthalmos (e.g. TORCH)
- Hypotelorism (holoprosencephaly)
- Upward slant (e.g. Down syndrome)
- Downward slant (e.g. trisomy 9)
- Epicanthic folds (e.g. trisomies)

Squint (e.g. TORCH, CP)

Nystagmus (e.g. TORCH, any cause of severe visual impairment, such as neurodegenerative disorders)

Corneal opacity (e.g. Cockayne's, congenital rubella, herpes)

Glaucoma (e.g. congenital rubella)

Visual acuity (impaired)
- Retinal causes (see below)
- Optic pathway causes (e.g. CP)

Visual fields: field defect (e.g. hemiplegic CP)

Eye movements: restricted upward gaze (HIV-1)

Pupils
- Anisocoria (e.g. congenital varicella)
- Unreactive to light (retinal or optic path causes of visual loss)

Lens: cataracts (e.g. TORCH, incontinentia pigmenti)

Fundi
- Chorioretinitis (TORCH)

Continued

Table 13.5 *(Continued)*

- Pigmentary degeneration (neurodegenerative disorders, e.g. ceroid lipofuscinosis, incontinentia pigmenti), Cockayne's, TORCH)
- Optic atrophy (e.g. disorders with pigmentary degeneration, TORCH, Krabbe's)
- Papillitis (e.g. incontinentia pigmenti)

Nose
Saddle shape (congenital syphilis)
Prominent (Cockayne's, Seckel's)
Midline groove (holoprosencephaly, hypopituitarism)

Face
Dysmorphism assessment of facies (syndromes)

Hearing
Hearing impairment (e.g. TORCH, Cockayne's, neuroaxonal dystrophy)

Neck
Goitre (hypothyroidism)

Back
Scoliosis (e.g. CP, neurodegenerative disorders)

Chest
Full praecordial assessment for congenital heart defects (congenital rubella, trisomies, other syndromes)

Abdomen
Hepatosplenomegaly (e.g. TORCH)
Dysmorphic features (e.g. umbilical, genital or anal anomalies in various syndromes)

Limbs
Dysmorphism assessment
- Hands (e.g. simian crease: Down syndrome)
- Joints (e.g. contractures: COFS)
- Proximal shortening (e.g. RCDP)

Gait, lower and upper limbs (older child)
Full assessment (excluding sensory) for:
- Upper motor neurone signs (CP, TORCH, neurodegenerative disorders)
- Lower motor neurone signs (neuropathies with some neurodegenerative disorders, e.g. Krabbe's)
- Cerebellar signs (CP, some neurodegenerative disorders, e.g. Pelizaeus-Merzbacher)

Gross and fine motor development (infants)
Full assessment for developmental delay (CP) or regression (neurodegenerative disorders)
Full lower and upper limb assessments (as above)

COFS = cerebro-oculo-facial skeletal syndrome; CP = cerebral palsy; PKU = phenylketonuria, RCDP = rhizomelic chondrodysplasia punctata; TORCH = toxoplasmosis, others (includes syphilis, *Listeria monocytogenes* and HIV), rubella, cytomegalovirus and herpes (both simplex and varicella-zoster).

trisomies), the lens for cataracts (e.g. TORCH and trisomies) and the fundi for chorioretinitis (TORCH).

After examining the eyes, check the hearing (impairment with various pathologies, e.g. TORCH, kernicterus). Complete the assessment of the face for dysmorphic features, and then proceed to examine the neck for goitre (hypothyroidism). Next, assess the praecordium for congenital heart defects (e.g. congenital rubella), the abdomen for hepatosplenomegaly (e.g. TORCH) and the genitalia for size (e.g. micropenis with hypopituitarism) and structure (e.g. cryptorchidism and/or hypospadias in various syndromal diagnoses).

Finally, assess the limbs, looking for dysmorphism such as joint contractures with cerebro–oculo–facial–skeletal syndrome (COFS), cicatricial skin lesions and limb deformity with congenital varicella, rhizomelia with rhizomelic chondrodysplasia punctata (RCDP).

Next, assess the gross- and fine-motor development. In an infant, perform the standard '180 degree examination' (see the short case on the floppy infant in this chapter). In an older child, a gait examination can be performed, followed by a neurological assessment of the lower and then the upper limbs, concentrating on the motor system.

At the completion of your examination, summarise the findings and give a differential diagnosis. You may then comment on investigations that you would find helpful. These will depend on your findings; the following may be of use. (Note that a few very rare conditions are mentioned, but only as examples to show the wide scope of conditions that can present with microcephaly.)

Investigations

Imaging

1. Skull X-ray for cerebral calcification, found in cytomegalovirus infection (periventricular) and in toxoplasmosis (diffuse), and to detect early closure of sutures.
2. CT scan or MRI for cerebral malformations, evidence of perinatal asphyxia or intrauterine infection. Also, these can define craniosynostosis.

Blood tests

1. Serological tests for intrauterine TORCH infections or HIV (HIV-1-related encephalopathy).
2. Chromosomal analysis for autosomal trisomy syndromes.
3. Neonatal screening tests for PKU and congenital hypothyroidism.
4. Metabolic studies (where clinically appropriate): e.g. galactocerebroside beta galactosidase deficiency in white blood cells in Krabbe's disease, increased plasma phytanic acid and decreased RBC plasmalogens in RCDP.

Urine

Metabolic screen to detect virus excretion with congenital cytomegalovirus infection.

CSF

To detect intrauterine or perinatal TORCH infections or HIV infection.

Electrophysiological studies

For example, electroretinogram (ERG) for infantile neuronal ceroid lipofuscinosis.

Tissue

(If the clinical picture indicates—rarely indicated.) Examples include electron microscopy of abnormal cytosomes (infantile neuronal ceroid lipofuscinosis) and nerve or muscle (infantile neuroaxonal dystrophy).

Examination procedure for craniosynostosis

Once craniosynostosis has been found, the examination is directed towards finding associated abnormalities and complications. In particular, abnormalities of the eyes and of the neurodevelopmental examination are sought.

Examine the eyes fully for signs such as proptosis (may occur with brachycephaly or with oxycephaly), hypotelorism (with trigonocephaly; may be associated with holoprosencephaly), colobomata (may occur with trigonocephaly), strabismus (especially sixth nerve palsy), and retinal findings of papilloedema or optic atrophy (with raised intracranial pressure). Next, check the hearing, as oxycephaly can be associated with auditory and vestibular impairments due to a narrowed internal auditory canal.

Then, assess the child neurodevelopmentally. Vision and hearing having been assessed already, proceed with evaluation of personal–social and language abilities, and gross- and fine-motor functions. Follow this with a full examination of the lower and upper limbs for long-tract signs, including assessment of balance and cerebellar function, in view of the possibility of vestibular dysfunction, as mentioned above.

Generally, scaphocephaly is associated with a normal intellectual and neurological examination, as is plagiocephaly. Brachycephaly may be associated with neurological abnormalities, especially eye signs, and oxycephaly may well be complicated by raised intracranial pressure and significant neurological sequelae. Trigonocephaly can be associated with intellectual impairment and midline defects such as cleft palate, so the palates of children with trigonocephaly should be examined using a torch. In cases with plagiocephaly, check for congenital torticollis as the cause of the asymmetric head shape, rather than craniosynostosis.

Seizures

Children with seizures may occasionally be encountered in the examination as short-case subjects. The introduction may direct the candidate to examine for the aetiology of the seizures. Less frequently the introduction may be directed towards finding more acute problems resulting in the current seizure activity.

Recurrent seizures

Begin by introducing yourself to the parent and patient. Stand back and inspect the patient carefully for any dysmorphic features. Look for diagnostic skin rashes, which occur in various neurocutaneous syndromes. Look for asymmetry by standing the child with hands and feet together. Limb asymmetry occurs in long-standing hemiplegia (due to relative growth arrest of the affected side).

Next check, or request, the blood pressure. Hypertension may itself be the cause, or may be a coincidental finding in a disease that causes seizures by another mechanism (e.g. neurofibromatosis type 1 [NF-1]). Trousseau's sign, for hypocalcaemia, can be mentioned at this point, but is best left until the end of the examination.

The head and neck are then examined as outlined in Figure 13.2. Start with the head (e.g. microcephaly with cerebral palsy, syndromes; macrocephaly with hydrocephalus, intracranial tumours). Examine the eyes fully, as this may give an indication of various conditions, including raised intracranial pressure (ICP) and cerebral palsy (CP). Hearing should be checked (e.g. impairment with CP, congenital rubella), and the lower motor cranial nerves examined.

Long tract signs are screened for by performing a gait examination. This can be followed by abbreviated lower and upper limb examinations (omit sensation testing to save time).

Any significant intracranial pathology may be identified by this stage.

Next, examination of the abdomen may be performed, to detect any hepatosplenomegaly due to neurometabolic disorders.

Finally, request the temperature chart and the urinalysis.

Figure 13.2 outlines this approach. Table 13.6 gives a more comprehensive listing of possible physical signs, for reference only.

Recent acute seizure

If the lead-in is 'This child has just had a seizure. Would you please examine him?', the approach is somewhat different. This is similar to the real-life situation of seeing a child

---

Figure 13.2 Recurrent seizures

1. Introduce self
Assess mental state

2. General observations
Dysmorphic features
Skin rashes
Posturing
Involuntary movements
Asymmetry

3. Sphygmomanometer
Blood pressure
Trousseau's sign

4. Head and neck
Head
   • Measure
   • Palpate
   • Auscultate
   • Transilluminate
Eyes (full examination)
Hearing
Lower cranial nerves

5. Gait and lower limbs
Full gait examination
Lower limbs: full motor examination

6. Upper limbs
Full motor examination

7. Abdomen
Hepatosplenomegaly (neurometabolic
   disorders)

8. Other
Temperature chart
Urinalysis

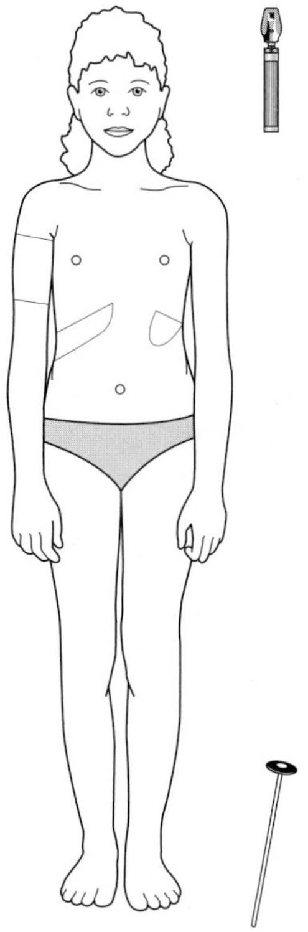

---

in the accident and emergency department who has just had a seizure (irrespective of a past history of recurrent seizures).

The examination should assess for the following:

1. Acute infections precipitating seizures (e.g. meningitis, encephalitis).
2. Evidence of recent trauma to the head (examine the head for bruising, fractures).
3. Hypertension (as in acute post-streptococcal glomerulonephritis).
4. Hypocalcaemia (Chvostek's and Trousseau's signs).
5. Long-tract signs (assess gait, lower and upper limbs).

Facial weakness

This is not an uncommon case. The lead-in may request examination of the face, or may be directed specifically: e.g. 'This child has had droopy eyelids since birth. Please examine the motor cranial nerves', or 'This child has facial weakness. Would you please assess?' Generally, the best approach to this case involves examining the motor cranial nerves (see the short case on motor cranial nerves in this chapter), and then, depending on those findings, going on to examine other areas of the nervous system. The

Table 13.6 Additional information: a more comprehensive listing of possible physical findings in children with recurrent seizures

General observations
Dysmorphic features (e.g. Angelman's, trisomy 13)
Skin rashes
- Facial port wine haemangioma (S-W)
- Facial naevus sebaceous (linear sebaceous naevus sequence)
- Forehead fibrous plaque (TS)
- 'Adenoma sebaceum' (facial fibroangiomatous lesions) (TS)
- Facial butterfly rash (SLE)
- Hypopigmented macules (TS)
- Pigmented flecks and whorls (incontinentia pigmenti)
- Café-au-lait spots (NF-1)
- Haemangiomata (K-T-W)
- Axillary freckling (NF-1)
'Neurometabolic' facies
- Coarse features (e.g. generalised gangliosidosis)
- Doll-like (Tay-Sachs)
Spastic posturing (e.g. CP)
Involuntary movements (e.g. CP)
Asymmetry (hands and feet together)
- Facial (Parry-Romberg, Proteus)
- Limbs (hemiplegia, K-T-W, NF-1, Proteus)

Sphygmomanometer
Elevated blood pressure (as cause, or coincidental: e.g. NF-1)
Trousseau's sign (hypocalcaemia)

Head
Size
- Small (e.g. TORCH, CP, syndromes)
- Large (e.g. IC tumour, hydrocephalus)
Shape
- Flat occiput (e.g. Angelman's)
- Prominent forehead (e.g. generalised gangliosidosis)
Scars (craniotomy for intracerebral haemorrhage, tumour; encephalocoele repair; bolt for ICP monitoring)
Scalp veins prominent (hydrocephalus)
Palpation
- Shunts (hydrocephalus)
- Sutures: separated (hydrocephalus)
- Skull bony defect (e.g. surgical removal, trisomy 13, encephalocoele)
- Fontanelles: delayed closure (e.g.

trisomy 13)
Percussion: 'cracked pot' sign (hydrocephalus)
Auscultation: bruit (arteriovenous malformation)
Transillumination
- Unilateral illumination (porencephalic cyst, subdural fluid)
- Bilateral illumination (hydrocephalus)

Hair
Lightly pigmented, broken, sparse, texture like steel wool (Menkes')

Eyes
Inspection
- Ptosis (e.g. linear sebaceous naevus, head injury with third nerve palsy)
- Squint (e.g. CP, raised ICP, congenital rubella)
- Nystagmus (e.g. Aicardi's, congenital rubella or herpes)
- Corneal enlargement (S-W)
- Iris: Lisch nodules (NF-1)
Function
- Visual acuity: impaired (e.g. CP, Aicardi's)
- Visual fields: field defects (e.g. IC tumour, haemorrhage, cyst)
- Visual neglect (e.g. parietal lobe tumour or haemorrhage)
External ocular movements
- Upward gaze palsy (pineal tumour)
- Lateral gaze palsy (e.g. IC tumour, haemorrhage)
- Sixth cranial nerve palsy (e.g. IC tumour causing raised ICP)
Pupil: dilated (third nerve palsy from IC tumour or trauma)
Ophthalmoscopy
Lens: cataracts (e.g. congenital rubella)
Retinae
- Papilloedema (IC tumour causing raised ICP)
- Optic atrophy (e.g. raised ICP)
- Haemorrhage (NAI)
- Chorioretinitis (e.g. congenital toxoplasmosis)
- Circular 'holes' (Aicardi's)
- Cherry red spot (Tay-Sachs)

Continued

Table 13.6 *(Continued)*

Hearing Impaired (e.g. CP, congenital CMV, or rubella, kernicterus) **Lower motor cranial nerves** Examination of the fifth, seventh, ninth, eleventh and twelfth nerves for signs of IC pathology (e.g. hemiplegic CP, tumour) Chvostek's sign (hypocalcaemia) **Abdomen** Injection sites (IDDM with recurrent hypoglycaemia) Hepatosplenomegaly (neurodegenerative disorders, e.g. Niemann-Pick type C,	Gaucher type II, generalised gangliosidosis) **Other** Temperature chart (precipitating fever) Urinalysis • Glucose (IDDM) • Protein (renal disease) • Blood (precipitating UTI, CRF) • Nitrites (precipitating UTI) • Specific gravity (high with SIADH, low with CRF) Cardiovascular examination: if evidence of long-tract signs, for underlying cyanotic congenital heart disease Hyperventilation to induce absence seizures can be mentioned

CP = cerebral palsy; CRF = chronic renal failure; IC = intracranial; ICP = intracranial pressure; IDDM = insulin-dependent diabetes mellitus; K-T-W = Klippel-Trenauney-Weber syndrome; NF-1 = neurofibromatosis type 1; SIADH = syndrome of inappropriate antidiuretic hormone excretion; SLE = systemic lupus erythematosus; S-W = Sturge-Weber syndrome; TS = tuberous sclerosis; UTI = urinary tract infection.

weakness may be bilateral, as in the case of myopathic diseases or neuromuscular junction disorders, or unilateral as in Bell's palsy (lower motor neurone) or as part of hemiplegia (most commonly upper motor neurone). This is detailed below.

There are three main groups of facial findings:

1. Ptosis and/or ophthalmoplegia with bilateral facial involvement: the differential diagnosis here includes Möbius' syndrome, myasthenia gravis (MG), infant botulism and myotonic dystrophy (MD).
2. No ptosis with bilateral facial involvement: possibilities include fascioscapulohumeral (FSH) dystrophy, bilateral lower motor neurone seventh cranial nerve palsy (LMN VII palsy) with Guillain-Barré syndrome, and occasionally cerebral palsy, which can produce bilateral upper motor neurone seventh nerve palsy (UMN VII palsy).
3. Unilateral involvement: unilateral facial weakness can be due to a unilateral LMN VII palsy, a unilateral UMN VII palsy or asymmetric crying facies (not really weakness, but hypoplasia of the depressor anguli oris muscle).

As with several neurological cases, examination of the mother or father is an essential part of the assessment (e.g. for myotonic dystrophy, or fascioscapulohumeral dystrophy). The following is a general approach to the case. Note that at certain points, depending on the findings, the examination may be redirected towards other aspects of the nervous system.

Begin by introducing yourself to the patient and parents. Engage the child briefly in conversation, noting any dysphasia (associated hemiplegia) or dysarthria (MD), and gaining an impression of mentation (decreased in MD and some causes of hemiplegia). Make a point of looking at the parents for any suggestion of a 'myopathic facies'. If this is present, remember to examine the parents after the child has been examined.

Next, with the child undressed above the waist, inspect the head for 'myopathic facies', ptosis and ophthalmoplegia, and note whether there is unilateral or bilateral involvement in the weakness. Visually scan the neck, trunk and upper limbs for wasting (e.g. FSH dystrophy), hemiplegic posturing, limb anomalies or hypoplastic fingers (Möbius' syndrome).

If there is bilateral facial involvement, and ptosis is demonstrated, examine the motor cranial nerves. If there is any abnormality of the external ocular movements, have the child look up for at least 30 seconds to elicit evidence of MG. Next examine the upper limbs, starting at the hands, looking for myotonia; percuss the thenar eminence. If this demonstrates myotonia, continue as outlined below for further signs and complications of MD. If there is no suggestion of myotonia, go on to examine for tone, power and reflexes, for evidence of neuropathy (e.g. in the Kearns-Sayre type of mitochondrial cytopathy).

If there is bilateral involvement and no ptosis, examine the motor cranial nerves. If the facies appears myopathic, say so, and go on to examine for myopathy (particularly FSH dystrophy). Describe muscle bulk, look for winging of the scapula and check tone, power and reflexes of upper limbs. Then check the gait, including having the child squat and rise from lying on the floor to elicit Gowers' sign. If the face is not myopathic (i.e. has bilateral LMN or UMN VII palsy), check the head circumference (cerebral palsy) and the remaining cranial nerves, followed by the gait (Guillain-Barré syndrome, cerebral palsy).

If there is unilateral lower motor neurone involvement, examine the eighth cranial nerve (acoustic neuroma) and the ears (for vesicles in Ramsay-Hunt syndrome), followed by gait (brainstem glioma), and request the blood pressure (hypertension as cause). If there is unilateral upper motor neurone involvement, examine the visual fields and gait (for hemiplegia).

If myotonia is suspected, examine for percussion myotonia at the thenar eminence and the deltoid. Have the child make a fist and then open the hand as fast as possible. After confirming myotonia, look for other associations (in older children), such as lens opacities, retinitis pigmentosa and choroid colobomata, and cardiomyopathy and conduction defects. After this, perform a functional assessment to assess the degree of impairment on the activities of daily living.

Floppy infant

This is a difficult case if not well practised. The introduction is commonly a variation on 'This baby has been found to be floppy. Would you please assess?' Other possibilities include combinations of 'apnoea and feeding difficulties' or 'feeding and respiratory difficulties'. Careful initial inspection in the latter situations should allow the approach outlined here to be followed as with the more obvious lead-in of 'floppy infant'.

Disorders that may be encountered include the following:

1. 'Hypotonic' cerebral palsy (CP).
2. Type 1 spinal muscular atrophy (SMA), i.e. Werdnig-Hoffmann disease.
3. Congenital myopathies.
4. Congenital myotonic dystrophy (MD).
5. Neonatal myasthenia gravis (MG).

The examination should first elicit whether the infant falls into the category of 'floppy weak' or 'floppy strong'. This is a very important point. Infants who are floppy and weak usually have disorders involving the lower motor unit. The pathology can be at the level of anterior horn cell, peripheral nerve, neuromuscular junction or muscle.

Infants who are floppy and strong usually have central neurological (upper motor neurone) causes, or non-neurological causes, such as connective tissue disorders (e.g. Marfan's syndrome).

Remember to look at the parents' faces for evidence of myotonic dystrophy. If this is suspected, the parent can be asked to make a fist and then open the hand quickly; this will detect myotonia more easily than a handshake. Look also for evidence of myasthenia gravis in the mother.

Commence inspection by noting any dysmorphic features, and describe the infant's posture, movements, head size, facial features, any interventions such as nasogastric tube, oxygen catheter, tracheostomy or gastrostomy, and any respiratory distress. The suggested procedure is outlined in Figure 13.3. A comprehensive listing of findings sought is given in Table 13.7.

When describing the posture, use appropriate terminology, commenting on the joint positioning in terms of 'external rotation at hips' and 'flexion at knees'. 'Frog-leg' posture is a well-recognised term, but should be supplemented with these more accurate terms.

Assessment of movement should focus on any difference between proximal and distal movement, and upper limbs versus lower limbs. Werdnig–Hoffmann disease (SMA type 1) may be associated with some degree of sparing of the hands and feet (e.g. finger and toe movement only), as well as face. Lumbar myelomeningocoele affects the lower limbs. Some congenital myopathies affect all limbs and face.

Describe any lack of movement with appropriate terms, such as 'paucity of movement'.

Inspection of the face can give many clues to the diagnosis. Infants with Werdnig–Hoffmann disease have alert, bright faces, whereas those with neuromuscular or muscular disorders may have ptosis, ophthalmoplegia, facial diplegia, a tented mouth and an expressionless 'myopathic facies'. Always check for tongue fasciculation, which is seen in Werdnig–Hoffmann disease. The presence of a nasogastric tube or gastrostomy suggests a feeding or swallowing problem, which may occur in several conditions, including SMA, some myopathies and intracranial ischaemia or haemorrhage.

An oxygen catheter in situ implies respiratory difficulties. Respiratory distress may be due to aspiration with SMA, CP or congenital MD, or diaphragmatic 'seesaw' breathing in SMA. A tracheostomy scar indicates previous intensive treatment for conditions that may improve with time, such as infant botulism, congenital MD or an intracranial catastrophe.

Next, the manoeuvres comprising the 180-degree examination may be performed to quantify the degree of hypotonicity. During these manoeuvres, signs such as scissoring with CP, or a posterior midline scar with myelomeningocoele may be noted.

Note that when assessing the ability of the infant to raise his or her head and trunk when placed prone, the infant's hands should be placed to either side of the shoulders (with the palms apposed to the bed and elbows flexed) to optimise the infant's ability to extend the upper limbs. If the child is positioned with the hands beneath the trunk, or with arms extended, an accurate assessment will not be possible.

Following the manoeuvres, the limbs are carefully examined; examine the lower limbs first. Confirm the hypotonia and check the joint mobility, noting any contractures and joint dislocations (especially at the hips). The strength should then be assessed. Note whether the child can raise the limb fully against gravity and sustain it in that position. The strength of a withdrawal response can be easily tested (tickle the feet).

At this point, it may be appropriate to indicate to the examiners your impression as to whether the child belongs in the 'floppy weak' (i.e. peripheral) or 'floppy strong'

Figure 13.3 Floppy infant

---

1. Introduce self
Look at parents' faces (myotonic
   dystrophy, myasthenia gravis)

2. General observation
Dysmorphic features
Head size
Facial features
Posture
Movement
Previous intervention
Respiratory difficulties

3. Manoeuvres: the 180-degree
   examination
a. Observe infant in supine position
To describe: posture, movement
b. Pull to sit
To detect: degree of head control/lag
c. Sitting
To describe:
  - Degree of head control
  - Degree of trunk control
  - Ability to sit unsupported
d. Attempted weight bearing
To detect:
  - Lower limb hypotonia/weakness
  - Lower limb scissoring (CP)
  - 'Advanced' weight bearing (CP)
e. Ventral suspension
To describe:
  - Posture of head, trunk and limbs
    (degree of hypotonia; infants with
    CP may have extensor posture)
f. Place infant prone and observe
To describe:
  - Degree of head control
  - Ability to lift head/trunk

4. Limbs
Inspect (small hands and feet in Prader-
   Willi)
Palpate
Tone
Power
Reflexes

5. Primitive reflexes
Test for:
  - Suck
  - Grasp
  - Stepping

- Placing
- ATNR
- Moro reflex

6. Head
Head
  - Inspect
  - Palpate
  - Auscultate
  - Transilluminate
Eyes
  - Full examination for evidence of
    intrauterine infection, CP,
    retinopathy of prematurity
Hearing
  - Test with bell and rattle for
    deafness from kernicterus,
    intrauterine infection, CP

7. Abdomen
Examine for hepatosplenomegaly due to
   intrauterine infection MPS (central),
   glycogen and lipid storage
   myopathies (peripheral)
Genitalia (hypoplastic in Prader-Willi)

8. Chest
Examine praecordium for cardiac
   enlargement and dysfunction due to
   glycogenoses types 2 or 3, or for
   congenital heart disease due to
   congenital rubella

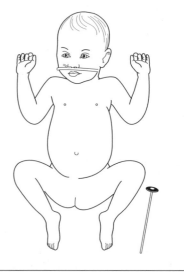

CP = cerebral palsy; MPS = mucopolysaccharidoses; PW = Prader-Willi syndrome; ATNR = asymmetric
tonic neck reflex.

Table 13.7   Additional information: details of possible findings on floppy infant examination

General observation

Dysmorphic features (e.g. Down, Prader-Willi, MPS, lipidoses)

Head size
- Microcephaly (e.g. CP)
- Macrocephaly (e.g. associated myelomeningocoele, congenital toxoplasmosis)

Facial features
- 'Ex-premmie' appearance (prematurity per se, CP)
- Alert (e.g. SMA)
- Expressionless (e.g. some congenital myopathies, MD, MG)
- Ptosis (as above)
- Ophthalmoplegia (as above)
- Nasogastric tube (e.g. hypotonic CP, some congenital myopathies, MD, MG)
- Oxygen catheter (e.g. hypotonic CP, SMA, some congenital myopathies, MD, MG)
- 'Fish' (triangular) mouth (e.g. congenital myopathies or MD)
- Tongue fasciculation (SMA)

Posture
- 'Frog-leg' lower limb posture (e.g. especially SMA, congenital myopathies)
- Fisted hands (CP)
- Arthrogryposis (e.g. congenital muscular dystrophy, MD)

Main areas affected
- Face (congenital myopathies, MD or MG)
- Lower limb (myelomeningocoele)
- Proximal limb (e.g. SMA)
- Distal limb (congenital MD)

Normal movement (e.g. connective tissue disorders)

Fasciculations (e.g. SMA)

Previous intervention
- Tracheostomy/scar (e.g. infant botulism)
- Gastrostomy/scar (e.g. hypotonic CP, congenital MD)

Respiratory difficulties

Upper airway noises (e.g. CP)
- Tachypnoea (e.g. aspiration with SMA, CP, congenital MD, Pompe's)
- Paradoxical breathing (e.g. SMA)
- Bell-shaped chest (e.g. SMA)
- Splayed lower ribs (e.g. SMA)

Limbs

Inspection
- Decreased muscle bulk (e.g. SMA, undernutrition)
- Fasciculation (e.g. SMA)
- Muscle biopsy site

Palpate
- Confirm hypotonia
- Contractures (causes of arthrogryposis)
- Joint hyperextensibility (connective tissue disorders)

Power
- Weak (e.g. SMA, congenital MD, muscular dystrophy or myopathies)
- Normal (e.g hypotonic CP, other central causes, connective tissue disorders)

Reflexes
- Absent (e.g. SMA)
- Decreased (e.g. neuropathies or, later, myopathies)
- Normal (e.g. connective tissue disorders)
- Increased (CP)

CP = cerebral palsy; MD = myotonic dystrophy; MG = myasthenia gravis; MPS = mucopolysaccharidoses; SMA = spinal muscular atrophy.

(i.e. central) group. This allows the remainder of the examination to be more directed. The more common causes of a floppy weak infant are Werdnig-Hoffmann SMA congenital myotonic dystrophy, and congenital myopathies. The more common causes of a floppy strong infant are hypotonic cerebral palsy and Down syndrome.

Tendon reflexes are helpful. If reflexes are very brisk, it is rare for the pathology to be a lower motor neurone lesion. Reflexes are always absent in the Werdnig-Hoffmann form of SMA.

If the cause appears peripheral, give a differential diagnosis at this stage. If a myopathy seems most likely, go on to examine the abdomen for hepatomegaly and the praecordium for cardiomegaly, for myopathy due to glycogenoses types 2 or 3. If a hereditary neuropathy seems most likely, request permission to examine the mother (e.g. for pes cavus). If a neuromuscular junction problem is likely, request permission to examine the mother for MG.

At the completion of the examination, request the reports on electromyography, nerve conduction velocity and muscle biopsy. Do not request the actual test, as if this is supplied interpretation is expected! Be prepared to tell the examiners the usual findings of the disease you suspect.

If the cause appears central, go on to check the primitive reflexes, which may provide evidence of CP. Then examine the head, eyes and hearing for evidence of intrauterine infection, and complications of prematurity which can lead to CP. Finally check the abdomen for hepatosplenomegaly (TORCH) and praecordium (for congenital heart disease due to congenital rubella). At the completion of the examination request relevant investigations (e.g. head ultrasound, head CT or TORCH screen).

Despite the fact that a number of diagnoses have been stressed, the important point is the method of examination. The candidate should aim to give an overall picture of the child, then categorisation and, lastly, actual diagnosis.

Hemiplegia

Children with hemiplegia are usually included in the short-case section under the introduction of 'Examine the gait'. The task is not just to identify the hemiplegia, but to ascertain the level of the problem and the aetiology. The examination can assess these factors sequentially as outlined here. The overall plan is as follows:

- Demonstrate the physical signs of hemiplegia in the lower and upper limbs.
- Demonstrate the level by assessing, as a minimum, the seventh cranial nerve (lower motor neuron [LMN] involvement implies pathology in the region of the pons; upper motor neuron [UMN] involvement implies a lesion above the pons), the visual fields (involvement implies site of lesion at internal capsule or above) and look for parietal lobe signs (cortical lesion).
- Look for the cause.

Cardiovascular causes

1. Hypertension.
2. Cyanotic congenital heart disease (CHD): before 2 years of age, usually cerebral thrombosis; after 2, cerebral abscess.
3. Subacute bacterial endocarditis (SBE).
4. Cerebral arteriovenous malformations (AVM).
5. Cerebral vaso-occlusive disease, e.g. moyamoya disease
6. Sturge-Weber syndrome (S-W): cerebral vessel anomalies.

Traumatic causes

1. Non-accidental injury (NAI).
2. Brain trauma: e.g. motor vehicle accidents (MVA).
3. Intraoral trauma.

Infective causes

1. Herpes simplex encephalitis (HSE).
2. Bacterial meningitis.
3. Cerebral abscess.

Systemic disorders

1. Systemic lupus erythematosus (SLE).
2. Sickle cell anaemia (SCA).
3. Homocystinuria.
4. Neurofibromatosis (NF), type 1.
5. Acute leukaemia, non-lymphocytic (ANLL) or lymphocytic (ALL).

Examination

In practice, there is a significant percentage of children with acute hemiplegia in which the cause is not yet known. A suggested approach is as follows.

General observations

Introduce yourself to the child and parent. Ask the child simple things, such as name, age and school. Note any dysphasia (dominant hemisphere) and note any obvious intellectual impairment (e.g. secondary to meningitis, HSE, NAI, MVA, homocystinuria).

Have the child adequately exposed, being sensitive to their modesty. Note the posture and describe it carefully. Note any asymmetry of the limbs (growth arrest). Assess the growth parameters. If tall or Marfanoid habitus, think of homocystinuria. Comment on whether the child is well or unwell, as she or he may be recovering from recent insults (e.g. encephalitis) or may be in distress from acute problems (e.g. SBE, CHD with cardiac failure). Check whether the child is cyanosed (CHD).

Examine the skin for the following:

1. Bruising/purpura (e.g. NAI, ANLL, ALL).
2. Pallor (e.g. SCA, ANLL, ALL).
3. Neurocutaneous stigmata (e.g. S-W syndrome, NF-1).
4. Cigarette or electric heater burns (NAI).

Gait (older child) or gross motor assessment (infant)

Now, after thorough inspection, take the child through a full gait examination (see the gait short-case approach in this chapter for details). In subtle cases of hemiplegia, manoeuvres such as the Fog test and 'reverse Fog' test may reveal the problem. Remember to check for sensory neglect when the child is standing up (when testing for Romberg's sign).

In infants too young to walk, where the introduction will obviously not be 'gait' but perhaps 'not using one side' or '6 months old and prefers the left hand', a gross–motor developmental assessment replaces the gait manoeuvres. Instead of the Fog test, use the 'cover' test, where the child's face is covered with a cloth, and each hand held in turn to see if the cloth can be removed equally well using either one. Also check the primitive reflexes for signs such as asymmetric Moro or parachute reflexes.

Lower limbs

Check tone, power and reflexes. Remember to test for clonus at both ankle and knee, crossed adductor response (abnormal after 9 months of age) and spread of reflexes. In view of time constraints, it is reasonable to omit, or postpone until later, sensory testing, if the examiners agree when you suggest this.

Abdominal reflexes

For a complete assessment of pyramidal tract function, these should be included. They correspond to spinal segments T7 to T12.

Upper limbs

As with lower limbs, just test tone, power and reflexes, and omit or postpone sensory testing.

Head

Inspect and describe facial features; there may be obvious facial asymmetry (e g. seventh cranial nerve lesion). In this case, it is best to examine the motor cranial nerves, starting with the twelfth nerve and working up. Check for tongue deviation (twelfth), asymmetry of shoulder shrugging (eleventh), asymmetry of palate elevation (ninth), eyebrow raising, tight closing of eyes, showing teeth and puffing out cheeks (all seventh), external eye movements (third, fourth and sixth; note that the third cranial nerve nucleus is in the midbrain, and the fourth is in the pons). At completion of motor cranial nerves, check the visual fields for field defects and for parietal visual neglect. A field defect implies a lesion at or above the internal capsule.

Now examine the higher centres for parietal lobe signs.

In older children, test for receptive dysphasia, agraphia ('write your name for me'), astereognosis (e.g. unable to recognise key in hand), ideomotor apraxia (e.g. 'show me how you brush your teeth') and left/right confusion. These occur when the dominant side is involved. Also test for constructional apraxia (e.g. ask the child to draw a clock), which occurs when the non-dominant side is involved, and finally examine for sensory extinction, which can occur with either side involved.

In younger children, the 'higher centres' part of the examination is more general, and works best if simple things are asked first, such as name, address age, sex ('Are you a boy or a girl'), naming parts of the body (e.g. pointing at nose, eyes, ears, arm and asking 'What's this?'). If the child is unable to succeed at the latter, point to something such as your watch, ask 'Is this a dog? A cat? A watch?' and note the responses.

Note that if there is no involvement of any cranial nerves or higher centres, then a spinal cord lesion is possible, and warrants a sensory examination being performed, as well as assessment of the spine itself.

By this stage the level will have been ascertained, and the cause can be sought. An approach is set out below.

Inspect and palpate the head for the 'S' signs:

1. **S**ize: head circumference may be increased with subdural haematoma, intracranial tumour.
2. **S**cars (e.g. craniectomy for repair of AVM, evacuation of subdural haematoma).
3. **S**utures and fontanelles (widened sutures, full fontanelle with raised intracranial pressure: e.g. with intracranial tumour, hydrocephalus).
4. **S**hunts (e.g. hydrocephalus, chronic subdural collection).

Auscultate the skull for bruits (AVM). Inspect conjunctivae for pallor (e.g. SCA). Examine the retinae for retinal haemorrhage (NAI), papilloedema (raised intracranial pressure), Roth spots (SBE). Inspect the oral cavity for haemorrhage from oral trauma.

Cardiovascular

Perform a full cardiovascular examination, looking for splinter haemorrhages (SBE), clubbing (cyanotic CHD), hypertension, central cyanosis (CHD), murmurs (CHD, SBE, SLE), carotid pulsation (decreased in arteritis), carotid bruits, hepatomegaly (SCA, ALL) and splenomegaly (SCA, SBE).

Spine

This is an essential part of the examination if there is no involvement of any cranial nerves or higher centres. If this is the case, the above head and cardiovascular assessments should be postponed.

Inspect for scoliosis (e.g. NF-1, spinal tumour) and scars (e.g. excised spinal tumour). Palpate for tenderness and masses. Auscultate for arteriovenous malformations or vascular tumours.

Urinalysis

This is for blood (e.g. SBE, post-streptococcal glomerulonephritis with hypertension, SCA) and protein (chronic renal disease with hypertension).

Intellectual impairment

The approach outlined here may be useful in assessing the aetiology for clinical problems such as developmental delay or developmental regression in the long- or short-case setting (the technique for performing a developmental assessment is discussed in a separate short case). It is imperative to differentiate between static and progressive causes of intellectual impairment. The examination procedure outlined here is quite comprehensive, covering multiple aetiologies of both groups of causes. Several neurodegenerative conditions (progressive causes) are mentioned. The examiners will not expect detailed knowledge of the individual conditions; they are simply mentioned for completeness, and of course many are relevant only in certain age groups.

You should still be able to assess in general terms for neurodegenerative conditions: remember that those predominantly affecting grey matter may present with dementia and seizures, while those affecting white matter tend to have problems of spasticity, cortical deafness and blindness.

Examination

Start by introducing yourself to patient and parent. Note the age and sex of the child, to allow age- and sex-appropriate neurodegenerative conditions to be borne in mind. Examples include: males with X-linked conditions such as fragile X, Menkes', Hunter's and Lesch-Nyhan syndromes; infants with conditions such as tuberous sclerosis (TS), Tay-Sachs disease, Leigh disease, infantile spasms, late infantile metachromatic leuko-dystrophy (MLD), infantile Gaucher's disease; older children with disorders such as juvenile Batten's disease, subacute sclerosing panencephalitis (SSPE), Wilson's disease, Huntington's chorea.

Stand back and scan for obvious dysmorphic features (e.g. Down syndrome, mucopolysaccharidoses), neurocutaneous stigmata (e.g. cutaneous findings of TS, ataxia telangiectasia, Sturge-Weber syndrome, incontinentia pigmenti) and other skin abnormalities, such as eczema with phenylketonuria (PKU) and thick skin with the mucopolysaccharidoses. Note any abnormal posturing, such as spastic quadriparesis with cerebral palsy (CP), late stages of white matter degenerations; hypotonic posturing in infants with atonic CP, Down syndrome, various degenerative conditions (Leigh's, Menkes', Pompe's, Zellweger's).

Note any involuntary movements, such as extrapyramidal movements (e.g. CP, Wilson's, Hallervorden-Spatz, Huntington's), static tremor (Wilson's, Hallervorden-Spatz), intention tremor (Wilson's, Friedreich's, some late-onset gangliosidoses, Leigh's, MLD), myoclonic jerks (e.g. Batten's, SSPE) or seizure activity (e.g. CP, TS, Zellweger's, degenerative conditions of the grey matter such as gangliosidoses, some white matter diseases such as adrenoleukodystrophy, Krabbe's).

Note the growth parameters, particularly the head circumference. This may be large with several inherited neurodegenerative disorders (e.g. Canavan's, Alexander's, Tay-Sachs, Gaucher's, generalised gangliodosis, mucopolysaccharidoses), as well as with hydrocephalus or chronic subdural effusion. Head circumference may be small with several syndromal diagnoses (e.g. Rubenstein-Taybi, Smith-Lemli-Opitz, Cornelia de Lange, and Seckel syndromes), intrauterine infections (TORCH) or autosomal recessive microcephaly. Make a point of measuring the head circumference yourself, and request progressive percentile measurements. The height is infrequently a useful guide, as most of the disorders can be associated with short stature. Marked obesity can indicate Prader-Willi syndrome, hypothyroidism or pseudohypoparathyroidism. Request the progressive percentiles of these parameters.

The systematic examination can be commenced at the head. After measuring it, inspect carefully for scars and shunts, palpate for fontanelle and suture patency in infants, shunts or bony defects (e.g. repaired encephalocoele). Transillumination is worth mentioning (for hydrocephalus, hydranencephaly, subdural effusion or porencephaly) so that the examiners know you have thought of it, although most candidates are probably not armed with an appropriate torch. Feel the hair in male infants (in Menkes' kinky hair syndrome, it feels somewhat like steel wool). Assess the face from a dysmorphic perspective. Note the size and position of the ears, and then make a detailed evaluation of the eyes, looking at external features (e.g. epicanthic folds, corneal clouding), function (e.g. blindness, squint) and ophthalmological findings (e.g. cataracts, optic atrophy, cherry red spot). Assess the nose, mouth, chin, neck and hairline for dysmorphic findings. Also examine the neck for goitre (hypothyroidism).

Next, a neurological assessment can be performed. Depending on the ability of the patient, this may be commenced with a full gait examination, including checking the back for scoliosis (e.g. CP, Friedreich's ataxia, ataxia telangiectasia), kyphosis (e.g. mucopolysaccharidoses), gibbus (GM1 gangliosidosis), or with a gross-motor developmental assessment.

This is then followed by examination of the lower and upper limbs, both for dysmorphic features and neurologically, especially for tone (e.g. hypertonia with CP, PKU, Gaucher's; hypotonia with hypotonic CP, Down, Leigh's) and reflexes (e.g. hyperreflexia with CP; hyporeflexia with MLD or Krabbe's, which cause peripheral neuropathy, Pompe's, Leigh's).

The abdomen can then be examined for hepatosplenomegaly (e.g. intrauterine TORCH infection, Gaucher's, Niemann-Pick, Hurler's, GM1 gangliosidosis, glycogen storage diseases) and the genitalia for dysmorphic features (various malformation syndromes) or large testes in the postpubertal male (fragile X).

Next the chest is examined for dysmorphic features and the praecordium for any evidence of cardiomegaly (e.g. Pompe's, mucopolysaccharidoses) or congenital valvular heart disease (e.g. congenital rubella, Down, Noonan's, other malformation syndromes).

After this, the hearing should be tested (e.g. impairment with intrauterine rubella, kernicterus, mucopolysaccharidoses).

With completion of this assessment for aetiology, the examiners may request an opinion regarding the level of impairment. If so, go on to perform a developmental assessment (see the separate case on this). This will give an approximation only of the true intelligence quotient.

The examiners will expect you to be familiar with the definitions of the various levels of intellectual handicap.

- IQ below 20: profound.
- IQ 20–34: severe.
- IQ 35–50: moderate.
- IQ 50–70: mild.

The examination procedure outlined here is thus primarily a neurological evaluation, but also incorporates a dysmorphology assessment, as numerous malformation syndromes are associated with intellectual impairment (e.g. Down syndrome, fragile X syndrome). Also sought are associated findings of both syndromal and neurodegenerative diagnoses. Note that prior knowledge is assumed regarding which conditions are degenerative and which are not, as with many physical signs, static and progressive causes are listed side by side.

The diseases listed in parentheses are scant examples only of most of the physical signs enumerated. Comprehensive lists of causes of each of these diagnostically helpful signs can be found in the standard textbooks of neurology. For reasons of space, many of the names of diseases are abbreviated, such that Down syndrome is listed as 'Down', Wilson's disease as 'Wilson's' and Huntington's chorea as 'Huntington's'.

At the completion of your examination, summarise your findings, give a brief differential diagnosis and then discuss which investigations would be relevant to this particular child; these obviously depend on the physical signs found.

This is clearly an enormous topic, but an attempt is given below to list, broadly, groups of investigations that may be useful.

Minimum investigations

All children with intellectual handicap should, as a minimum, have the following investigations.

Blood

1. Thyroid function tests (hypothyroidism).
2. Karyotype (e.g. Down, fragile X).
3. TORCH serology in infants.
4. Creatine phosphokinase in boys (Duchenne's muscular dystrophy).
5. Vitamin B_{12} (in vegetarian families).

Urine

Metabolic screen.

Imaging

Cranial CT or MRI scanning is often useful, both to exclude space-occupying lesions such as intracranial tumours, hydrocephalus and chronic subdural effusion, and to diagnose degenerative conditions such as the leukodystrophies (hypodensity of white matter) and grey matter disorders.

Neuropsychological assessment

A formal neuropsychological assessment by a psychologist will also be appropriate. The following is a brief selection of some of the psychometric tests in common use for general aptitude (intelligence).

1. Stanford–Binet Intelligence Scale: age range 2 years to adult.
2. Wechsler Intelligence Scale for Children—Revised (WISC-R): age range 6–16 years.
3. Wechsler Preschool and Primary Scale of Intelligence (WPPSI): age range 4–6½ years.
4. McCarthy Scales of Children's Abilities: age range 2½–8½ years.

Further investigations

Further tests are determined by the clinical picture. The following is a more comprehensive listing of groups of investigations that may be relevant.

Blood

1. Organic acids (organic acidurias), lactate and pyruvate (Leigh's), ammonia (urea cycle disorders), HIV serology (HIV encephalopathy), uric acid (Lesch-Nyhan), caeruloplasmin (Wilson's), measles serology (SSPE).
2. White cell lysosomal enzymes:
   a. Lipidoses (e.g. Gaucher, Niemann-Pick, gangliosidoses).
   b. Leukodystrophies (e.g. MLD, Krabbe).
   c. Mucopolysaccharidoses (e.g. Hurler, Hunter).
   d. Mucolipidoses (e.g. mannosidosis, fucosidosis).
   e. Long chain fatty acids (e.g. peroxisomal disorders, adrenoleukodystrophy).

CSF

1. Protein (elevated in MLD, Krabbe's).
2. Gammaglobulin (elevated in SSPE).
3. Measles antibody titre (SSPE).
4. HIV antibody titre (HIV encephalopathy).

Tissue biopsy and electron microscopy

Muscle, nerve, brain, rectal tissue, bone marrow, skin, liver or leucocyte may be required, depending on the disease suspected.

Neurophysiological studies

1. EEG (e.g. specific for SSPE; helpful for Lafora's, Batten's).
2. Nerve conduction studies and electromyelography (e.g. MLD, Krabbe's).
3. Visual evoked response (VER) and electroretinography (ERG). VER tests the function of the optic nerve pathways (i.e. white matter), while ERG evaluates the retina (i.e. grey matter). They are useful in differentiating grey from white matter disorders (e.g. Batten's, Lafora's).
4. Brainstem auditory evoked response to detect hearing loss.

Other

In children with dysmorphic features, a computerised searching system may be very useful in pinpointing a syndromal diagnosis.

Involuntary movements

This is a somewhat infrequent case. The approach outlined here covers the following four types of involuntary movement: chorea, athetosis, dystonia and tremor. Hemiballismus, tics, myoclonus and seizure activity are mentioned briefly.

Background information

The following are brief descriptions only of the types of involuntary movements. Comprehensive descriptions are in all standard neurology texts.

Chorea. This describes irregular rapid movements involving any muscle group, especially distal. Causes include cerebral palsy (CP), Sydenham's chorea, Wilson's disease, systemic lupus erythematosus (SLE), moyamoya disease and degenerative conditions such as ataxia telangiectasia, Huntington's chorea, Lesch-Nyhan syndrome and phenylketonuria (PKU). Chorea is due to pathology affecting the corpus striatum.

Athetosis. This describes slow writhing movements of proximal extremities. It can accompany chorea, as in dyskinetic CP, Wilson's disease, Lesch-Nyhan and ataxia telangiectasia. Athetosis is due to pathology affecting the outer region of the putamen.

Dystonia. This comprises sustained abnormal posturing, which may be brought on rapidly in 'dystonic spasms'. Causes include drugs (tardive dystonia), degenerative disorders such as Wilson's, Hallervorden–Spatz and Huntington's diseases and posthemiplegic.

Tremor. There are three basic types:
1. Static tremor: present at rest, disappears with action. Causes include Wilson's, Parkinson's, Huntington's and Hallervorden–Spatz diseases.
2. Postural tremor is most notable when the arms are outstretched in front of the body, but can occur through a range of movement. Causes include thyrotoxicosis, phaeochromocytoma, familial tremor, physiological tremor and Wilson's disease.
3. Intention tremor is marked at end points of movement, but is not present during the course of movement. Causes include many disorders affecting the cerebellar hemispheres and pathways, including Wilson's disease. Note that asterixis, or 'flapping tremor', is not actually a tremor, and should be differentiated from this. Causes include liver failure and hypercapnia.

Hemiballismus. This is unilateral random gross rotatory movements of the proximal portion of a limb. Exceptionally rare in paediatrics, it is due to pathology in the subthalamic region on the side opposite to the affected side.

Tics. These are brief, separate, defined movements, usually involving the head and face, that can be voluntarily suppressed. Causes include benign childhood tics, and the Gilles de la Tourette's syndrome.

Myoclonus. This is sudden, disorganised, irregular contraction of a muscle or muscle group (distinguished from fasciculations, which cannot cause movement of a complete muscle group). Causes include seizure disorders (e.g. infantile spasms, benign juvenile myoclonic epilepsy), degenerative conditions (e.g. neurocutaneous syndromes, Menkes',

Tay-Sachs, Wilson's), structural brain anomalies (e.g. Aicardi's syndrome, porencephaly), cerebrovascular accidents, anoxic brain injury, infections (e.g. SSPE, HIV encephalopathy) and metabolic disorders (e.g. aminoacidopathies).

It is clear from surveying the aetiologies of the various disorders above that Wilson's disease and CP can cause choreoathetosis, tremors, dystonia or myoclonus, so the examination needs to evaluate thoroughly for these two conditions, irrespective of the type of movement disorder.

It is often difficult to differentiate between the types of movement: e.g. between hemiballismus and chorea. It does not matter if the candidate is unable to decide. What is important is to describe what is seen accurately and to have an approximate idea of the likely region of the pathology (e.g. basal ganglia). For this reason, the outline given below is essentially similar, whether the problem is chorea, athetosis, dystonia or tremor.

Remember that movement disorders can coexist: for example, dystonic spasms can be accompanied by tremor and myoclonus. If myoclonus or seizure activity seems most likely, indicate this to the examiners, and then proceed as outlined in the case on recurrent seizures, as myoclonus may be associated with primary seizure disorders, as well as with degenerative or other disorders that can be associated with seizures (as noted above). Any accompanying change in consciousness should help decide if the myoclonus is seizure related.

Examination

Begin by introducing yourself to the patient and parent. Try to gain an impression of whether there is any intellectual impairment (e.g. CP, Huntington's, PKU) or hearing impairment (e.g. kernicterus) and note the speech (e.g. cerebellar dysarthria, palilalia with Parkinson's disease).

Stand back and inspect for evidence of stigmata of chronic liver disease (Wilson's disease), telangiectasia (ataxia telangiectasia), facial butterfly erythema (SLE), fair complexion with blond hair (PKU), mask facies (Parkinson's disease), prominent eyes (thyrotoxicosis), evidence of self-mutilation (Lesch-Nyhan) or spastic posturing (CP).

Make a point of looking at the parents (e.g. Huntington's). Describe the quality and distribution of the movements: whether they are unilateral or bilateral; involve face, arms, trunk, or legs; are fast or slow, regular or irregular, distal or proximal.

A series of manoeuvres can then be performed to establish more clearly which sort of movement is occurring.

Have the child shake hands with you and then squeeze your finger. This is to detect a 'milkmaid grip', which occurs with chorea. Then ask the child to hold out his or her hands, first with palms up, and then with palms down. This may detect static tremor or chorea. Ask the child to hold the arms outstretched to either side of the body. Then have the child try to put both index fingers to either side of the nose, as close as possible to the nose without touching. This is a sensitive test for several involuntary movements including intention tremor. Finally, have the child hold his or her wrists back in extension to exclude asterixis.

Have the child hold both arms up above the head. Look for the development of pronation (pronator sign) with chorea. Check for dysdiadochokinesis if there is any suggestion of intention tremor. Check the upper limb tone (decreased with chorea, increased with CP, rigidity as in Hallervorden-Spatz), power and reflexes. A rapid functional assessment (e.g. write name, drink from a cup) may be performed at this stage to assess the degree of incapacity caused by the movement.

By this stage it may be clear whether the problem is (most probably) chorea or tremor. This will allow much of the following to be omitted, as it will not be relevant.

If the type of movement is not yet clear, a full gait examination can be performed, looking for evidence of CP, cerebellar disease, and Wilson's or Huntington's diseases. Take note of heel–toe walking (cerebellar disorders), squatting (thyrotoxicosis), and also have the child walk, turn quickly, stop and recommence walking (Parkinson's disease). This can be followed by a neurological lower limb evaluation for tone, power, reflexes and cerebellar function.

The head may then be examined. Measure the head circumference (decreased with CP). Inspect the face for malar flush (SLE). Look at the eyes for lid retraction or proptosis (thyrotoxicosis), telangiectasia (ataxia telangiectasia), Kayser-Fleischer rings (Wilson's disease), nystagmus (cerebellar disease, ataxia telangiectasia), oculomotor dyspraxia (ataxia telangiectasia). Test the extraocular movements, looking for nystagmus, and check for lid lag (thyrotoxicosis). Check the ears for telangiectasia (ataxia telangiectasia) and test the hearing (kernicterus, CP), and if it is abnormal perform Rinne's and Weber's tests. Have the child poke out the tongue, to detect a 'Jack-in-the-box' tongue, which may occur with chorea. Check the neck for goitre (thyrotoxicosis).

Next, the cardiovascular system can be examined for evidence of rheumatic heart disease (Sydenham's chorea). Check the pulse for abnormal wave form (e.g. aortic incompetence) and tachycardia (thyrotoxicosis). Request or take the blood pressure (for phaeochromocytoma as the cause of tremor). Palpate and auscultate the praecordium for valvular disease.

Examine the abdomen for prominent abdominal wall veins, hepatosplenomegaly or ascites (Wilson's disease) and look for peripheral signs of chronic liver disease. If tremor is the problem, also look for abdominal wall needle marks (diabetic hypoglycaemia as the cause of tremor) and palpate for the adrenal glands (but check with the examiners that there is no contraindication to deep palpation as palpating a phaeochromocytoma can cause an acute hypertensive crisis).

At the completion of the case, summarise your findings, present a differential diagnosis and discuss which investigations would be in order.

Neurofibromatosis, type 1 (NF-1)

As children with NF-1 often appear in both the long- and the short-case sections of the examination, it is worth having a systematic approach to examining for the myriad complications of this condition.

The short-case approach to NF-1 should include assessment of the growth parameters, eyes, blood pressure and spine in particular, just as should occur with each review of any patient with NF-1 in the outpatient clinic setting.

Begin by introducing yourself to the patient and parents. Ask the child her or his age, school and grade: you may gain an impression of any significant intellectual impairment. General observation should commence with growth parameters: patients with NF-1 often have macrocephaly and short stature. Macrocephaly in this context usually reflects a large brain, but may also be due to an intracranial tumour mass or hydrocephalus secondary to aqueductal stenosis or to a tumour, such as astrocytoma, causing obstruction to CSF flow. Measure the head circumference, height and lower segment (LS) yourself. Calculate the US:LS ratio (may be decreased with scoliosis) and request progressive percentile charts for head circumference, height and weight. The weight can decrease rapidly, with diencephalic syndrome from chiasmal glioma compromising the hypothalamic function.

Inspect the skin for café-au-lait (CAL) macules: count them (and measure their maximal diameter with a tape measure if there is any doubt about fulfilling the diagnostic criteria). Make a show of looking for axillary and inguinal freckling. Look also for neurofibromas, and note any associated scratch marks (due to excessive pruritis: neurofibromas have a high mast cell content).

It is worth knowing at what age certain skin manifestations appear:

1. Café-au-lait spots are usually present at birth; they are obvious by the end of the first year of life.
2. Axillary freckling develops in mid-childhood.
3. Peripheral neurofibromas usually appear at the onset of puberty.

Next, perform a Tanner pubertal staging (can be precocity or delay).

Request the blood pressure. Hypertension in NF-1 may be due to a number of causes: renal artery stenosis, phaeochromocytoma, coarctation of the aorta, noradrenaline-producing neurofibromas (usually paraspinal, of autonomic ganglia) or essential hypertension.

A series of manoeuvres can then be performed to assess for scoliosis and other skeletal anomalies. First, look at the child's back in the standing position. Have the child bend forwards and touch their toes: look at the back from all angles for kyphoscoliosis or scars (e.g. posterior fusion and insertion of metal rod). Describe in detail any abnormality found (e.g. scoliosis: site, convexity to which side, associated scapular and iliac crest positions—see the short case on scoliosis in this chapter for details). Then, inspect the chest from the front and side for pectus excavatum. Have the child stand with the legs together and hands together with arms extended, and inspect the entire body for asymmetry (e.g. hemihypertrophy or segmental hypertrophy due to plexiform neurofibromas). Focus on the lower limbs for any evidence of tibial bowing (usually congenital, directed anterolaterally, at the lower third of tibia; secondary to bony dysplasia), genu varum or valgum, or pes cavus (secondary to spinal cord involvement: e.g. compression by neurofibromas, untreated kyphoscoliosis or vertebral collapse from erosions associated with neurofibromas).

Next examine the head. Look for scars (e.g. resection of intracranial tumour, shunt insertion for hydrocephalus). Feel for suture separation, shunts and their tubing, or bony defects (especially occipital, associated with cerebellar hypoplasia). Note any facial asymmetry, or disfigurement due to soft-tissue masses (especially in the periorbital area). Note that large plexiform neuromas of the head and neck are almost always obvious by 12 months of age and do not develop after this time.

A full eye examination can then be performed, looking in particular for proptosis, which may be non-pulsating due to neurofibromatous tissue within the orbit (e.g. optic glioma), or pulsating (transmitted brain pulsation) when associated with a congenital bony defect (sphenoid wing dysplasia) of the posterior orbital wall, ptosis (plexiform neuroma can cause 'S-shaped' lid) and Lisch's nodules (small, light brown, dome-shaped iris hamartomas, seen in 90% of patients by 5 years of age by slit lamp examination). Make the examiners aware that they are only very occasionally visible to the naked eye. Assess visual acuity and external ocular movements. Presenting signs of optic nerve or chiasmal gliomas can include diminished visual acuity or strabismus.

Hearing should be tested, as impairment may be treatable. However, if this is done at this stage, it may give the examiners the impression that the candidate does not appreciate the difference between NF-1 and NF-2. Acoustic neuromas are particularly unusual in NF-1. The author would defer checking the hearing at this stage, and perform it at the end of the examination.

In the child over 2 years of age, a gait examination can next be performed (in those under 2, a neurodevelopmental assessment is more appropriate at this point), followed by a full neurological assessment of the lower limbs. Look for long-tract signs reflecting cerebral involvement (e.g. tumours, cerebrovascular accidents due to hypertension or berry aneurysm rupture) or spinal cord involvement (e.g. spinal neurofibroma). Also examine for cerebellar signs (e.g. cerebellar astrocytoma, asymmetrical cerebellar hypoplasia).

Next, a thorough neurological examination of the upper limbs can be performed, again looking for evidence of long-tract and cerebellar involvement (e.g. neurofibromas arising from cervical or brachial plexuses; intracranial tumour or haemorrhage). If time permits, a higher functions assessment may be performed (mild intellectual impairment occurs in up to one-third of NF-1 patients).

The abdomen can next be examined, particularly for large visceral neurofibromas (may be evident in the loin) and renal artery stenosis.

At the completion of your examination, summarise your findings and outline the investigations you would perform.

Neuromuscular assessment

The request to perform a neuromuscular assessment does not mean that the problem is neuromuscular disease. A common error is to assume that there is neuromuscular pathology, even when the patient has an obvious problem such as hemiplegia or spastic paraparesis. The candidate should first form an opinion as to whether the problem is neuromuscular. Having determined that it is, another common problem in differential diagnosis is to fail to think of major levels of lesion (i.e. anterior horn cell, peripheral nerve, neuromuscular junction and muscle fibre).

There are several possible introductions: for example, 'This boy has increasing difficulty climbing stairs' or 'This girl has been having trouble with increasing tiredness and weakness'.

Essentially, a neuromuscular assessment is a modified neurological examination. Specific manoeuvres are included that aim at eliciting relevant signs of various neuromuscular disorders. The procedure outlined below describes several of these.

Start with general observations. Enquire whether the child can stand for you. Then, focus your attention systematically on the following.

1. Posture (e.g. as in Duchenne's muscular dystrophy; see long case).
2. The face: for myopathic facies, ptosis, presence of nasogastric tube or oxygen catheter, tongue fasciculations (spinal muscular atrophy).
3. The neck: for tracheostomy tube, or scars from a previous tracheostomy, goitre (hyperthyroidism and hypothyroidism can both cause myopathy), muscle bulk (for facioscapulohumeral dystrophy), contractures (Emery-Dreifuss muscular dystrophy).
4. Upper limbs: for horizontal axillary skin folds (Duchenne's muscular dystrophy), proximal muscle wasting (most myopathies), distal muscle wasting (myotonic dystrophy, neuropathies), fasciculations (spinal muscular atrophy), scars (tendon releases or transfers), contractures.
5. The back: for scoliosis, kyphosis, lordosis.
6. Lower limbs: for proximal or distal wasting, fasciculations, scars (tendon releases or transfers), contractures, foot deformity such as pes cavus.

Remember to glance at the parents for any evidence of myopathic facies, peroneal atrophy or pes cavus.

After this, ask whether the child can walk for you. Have the child go through a full gait examination (i.e. walking normally, walking on toes, walking on heels, walking heel to toe, running, hopping, jumping, using stairs, stepping up onto a chair or stool, squatting and rising, lying on floor and rising, performing push-ups). This may give very valuable clues to help differentiate between neuropathy and myopathy.

Next, ask the child to hold up both arms above the head, to test for proximal upper limb weakness. Have the child make a fist and then quickly open the hand (easier to assess than a handshake) and finally percuss the thenar eminence (these manoeuvres involving the hands are to detect myotonic dystrophy). If positive, go on to tap the deltoid muscle with a tendon hammer, for myotonia, and ask the mother to make a fist and then open her hand quickly and percuss over her thenar eminence as well.

Next, ask the child to look upwards at the roof (unless there is already ptosis) for a full thirty seconds (screening for myasthenia gravis).

Following these screening tests, perform a standard neurological examination of the lower limbs and upper limbs (including palpating for hypertrophied lateral popliteal, ulnar and greater auricular nerves), followed by the motor cranial nerves. By this stage, the type of problem should be apparent and will allow guidance as to what else should be examined.

If a myopathic process is most likely, then at the completion of the neurological examination, it may be wise to examine the cardiorespiratory system next (cardiac muscle can be involved in Duchenne's muscular dystrophy, Pompe's disease [in infants]; conduction defects can occur in myotonic dystrophy, Emery-Dreifuss muscular dystrophy and mitochondrial cytopathies) and the abdomen (for storage diseases).

Scoliosis

Candidates may seldom consider this case, and as such it can prove difficult. The first thing to determine is the classification of the scoliosis: whether it is postural, compensatory or fixed (structural). Most often it will be the latter group, which can itself be conveniently subdivided into three major groups of causes.

1. Idiopathic (congenital and later onset).
2. Paralytic (i.e. neuromuscular causes).
3. Bony or ligamentous (e.g. connective tissue disorders).

Thus, the examination focuses firstly on manoeuvres to assess classification.

Once classified as fixed, the numerous causes of this are sought. Inspection will give valuable clues to several groups, such as skeletal dysplasias, neurocutaneous stigmata and malformation syndromes. A thorough neurological evaluation is essential, as there are potential causes at most levels of the neuraxis. Examples include cerebral palsy (CP), spinocerebellar degenerations (e.g. Friedreich's ataxia), anterior horn cell disease (e.g. Kugelberg-Welander disease), peripheral neuropathies (e.g. Charcot-Marie-Tooth disease), myopathies (e.g. mitochondrial cytopathies), muscular dystrophies (e.g. Duchenne's muscular dystrophy), myotonic disorders (e.g. myotonic dystrophy). Finally, the child should be evaluated for complications of the scoliosis itself, such as cardio-respiratory compromise.

Begin by introducing yourself to the patient and parent. Try to gain an impression of the child's intelligence (impairment with Coffin-Lowry syndrome, homocystinuria). The child should be undressed down to the underwear. Inspect for any dysmorphic features (e.g. Turner's, Noonan's, Coffin-Lowry syndromes) or other obvious signs of underlying disease (e.g. disproportionate short stature, limb bowing, Marfanoid habitus, neurocutaneous stigmata). Note the growth parameters, in particular height. Short stature may be due to the scoliosis per se or an underlying problem (e.g. skeletal dysplasias, metabolic bone diseases such as X-linked hypophosphataemic rickets, neurofibromatosis type 1 (NF-1), Turner's or Noonan's syndromes). Tall stature may be due to Marfan's syndrome or homocystinuria. Macrocephaly may occur with NF-1 or hydrocephalus. For completeness, the height, arm span and lower segment can be measured by the candidate, the upper segment:lower segment ratio calculated, and the degree of trunk shortening (or limb shortening in skeletal dysplasias) quantified. Inspect thoroughly for neurocutaneous stigmata such as café-au-lait spots and axillary freckling with NF-1, which can cause scoliosis by several mechanisms including muscle imbalance, hemihypertrophy, hemivertebrae and 'dumbbell' tumour. Other rarer neurocutaneous syndromes that may lead to scoliosis include incontinentia pigmenti and hypomelanosis of Ito.

Next, focus on the back itself; look for thoracotomy scars (e.g. from repair of associated abnormalities such as congenital diaphragmatic hernia or congenital heart disease) or posterior midline scars (myelomeningocoele repair), hairy patches or lipomas. Describe in detail the following features (mnemonic: all starting with 'S'):

- **S**coliosis (site and convexity to which side).
- **S**houlders and hands (higher on side to which primary curve convex).
- **S**capulae (prominence on which side).
- **S**kin (loin) crease symmetry.
- **S**uperior iliac spine position.
- **S**pare ribs (rib cage rotation posteriorly or anteriorly).
- **S**pace between arms and body (asymmetry).

Look for any limb bowing (e.g. rickets). Inspect for evidence of neuromuscular problems, such as pes cavus (e.g. Charcot-Marie-Tooth disease, Friedreich's ataxia), 'champagne bottle legs' (Charcot-Marie-Tooth), or prominent calf muscles (Duchenne's muscular dystrophy).

Note whether the occiput aligns directly over the buttock crease. To be more accurate, a 'plumb-line' can be dropped from the occiput to ascertain whether there is failure of alignment.

Following this initial inspection with the child standing, there are three manoeuvres to assess the degree of correctability of the curve.

1. Have the child bend forwards and touch the toes. Reassess the curve, look at the rib hump, and describe these. This manoeuvre can confirm a fixed scoliosis or exclude a postural scoliosis.
2. Sit the child down on a chair and re-evaluate the curve. Sitting will eliminate any contribution of unequal leg length to the curvature.
3. Applying upward traction on the proximal upper limbs (lifting under the axillae) should straighten any mobile component of the curve.

Next, palpate and percuss over the spine for tenderness from metabolic disorders (e.g. rickets), inflammatory disorders (e.g. chronic tuberculosis) or tumour, and then auscultate over the apex of the curve (for vascular tumour such as haemangioma as underlying cause).

Now examine the back movements. Forward flexion should cause a measurable increase of 10 cm between C7 and S1 in postpubertal patients, and fingers should be able to reach the toes (with knees extended). Extension to 30 degrees is normal, with lateral flexion to 35 degrees, and rotation (sitting, which anchors the buttocks) to 45 degrees.

The next part of the examination assesses for neuromuscular causes or consequences of the scoliosis. Perform a standard gait examination, followed by a lower limb examination. Measure the actual lower limb lengths (anterior superior iliac spine to medial malleolus), inspect for scars, muscle wasting, contractures and foot deformities (e.g. pes cavus), and then test power, tone and reflexes, cerebellar function, and sensation (can omit the latter, as it is time consuming). Then, percuss the bladder (for neurogenic storing bladder) and offer to test the anal wink.

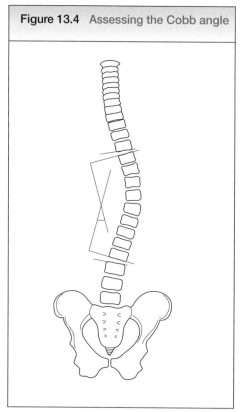

Figure 13.4 Assessing the Cobb angle

It is important not to overlook evidence of weakness of intrinsic muscles of the feet, decreased ankle jerks and evidence of bladder involvement, as these may be the only clues to tethering of the spinal cord.

Examination of the upper limbs, again for neurological causes, is followed by evaluation of the head for macrocephaly (e.g. NF-1, hydrocephalus), the eyes for evidence of NF-1 (e.g. Lisch nodules of iris, strabismus from optic glioma, proptosis), or Friedreich's ataxia (nystagmus), Marfan's syndrome (dislocated lenses) or osteogenesis imperfecta (blue sclerae).

After the neurological assessment, examine the chest for cardiorespiratory complications. Examine the heart for evidence of cor pulmonale, a complication of scoliosis per se, and for heart disease associated with possible underlying aetiologies (e.g. congenital heart disease associated with congenital thoracic scoliosis, mitral valve prolapse in Marfan's syndrome, pulmonary valve stenosis with NF-1). Do not forget to take the blood pressure (may be elevated in NF-1, Marfan's syndrome, spina bifida, or with congenital renal anomalies in association with thoracolumbar scoliosis). Finally, check the chest expansion, and request a peak flow reading, to give some indication as to whether restrictive lung disease is present.

Figure 13.4 shows how to assess the Cobb angle. First find the upper and lower vertebrae of the curve by erecting tangents to the vertebral bodies and identifying where the disc spaces first become widened on the concavity of the curve. Next, draw perpendiculars from the tangents at the top of the upper vertebra and the bottom of the lower vertebra, and measure the angle between them. Note that if the tangents of the upper and lower vertebrae are extrapolated, they intersect at a point which is the centre of a circle of which the curve is an arc. This method can be repeated for each of multiple curves.

Spina bifida

A comprehensive short-case approach to spina bifida is very useful in both long- and short-case contexts. It is one of the few cases where it can be better to start at the bottom and work up. It is important to have a good knowledge of sensory dermatomes, and to know the motor root values, of the entire body (not just the lower limbs).

The general plan for this case is as follows:

1. Demonstrate the level of the lesion.
2. Functional assessment.
3. Look for associated abnormalities/complications.

This case may be introduced in several ways: for example, 'This boy has spina bifida. Would you please assess him/his function above the level of the lesion?' Other introductions (e.g. big head, scoliosis, talipes) may have spina bifida as the underlying diagnosis. When the diagnosis is reached, the candidate may then proceed with assessment of function (e.g. ability to walk) and disease complications (e.g. hydronephrosis, hydrocephalus).

Thorough inspection is crucial in this case, particularly when the patient is an infant. Much can be gleaned from simply taking one minute to stand back and look. In particular, the child's posture and spontaneous movement is valuable in indicating the level of the lesion before the back is inspected directly.

A few points worth noting are outlined below. The positions described refer to those seen with the child supine.

1. Hip flexion corresponds to L1 and L2, so is affected in high lesions.
2. Lesions above L1 cause total paraplegia, as hip flexion is absent. Thus, in thoracic lesions, the lower limbs are flaccid, in a 'frog leg' position of external rotation, with some degree of passive abduction and flexion at the hips, and the knees slightly flexed, the ankles plantar flexed.
3. Lesions in the high lumbar zone cause the child to lie in a position of flexion and adduction at the hips.
4. Lesions with L3 preserved allow an infant to exhibit some kicking movements when upset, with some knee flexion and extension.
5. Lesions in the low lumbar zone result in a position of hip flexion and adduction, good knee flexion and extension, and ankle dorsiflexion, due to unopposed action of the tibialis anterior (L5).
6. Hip extension corresponds to L5, S1 and S2, and so is affected in all but the lower sacral lesions.
7. Lesions at S3 or below completely spare lower limb sensory and motor function, but cause paralysis of bladder and anal sphincters, and 'saddle anaesthesia'.

The examination procedure given here covers children of any age, and is thus quite detailed. It should of course be modified to suit the individual patient. If it were followed as it stands, it would certainly appear too rigid and would obviously reflect rote learning, which is not the idea of this book, nor will it meet with approval from the examiners.

The introduction, and the child's age and degree of cooperation, will determine the best order to perform the examination. If the lead-in is a functional assessment above the level of the lesion, don't start by describing the foot deformities.

Examination

Begin by introducing yourself to patient and parents. The child should be undressed down to nappies or underpants. Interact with the child: if old enough, ask name, age and school to gain an impression of their development. In infants, note the degree of alertness, the pitch of the cry, which is high-pitched with raised intracranial pressure in cases with the Arnold-Chiari malformation (ACM) and resultant hydrocephalus. The presence of a nasogastric tube, stridor or apnoea and, in older children, a hoarse voice may all occur with lower cranial nerve palsies due to brainstem compression with severe ACM. Note the respiratory rate: tachypnoea may be a sign of aspiration pneumonia (due to lower cranial nerve palsies) or of cardiac failure (due to hypertension, or cor pulmonale in patients with severe kyphoscoliosis).

Stand back and inspect carefully the child's posture and spontaneous movement. Describe the posture in detail, focusing on each joint systematically (e.g. 'flexed at hips, hyperextended at the knee') and noting any deformities (e.g. talipes equinovarus). Note

---

Figure 13.5 Spina bifida

---

1. Introduce self
Interact with child, gain impression of
   development

2. General inspection
Alertness
Cry (high-pitched with ACM)
Nasogastric tube (severe ACM)
Respiratory distress
Hoarse voice (severe ACM)
Posture
   • Deformity (e.g. TEV, dislocated
     hips)
Muscle bulk
   • Lower versus upper limb
Movement
   • Lower versus upper limb
   • Ataxia (with ACM)
Head
   • Size
   • Shunts
   • Eye signs
Skin

3. Back
Lesion
   • Site: closure scar (describe)
   • Spinal deformity: scoliosis,
     kyphosis
Scars (e.g. fixation rod)

4. Lower limbs
Inspect
Palpate
Tone
Power
Reflexes
Joint movement
Sensation

5. Abdomen and pressure areas
Inspect
   • Scars (e.g. VP shunt)
   • Distension (lax muscles)
   • Ileal conduit
   • Patulous anus
   • Dribbling of urine
   • Tanner staging (precocity)
   • Pressure sores
Palpate
   • Kidneys (hydronephrosis)
Percuss
   • Bladder (urinary retention)
Check
   • Abdominal reflexes

   • Anal wink
   • Anal tone
Urinalysis
   • To detect CRF, shunt nephritis,
     UTI

6. Head
Inspect
   • Size
   • Shape (e.g. frontal prominence
     with ACM)
   • Signs of hydrocephalus (scalp
     vein prominence, shiny skin, sun-
     setting eyes, shunt scars)
Measure head circumference
Request progressive percentiles
Palpate (sitting up)
   • Fontanelles
   • Sutures
   • Shunt, trace tubing

7. Eyes
Inspect
   • Nystagmus (severe ACM)
   • Squint (e.g. with ACM)
Visual acuity
External ocular movements
   • Sixth nerve palsy (raised ICP)
   • Impaired upward gaze (Parinaud's
     syndrome with hydrocephalus)
Fundi
   • Papilloedema (raised ICP)
   • Optic atrophy (long-standing
     raised ICP)

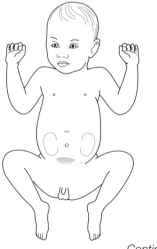

Continued

Figure 13.5 *(Continued)*

8. **Hearing and bulbar function**
Assess hearing
Check lower cranial nerves (nine, ten, eleven, twelve)
Suck and swallow
Gag reflex (if cannot swallow)
Tongue atrophy

9. **Upper limbs**
Full examination, for signs of syringomyelia

10. **Blood pressure**
Hypertension (CRF)

11. **Chest**
Full examination of praecordium and lung fields for signs of cardiac failure due to:
- Hypertension (CRF)
- Cor pulmonale (kyphoscoliosis)

12. **Functional/developmental assessment**
Assess ADL in older children
Perform developmental assessment in infants

ACM = Arnold-Chiari malformation; ADL = activities of daily living; CRF = chronic renal failure; ICP = intracranial pressure; TEV = talipes equinovarus; UTI = urinary tract infection; VP = ventriculoperitoneal.

the muscle bulk, comparing lower limbs with upper limbs. Observe the child's movements, again lower limbs versus upper. If the child's movements seem unsteady, this may be due to weakness in higher lesions, or severe ACM which may cause ataxia. Do not hurry your description of posture and movement.

Next, inspect the head, noting its size (hydrocephalus from ACM) and any obvious shunts. Look at the eyes for squint or nystagmus (either can occur with ACM). Scan the

---

Table 13.8 Additional information: details of possible findings on spina bifida examination

General inspection
Respiratory signs
- Stridor (severe ACM)
- Apnoea (severe ACM)
- Tachypnoea (aspiration pneumonia, cardiac failure)

Skin
- Pressure sores
- Scars (e.g. of VP shunts, tendon releases)

Growth parameters
- Head circumference: increased (hydrocephalus)
- Height: usually decreased
- Arm span (use instead of height): may be normal for age
- Weight: obese for height, not for arm span

Lower limbs
Inspection

- Muscle bulk, wasting
- Joint deformity (e.g. dislocated hips, talipes)
- Contractures
- Scars (e.g. tendon releases, transfers or osteotomies)
- Spontaneous movement

Palpation: muscle bulk (each muscle compartment)
Check tone, power, reflexes (including with reinforcement)

Joint movement
- Hip (e.g. fixed flexion deformity; check for dislocation last)
- Knee (e.g. fixed hyperextension)
- Ankle (e.g. fixed dorsiflexion)

Check hips for dislocation
Sensation: demonstrate the sensory level (may use a new pin in infants; full examination in older children)

ACM = Arnold-Chiari malformation; VP = Ventriculoperitoneal.

abdomen for any scars (e.g. ventriculoperitoneal shunt). Note the child's growth para-meters: the head may well be enlarged due to hydrocephalus, so measure it yourself. Request the other growth parameters. The height is usually decreased, due to a short trunk (associated kyphoscoliosis) and short lower limbs (decreased growth and contrac-tures). The weight for the actual height implies obesity, but should be compared to the arm span instead, to give a more accurate indication of true obesity. Generally these children are not obese for their arm span.

Next, focus your attention on the back. Note the site of the lesion, the size of the repair scar and look for any kyphosis, scoliosis or scars (fixation rods for kyphoscoliosis).

Then, the examination proceeds well if started at the lower limbs. A thorough neurological examination is necessary. In an infant with no spontaneous lower limb movement, a pinprick stimulus may still result in a flexion withdrawal of the legs. This is a spinal reflex due to elements of the spinal cord, distal to the clinical level of the lesion, that are preserved. The fact that the child makes no facial or emotional response from which to infer a painful sensation should prevent misinterpretation of this response.

Examination of the abdomen may then be performed, followed by the head and the upper limbs. Next, take the blood pressure and examine the chest. After this, you may perform a functional assessment in older children, looking at the activities of daily living, such as reading, writing, using a knife, fork, spoon, comb, toothbrush, and ability to attend to personal hygiene (i.e. toileting, insertion of tampons). In younger children, perform a developmental assessment (see the short-case section on this in this chapter). Several of the findings sought at each step are outlined in Figure 13.5 and additional detail is listed in Table 13.8.

14

Oncology

Long case

Oncology

The oncology long case provides an opportunity for a general paediatrician to display competence in handling a child with cancer, and his or her family, in the context of the domestic situation, schooling needs and wider social relationships, as well as within a medical framework representing different levels of care, characterised by the general practitioner, the general paediatrician, the paediatric oncologist and other consultants whose help may be required from time to time.

The general paediatrician (the candidate) should be able to demonstrate that he or she can handle the medical aspects of a child with cancer as easily as the complex professional interrelationships which are involved in each case. The candidate should also be familiar with any recent advances that could affect the management of the patient.

The last few years have seen many advances and improvements in most areas of oncology, including: molecular genetic diagnosis, with newer emerging tests such as comparative genomic hybridisation, spectral karyotyping and gene expression micro-arrays; radiation delivery techniques, such as three-dimensional conformal therapy and intensity-modulated radiotherapy, stereotactic radiosurgery, proton therapy, intraoperative radiotherapy and brachytherapy (placing of radioactive substances in contact with target tissue); development of cancer-targeted therapies, such as biologic retooling (this term includes immunotargeting and monoclonal therapy, antitumour immunostimulatory therapies, cancer vaccines and oncolytic microbes); and molecular targeting of tumour cells, such as the development of inhibitors (e.g. STI-571) to the cytoplasmic tyrosine kinase that is found in chronic myeloid leukaemia (CML).

An ongoing major study, the Childhood Cancer Survivor Study (CCSS), supported by the US National Cancer Institute, is now following 14,000 long-term survivors of childhood cancer. A web-based comprehensive set of guidelines for management of such survivors, the *Children's Oncology Group (COG) Long-Term Follow-Up Guidelines for Survivors of Childhood, Adolescent, and Young Adult Cancers*, can be found at <http://www.survivorshipguidelines.org>. Both these initiatives have expanded the literature significantly and are very useful.

In Australia and New Zealand, all major paediatric centres are full members of the US-based Children's Oncology Group (COG), a consortium of childhood cancer centres that aggressively promotes clinical and laboratory research trials in paediatric oncology.

The general principles of care are similar for patients with haematologic malignancies, solid tumours or brain tumours. The principal difference between these three categories is the level of professional collaboration in optimising each patient's care.

An approach to any oncology long case could potentially fit into the following scheme.

History: an overview

At the outset of the interview it is important to identify clearly the primary and secondary diagnoses, as well as important historic landmarks such as date of diagnosis, date of completion of therapy, history of relapse, or major secondary events such as significant endocrinopathies or second tumours. An overview of the child's condition lasting 2–3 minutes is important in order for the candidate to spend time gathering data relevant to the presentation. Unfortunately, parents of oncology patients have frequently had excessive medical contact and could fill hours recounting 'what the doctor said'. This approach is very time consuming and often unhelpful.

Before diagnosis

1. Initial symptoms (with particular reference to the usual non-specific nature of oncology symptoms). A notable difference from adult presentation is the paucity of these symptoms. Unlike adults with cancer, it is very unusual for a child to present with weight loss, haemoptysis or haematemesis and melaena. Symptoms that may present in children include a mass, and the eight 'Ps': **P**yrexia, **P**ain, **P**allor, **P**urpura, **P**ersistent squint, **P**ersonality change, **P**osterior fossa symptoms, and do not forget the **P**retenders (i.e. ALL or neuroblastoma impersonating arthritis, or mediastinal lymph nodes impersonating asthma).

2. Symptom duration (may give a guide to disease 'tempo'). For example, patients with B-cell lymphoma may present as extremely ill, with a history of illness spanning a few days, compared to a patient with a brain tumour or other solid tumour who may have experienced symptoms for many months.

3. Parental guilt about acts of commission or omission that may have contributed to their child developing cancer.

4. An enquiry about the parent's feeling towards the diagnosis is often revealing. Most parents are initially very angry, an anger which may be self-directed and related to guilt, or directed at doctors or others who they perceive as having failed in their duty to provide an early diagnosis, although, at the time, the non-specific symptoms may not have suggested malignancy as a likely possibility.

Factors 3 and 4 (above) will impact on the family's approach to their sick child and possibly bias the relationships they establish subsequently with people entrusted with the care of their children, particularly as the care of a child with cancer nowadays can be expected to span in excess of 10 years among those patients (over 70% of cases) whom we expect will survive.

Post-diagnosis phase

Important aspects in the history include an appreciation of the parents' understanding of the details and significance of the diagnosis, or even whether the family knows what the exact diagnosis is. The candidate should enquire about the level of knowledge of treatment-related details that the family has acquired in the interval from diagnosis, as well as their perception of prognosis, which falls into two broad categories: what they have been told by their doctor, and what they believe. The level of parental awareness and understanding of the condition is important as this affects the parents' level of care for the child and compliance with medication requirements and appointments. It also influences whether they strive to maintain a near-normal lifestyle for the child, or withdraw him or her from society in anticipation of early death, perceived needs of additional protection, and such like. The candidate should enquire about the impact of the diagnosis on siblings, the marital relationship, the financial situation for the family and job stresses. Parents may respond inappropriately in the post-diagnosis phase, by selling their house to relocate closer to the hospital, resigning from stable employment, or moving away from familiar and supportive communities, because they believe they are acting in the best interests of the child.

Current status of the patient

The details of the therapy received in the specific treatment protocol for that patient should be sought. The details should be general. Is most medication oral, IV or IM? Is there a central line? How many visits to the hospital for treatment? Can the local doctor or local hospital give any chemotherapy? No candidate will be expected to be familiar with all protocols.

Enquire about problems such as infections (especially pulmonary), marrow suppression and problems secondary to it (such as febrile neutropenic episodes and thrombocytopenia), compliance with oral chemotherapy and pneumocystis prophylaxis with cotrimoxazole (or similar drug), and any other side effects from therapy, including nausea, vomiting and rashes. Then concentrate on the current status, particularly the immediate (rather than late) effects of treatment and their consequences, such as: lethargy and easy fatigability from anaemia; nausea, vomiting and anorexia resulting in weight loss; alopecia; limitation of activities (e.g. swimming) because of the presence of central lines, or ostomies involving the gastrointestinal or genitourinary tracts.

Other

The impact on daily activity of amputation of a lower extremity for bone tumour should be explored (and secondary consequences such as kyphoscoliosis sought during physical examination). Growth and development should be explored with the families. Social issues and schooling can then be discussed in the light of the foregoing information.

Finally, details of late effects of treatment and underlying illness should be sought.

Any family history of conditions associated with a predisposition to malignancy should be noted (e.g. immunodeficiencies, neurofibromatosis type 1).

From the above, the candidate should be able to formulate a comprehensive problem list, picking up items from each of the sections, prioritising these and being ready to discuss them.

Examination

See the short-case section in this chapter on late effects of oncology treatment.

Management plan

The following is an outline of the major issues that the general paediatrician may need to address, divided into general and specific problem areas.

Discussion points

1. Relapse of primary disease.
2. Growth and development.

3. Development of second tumour.
4. Social issues.
5. Schooling.
6. Infection.
7. Immunisation.
8. Issues related to ongoing chemotherapy (e.g. crisis intervention for bone marrow suppression).
9. Supportive care.
10. Stem cell transplantation (bone marrow, peripheral blood, cord blood).
11. Therapeutic modifications: risk-adapted therapy.
12. The dying child.

Relapse of primary disease

Note that patients who relapse are unlikely to be selected for an examination. However, this does not diminish the importance of properly assessing the issues regarding relapse.

In seeking symptoms from parents or patient, the candidate ought to enquire whether any new symptoms resemble those present before the diagnosis, and determine the level of anxiety that these new symptoms are causing. Progressive symptoms such as weight loss, unexplained anorexia, nausea, fever or the appearance of lymphadeno-pathy, organomegaly, excessive bruising, bleeding, gum oozing, knotty palpable masses or painful bony masses all warrant further investigation.

Growth and development

Irradiation is the single most important factor in determining long-term growth and development. The candidate should know which structures were within the treatment portal, and the total dose used. Patients treated with craniospinal irradiation will be at the combined risk of hypopituitarism and relative shortening of the vertebral column. Any irradiated area may demonstrate relative soft-tissue atrophy.

In the past cranial radiotherapy was used for CNS prophylaxis in a majority of patients with ALL. Modern treatment regimens now restrict the use of cranial radiation to 10% or less of patients with ALL. Up to 50% of children treated for acute leukaemia with cranial radiotherapy can have decreased growth hormone secretion. Loss of final height can also be influenced by early (rarely precocious) onset of puberty, or (too) early institution of testosterone therapy for hypogonadism in boys. The management usually comprises growth hormone, delaying treatment with testosterone. There have been reports in the literature linking use of growth hormone with subsequent brain tumour development. However most investigators do not believe currently that the risk is enhanced.

If there has been a bone marrow transplant, the eyes should be checked by a paediatric ophthalmologist regularly (say 12–24 monthly) for cataracts from total body irradiation (or from steroids). Hearing may be impaired by drugs such as cisplatin or aminoglycosides, and requires regular review and audiological assessment. Ideally, a formal psychological assessment should be carried out before any cranial irradiation. After treatment, psychological assessment may be repeated on a regular basis, in conjunction with neurological examination, CT scanning and assessment of school performance, to monitor neuropsychological outcome and provide early rehabilitative intervention if needed. The spectrum of central nervous system damage varies from decreased performance at school, to frank leukoencephalopathy, spasticity and significant intellectual impairment. Intravenous methotrexate may result in leuko-encephalopathy in children with ALL, especially after irradiation. Pubertal development may be precocious; however, most children treated for ALL have delayed puberty, with high gonadotropin levels from end-organ gonadal damage.

The other issue to address in adolescent patients is future reproductive potential. In boys with tumours such as Hodgkin's disease, sperm storage should be considered before irradiation and chemotherapy. In girls, ovarian tissue storage is available.

Development of second tumour

The risk of developing a second malignancy may approach 15–20% at 20 years in long-term survivors of childhood cancer, and appears related to the original diagnosis and treatment modalities. In ALL, children who have received cranial irradiation when under 6 years of age are susceptible to brain tumours, and children who have had extensive treatment with epipodophyllotoxins (teniposide and etoposide) are at greater risk of developing acute myeloid leukaemia (AML).

Social issues

Some long-time survivors have trouble adjusting to the stress of normal life. This can be assessed by simple interview and psychometric testing. Potential problems include diminished school performance, behavioural problems, impaired attainment of social skills, ongoing anxiety regarding relapse and the financial burden of the child's treatment on the family. These areas should be explored so that appropriate intervention can occur.

School

Survivors of ALL in particular are at risk of school-related problems, including repeating grades and a need for special education. This may relate to neurological damage from CNS prophylactic therapy. Assessment of school performance allows evaluation of problems with memory, concentration and attention span: all well-recognised sequelae. The amount of schooling a child missed during treatment should be noted. Has the trend of school absence continued after therapy was completed? If so, determine the reasons. Is it excessive concern about infections such as varicella or measles (exposures to which are not relevant more than 6 months from the end of treatment)? The school situation must always be explored at follow-up.

Infection

The child on chemotherapy

Common childhood infections occur in leukaemic children just as in normal children, and many can be managed in the usual way, provided that the child does not appear toxic, there is an identifiable localised infection, the neutrophil count is greater than 1.0×10^9/L, and regular follow-up is provided. Often chemotherapy may be continued, after consultation, through the course of mild infections, be they bacterial or viral. If a child is unwell at home, with a fever and rhinorrhoea, the parents should be advised to contact the paediatrician. If the temperature is above a previously agreed level (e.g. 38 degrees Celsius), then the child should be seen either in hospital or at the surgery.

A general rule is that there should be no treatment (including antipyretics) given for infection, unless a full blood count and blood cultures (as a minimum) have been performed.

If the neutrophil count is low (below 0.5×10^9/L), the child should be admitted to hospital. The management of febrile neutropenia should include broad-spectrum parenteral antibiotic therapy (e.g. ceftriaxone, tobramycin, teicoplanin). Antibiotics ideally should be commenced within 1–2 hours of the child reaching the emergency room. It is inappropriate to wait for the results of the blood count before starting therapy with antibiotics, especially if there is any delay in processing the sample in the laboratory. In such circumstances antibiotics should be started. If the count is normal there is less cause for concern. Remember, however, that many patients have central venous access devices in place which can be the cause of serious infections despite normal neutrophil numbers. *Always* remind the family that fevers occurring within 6–8 hours of flushing a central line may be due to the introduction of bacteria into the patient from an infected CVL. See below for more details.

Granulocyte colony stimulating factor (G-CSF) can decrease duration of hospitalisation for prolonged febrile neutropenia after intensive remission induction chemotherapy. G-CSF can be started 24 hours after cytotoxics and is given subcutaneously daily for 10 days. G-CSF may be ceased when the neutrophil count is greater than $1.0 \times 10^9/L$, and beyond the nadir. A new long-lasting form of G-CSF is now available—Peg-G-CSF—which is administered as a single dose 24 hours after completing the chemotherapy course.

Exposure to certain viruses requires specific intervention. In the case of varicella contacts, varicella zoster immune globulin should be given within 96 hours of exposure, and is more efficacious the earlier it is given. With measles contacts, standard immunoglobulin is recommended. In patients who are at risk of significant infection with herpes simplex virus (HSV), valacyclovir can be used (this has a longer half-life than aciclovir). Ganciclovir is often used for CMV prophylaxis in the setting of stem cell transplantation.

For prophylaxis against oral candidiasis, oral nystatin or amphotericin B lozenges can be given. In patients with prolonged neutropenia and/or lymphopenia, fluconazole may be used (covers *Candida* but not *Aspergillus*), or itraconazole (covers aspergillosis, e.g. post-transplant). Cotrimoxazole is recommended as prophylaxis against *Pneumocystis carinii*, particularly in patients with prolonged lymphopenia (lymphocytes less than $1.0 \times 10^9/L$ or CD4 count below 400). In patients where cotrimoxazole causes neutropenia, or there are unacceptable side effects, pentamidine may be considered.

Mouthcare is important in children with mouth ulceration or mucositis, or in those at risk of these if they are neutropenic ($<1.0 \times 10^9/L$). Chlorhexidine mouthwash is useful, as it is bacteriocidal.

The child off chemotherapy

For the first 6 months after completion of chemotherapy there is a continued susceptibility to infection. After this time, the risk diminishes unless there is coexistent chronic graft-versus-host disease (GVHD). Children with chronic GVHD are immunosuppressed as they are generally receiving steroids and anti-T-cell medications (cyclosporine or mycophenolate). They are often relatively neutropenic. Patients with active GVHD should not attend school. It is advisable for the schoolteacher to notify the parents, within the first 6 months of ceasing chemotherapy, of any outbreaks of chickenpox or measles in the class.

Immunisation

Susceptibility to live vaccines is maximal during chemotherapy and for the first 6 months after chemotherapy. Thus avoidance of live vaccines is recommended, with the exception of live varicella vaccine, which can be given safely during the maintenance therapy for ALL (but not during the early intensive phases—the first 6 months of treatment). Killed virus vaccines (e.g. Salk vaccine) can be given. In the case of polio immunisation, patients should be kept away from other children who have had the live

Sabin vaccine for about 6–8 weeks, and their siblings should receive the killed polio vaccine. Some authorities avoid administering live measles and mumps vaccine to siblings, as there is a small risk of transmission. Other authorities consider this risk minimal and the vaccine safe. Influenza vaccine is safe and may have a place in patients with chronic chest symptoms. Hepatitis B recombinant vaccine is safe, but as these patients are immunosuppressed, adding a further booster dose is recommended. Titres may be checked 12 months later to assess efficacy.

Issues related to ongoing chemotherapy

For oncology patients receiving chemotherapy, there are misconceptions about how to best 'protect' children. In general, the following advice is standard in Paediatric Oncology Centres:

1. Check that relatives are well before visits.
2. Patients can swim in swimming pools (even with central lines, but they require prompt cleaning after the swim).
3. Children can go shopping in supermarkets, attend group gatherings (e.g. church, birthday parties).
4. Prophylactic cotrimoxazole is essential.

Crisis intervention

The candidate should be familiar with medical practices in his or her own teaching hospital's oncology unit. For example, prophylactic platelet transfusions for severe thrombocytopenia (platelet count is below 20×10^9/L) is not standard practice in all units.

Drug toxicities

The paediatrician must be aware of the various side effects of the many drugs used in the treatment of the malignancy, and be cognisant of a confusing complaint, e.g. ataxia in a child with leukaemia, being possibly due to drug toxicity (e.g. vincristine neuropathy) rather than necessarily meaning CNS relapse.

Thrombocytopenia is one of the more common drug side effects. If the platelet count is below 20×10^9/L, spontaneous bleeding can occur. If the platelet count is below 50×10^9/L, minor trauma can result in bleeding. If there is no overt bleeding, then simple precautions suffice, such as avoiding injurious activities or invasive procedures (unless essential, which may require them to be covered by platelet transfusion), body-contact sports, strenuous exercise or hard-bristled toothbrushes. Note that severe headaches may indicate CNS haemorrhage. Avoidance of drugs such as aspirin or antihistamines (which can interfere with normal platelet function) is important.

Febrile neutropenic episodes

Neutropenia means a neutrophil count of below 1.0×10^9/L, but most infections occur with a level below 0.5×10^9/L, and most of those are below 0.2×10^9/L. Clinically, the problem can be very difficult to assess, as there are no classic signs or symptoms. Particular areas on which to focus include the skin, mucous membranes (ulceration, candida, herpes), chest, central-line site and perianal region (ischiorectal abscesses can be very subtle).

Management usually includes admission to hospital, culture of the potential sites outlined, blood cultures, and administration of broad-spectrum parenteral antibiotic therapy. Most units withhold chemotherapy until the child is afebrile for more than a day and the neutrophil count returns to above 1.0×10^9/L.

Pulmonary infections

These are among the most common form of severe infection seen in oncology patients, and there are many possible pathogens. The neutrophil count plus the chest X-ray may be useful guides in management. Note that in the presence of neutropenia, pulmonary markings may not be prominent, despite significant infection. Approximately 50% of bacterial infections are due to gram-positive bacteria and the remainder are due to gram-negative organisms: thus broad-spectrum antibiotic therapy cover is advisable. Opportunistic infections can occur, such as *Pneumocystis carinii* (although most patients are on cotrimoxazole prophylaxis for this), opportunistic viruses (e.g. cytomegalovirus), fungi, *Mycobacterium* or *Mycoplasma*. Note that radiological findings may be due to noninfectious causes (e.g. leukaemic infiltration or toxicity from chemotherapy or radiotherapy).

Central venous access devices

These may be central lines or totally implantable venous access devices, such as Port-a-Cath and Infuse-A-Port. These devices are routinely used in most conditions encountered in oncology. They require regular heparin flushes to avoid clots forming, and may on occasion become infected, particularly with *Staphylococcus* species.

Supportive care

Mouth care

Mouth care is important in children with mouth ulceration or mucositis, or in those at risk of these if they are neutropenic ($<1.0 \times 10^9$/L). Chlorhexidine mouthwash is useful, as it is bacteriocidal. In very young patients, chlorhexidine gel is appropriate, and before meals xylocaine viscous is useful.

Antiemetics

All chemotherapy protocols include the use of 5-HT$_3$ antagonists such as ondansetron, as vomiting occurs predictably after many specific chemotherapeutic agents. Ondansetron can be given intravenously or orally, the latter being significantly cheaper and available in the form of wafers or syrup. If ondansetron is not enough, metoclopramide or dexamethasone provide additional antiemetic effect.

Many of the drugs used in solid tumour protocols are very emetogenic. These include adriamycin, carboplatin, cisplatin, cyclophosphamide (CPA) and ifosphamide. Ondansetron is usually given before, during and after each chemotherapy infusion.

Bone marrow transplantation (BMTx)

In the weeks leading up to BMT, especially in late autumn/early winter, isolating the children is a good idea because if they get RSV, parainfluenza, adenovirus or influenza, this will delay the BMT.

Candidates should know that pre-transplant preparative regimens usually combine very high-dose cytotoxic agents and immunosuppressive agents (e.g. CPA, cytosine arabinoside [ara C], etoposide [VP-16], thiotepa, melphalan, busulphan) with total body irradiation.

After BMTx

All recipients of allogeneic marrow are at risk of GVHD post-engraftment. Agents used to prevent this occurring include methotrexate (MTX), cyclosporine (CSA), prednisolone, tacrolimus and mycophenylate mofetil. The main target organs of acute GVHD are skin (maculopapular rash), liver (cholestatic jaundice) and gut (anorexia/diarrhoea).

Acute GVHD may require treatment with prednisolone, antithymocyte globulin, tacrolimus, psoralin plus ultraviolet light (PUVA).

In the first 6 months after transplant, the child should not attend school, and social contacts should be limited (especially with GVHD). There are no firm recommendations regarding use of live viral vaccines for these patients. If the child is well, and has no GVHD, then after 12 months live viral vaccines are safe.

Late effects

Chronic GVHD appears around 80 days post-BMTx. The main target organs are skin (epidermal atrophy, focal dermal fibrosis, scleroderma, loss of hair and nails), liver (cholestatic jaundice), eyes (keratoconjunctivitis sicca), mouth (erythema, lichenoid lesions of buccal mucosa). Less often the lungs, gut and neuromuscular system may be involved. If GVHD is extensive, treatment may involve use of prednisolone with CPA, prednisolone with tacrolimus, azathioprine, PUVA.

Other effects related to the BMTx process include graft rejection and immunologic dysfunction (short-lasting donor-derived T- and B-lymphocyte immunity (TBI); reimmunisation of patients should occur 12 months post-BMTx).

Complications of the preparative regimen include lung disease (both restrictive and obstructive defects can occur long term), development of second malignancies (at 15 years, around 6% if no TBI, but 20% if received TBI), endocrine dysfunction (growth hormone deficiency, gonadal dysfunction, hypothyroidism) and neuropsychological problems.

Cord blood transplantation (CBT)

Umbilical cord blood (CB) is an alternative source for transplantable stem and progenitor cells. CB can be collected from the placenta via the umbilical vein after the baby is delivered. GVHD occurs at lower rates than matched sibling BMTx. Cord blood is available at short notice. Disadvantages include potential for unknowing transmission of genetic diseases (e.g. immune deficiency and storage diseases), and the limitation of volume and cell content of what is collected (i.e. the finite number of stem cells in the CB unit). CBT may be very useful for those without a matched donor for BMTx.

Therapeutic modifications: risk adapted therapy

As the number of survivors has increased, so has there been heightened awareness of potential consequences of treatment. This has led to modifications to therapy to enhance the quality of life for survivors. The following brief summary outlines risk-adapted therapies aimed at diminishing complications, the latter grouped according to the organ system involved.

Cardiopulmonary

Decreased dose of radiation; improved shielding of heart and lungs; decreased doses of anthracyclines (cardiotoxic), bleomycin (pulmonary toxicity); newer anthracyclines with decreased cardiotoxicity; use of cardioprotective agents (dexrazoxane); routine monitoring (e.g. echocardiography, pulmonary function tests).

Endocrine

Lower doses and volumes of radiotherapy; routine oophoropexy during pelvic radiotherapy; reducing doses of alkylating agents in patients with good prognoses; routine testing for deficiencies of various hormones (e.g. growth hormone, oestrogen, thyroid hormone) and replacement thereof; ovarian tissue and sperm storage.

Genitourinary

Use of mesna, a uroprotectant drug that binds to toxic metabolites in the urine, after CPA or ifosfamide, decreases haemorrhagic cystitis; new analogues with less renal toxicity (e.g. carboplatin compared with cisplatin); routine monitoring (e.g. blood testing for electrolytes, including phosphorus, and magnesium).

Neurological

Elimination of intrathecal and intravenous methotrexate after cranial irradiation has decreased leukoencephalopathy; delaying therapeutic radiation until older (aiming for over 3 years) by utilising systemic chemotherapy; routine monitoring of neuropsychological status.

Second malignancy

Decreased exposure to alkylating agents, plus limiting volume of radiation in Hodgkin's disease; greatly diminished use of epipodophyllotoxins in leukaemia; increased education of survivors about potential of late effects of their specific therapy.

The dying child

There are many issues that need to be addressed in a child for whom no further beneficial therapy is possible. Most children nowadays die at home. Palliative treatment involves issues of control of pain, nutrition and appreciation of the psychosocial dynamics of the family. These children may show an inability to cope by features such as denial of their illness, withdrawal, unwarranted anger.

The family's mourning can include, again, denial, anger and depression, and very often seeking further opinions or considering alternative forms of therapy. These processes should be understood and accepted by the paediatrician. For the child who dies in hospital, the major objective is ensuring maximum comfort. This can be aided by surrounding the child with familiar possessions from home and having no restriction on visitors. Invariably other children on the ward become aware of the change in the management of these patients, and frank discussion should be encouraged as well as permitting interaction with the dying child.

The death of the child invariably is associated with confusion and shock, irrespective of the degree of expectation and preparation. Prior discussions regarding issues of post-mortem examination and, if the child dies at home, transport of the body to the hospital, are usually beneficial to the family. The role of the paediatrician extends beyond the death of the child to helping the family cope with caring for siblings, discussing unresolved issues, intervening, by appropriate referral, where an abnormal grief reaction is apparent, such as acting out by siblings, or severe depression and contemplation of suicide in the parents. As the most severe grief may occur some months after the child's death, follow-up should be for many months rather than weeks.

Short case

Late effects of oncology treatment

Later effects of oncology treatment plus common signs of disease relapse (in particular, acute leukaemia) are outlined in Table 14.1. This is incomplete, of course, by nature of the wide range of tumours and their individual modes of relapse. Some of the findings mentioned will be relevant only to children still on chemotherapy. This approach may be found useful in assessing children in follow-up clinics.

Table 14.1   Late effects of oncology treatment

General observations

Introduce yourself: ask name, age, school; assess intelligence (is child alert, conversant?) (leukoencephalopathy secondary to treatment; subnormal IQ with intracranial tumours). Note any deformities /amputations.

Parameters

- Height: (short stature: growth hormone deficiency, panhypopituitarism from cranial XRT, hypothyroidism from thyroid XRT, steroid therapy, skeletal changes from radiation of spine)
- Upper segment:lower segment ratio (skeletal changes from radiation of spine)
- Weight
- Head circumference
- Percentile charts, noting trend since treatment

Tanner staging (delayed from alkylating agents or radiation to gonads)

Cushingoid features (steroid therapy)

Tachypnoea, cyanosis or cough (radiation or chemotherapy-induced pneumonitis, or pulmonary infection)

Skin

- Pallor: anaemia from marrow suppression (most agents), or bone marrow relapse of leukaemia (or development of secondary leukaemia)
- Bruises: thrombocytopenia from marrow suppression (most agents) or (rare) coagulopathy from L-asparaginase, or bone marrow relapse of leukaemia
- Dermatitis (MTX, 6-MP, 6-TG)
- Hyperpigmentation (chronic GVHD from BMT)
- Desquamation (bleomycin)
- Jaundice (MTX, 6-MP, 6-TG, bleomycin, radiation to liver)
- Pigmented naevi (increased by most agents)

Manoeuvres

Stand with hands and feet together (asymmetry from XRT to limbs or hemihypertrophy with Wilms' tumour; do not confuse the two)

Gait: for evidence of neuropathy (VCR), spasticity (leukoencephalopathy), cerebellar ataxia (L-asparaginase), or antalgic limp (marrow relapse of leukaemia); also may detect evidence of cerebral tumour (second malignancy)

Romberg's test (neuropathy from VCR)

Back

Inspect; look for scars, any vertebral masses (secondary malignancy)

Bend forward and touch toes (to assess for scoliosis or kyphosis from spinal irradiation, particularly if unilateral)

Palpate for tenderness (steroids; rickets from ifosfamide)

Upper limbs

Asymmetry (limb radiation, hemihypertrophy)

Contractures (limb XRT, chronic GVHD)

Peripheral stigmata of chronic liver disease (MTX, 6-MP, radiation to abdomen)

Palmar crease pallor (marrow suppression)

Pulse (untreated hypothyroidism from radiation to thyroid)

Peripheral neuropathy (vinca alkaloids, usually reversible; test reflexes and sensation to document this)

Functional assessment if:

- any asymmetry or contractures suggestive of radiation to limb, *or*
- scars from resection of tumour with potential neurological or vascular complications, *or*
- amputation: examine function with prosthesis; check how well it fits, any loosening or sign of infection

Blood pressure (elevated from steroids, bleomycin, MTX nephrotoxicity, radiation nephritis)

Head and neck

Alopecia (reversible—can occur with ADR, bleomycin, CPA, daunorubicin, VCR; irreversible—can occur post-BMTx, secondary to busulfan, or if cranial radiotherapy and anthracycline given close together)

Midfacial hypoplasia, with small nose, chin (radiation to head and neck causing altered growth of bone and soft tissue)

Continued

Table 14.1 *(Continued)*

Eyes
- Aniridia (association with Wilms' tumour)
- Conjunctival pallor (marrow suppression, various agents)
- Scleral icterus (bleomycin, MTX, 6-MP, 6-TG, radiation to liver)
- External ocular movements for evidence of cranial nerve palsy (CNS relapse of leukaemia, VCR neuropathy)
- Cataracts (corticosteroids, radiation to eyes)
- Papilloedema (CNS relapse of leukaemia)

Mouth
- Dry (salivary gland dysfunction from XRT)
- Mucositis (MTX, 6-MP, 6-TG, actinomycin D)
- Dental abnormalities: poor enamel and root formation (radiation to head)
- Dental caries (most agents)
- Thyroid: look and palpate for nodules (thyroid carcinoma from craniospinal XRT)

Chest

Praecordial assessment for cardiomegaly (cardiomyopathy) from anthracyclines (the 'rubicins') or radiation (mediastinal XRT), pericarditis (reversible—from mediastinal XRT), evidence of congestive cardiac failure (from cardiomyopathy).

Full respiratory examination for tachypnoea, cough or crackles due to interstitial pneumonitis or pulmonary fibrosis (bleomycin, busulphan, MTX, CPA or radiation), pulmonary infection (opportunistic viruses, bacteria/fungi if still on chemotherapy)

Assess bony tenderness at sternum, clavicles, spine (marrow relapse: leukaemia, secondary leukaemia)

Abdomen

Scars (previous diagnostic, curative or debulking surgery)

Prominent veins (chronic liver disease from MTX, 6-MP or XRT to abdomen)

Hepatomegaly (MTX, 6-MP or relapse of leukaemia or lymphoma)

Splenomegaly (relapse of leukaemia or lymphoma)

Genitals: Tanner staging (delay from alkylating agents or gonadal XRT); ambiguous genitalia with Denys-Drash syndrome

Testicular enlargement (relapse of leukaemia)

Undescended testes (association with Wilms')

Lower limbs

Asymmetry (limb radiation, hemihypertrophy)

Contractures (limb XRT, chronic GVHD from BMT)

Ankle oedema (from cardiac failure or liver disease; see above)

Bony (tibial) tenderness (marrow relapse of leukaemia)

Peripheral neuropathy (vinca alkaloids; usually reversible; test ankle and knee jerks and sensation to document this)

Delayed relaxation of ankle jerks (hypothyroidism from thyroid radiation)

Functional assessment if:
- any asymmetry or contractures suggestive of radiation to limb, *or*
- scars from resection of tumour with potential neurological or vascular complications, *or*
- amputation: examine function with prosthesis; check how well it fits, any loosening, or sign of infection

Other

Temperature chart: fever with intercurrent infection (myelosuppression with various agents) or (rare) radiation pneumonitis

ADR = adriamycin; BMT = bone marrow transplantation; CNS = central nervous system; CPA = cyclophosphamide; GVHD = graft-versus-host disease; MTX = methotrexate; 6-MP = 6-mercaptopurine; 6-TG = 6-thioguanine; VCR = vincristine; XRT = radiotherapy.

The respiratory system

Long cases

Asthma

Recent advances in management have included improved understanding of the underlying pathophysiology of asthma as follows:

- The roles of T helper lymphocytes Th1: generate interleukin (IL)-2, interferon-gamma; defend against infection; early Th1 predominance from exposure to child care, siblings, viruses and endotoxins may inhibit airway inflammation and atopic sensitisation.
- The roles of T helper lymphocytes Th2: produce mediators of allergic reactions, including IL-4, -5, -6, -7 and -13; Th2 predominance may promote ongoing airway inflammation.
- The Th1/Th2 relationship to the 'hygiene hypothesis'.
- Introduction of new medications: e.g. omalizumab, a murine recombinant monoclonal humanised antibody that blocks IgE (and skin allergy tests in atopic patients), suppresses early- and late-phase allergic responses (EPR and LPR) and sputum eosinophilia.
- Better understanding of long-term effects of inhaled corticosteroids (they cause very little, if any, long-term effect on growth).
- Better understanding of the place of leukotriene modifiers in the asthma armamentarium (second-line agents in mild or moderate asthma).

Recent trends in management have included increased prescribing of combination therapies: long-acting beta-2 adrenoreceptor agonists (LABA) with inhaled corticosteroids (ICS). By August 2004 combination therapy with LABA/ICS claimed over 40% of the 'preventer' market in Australia, raising the question as to whether overprescription of combination therapy may be occurring. Candidates should be familiar with this issue.

The long-case management aims remain: control of cough and wheeze, enabling the child to participate in normal daily activities and educating both child and parents to manage asthma within the family's lifestyle. One should not underestimate an asthma long case, as important issues could be omitted, such as: the child's technique of using aerosols, spacers and peak flow meters; what treatment is taken during holiday trips to remote areas in a severe asthmatic with previous life-threatening episodes; whether the adolescent is actually taking his/her recommended steroids twice daily (or at all); or whether he/she smokes actively.

History

Presenting complaint

Reason for current admission.

Symptoms

Dyspnoea, wheeze, cough, exercise tolerance (last in races?), nocturnal symptoms (cough, wheeze, wakening), morning symptoms (tightness, wheeze), use of bronchodilators, viral upper respiratory tract infections, cyanosis, syncope. Provide a detailed expansion of important or specific symptoms: e.g. for cough, note duration, nature (e.g. productive/loose), frequency, timing (day/night), effects (vomiting, awakening, family disruption), sputum (amount, colour, blood), associated symptoms (fever, wheeze, shortness of breath, upper airway obstructive symptoms), responsiveness to beta-2 agonists/antibiotics).

Pattern of episodes

Frequency of attacks (infrequent [less than every 4–6 weeks] or frequent [more than every 4–6 weeks], episodic, chronic), severity (e.g. how often needing bronchodilators or oral steroids at home), time of year (perennial, seasonal), diurnal variation, geographic variation.

Precipitants

Usual triggers: weather, temperature change, humidity, viral upper respiratory tract infection, exercise, tobacco smoke, allergic precipitants, animals (e.g. birds, furry animals such as cats), food (e.g. Chinese food with MSG, pickled onions, juices), inhalants, pollen, dust (house dust mite), mould, emotion, aspirin.

Typical acute exacerbation

Initial symptoms, precipitants, tempo of progression, rate of recovery, how child handles the illness, usual outcome, treatment required.

Social history

Disease impact: on child (school missed, limitation of activities, effect on development, education, behaviour, peer interaction); on family (financial issues such as costs of nebuliser, peak flow meters, oxygen cylinders, frequent hospitalisation, private health insurance; disruption of family routine); on siblings (changed holiday plans to allow nebulisation or hospital access for emergencies); social supports (e.g. Asthma Foundation, local parent groups).

Past history

Age at onset, diagnosis, the number of hospitalisations, treatment required, changes in clinical course, previous investigations, past complications (e.g. pneumothorax, intensive care admissions).

Family history

Asthma, 'wheezy bronchitis', hay fever, allergies, eczema.

Management

Present treatment in hospital, usual treatment at home (inhaler/spacer; technique used), school, before exercise, previous medications tried, side effects (e.g. steroids), levels (e.g. theophylline), physical activity (e.g. swimming), holiday camps, compliance, alternative therapies tried, allergen avoidance, immunotherapy, dietary manipulation (appropriate or not), use of Medicalert bracelet, home monitoring with peak flow meter, crisis plan.

Understanding of disease

By child and by parents. Ask degree of previous education (by doctors, by reading, attending lectures). Ask if they know the differences between preventers and relievers.

Examination

General impression

Note any facial features suggesting Cushing's syndrome (flushed cheeks, moon face) or atopy (swollen, discoloured eyelids; transverse nasal crease from 'allergic salute'). Check percentiles (decreased weight and height from disease or its treatment), Tanner staging (delayed puberty), sick or well, tachypnoea at rest, use of accessory muscles. Note the skin (e.g. dry skin, atopic eczema at elbows, knees). Note any clubbing (e.g. obliterative brochiolitis with bronchiectasis mimicking asthma). If cough is a current symptom, ask older patients if they can produce sputum, as it may indicate a complicating factor such as chronic bronchitis or bronchiectasis.

Vital signs

Pulse (rate, palpable paradox), blood pressure (side effects of steroids or beta-2 agonists), temperature (precipitating viral upper respiratory tract infection).

Respiratory examination

1. Hands: tremor (beta-2 agonists).
2. Chest: deformity, increased antero-posterior diameter, Harrison's sulcus, expansion, tracheal position, apex position, palpable pulmonary valve closure, right ventricular overactivity, percussion, auscultation. If age appropriate, peak flow (ideally before and after nebulised salbutamol; impractical in exams).
3. ENT: ears—serous otitis media; nose—allergic rhinitis; pale, swollen, nasal mucosa, visible inferior turbinates, green/clear discharge; throat—redness or exudate. Cervical nodes: lymphadenopathy.

General examination

Steroid side effects (e.g. proximal muscle weakness, dermopathy, cataracts), accurate Tanner staging, and the remaining systems involved in the child with multiple problems.

Diagnosis and investigations

Generally a clinical diagnosis; on occasion some investigations may be warranted.

Peak expiratory flow rate (PEFR) measurements and spirometry

PEFR monitoring is unreliable in children under 7 years and is easily manipulated by older children and adolescents. It adds little to noting symptoms and use of bronchodilators in those with severe asthma. Spirometry in those over 7 years can be measured, as this gives a more sensitive measure of airways obstruction.

Chest X-ray

Helpful if there is doubt about diagnosis. Inspiratory and expiratory films may exclude an inhaled foreign body or other structural lesions. In acute asthma, the only indications are suspected pneumothorax or first-ever presentation (to exclude other diagnoses).

Other investigations

Provocation inhalation challenge testing (methacholine, histamine) may be useful to confirm bronchospasm in cases with diagnostic difficulty, recurrent cough or recurrent breathlessness. Tests to exclude other diagnoses that may present with cough or wheeze include: (a) sweat test; (b) $alpha_1$-antitrypsin phenotype; (c) sputum microscopy and culture; (d) immunoglobulins, including IgG subclasses; (e) bronchoscopy (may detect congenital tracheomalacia or bronchomalacia), especially if wheeze and hyperinflation commenced early in life, and are unresponsive to anti-asthma treatment; (f) high-resolution CT scan of thorax is useful if looking for parenchymal lesions (e.g. bronchiectasis, or congenital structural lung lesions); helical CT scan of thorax if checking mediastinum or for vascular lesions; (g) electrocardiogram—occult cardiac disease.

Treatment

Acute

1. **Position**. Sit child up, for ease of chest expansion, and diaphragmatic excursion.
2. **Oxygen**. All children with acute severe asthma are hypoxic. Always check pulse oximetry. Aim is maximum inspired oxygen; keep the SaO_2 above 90%.
3. **Beta-2 agonists** (e.g. salbutamol). Nebulised for severe, life-threatening asthma; for mild and moderate asthma, pMDI with spacer. For very severe asthma, continuous nebulised therapy (dose 0.3 mg/kg/hour; prevents rebound bronchospasm); for moderately severe cases, either intermittent nebulised therapy (dose 0.15 mg/kg/dose [to maximum of 5 mg] or 6–12 puffs pMDI via spacer, every 20 minutes, initially). If nebulised therapy is needed, the optimum volume of drug in the 'acorn' of the nebuliser is 4 mL, with the driving oxygen rate being 8 L/min; can give with ipratropium bromide (see below).
4. **Intravenous beta-2 agonists.** If nebulised therapy is not working, when inspiratory flow rates are very low, or the need for high-flow oxygen precludes nebuliser. An initial salbutamol bolus is followed by an infusion, incrementally increased until there is a good response. Toxicities: hypokalaemia, tachyarrhythmias, metabolic acidosis.
5. **Nebulised anticholinergics.** Ipratropium bromide augments actions of beta-2 agonists. Dose is 250 mcg each 20 minutes initially.
6. **Corticosteroids (CS)** (oral prednisolone, IV hydrocortisone or methylprednisolone). Used in all moderate to severe episodes; decreases morbidity. High dose for 4 days, then stop. Treatment for any longer duration should be slowly weaned.
7. **Other medications**
   a. Theophylline preparations are used less, due to concerns regarding efficacy and toxicity. There is a narrow therapeutic/toxic margin. Toxicities include vomiting, arrhythmias and, in cases of inadvertent overdosage, intractable seizures. IV aminophylline still has use in the child not responding to other treatments.
   b. Other 'back to the wall' treatments include IV adrenaline ('God's own inotrope'), isoprenaline, magnesium sulphate, or bicarbonate.

c. Non-conventional therapies in acute severe asthma include general anaesthesia with halothane or ether, helium–oxygen (Heliox), extracorporeal membrane oxygenation (ECMO), or even bronchial lavage.

8. **Face mask continuous positive airway pressure (CPAP).** Safer than ventilation, CPAP decreases resistance to air flow, inflates the lungs, decreases the work of respiratory muscles and recruits expiratory muscles. This can reverse deterioration such that children will request it once they have experienced it. Pressures of 5–10 cm H_2O for 10 minutes every hour can be effective. It can be nebulised through the circuit.

9. **Mechanical ventilation.** A last resort. Indications are respiratory arrest, extreme fatigue or relentness hypercapnia. A treacherous path, with morbidity risks including barotrauma, gas trapping (compromised cardiac function), dysrhythmias, atelectasis, nosocomial pneumonia. Strategies to minimise these include: initial rapid sequence induction, oral intubation, sedation, paralysis; permissive hypercapnia, minimal positive end expiratory pressure (PEEP), prolonged expiratory time, low rate, limitation of peak inspiratory pressure (PIP).

Preventative

1. Modification/avoidance of precipitants

Use of beta-2 agonist or cromolyn before exercise, initiating regular inhaled therapy at home at the onset of viral upper respiratory tract infections (URTIs). Avoid cigarette smoke (active and passive), known allergens. For house dust mite avoidance, simple measures: minimise soft furnishings, soft toys in the sleeping areas; cover mattresses and pillows with barrier materials; keep house well ventilated, free of damp and mould (avoid vaporisers; fix leaky taps, pipes), cockroach allergens (use boric acid cockroach traps) and pets (remove pet from home; if this is unacceptable, at least out of bedroom). No carpet is best in the bedroom. Acaricides are not recommended. House dust mites are killed by direct sunlight, hot water washing (>55°C) or extreme cold (can put soft toys in deep freeze overnight, once a month). For atopy, cetirizine was trialled in the ETAC (Early Treatment of the Atopic Child) study. It did not alter the asthma 'rate' compared to placebo, but it reduced the prevalence of asthma in children who were RAST positive to house dust mite, or grass pollen; benefits were applicable to 20% of children only.

2. Inhaled corticosteroids (ICS): fluticasone propionate [FP], budesonide [BUD], beclomethasone diproprionate [BDP], triamcinolone acetonide, flunisolide, mometasone

ICS are the mainstay of treatment in persistent asthma. FP, BUD and BDP are used in most countries; in addition, triamcinolone acetonide and flunisolide are used in the USA, and mometasone is used in the UK. The most appropriate dosage is the lowest that gives symptom control. Side effects are minimal in doses below 400 mcg of BDP or equivalent daily in children over 5, for periods of at least 24 months. If doses above 400 mcg are used, side effects may include short-term growth suppression, and adrenal suppression. Clinical adrenal suppression has been described in children receiving over 400 mcg ICS daily presenting with hypoglycaemia. At higher doses, add-on agents (such as long-acting beta-2 agonists [LABAs]) should be used. There are insufficient data to comment on the safety of ICS in those under 5 years. Once the dosage exceeds 800–1000 mcg daily, side effects increase but the clinical effect does not: it plateaus (flat dose–response curve). ICS given as metered dose inhaler (pMDI) should always be given through a spacing device (increases amount delivered to airways and decreases oral candidiasis from pharyngeal deposition from aerosol).

As above, there is a risk of hypothalamic pituitary axis (HPA) suppression. Doses causing this depend on weight and age. Approximately 36 mcg/kg/day of BUD or BDP will cause some HPA suppression. After taking ICS, children should rinse the mouth and spit (can do when cleaning teeth); it decreases oral candidiasis and systemic absorption. ICS potential side effects include decreased bone mineralisation and cataracts. Fluticasone propionate (FP) has a topical potency approximately double that of BUD or BDP (FP 200 mcg daily = BUD 400 mcg daily). Mometasone has similar potency to FP (double that of BUD or BDP). FP and BUD have high topical potency, fast clearance, low oral bioavailability, high affinity for glucocorticoid receptors, fairly inactive metabolites, but systemic effects can occur with high doses, due to absorption from the lung. Once a child needs more than 400 mcg daily of BUD or BDP, fluticasone should be considered.

3. Long-acting beta-2 agonists (LABAs): e.g. salmeterol xinofoate, eformoterol fumarate dihydrate

Although not preventers, LABAs are most often prescribed in combination medications with ICS, and as such make up a large percentage of the medications taken for 'prevention'. These are symptom relievers, providing bronchodilation for up to 12 hours. Eformoterol has an onset of action similar to that of salbutamol, faster than that of salmeterol: not for acute asthma; useful for symptomatic poorly controlled asthma, especially nocturnal waking. Eformoterol was initially promoted as protective against exercise-induced asthma for up to 9 hours, but tachyphylaxis can occur. Eformoterol is banned by the IOC, in contrast to salmeterol. Addition of either LABA should be considered with sleep disturbance due to asthma, or in those using regular short acting beta-2 agonists (SABAs) despite taking high-dose ICS. Adding a LABA to ICS leads to improved symptom control, less rescue or reliever use and no increase in exacerbations. No child should receive LABAs without ICS. For breakthrough symptoms or as prophylaxis against exercise-induced asthma, SABAs are preferred.

4. Combination therapies: ICS + LABAs: fluticasone propionate (FP) + salmeterol xinofoate (SX); budesonide (BUD) + eformoterol fumarate dihydrate (EFD).

In Australia, these are available as follows:

- FP dose/SX dose (mcg)—Accuhaler (powder for inhalation): 100/50, 250/50, 500/50. SX dose fixed (50); FP dose varies. FP dose/SX dose (mcg): pMDI 50/25, 125/25, 250/25; SX dose fixed (25); FP dose varies.
- BUD dose/EFD dose (mcg)—100/6, 200/6, 400/12 (not recommended under 18).

These combination medications have been promoted effectively by the pharmaceutical companies. They can be useful in severe persistent asthma, and moderately severe asthma. However, given that around 25% of asthmatic children have persistent asthma, and given that most of these patients have mild persistent asthma, it is of some concern that so many physicians are prescribing ICS + LABA so often.

5. Cromolyns (sodium cromoglycate, nedrocromil sodium)

Effective in 70% of asthmatic children; useful as first-line preventers, for exercise-induced asthma, as steroid-sparers or for asthmatic cough (nedrocromil is particularly useful here).

6. Leukotriene modifiers (LTMs)

There are two classes:

1. Leukotriene receptor antagonists (e.g. montelukast, zafirlukast).
2. 5-lipoxygenase inhibitors (e.g. zileuton).

These improve FEV_1 of 10–20%, who show greatest improvement within first 4 weeks of starting treatment. Given orally, once or twice daily. As effective as cromolyns or around 300 mcg of BEC. Particularly useful in aspirin-induced asthma. Also used as steroid sparer and for prevention of exercise-induced bronchoconstriction. Well tolerated. Specific side effects described include raised liver enzymes with higher than recommended dosage (zileuton), and 'unmasking' of eosinophilic vasculitis (Churg-Strauss disease) suppressed by steroids, becoming evident as steroids withdrawn. LTMs are second-line agents in mild asthma (if inhaled therapy is not viable) and can be given with a low-dose ICS in moderate persistent asthma, but LTM + ICS is less effective than ICS + LABA. They have little place in severe asthma.

7. Theophylline

This has anti-inflammatory effects and may have a place in persistent asthma, particularly in children receiving high-dose steroids. As noted previously, it should be borne in mind that theophylline's therapeutic range is quite close to its toxic range. Theophylline has the dubious distinction of being the drug prescribed most commonly by doctors subsequently taken to court, successfully, for medical negligence. Those cases involved (you guessed it) inadvertent theophylline overdosage, leading to seizure activity and subsequent brain damage.

An overdose of theophylline can cause ongoing seizures that can be resistant to all forms of anticonvulsive therapy including thiopentone and general anaesthesia.

8. Omalizumab

This is a monoclonal antibody produced by recombinant DNA technology, given as a subcutaneous injection, 2- to 4-weekly, for an extended period. In Australia, it is approved for children aged 12 years and over. It is known to be effective in the treatment of allergic rhinitis, and is being assessed for therapy and prevention of anaphylaxis, food allergy and atopic dermatitis. It decreases free IgE, it suppresses both EPR and LPR. In asthma, it improves symptoms and reduces the need for ICS. It is as yet unclear as to the best selection of patients for treatment, what duration of treatment is of most benefit, and whether it can arrest disease progression. It can be considered in children requiring unacceptably high doses of ICS or oral CS, or those with CS-induced side effects. A disadvantage is its expense.

9. Other treatments

Candidates should be aware of anecdotal reports in the use of anti-inflammatory drugs (AIDs) and immunomodulator approaches. It has been noted that asthma symptoms in children with cancer are less with chemotherapy. Methotrexate, gold, cyclosporin, hydroxychloroquine, intravenous gammaglobulin have been used in very problematic asthmatics. Research continues into various treatments, including platelet-activating factor antagonists, prostanoid inhibitors, bradykinin antagonists, antioxidants, nitric oxide synthase inhibitors, NSAIDs, and 'dissociated steroids' with AID efficacy (inhibition of transcription factors) but fewer systemic side effects.

Delivery methods

The child must have an age-appropriate mode of drug delivery. Most anti-asthma drugs can be given by pMDI + spacer ± mask; pMDI + spacing devices have replaced nebulisers in all but life-threatening asthma.

417

Spacing devices

These can be used at all ages. Small volume (150 mL) spacers with face masks (e.g. Aerochamber, Breath-A-Tech) are useful in young infants and children up to 4 years. Large volume (750 mL) devices (e.g. Volumatic, Nebuhaler) are ideal for those over 4. They are very useful and effective in acute asthma if no nebuliser is available; can give 6–12 puffs pMDI via spacer, on the way to hospital. Three important points in daily use (not rescue use) of spacer:

1. Load with one puff pMDI at a time.
2. Allow 30 seconds (timed) for inhalation of drug from loaded spacer.
3. Do not clean the spacer until the valve 'clogs up', as cleaning can cause static electricity, and the minimally charged medication particles of the pMDI 'stick' to the walls of the spacer. In short, 'One puff, 30 seconds, don't clean it'. When cleaning is needed, use detergent and leave to dry.

Nebuliser therapy

This is very useful in life-threatening and acute severe asthma. There are still parents who prefer their child under the age of 2 years to have nebuliser therapy, as they find it more effective, or because their child struggles with spacers.

Powder inhalers (e.g. Turbuhaler, Accuhaler, Aerolizer, Diskhaler)

These are useful from 7 years of age.

pMDIs (e.g. salbutamol, terbutaline)

These can be used alone in children over 8 years, but only 7% reaches the lungs. pMDIs should always be used with spacers, as this can triple the amount of drug delivered. Newer pMDIs (e.g. Autohaler) can automatically administer the dose on commencement of inspiration. CFC propellants have been phased out and replaced with hydrofluoroalkane (HFA) propellants, subsequent to the internationally agreed Montreal Protocol to protect the ozone layer.

Optimum management for the child

The Australian National Asthma Campaign's six-point plan is as follows:

1. Assess asthma severity.
2. Achieve best lung function.
3. Maintain best lung function—avoid trigger factors.
4. Maintain best lung function with optimal medication.
5. Develop an action plan.
6. Educate and review regularly.

This plan is available at <http://hna.ffh.vic.gov.au/asthma>. In keeping with this plan remember the following points:

1. Every child should have a written asthma treatment program, fully explained, and an appropriate crisis management plan.
2. Every child requires regular monitoring of her/his disease and its treatment, plus the complications of each, including growth (failure of linear growth can be due to undertreatment, or to overtreatment with steroids). Other treatment complications should be sought: tremor, hyperactivity (LABAs, SABAs), Cushingoid features (ICS, oral steroids), nausea, vomiting (theophylline).
3. Every child should be assessed for any inadequacy in current treatment, suggested by the following:

a. Frequent waking to use inhaled bronchodilators.

b. Need for inhaled treatment immediately upon awakening.

c. Evidence of bronchospasm during physical activity, and limitation of activity.

d. Using more than one pMDI per month.

e. Conversely using less than one pMDI per 3 months (non–compliance), particularly preventative therapy.

f. Using SABAs more than three times a week for relief of symptoms.

g. Time off school/work.

Common management issues

In the long case, the medical therapy may well be adequate, and the 'big opening' for discussion may be social and psychological issues related to asthma. The following headings include many of the more common problems encountered.

Is control optimal at home?

The child should be able to participate in all ordinary daily activities. The symptoms outlined above should be sought, and the treatment considered with respect to the child's age and ability. Maintaining physical fitness with exercise (e.g. swimming) and the treatment of exercise-induced asthma are very important. Allergen avoidance and removal from exposure to cigarette smoke also should be addressed, if relevant.

Is the crisis plan appropriate?

Is a nebuliser, or spacer, available for emergencies. How far away is the local doctor (is there a nebuliser there?), where is the nearest ambulance station, where is the nearest hospital? Has this child's asthma received appropriate priority triage in the past (both for ambulance and the department of emergency medicine at the nearest hospital)? The candidate should stress the importance of ensuring appropriate triaging of this child with severe asthma. Does the disease severity warrant home oxygen, subcutaneous terbutaline or adrenaline? Do the parents know when to 'bail out' nebulising at home, and bring child to the hospital? Parents should know to seek medical aid if they are worried by their child having a bad attack, if the child needs beta-2 agonists 2-hourly, if wheezing is not settling and continuing for over 24 hours, if symptoms worsen quickly, or there is little relief from beta-2 agonists.

Is there adequate education of those involved?

This includes education of the child, parents and teachers:

1. *The child.* Should know to take beta-2 agonist before exercise.
2. *The parents.* Need to understand the treatment and know when to initiate more frequent treatment, how to monitor the child. Do they understand that the child should not avoid sport at school? Are they aware of the prognosis?
3. *The teachers/school.* Is a pMDI with spacer available to the child at all times? Do teachers appreciate the need for treatment? Do sports instructors inappropriately exclude the child from games?

What is the main worry of the parents?

Uncertainty regarding the nature and outcome of asthma, effects on schooling, and home management of acute exacerbations are common causes for parental anxiety. Sometimes their fears are based on hearing about a severely affected patient, and then incorrectly extrapolating this to their child. The management of these parents is through education. However, in other children the approach is quite different. The risk of dying can be the major concern of the mother (and a realistic one) of a 10- to 14-year-old steroid-dependent asthmatic, who is exactly the sort of patient you may encounter in the examination. This issue should be addressed. In children with life-threatening asthma, the crisis plan must be clear, with consideration given to home oxygen, parenteral treatment, wearing an identification bracelet with medical details, even moving closer to the hospital.

Is there a problem with adherence to treatment?

Adherence to treatment in adolescence is often a problem, and there may also be parental concern about long-term corticosteroid usage, which can lead to non-adherence on their behalf. The added risk of peer pressure-induced smoking or medication avoidance is not an uncommon management problem. Another compliance issue is parents' almost invariable inability to stop smoking or, in many cases, even smoke away from the child, despite constant requests. This has been documented by testing the urine of the child for cotinine levels before and after education about smoking. The other point to explore is the responsibility of care—whether it belongs predominantly to the patient or parent—as this is a key issue in adolescence.

Is there an inappropriate amount of school being missed?

If long periods of school are being missed, the reason may not just be hospitalisation, and this area should be explored. There can be parent–child interdependence, or school avoidance, related to asthma. Parents not infrequently fear that school may aggravate the disease (related to exposure to viral illnesses, or assuming that rest at home is somehow beneficial). Treatment is planned around normal schooling.

Are social supports sufficient?

The family needs to be aware of the many supportive groups and services available (e.g. the Asthma Foundation), where to get printed information regarding asthma and the benefits and financial assistance to which they may be entitled, and should have access to a social worker to assist in these areas. Whether the family is coping, with the current supports, needs to be explored.

Other

There are of course many other issues, but they are beyond the scope of this section: it would require an entire book to cover the area adequately.

Neonatal intensive care unit graduate: chronic lung disease

Chronic lung disease (CLD) in the neonatal intensive care unit (NICU) graduate has two commonly used definitions:

1. Oxygen requirement beyond 28 days with abnormal chest X-ray (CXR).
2. Oxygen requirement beyond 36 weeks post-conceptual age.

The term describing the pathology of the condition, bronchopulmonary dysplasia (BPD), is often used interchangeably with CLD. CLD results predominantly from positive pressure ventilation of functionally immature lungs.

An increasingly large number of children with CLD are available for long-case participation. Many have had postnatal steroid therapy for prevention and/or treatment of CLD. Recently, evidence has accumulated that suggests that the risks of steroid therapy used postnatally in babies with CLD may outweigh the possible benefits.

In 2002, the American Academy of Pediatrics (AAP) and the Canadian Pediatric Society (CPS) issued guidelines for postnatal steroid therapy for CLD. In summary, they found that systemic administration of dexamethasone to preterm infants who are mechanically ventilated decreased the incidence of CLD and extubation failure, but did not decrease overall mortality; that treatment of infants with very low birth weight (VLBW) with dexamethasone is associated with an increased risk of short- and long-term complications including impaired growth and neurodevelopmental delay; and that no substantial short- or long-term benefits were demonstrated from the use of inhaled corticosteroids in the prevention or treatment of CLD. The short-term adverse effects included hyperglycaemia requiring insulin, hypertension, gastrointestinal bleeding, intestinal perforation, hypertrophic obstructive cardiomyopathy, poor weight gain, poor growth of head circumference, a trend towards a higher incidence of periventricular leukomalacia (PVL), and adrenal suppression.

Recommendations made by the AAP and CPS advised against the routine use of systemic dexamethasone for the prevention of CLD in infants with VLBW, and suggested that more trials were needed to evaluate other aspects (e.g. long-term neurodevelopmental assessment, alternative anti-inflammatory agents), but noted that corticosteroid use should be limited to exceptional clinical circumstances only (such as a baby on maximal ventilatory and oxygen support), after informed parental consent.

Advances have occurred in understanding that the pathogenesis of CLD is associated with an inflammatory cascade, with the involvement of cytokines in lung maturation and injury. Before the widespread use of antenatal steroids and surfactant, chorioamnionitis (CA) was associated with the occurrence of CLD. Recent studies suggest that CLD is not increased following exposure to CA. These studies have been in the current context of antenatal steroid and surfactant use.

The single most significant predictor of CLD developing is low gestational age. Complications of CLD may include pulmonary hypertension (if oxygenation not maintained), recurrent hospitalisation with lower respiratory infections such as RSV, and bronchial hyper-reactivity. The lungs of a baby with CLD have low compliance, with increased work of breathing.

History

Presenting complaint

Reason for current admission: commonly a deterioration associated with an intercurrent viral illness, or related to other complications of prematurity.

Past history

1. Pregnancy, gestation, delivery, birth weight, Apgar scores.
2. Initial resuscitation required, when intubated, underlying respiratory diagnosis (e.g. hyaline membrane disease, meconium aspiration), duration of ventilation, continuous positive airways pressure (CPAP), oxygen requirement.
3. Complications of ventilation (e.g. air leaks, subglottic stenosis, tracheal stenosis, tube blockage), apnoeic episodes, associated problems (e.g. patent ductus arteriosus [PDA], intraventricular haemorrhage [IVH], PVL, retinopathy of prematurity [ROP]).
4. Drugs/treatments used (e.g. salbutamol, ipratropium bromide, theophylline, corticosteroids, diuretics, RSV intravenous immune globulin [RSV-Ig], palivizumab).

5. Monitoring since extubation, discharge details (e.g. age, weight, treatment).
6. Hospitalisation details (frequency, duration, usual treatment).
7. Outpatient clinics attended (where, how often, usual tests: e.g. chest X-ray, pulse oximetry).
8. Any recent change in symptoms or management.

Current status

1. Symptoms:
   a. Respiratory-specific: e.g. tachypnoea, poor feeding, poor weight gain, fatigue, wheeze, cough, fever, cyanosis, apnoea, plus symptoms related to O_2 use (epitaxis, nasal problems: discharge, obstruction).
   b. Non-respiratory-specific for conditions the child is at risk of: gastro-oesophageal reflux (GOR), vomiting, feeding difficulties, aspiration.
2. Home management: e.g. nasal oxygen, nebulised bronchodilators, oral theophylline, diuretic (e.g. frusemide), antibiotics.
3. Status of other systems where ex-premmies have increased risk of dysfunction: e.g. ears, eyes, development, renal, cardiac, gut from necrotising enterocolitis (NEC).

Social history

Disease impact on family, financial consideration (e.g. nebuliser, oxygen cylinders, oxygen 'concentrator'—actually a blender), social supports, understanding of disease, expectations for future, access to paediatrician, hospital, any exposure to tobacco smoke.

Immunisation

Routine (what age given). Specific (RSV-Ig; palivizumab).

Examination

Table 15.1 gives an approach to the cardiorespiratory examination (specifically) of the NICU graduate. It does not include looking for other complications of prematurity (e.g. IVH), but does include toxicities relating to ventilation and oxygen.

Management

Prevention

No data confirms unequivocally the efficacy of any preventative strategy. Antenatal corticosteroids do not alter the rate of CLD (although they do decrease mortality and development of hyaline membrane disease [HMD]). However, guidelines used include the following:

* Avoidance of excess fluid intake, early administration of surfactant to babies with HMD requiring assisted ventilation.
* With conventional ventilation, avoidance of overdistension and hypocarbia, use of higher rates (60 breaths per minute) and lower inspiratory times (0.3–0.35 seconds) (reduces incidence of airleak).
* With high-frequency oscillatory ventilation (HFOV) use of high-volume strategy (decreases incidence of oxygen requirement at 36 weeks post-menstrual age). Note that the benefits of HFOV in preventing CLD are outweighed by risks of air leaks and IVH.

Table 15.1   An approach to the cardiorespiratory examination of the NICU graduate

General observations
Parameters
- Weight
- Height
- Head circumference
- Percentiles

Sick or well, pallor, cyanosis, alertness, movement
Nutritional status: visual scan for muscle bulk, fat
Respiratory
- Distress (tachypnoea, tracheal tug, intercostal, subcostal recession)
- Audible wheeze
- Stridor (subglottic stenosis, vocal cord damage from intubation)
- Cough
- Cyanosis
- Oxygen cannula

Chest
Inspection
Breathing pattern
Respiratory rate
Chest deformity
- Pectus carinatum
- Increased anteroposterior diameter (hyperinflation)
- Rib rosary (vitamin D deficiency)
Scars
- Previous tracheostomy
- Intercostal catheters
- Repair of patent ductus

Palpation
Tracheal position
Apex position
Palpable pulmonary valve closure
Right ventricular overactivity
Percussion can be deferred until after auscultation, as it may cause crying in younger infants.

Auscultation
Lungs
- 'Air entry'

- Breath sounds
- Vocal resonance
- Crackles
- Wheezes
Heart
- Loudness of second heart sound (pulmonary hypertension)
- Murmur of PDA

Percussion
For hyperinflation, consolidation
After the above, palpate the liver for ptosis (hyperinflation) and percuss for liver span (hepatomegaly from congestive cardiac failure [CCF])

Upper limbs
Hands: scars of previous intravenous cannulae
Nails
- Clubbing
- Cyanosis
Pulse
- Rate
- Paradoxus
- Hyperdynamic (PDA)
- Pulsus alternans (CCF)
Blood pressure: hypertension (renovascular hypertension due to umbilical catheter, corticosteroid use or renal dysfunction)

Head
Eyes
- Nystagmus (ROP)
- Visual acuity (ROP)
- Fundi: ROP (and grading of this)
Nose: deformity due to prolonged intubation

Lower limbs
Palpate for ankle oedema (CCF)

Other
Temperature chart (infection)

CCF = congestive cardiac failure; PDA = patent ductus arteriosus; ROP = retinopathy of prematurity.

Oxygen therapy

Adequate oxygenation is the most important factor for growth and development. Home oxygen is usually administered via nasal prongs. Low-flow oxygen (less than 2 litres/min) can be provided via various different-sized cylinders, or by an oxygen 'concentrator' (actually it is a blender), which is electrically powered, so requires a power point. All families must be supplied with cylinders (usually one size E, which is small and portable, and two size C, which are larger to be kept at home) in case a power cut makes the concentrator inoperative. If the flow of oxygen needed is above 1 litre/min, a concentrator is cheaper than cylinders. Concentrators are rarely used in infants; respiratory physicians rarely use subnasal O_2 >1–1.5 litres/min, as nasal problems become a major issue. Concentrators do not deliver 100% O_2 as cylinders do.

Oxygen is needed if the child's PO_2 in air is below 60 torrs. The aim is for the oxygen saturation (SaO_2) to be between 94% and 98% in the awake and asleep phases. Aiming for higher levels may worsen lung disease and does not necessarily improve long-term growth or development. The actual range is controversial. Neonatologists generally use a lower limit of 90%, but respiratory physicians generally use a higher range (>94%), which is probably reflective of the age of infants and hence the risk of ROP. In the early phase, a lower SaO_2 is usually accepted, but upon discharge when infants are well over the corrected term of gestation, a higher minimal SaO_2 is usually used. Oxygen administration is associated with increased weight gain, decreased pulmonary hypertension, decreased SIDS-like events and decreased morbidity and mortality. Home oxygen therapy avoids prolonged and expensive hospitalisation.

At discharge from NICU, the average requirement for CLD is low-flow subnasal oxygen at 250–1000 mL/minute. The median duration of oxygen requirement is 6–10 months. Weaning should occur very slowly, over about 12 weeks, guided by regular saturation monitoring. An intercurrent acute respiratory tract infection may require reinstitution of oxygen.

Increased oxygen is needed during increased activity, feeding and sleeping (rapid eye movement sleep is associated with increased activity, irregular breathing and carries a risk of hypoxia), so that monitoring of these times indicates when the child is able to cope in air. Oxygen is discontinued first when awake, then eventually when asleep. These children may be admitted to hospital overnight, for oximetry off oxygen while asleep. If the saturation level is consistently below 94%, oxygen therapy is still required; if it stays at or above 97%, then oxygen can probably be discontinued. Alternatively, as an outpatient, a period of oximetry for one hour when awake demonstrating saturations consistently above 97% indicates supplemental oxygen is no longer required. Once oxygen is discontinued, weight gain is watched closely over the ensuing few weeks to ensure adequate growth is occurring. As above, note variation of acceptability of minimum SaO_2.

Growth and development

Children with CLD are at high risk of associated neurodevelopmental and growth problems. Much of the child's energy expenditure is related to the work of breathing, and this contributes to failure to thrive unless nutritional supplementation to 120–150% of usual requirements is achieved. Motor delay is not uncommon (e.g. poor muscle bulk, general debility) and, if not associated with intellectual impairment, may improve with time. Developmental assessment (intellect, vision, hearing) is regularly performed to enable appropriate intervention.

Nutrition

As mentioned above, adequate nutrition is of paramount importance. Tachypnoeic infants do not feed well, the time they take for a breastfeed or bottle being proportional to the severity of their CLD. As these children may need to avoid fluid overload, the quality of feed should be altered, not the quantity. Usual requirements are around 140–180 kilocalories/kg/day, but the real test is whether the child grows, and these figures are guides only. Calorie supplementation may be achieved by increasing the caloric content of infant milk formulae to 24–32 kcal/30 mL. Added calories may comprise increased measures of milk powder (extra scoops), glucose polymers, vegetable oil or medium-chain triglyceride oil. In breastfed infants, small-volume high-calorie supplements can be given. Calorie wastage must be avoided; this occurs when too many calories are given.

Another problem is the lack of oral intake early (while in NICU), with poor tolerance to and lack of interest in feeds, which may persist. Some children require feeding at night via gastrostomy (often with fundoplication), particularly infants with gastro-oesophageal reflux. Nasogastric tube feeding is generally avoided (it can aggravate reflux and cause increased nasal problems), but is sometimes necessary. Provision of adequate vitamins and minerals (especially iron, folate and fluoride) is important. Supplemental oxygen can improve nutrition.

Obstructive airways disease and bronchodilators

These patients have obstructive lung disease, with variable airway hyperactivity, but are not uniform in their response to drugs. Many have hypertrophied lung smooth muscle and respond to bronchodilators (even when preterm) earlier than true 'asthmatics'. Combinations of inhaled beta-2 agonists, ipratropium bromide, ICS, sodium cromoglycate (given by nebuliser or pMDI with spacer), oral corticosteroids or oral theophylline are widely used with variable success. Most units try these medications for at least some weeks to ascertain efficacy. Theophylline stimulates the respiratory centre (useful for treating central apnoea) and increases diaphragmatic contractility; serum levels are checked regularly. Oral dexamethasone side effects may include hyperglycaemia, myocardial hypertrophy, hypertension, gastrointestinal bleeding or perforation, and adrenal suppression. Despite the common usage, there is inadequate long-term data to recommend the use of any beta agonist, ipratropium bromide, or theophylline in CLD.

Fluid balance and diuretics

These infants tend to accumulate interstitial lung fluid; fluid overload should be avoided. Fluid intake of up to 180 mL/kg/day are usually well tolerated. Diuretics may need to be used (especially in children with some degree of cor pulmonale). Diuretics may act as pulmonary vasodilators. Initially, frusemide with potassium supplementation is used for short periods. For longer-term use, hydrochlorothiazide and spironolactone may be used (fewer side effects than frusemide). Serum urea and electrolytes should be monitored to avoid side effects (hypokalaemia, hyponatraemia, metabolic alkalosis). Prolonged frusemide therapy (over 2 weeks) can cause renal calcification, detectable on ultrasound. Although diuretics improve lung mechanics and oxygenation in the short term, no long-term benefits have been demonstrated.

Immunisation and RSV immune prophylaxis

Routine immunisation is particularly important in these children. Often allowed to lag behind because of their prolonged stay in the NICU, immunisation should be given at the appropriate chronological age, uncorrected for prematurity. Some units use RSV Ig. Prophylaxis with IV or IM RSV Ig (which is very expensive) significantly decreases incidence of RSV infection and subsequent hospitalisation by about 50%. It can be given on an individual needs basis on discharge from hospital, and then monthly during the peak RSV season. The other preparation used for immune prophylaxis is palivizumab, a humanised RSV monoclonal antibody given intramuscularly. Infants with a gestational age below 28 weeks can benefit from prophylaxis up to 12 months of age, whereas infants with a gestational age of 29–32 weeks may benefit up to 6 months of age. Treatment is for children under 2 years of age who are still having oxygen, and is used in the anticipated RSV season for 4–6 months of the year.

Avoidance of tobacco smoke

Smoking in the house is forbidden if a baby is receiving oxygen, because of the fire hazard. However exposure to smoke still occurs. Exposure to smoking increases pulmonary inflammation, worsens lung function, increases the risk of developing respiratory tract infections and increases the risk of cot death. Parents should be encouraged to stop smoking, but this is rarely successful, and this is a difficult issue.

Social issues

The degree of psychosocial difficulty depends to some extent on the associated problems the child has. If there is severe neurological impairment, there is a parental separation rate approaching 50%. There tend to be three phases after the initial discharge of the child from hospital: first, a 'euphoric' phase, which may last about 6 weeks; then a period of despair and exhaustion, lasting from around 6 weeks to 6 months post-discharge; and finally the stage of acceptance. Another common problem is the 'vulnerable child syndrome', a parent–infant behaviour disorder that may include problems with feeding, difficulty separating from the mother, overindulgence and over-protection, leading to the child 'running the household'. This may be prevented by spending more time with the parents, educating them in potential problem areas that are well recognised, by normalising the management of the baby, and by normal and appropriate discipline.

Associated apnoea and bradycardia

Children with CLD appear to be at higher risk of apnoea and sudden death than other infants. Some units provide monitors for the first few months after discharge home. Sleep laboratory studies may show unrecognised bradycardia/apnoea and may guide therapy (e.g. theophylline), but are not useful in prognosis. Adequate oxygenation by low-flow oxygen is the most important aspect to prevent unrecognised hypoxia and bradycardia.

Other problems

Excluding the numerous other complications of prematurity, the other common problem these children experience is that of intercurrent viral illnesses, which can become complicated by bacterial superinfection, which is life-threatening. Early insti-tution of antibiotic therapy for respiratory infections is recommended. If these children become acutely unwell, with respiratory distress, the parents should have the child checked, preferably by a doctor familiar with them, or at the nearest hospital. They should be told to resist the temptation to just 'turn up the oxygen', or recommence it if discontinued previously.

Prognosis

Most problems with CLD occur in the first year of life. Long term, most children with CLD have minimal functional abnormalities, mainly due to the increase in the number of alveoli that occurs from birth (20 million saccules at term; air–tissue interface 2.8 m^2), producing new alveoli up to the age of 8 years (300 million alveoli; air–tissue interface 32 m^2).

Cystic fibrosis

This is a common long case and is expected to be handled well. Survival continues to increase, with overall median survival in Australia at the time of writing (2005) at over 36 years (males 44, females 28). Progress in the evolution of gene therapy is slower than expected, but a side effect of gene research has been better understanding of airway biology and airway defence systems. Lung and liver transplantation have become standards of care, and their number increases each year. Longer survival has led to more patients developing cystic fibrosis–related diabetes (CFRD) and musculoskeletal complications.

Genetics

Cystic fibrosis is autosomal recessive. Molecular genetics: cystic fibrosis (CF) is caused by mutations in the **c**ystic **f**ibrosis **t**ransmembrane conductance **r**egulator gene (CFTR); the locus is on the long arm of chromosome 7 (7q31.2); the protein is called CFTR. Over 1300 different mutations in the CFTR gene are known; almost all are point mutations or small (1–84 base pair) deletions. The CFTR gene codes for a 1480-amino acid integral membrane protein of 170 kDa, a cyclic-AMP-regulated chloride channel on the apical surface of epithelial cells. The deficiency of CFTR function leads to abnormal regulation of chloride channels and decides the phenotype of the epithelial cells. The most common mutation worldwide is delta-F508, where there is deletion of phenylalanine at the 508th amino acid within the CFTR protein; this accounts for 30–80% of mutant alleles, depending on the ethnic group.

There are five functional classes of mutation in CF:

- Class I mutations cause *reduced or absent synthesis* of CFTR, and are associated with nonsense, frameshift or splice junction mutations (e.g. G542X: 2.5% of cases; no synthesis of CFTR).
- Class II mutations cause a *block in protein processing*, and are associated with missense mutations and amino acid deletions (e.g. delta-F508: 70% of cases in Australia; blocked processing of CFTR).
- Class III mutations cause a *block in the regulation of the CFTR chloride channel*, and are associated with missense mutations (e.g. G551D: 1.6% of cases; blocked regulation of CFTR).
- Class IV mutations cause *altered conductance of CFTR chloride channel*, and associated with missense mutations (e.g. R117H: 0.3% of cases).
- Class V mutations cause *decreased splicing of normal CFTR*, which decreases membrane CFTR function and can act concurrently with other mutations on the same allele.

Different mutations are more common in different countries. It is not necessary to be homozygous for the same mutation to have CF. The most common defects can be detected within hours by polymerase chain reaction (PCR). Gene mutations are weakly correlated with clinical severity: genotype/phenotype correlations are strongest for pancreatic insufficiency with patients homozygous for the delta-F508 mutation being almost always pancreatic insufficient (99%). Classes I–III mutations tend to produce more severe disease than IV–V mutations. Gene frequency in most Caucasian populations is

1 in 25, giving an incidence of 1 in 2500. In contrast, incidence in African-Americans is 1 in 15,000 and in Asian populations approximates 1 in 31,000.

History

Presenting complaint.

Reason for current admission: often a combination of loss of weight, appetite and energy, and an increase in cough, sputum and school/work missed, warranting a 'tune up'. This is timed to fit in with the family, e.g. before holidays.

Current status

Respiratory disease

1. Symptoms: upper respiratory tract infection (URTI) symptoms, impaired exercise tolerance (important but relatively uncommon in children); cough frequency, severity (cough syncope extremely rare), nocturnal or exercise-induced wheeze or asthma, recent change in pattern; sputum volume, colour, blood, and any recent change in these; fatigue, dyspnoea, wheeze, response to bronchodilators, peak flow pattern (limited value); need for home oxygen; chest pain; chronic sinusitis; glue ears; nasal polyps (nasal polyps produce symptoms of rhinorrhea, nasal blockage, snoring and even occasionally have protruded from the nose).
2. Infective agents: acquisition of chronic infection with *Pseudomonas* is an important prognostic factor, with early acquisition (under 5–6 years) of mucoid *Pseudomonas* being associated with increased mortality, especially in females, and increased morbidity. Also *Burkholderia cepacia* acquisition is important.
3. Past complications: e.g. pneumothorax, moderate-large haemoptyses, allergic bronchopulmonary aspergillosis (ABPA).
4. Investigations: e.g. sputum colonisation, chest X-ray, pulmonary function tests, overnight oximetry.
5. Home management: e.g. exercise, physiotherapy (frequency, type and by whom), PEP mask; nebulised antibiotics, saline, bronchodilators, or dornase alpha; pMDIs (bronchodilators, ICS); oral antibiotic or corticosteroid; venous port access for parenteral antibiotics.
6. Future therapy plans: use of newer antibiotics, oral or nebulised; corticosteroids; consideration of lung transplant, gene therapy, experimental therapies.

Gastrointestinal disease

1. Symptoms: e.g. growth, weight loss, appetite, dietary history, stool pattern (oily, pale, bulky or offensive, blood, melaena), passing wind and burping (may not be popular but can have an impact on kids at school), abdominal pain, vomiting, haematemesis, heartburn.
2. Past complications: e.g. meconium ileus or equivalent (this is termed DIOS [distal intestinal obstruction syndrome] now), rectal prolapse, jaundice, portal hypertension, fibrosing colonopathy, gastrostomy.
3. Investigations: e.g. faecal fat studies, liver function tests, hepatobiliary ultrasonography or Tc-99m scintigraphy.
4. Home management: e.g. pancreatic enzymes, vitamins, salt tablets.
5. Future plans: e.g. gastrostomy, sclerotherapy, liver transplantation.

Other systems

Symptoms, past complications including episodes of dehydration (which is a significant problem in warmer climates, and which increases the risk of pneumonia and DIOS), investigations, home management and future plans regarding diabetes mellitus, cardiac disease, growth failure, pubertal delay, arthropathy.

Past history of CF

Initial symptoms, investigations and management prior to diagnosis, diagnosis (when, where, how), subsequent investigations and management, progress of disease, hospitalisation details (frequency, duration, usual treatment), complications of disease and treatment, outpatient clinics attended (where, how often, routine tests performed), any recent change in symptoms or management.

Immunisations (especially pneumococcal, influenza vaccines).

Venous access is a serious issue, especially as aggressive treatment now starts earlier. Complications of totally implantable venous access devices can be serious.

Allergy may be an important issue, with some children requiring desensitisation.

Social history

Disease impact on patient

Growth, development, self-image (may have short stature, intravenous access ports, offensive flatus, decreased ability for physical activity), independence, requests for transfer to adult care, compliance (reluctant to take medications in front of peers), schooling (attendance, performance, teacher awareness of disease and its treatment, peer interactions), employment prospects, limitation of activities of daily living (including sport), depression (inevitability of death), consideration of marriage, prevention (smoking). Fertility must be discussed: what has been said and to whom? Many units normally talk with boys around 14 years of age and discuss all health-related issues, including normal sexual function, reduced ejaculate, choices for future with microaspiration sperm and IVF techniques. Smoking must be discussed. Alcohol is another discussion area for the pancreatic-sufficient children, as they have an increased risk of pancreatitis.

Disease impact on parents

Restricted social life, marriage stability, maternal depression, denial, fears for the future, requirement to stop smoking, financial considerations (medical treatment, food, travel, awareness of benefits available, modifications of holiday plans).

Disease impact on siblings

Sibling rivalry, hostility, effect of family's financial burden, genetic counselling.

Social supports

Social worker, Cystic Fibrosis Association, community nurse, extended family, close friends, CF 'social network', respite from managing child, financial support.

Coping

Who attends with patient, who gives treatment, confidence with management, parents' main concerns, degree of understanding of disease, expectations for future, understanding of prognosis (by patient and parent).

Access

To local doctor, paediatrician, cystic fibrosis clinic sister, Cystic Fibrosis Association, hospital.

Family history and genetic aspects

Other members with CF; whether other siblings screened, more children planned, prenatal diagnosis (and subsequent management for positive result) discussed; patient's fertility, female patient's contraception, pregnancy risk (have these been addressed?).

Immunisation

Routine, early measles immunisation, gammaglobulin for measles contacts, requesting yearly influenza vaccine.

Examination

The approach given in Table 15.2 assesses patients with CF for disease progression, severity and current status of disease. It looks particularly at clubbing, flap, chest deformity, cor pulmonale, nutrition, puberty, diabetes, chronic liver disease, hypertrophic pulmonary osteoarthropathy. Two very important signs are the cough and the sputum, and these may give a better indication of the state of the lungs than any other finding on physical examination.

Table 15.2   Examination of the child with cystic fibrosis

General inspection
Position patient: standing, with adequate exposure, for a complete examination, but sensitive to the patient's modesty. Although ideal, the patient being fully undressed (as stated in previous editions) is neither practical nor sensitive in most patients, and should not be encouraged.
Parameters
- Weight
- Height
- Head circumference
- Percentiles

Sick or well
Pubertal status (delay)
Vital signs
- Respiration
- Pulse
- Temperature
- Urinalysis (glucose)

Nutrition
- Muscle bulk (protein): e.g. biceps, quadriceps
- Subcutaneous fat: e.g. mid-arm, subscapular
- Pallor (anaemia)

Peripheral stigmata of CLD
Oedema (hypoproteinaemia)

Upper limbs
Nails
- Clubbing
- Cyanosis
- Leukonychia (CLD)

Fingers
- Fingertip prickmarks (BSL testing)
- HPOA

Palms
- Erythema (CLD)
- Crease pallor (anaemia)

Pulse
- Paradoxus (severity of airway obstruction)
- Alternans (CCF)
- Bounding (hypercarbia)

Flap
- Hypercarbia
- Liver failure (rare)

Joints: arthropathy
Skin
- Bruising or petechiae (CLD, vitamin K deficiency)
- Spider naevi (CLD)
- Scratch marks (cholestasis)

Muscle: bulk (palpate, if not done already)
Axilla: hair, odour (Tanner staging)

Head
Eyes
- Conjunctival pallor
- Scleral icterus
- Retinal venous dilation (hypercarbia)

Ears
- Secretory otitis media
- Hearing (aminoglycosides)

Continued

Table 15.2 *(Continued)*

Nose: nasal polyps

Mouth

- Angular cheilosis
- Central cyanosis (lips, tongue)
- State of teeth, dental hygiene
- Oral thrush

Face

- Cushingoid (systemic corticosteroids)
- Acne and facial hair (pubertal status)

Chest

Inspection

- Chest deformity: pectus carinatum, increased AP diameter (hyperinflation), thoracic kyphosis
- Scars: previous pneumothorax, bilateral lung transplant, venous access port (e.g. Port-A-Cath, Hickman)
- Tanner stage of breast development
- Harrison's sulcus
- Chest expansion

Cough: moist, productive, request sputum

Perform peak flow measurement if meter available (limited usefulness)

Palpation: tracheal position, apex position, palpable pulmonary valve closure, right ventricular overactivity.

Percussion for hyperinflation, consolidation

Auscultation (note: may be normal even in moderately severe CF)

- Air entry
- Breath sounds
- Vocal resonance
- Adventitious sounds
- Crackles
- Wheezes
- Loudness of second heart sound (pulmonary hypertension)
- Gallop rhythm (cor pulmonale)

Abdomen

Inspection

- Distension (poor abdominal musculature with protein-calorie malnutrition, ascites with CLD)
- Scars (e.g. gastrostomy, previous meconium ileus, hepatobiliary surgery for common bile duct stenosis, fundoplication)
- Venous access port (e.g. Infuse-A-Port),
- Prominent abdominal wall veins (CLD)
- Needle marks (diabetes mellitus)
- Tanner stage of pubic hair
- Striae (corticosteroids)

Palpation

- Liver ptosed (chest hyperinflation); liver edge—is it firm, or is it bumpy (cirrhotic)?
- Hepatomegaly (fatty liver with malabsorption or corticosteroid use, CCF with cor pulmonale)
- Splenomegaly (portal hypertension)
- Faecal masses (DIOS can present as a right iliac fossa mass)
- Herniae

Assess for ascites (fluid thrill, shifting dullness)

Examine genitalia

- Tanner staging
- Hydrocoele

Inspect anus for rectal prolapse

Lower limbs

Inspection

- Toe clubbing
- Bruising (vitamin K deficiency, CLD)
- Joint swelling (arthropathy)

Palpation: ankle oedema (hypoproteinaemia)

Gait examination

- Peripheral neuropathy (vitamin E deficiency)
- Cerebellar ataxia (vitamin E deficiency)
- Proximal muscle weakness (corticosteroids)

(Note that clinically evident vitamin deficiencies are very rare in CF, so signs of vitamin A and D deficiencies are extremely unlikely to be seen.)

BSL = blood sugar level; CCF = congestive cardiac failure; CLD = chronic liver disease; HPOA = hypertrophic pulmonary osteoarthropathy.

Investigations

Diagnostic

Neonatal screening

Most infants with CF are detected in this way in Australia at present (2006), as neonatal screening is now universal across Australia and New Zealand. Each Australian state performs this slightly differently, although all check immunoreactive trypsin (IRT) on the neonatal screening blood test, followed by gene analysis on the top 1% IRTs. Blood immunoreactive trypsin (IRT) levels are measured in the Guthrie blood sample. IRT levels in CF are 2.5–7.5 times the normal range. Samples with IRT levels above the 99th centile are tested for the delta-F508 mutation. Homozygotes are detected directly. Heterozygotes are recalled for sweat testing. Making the diagnosis when children are presymptomatic does have a significant positive impact on prognosis.

The critical aspect is accurate diagnosis; it needs to be confirmed. Sweat tests should be done only in centres that do at least 50 per year (so private pathology laboratories may not be appropriate places to do it). The diagnosis is made based on two mutations plus a positive sweat test, or consistent clinical features, or one mutation plus a positive sweat test. It is possible to have two mutations, but a normal sweat test and no clinical manifestations (except probably male infertility). Also, there can be difficult scenarios with borderline sweat test results. Two mutations alone does not equal diagnosis; these children are at risk of CF-related disease over time.

Sweat testing

The Gibson-Cooke classic technique requires 100 mg of forearm sweat obtained by pilocarpine electrophoresis. In 98% of CF patients, sweat chloride is >60 mmol/L, and this is diagnostic. However, 2% of patients have sweat chlorides below this level, usually between 50 and 60 mmol/L (the equivocal range), but about 1 in 1000 will have a value in the 40s, and may require direct gene probing or pancreatic stimulation testing. False-negative results can occur in children with pancreatic sufficiency or oedema. False-positive results can occur in children with malnutrition (e.g. due to coeliac disease or emotional deprivation), immune deficiency (e.g. AIDS, hypogammaglobulinaemia), eczema, adrenal insufficiency and hypothyroidism.

Other

Pancreatic stimulation testing can diagnose CF in cases with normal or borderline sweat tests; it will always reveal abnormal ductal function in CF. At diagnosis, patients need a faecal sample to check for fat globules, chymotrypsin, or elastase, to document presence and severity, or absence, of steatorrhoea. Eighty-five per cent of CF patients have fat malabsorption (stool fat output over 7% oral fat intake), i.e. they have pancreatic insufficiency (PI). Serum vitamin levels are checked early, as vitamin E deficiency can be corrected and may result in improved IQ (compared to loss of IQ with persistent vitamin E deficiency).

Monitoring of disease

Not many routine tests are done in CF:

1. Routine clinic visits, usually at least every 3 months: note weight, nutrition, sputum, spirometry.
2. Documentation of disease progression at intervals of 6 months to 1 year. The following may be done: chest X-ray (CXR), pulmonary function tests, liver function tests, full blood count, measurement of skin fold thickness. Vitamin

levels and work up for ABPA with total IgE can be performed annually. A high-resolution CT scan of the thorax in primary and secondary school can assess progress of bronchiectasis.

Other investigations as indicated

1. Cardiac: electrocardiography, echocardiography (right ventricular hypertrophy) usually only done when heading for transplant.
2. Gastrointestinal: serum protein and albumin, liver function tests, coagulation studies, abdominal X-ray (meconium ileus, equivalent or peritonitis), abdominal ultrasound (gall bladder, liver), hepatobiliary Tc-99m scintigraphy (common bile duct strictures), percutaneous transhepatic cholangiogram (PTC) and endoscopic retrograde cholangiopancreatography (ERCP) to detect strictures, pancreatic function tests.
3. Other. Whether CFRD should be screened for, with an oral glucose tolerance test (GTT) in children over 10 years, is debatable. A fasting blood glucose is not particularly useful in this context, as it does not exclude diabetes and can be normal in patients with significant CFRD; a GTT is a better test. Urea and electrolytes may be used to assess salt loss, and dye studies in patients with venous access ports can be used for assessment of port function.

Management

The aims of management include: (a) ensuring optimal growth and development; (b) delaying progress of pulmonary disease; (c) preventing/treating complications; (d) normal lifestyle; (e) patient and family education; (f) recognition and treatment of psychological problems.

Hospitalisation

Parameters used in assessing the need for hospitalisation (usually patients are seen in clinic every 2–3 months) include decreasing weight (or poor appetite), diminished exercise tolerance or deteriorating lung function test results, increased cough and sputum production. School holidays are usually chosen (if possible), as this interferes less with lifestyle, although the reality of hospital bed shortages often means patients are admitted when a bed is available rather than when it is convenient to the child.

Treatment of lung disease

Antibiotics

The following is a general guide. Intermittent oral antibiotics can be used for exacerbations of disease with minimal respiratory symptoms. Ciprofloxacin plus nebulised antibiotics such as tobramycin or colistin may be used in patients with chronic *Pseudomonas aeruginosa* infection. Continuous oral antibiotics may be appropriate with persistent sputum production or deteriorating lung function. Nebulised antibiotics can be cycled one month on, one month off, or alternate tobramycin/colistin month by month. Intravenous (IV) therapy is reserved for a sick child or deterioration in status on appropriate home treatment, or specifically for eradication-type therapy, if that is required. Occasionally regular admissions are booked for children with very severe lung disease.

Microbiology of lung pathogens dictates usual treatment plans. Initially, the main organisms encountered are: *Staphylococcus aureus, Streptococcus pneumoniae, Haemophilus influenzae, P. aeruginosa* non-mucoid (probably cause of at least 30% exacerbations in children under 2 years of age), mucoid strains of *P. aeruginosa* (in >50% of CF patients). *Burkholderia cepacia* infection may be associated with rapidly progressive lung disease. Approximately one-third of CF patients have precipitating antibodies to *Aspergillus fumigatus*, and two-thirds have positive skin tests for this. Infection-control issues are important. Cross-infection must be minimised, avoiding risk of transmission of *B. cepacia* or *P. aeruginosa* between infected and noninfected patients. Some clinics cohort by strain of *P. aeruginosa* as well.

The following points should be noted:

1. **Sputum cultures** do reflect lung flora in CF (but only in children who can produce sputum easily). Oropharyngeal cultures have poor sensitivity and positive prediction (around 55%), and better specificity and negative prediction (around 85%).

2. **Choice of antibiotic** for hospital treatment is usually an antipseudomonal penicillin (e.g. ticarcillin with clavulate, piperacillin) and an aminoglycoside (e.g. tobramycin), plus oral flucloxacillin. Cephalosporins such as ceftazidime, nalidixic acid derivatives and polymyxins may also be used.

3. **Dose of antibiotic.** Abnormal metabolism, and rapid excretion, of antibiotics occurs. 'Double dose' antibiotics are needed, especially aminoglycosides (e.g. tobramycin, gentamicin). Adult-dose IV antibiotics can be given from 7 years of age, in general, but this does depend on the antibiotic. As patients get older, tobramycin dose may need to be wound back. Aminoglycosides are given as single daily doses.

4. **Route of antibiotic:**

    a. *Intravenous (IV)*. Issues include the problem of venous access: peripheral lines (standard and 'long') versus implantable devices (Infuse-A-Port, Port-A-Cath).

    b. *Inhaled*. Many units use nebulised antibiotics (e.g. gentamicin, colistin, ticarcillin, tobramycin) at home in some children. Their use is associated with a dramatic decrease in hospital admissions. Disadvantages include allergy, resistance, expense, bronchoconstriction (infrequent) and time required for nebulisation (compliance problem). The last of these can be aided by using a 'Miser' attached to the nebuliser, which allows increased drug delivery; it is important to have the appropriate nebuliser device for the drug.

    c. *Oral*. For mild-to-moderate exacerbation of lung disease (outpatient management), directed against the most likely (non-pseudomonal) flora. Cotrimoxazole or amoxycillin with clavulanic acid can be used. If no improvement occurs with first choice, change antibiotics based on sputum sensitivities. Some centres give oral flucloxacillin prophylactically in the first year. Ciprofloxacin, an oral antipseudomonal quinolone, can be used in older children for a short period, usually 2–3 weeks. However, resistance can develop quickly. Longer courses are used for eradication of *P. aeruginosa*, usually one month of oral ciprofloxacin plus two months of nebulised colistin.

    Any of these modes of delivery can be used at home.

Most exacerbations of chest disease are probably due to viral infections.

Azithromycin is used as an adjunct treatment, particularly with the aim of reducing the number of days of IV antibiotic use required. It has a long intracellular half-life and can be given three times a week, but is quite expensive.

Chest physiotherapy
Parents and patient are educated in home physiotherapy from the time of initial diagnosis. 'Classical' physiotherapy comprises postural drainage, percussion and vibration,

and requires the assistance of a partner. It is usually performed for 10–20 minutes, once or twice a day. It is most useful in children with chronic sputum production, but its value is uncertain in older children with 'dry' chests. It remains useful in acute exacerbations of disease. Tips are no longer used as they are known to increase gastro-oesophageal reflux disease and can be associated with worsening lung disease.

Other methods encourage independence and may be used in combination with the above. Positive expiratory pressure (PEP) masks are used by several centres. The resistance of the mask is variable; the appropriate value can be chosen by lung-function testing to document the highest increase in forced vital capacity achieved. It is usually used for 10 minutes at a time, once or twice a day. Forced expiratory technique can be taught from 8–9 years. Exercise should be encouraged from a very young age and especially encouraged to continue in the teenage years.

Nebulised treatment
Bronchodilators, saline, hypertonic saline, mucolytics may be used, and are best given before chest physiotherapy. Antibiotics, cromolyn or corticosteroids, when used, are best given immediately after physiotherapy. Hypertonic (6%) saline can achieve improvement comparable to that with dornase alpha (see below). Nebulised amiloride (a sodium channel blocker) has been trialled without great success. Nebulised uridine triphosphate (UTP) and other stimulators of calcium-dependent non-CFTR-activated chloride channels have been trialled with equivocal results. Other inhalation-based treatments trialled have included the antiprotease proteins, recombinant alpha-1-anti-trypsin, and recombinant human secretory leukoprotease inhibitor (rhSLPI).

Bronchodilator treatment
Increased bronchial reactivity is found in 40–75% of CF patients. Standard anti-asthma treatment may be used, including inhaled (nebulised or pMDI) beta-2 agonists (e.g. salbutamol). Note that the condition of some patients can deteriorate following bronchodilators, with a loss of airway wall tone, and dynamic airway compression.

Anti-inflammatory treatment
Long-term use of oral corticosteroids (OCS) and of ibuprofen has been shown to slow the progress of CF. Inhaled corticosteroids (ICS) have yet to be studied adequately, but despite this are the most widely used. Asthma should be appropriately managed. Ibuprofen is not often used, as drug levels need to be monitored and a particular range adhered to; also, some adverse events can occur, including GI bleeding.

Mucolytic treatment: dornase alfa (recombinant human deoxyribonuclease 1)
Dornase alfa (rhDNase 1) is an enzyme that cleaves extracellular DNA and decreases viscoelasticity of purulent lung secretions. It is expensive, and used in children with chronic suppurative disease or obstructive disease, with forced vital capacity (FVC) at least 40% of predicted. It is impossible to predict who will respond to it. A small number of patients may get worse or show no change, and a third will show a marked improvement in lung function. In most cases response can be judged within 2 weeks of starting treatment. Given once daily through an approved nebuliser (not ultrasonic; preferably with a mouthpiece), a 1-month trial is used to assess the change in lung function. It is stopped if FEV_1 decreases or there is less than 10% improvement in FEV_1. There are few long-term data regarding any influence on overall progression of disease. Many patients may feel symptomatically better, but hospital admission rates are not reduced. It has no place in acute respiratory tract infections.

Alternative therapies

These are frequently used, often cost large amounts of money and can be dangerous. Occasionally unscrupulous operators have tried to sell household bleach as something that kills germs and can be nebulised. There was a fad for nebulising tea tree oil as well. Silver is used by many and can cause severe discolouration of the skin and anaemia. It is always worth asking about alternative therapies.

Allergic bronchopulmonary aspergillosis (ABPA)

This is difficult to diagnose in CF, as the features of ABPA (CXR findings, increased serum immunoglobulins) occur in CF, except for IgE. A high IgE level is suggestive of ABPA if other features are present. Despite no conclusive prospective trials, management often includes steroids (e.g. orally, daily, for 1–6 weeks, then alternate daily for a total of 4–6 months), physiotherapy and antibiotics. Antifungals may be effective, and should be considered; long-term use is advocated by some units. Progress may be monitored by IgE levels. ICS may ease the asthma symptoms.

Haemoptysis

A common complication of moderate to severe lung disease. No specific treatment is needed for minor haemoptysis; treat infection and reassure the child. Any haemoptysis over 15–20 mL probably warrants hospital admission, and may need oxygen, vitamin K or transfusion with larger bleeds. Massive haemoptysis (over 300 mL blood loss in 24 hours, with falling haematocrit and hypotension) can occur from bronchial collateral vessels (usually upper lobe). Treatment includes upright position, stopping chest physiotherapy, arranging cross-match, treating with intravenous antibiotics, vitamin K and reassurance. Bronchial artery embolisation or, in severe cases with respiratory failure, intubation with balloon tamponade and emergency lobectomy may be needed. For frequent life-threatening haemoptyses, lung transplantation may be needed.

Pneumothorax

A complication of severe lung disease. Generally the more severely affected lung collapses. A poor prognostic indicator (75% die within 3 years), recurrence is common.

Acute management: oxygen—a conservative approach if possible, but each case should be treated on its merits. The prospect for future lung transplantation is adversely affected by more aggressive intervention, such as tube thoracostomy (can scar pleura, and also may cause bronchopleural fistula), chemical pleural sclerosis or surgical pleural abrasion. Needle aspiration may bring symptomatic relief.

Cor pulmonale or right heart failure

This is a poor prognostic indicator (median survival 6 months). Treat hypoxia with home nocturnal oxygen. Diuretics may be needed. Treat any infection. BiPAP can be used in patients with respiratory failure to maintain them and avoid heart failure. Cor pulmonale can resolve with lung transplantation (see below).

Lung transplantation

CF is the most common indication for paediatric lung transplant. CF does not re-occur in transplanted lungs. Bilateral sequential single-lung transplantation is now the operation of choice, the sole option for long-term survival of terminal patients. The mainstem bronchus and pulmonary artery are connected by end-to-end anastomoses; the two pulmonary veins from each lung are harvested intact with a patch of the left atrium of the donor, and then each left atrial patch is sewn to the recipient's left atrium. This is performed using cardiopulmonary bypass. Living-donor lobar transplantation

(LDLT) is another option, which is rarely performed because of technical and ethical complexities: it requires two donors, each undergoing a lower lobectomy to provide a right and left lower lobe to serve as right and left lungs for the recipient; for adolescents taller than 152 cm, donors need to be tall enough to provide adequate lung tissue.

The main indications are: life expectancy less than 2 years (usually corresponds to FEV_1 below 30% predicted), quality of life impaired (oxygen dependent at home, doing nothing), or frequent life-threatening haemoptysis. Ideal clinical status includes no major systemic disease (and preferably no surgical procedure to chest), optimal nutrition (between 70% and 130% of ideal body weight), not on ventilator and on no more than low-steroid dose (5 mg or less of prednisolone per day), adequate psychological status, adequate social supports, no major psychiatric illnesses.

There are virtually no contraindications to transplantation. Advice from local tertiary centre transplantation centres should be sought for each case considered. There are, however, areas for discussion in cases with progressive neuromuscular disease, previous malignancy in the last 2 years, pleural space disease, active infection with *Aspergillus*, *Mycobacterium*, or multiply resistant bacteria like some strains of *B. cepacia*, high-dose steroids, gross malnutrition, and some psychosocial areas (noncompliance with recommended treatment, major psychoaffective disorders). Donor–recipient matching is based on ABO blood group incompatibility, CMV antibody status and size of thoracic cage. Immunosuppressive regimes may include a calcineurin phosphatase inhibitor (e.g. tacrolimus), a purine synthesis inhibitor (e.g. mycophenolate mofetil) and prednisolone.

Complications fall into three groups:

1. Immediate phase (first few days post-transplant)

Subgroups include the following:

a. Hyperacute rejection (due to prior exposure to foreign tissue antigens, complement-mediated vascular injury and thrombosis that can lead to loss of the graft; rare).

b. Early graft dysfunction due to ischaemic injury during harvesting and reimplanting the lungs; occurs in 13–35%; manifests as pulmonary oedema (noncardiogenic), with decreased lung compliance, poor oxygenation; managed supportively (ventilation, extracorporeal membrane oxygenation [ECMO], nitric oxide).

c. Surgical complications (airway and vascular anastomoses can break down; bleeding from vascular anastomoses or chest cavity can be persistent; vocal cord and hemidiaphragm paresis or paralysis can occur, but usually resolve in a few months; early re-operation needed in around 10% of cases).

d. Infection of pulmonary allograft, secondary to poor mucus clearance (impaired cilial function), poor cough (pain), impaired diaphragm function (phrenic nerve injury), low IgG (from cardiopulmonary bypass) and immune suppression.

2. Early phase (first few weeks post-transplant)

Subgroups include the following:

a. Acute rejection (common; may present with dyspnoea, fever, hypoxia, abnormal chest X-ray with perihilar infiltrates or effusions, obstructive-pattern spirometry); diagnosed on bronchoscopy, bronchoalveolar lavage, transbronchial biopsy; treated with high-dose IV methylprednisolone; if persists, treated with mono- or polyclonal T-cell antibody preparation (e.g. OKT3, or antithymocyte globulin [ATG]).

b. Infection: CMV—treat with valganciclovir; bacterial lower respiratory tract infection—treat with IV antibiotics.

c. Side effects of surgery (narrowing at suture line of airway anastomosis): treated with bronchoscopic balloon dilatation; distal intestinal obstruction syndrome [DIOS], see below; arrhythmias, usually atrial, from interference with integrity of muscle along suture lines, where donor atrial patches with pulmonary veins are attached (see above).

d. Side effects from medication (triple immunosuppression with calcineurin phosphatase inhibitor [e.g. tacrolimus], a purine synthesis inhibitor [e.g. mycophenolate mofetil], and prednisolone; see other sections on organ transplantation (e.g. renal, liver, heart) for discussion of these drugs).

e. Seizures (can be due to tacrolimus or cyclosporine, secondary to cerebral vasoconstriction).

f. Hypertension (in 36% of cases at 1 year, 71% at 5 years; may be due to tacrolimus or cyclosporine, or steroids): treat with calcium channel blockers or angiotensin converting enzyme (ACE) inhibitors.

g. Diabetes mellitus (occurs in 20% at 1 year, 28% at 5 years) can be precipitated by steroids, or tacrolimus.

h. Renal dysfunction (hypomagnesaemia, renal tubular acidosis, chronic renal insufficiency; more common in re-transplantation).

3. Late phase (months post-transplant)

Subgroups include the following:

a. Bronchiolitis obliterans (OB) (the main reason that lung transplantation is not as successful as solid organ transplantation); treatment difficult—tried treatments include ATG, cyclophosphamide, methotrexate, total lymphoid irradiation; better management of rejection has led to improved rates of OB.

b. Malignancy (most often post-transplant lymphoproliferative disorder (PTLD); in 6.5% at 1 year, 8.2% at 5 years): treatment—reduced immunosuppression plus CD20 antibodies.

c. Renal failure (due to calcineurin inhibitors and other nephrotoxic drugs [e.g. aminoglycosides]; occurs in 7.7% at 1 year, 26% at 5 years).

Post-transplant, any acute respiratory illness or acute febrile illness should be investigated and treated aggressively. One needs to be aware that many medications (anticonvulsants, macrolides, antifungals) can interact with the main immunosuppressive agents used (tacrolimus, cyclosporine); MIMS or similar reference should be checked each time a new medication is contemplated.

The drug levels of antirejection therapy such as cyclosporine must be closely monitored, as inadequate pancreatic enzyme supplementation and erratic absorption of medication can decrease the levels, allowing rejection to occur. If there are many episodes of graft rejection within 2 months of lung transplantation, there is a high frequency of post-transplant lymphoproliferative disease (PTLD).

Females may require transplantation earlier than males as they have a median survival of 28 years, compared to males' 44 years. Suggestions are that females should be assessed and transplanted at a different lung function compared with males, but this varies with different centres. The survival rate approaches 80% at 1 year, 70% at 2 years, 50% at 5 years. The three most significant factors for poor outcome are repeat transplant, mechanical ventilation at transplant and coexistent congenital heart disease. The three main causes of death are early graft dysfunction (most deaths in the first 30 days post-transplant), infection (first year post-transplant), and bronchiolitis obliterans (beyond first year post-transplant, for cadaveric transplant recipients; rare in LDLT). Preoperatively, a 2-week assessment in hospital in necessary. Usual age has been around

17–19 years. The rate-limiting factor for this treatment is the scarcity of donor organs. To overcome this, as well as LDLT, reduction surgery and xenograft transplantation from genetically engineered porcine donors have been developed.

Immunisation

As well as routine vaccination, many paediatric respiratory units actively encourage influenza vaccination, particularly for very young patients and for those with severe lung disease. Illnesses resembling influenza may be treated with antiviral agents, e.g. oseltamivir oral preparation makes it suitable for children from 12 months of age. *Pseudomonas* vaccines are being trialled.

Burkholderia cepacia *infection*

This can be associated with rapid decline in lung function, and increased mortality. It is now recognised that this organism can survive in respiratory droplets on environmental surfaces for prolonged periods, such as in CF clinics. Person-to-person spread occurs. Patients with *B. cepacia* infection are usually seen separately in outpatient clinics and are nursed in isolation as inpatients. Cohorting of patients with *B. cepacia* infection cannot be done. Nine genomovars are recognised. The organism is found in the environment and sporadic infections are seen. In Australia there was one outbreak of 'epidemic' *B. cepacia* in Newcastle. It is important to strain type *B. cepacia* and to ensure that there is no person-to-person spread; vigilance is required with all aspects of care including healthcare professionals' hand washing, equipment use and cleaning in pulmonary function laboratories. Colonisation with *B. cepacia* is a relative contra-indication for lung transplantation in Australia, but not in Canada (where a higher percentage [up to 50%] of patients are infected with this organism).

Treatment of gastrointestinal disease

Pancreatic insufficiency (PI)

The degree of PI is determined by the specific nature of the CF mutation. Certain mutant alleles are associated with PI or pancreatic sufficiency (PS). Fat absorption improves from about 60% without therapy, to 85–90% with pancreatic enzyme replacement therapy (PERT). Dosage regimens have been revised since recognition of the association between high-strength PERT and the development of fibrosing colonopathy.

PERT doses should be derived from a ratio of lipase units per gram of dietary fat ingested; an upper limit of 10,000 units lipase/kg/day has been suggested.

Pancreatic enzyme supplements contain lipase, amylase and proteases. Most units use enteric-coated microspheres. Adjusting PERT to the fat content of foods ingested can lead to increased absorption of fat, despite no change on total capsule number. PERT guidelines for infants suggest 500–1000 units lipase per gram of dietary fat, starting with a minimum dose (2500 units lipase per 120 mL formula/breast feed), increasing the dose according to weight gain and bowel signs. For children, 500–4000 units lipase per gram of dietary fat. Adjustment should be in concert with medical staff, not independently. The contents of the capsules should be mixed with fruit gel or yoghurt, not chewed, and the oral cavity should be cleared with a finger after the feed to remove residual microspheres, as enzymes work for up to 30 minutes after ingestion. PERT should be given with all foods and fluids that contain fat. The aim is for normal growth and normal stools.

Some patients appear refractory to PERT (i.e. stool fat output persistently above 25% of fat intake), related in some to duodenal acidity. Treatment for these patients may include gastric acid suppression with antacids, H_2 receptor blockers (e.g. ranitidine), proton pump inhibitors (e.g. omeprazole), or prostaglandin analogues (e.g. misoprostol) to aid fat digestion. An alternate pancreatic enzyme preparation may be tried, as dissolution profiles may vary, or preparations may be given at the start of the meal, for earlier onset.

Nutrition

A high-energy diet is recommended. CF patients require approximately 120% of normal energy requirements because of increased energy use (due to the effort of breathing, infection), decreased protein synthesis with acute exacerbations of chest disease, nutrient loss with malabsorption, anorexia and raised basal metabolic rate. Less than optimal nutrition may lead to poor growth, impaired respiratory function and decreased exercise tolerance.

Diet should be liberal, with a high intake of a variety of foods, rich in fat (extra margarine, butter, ice-cream, cream), sugar (unless diabetic), salt, milk products, protein foods, cereals and bread. Breastfeeding is desirable for babies with CF; soy milks are not recommended.

In advanced lung disease, with loss of weight and anorexia, despite optimal oral intake, long-term supplementation of nutrition may be appropriate by invasive means (e.g. nasogastric tube or gastrostomy). Caloric supplementation may result in improvement in growth and well-being. Nutritional and respiratory status influence each other; if one should deteriorate so will the other.

Patients are at risk of deficiencies of fat-soluble vitamins A, D, E and K, especially at diagnosis. Recommendations vary on vitamin supplementation. Most units give a standard multivitamin preparation daily.

Salt

Many units use oral rehydration solutions (e.g. Glucolyte or Gastrolyte) as a source of salt, as fluid as well as salt is useful, particularly in young children. Guidelines for recommended amounts of salt are as follows:

1. Under 6 months: 0.5 g/day (1 g/day in hot weather).
2. 6–12 months: 1 g/day (1.5 g/day in hot weather).
3. 1–5 years: 2 g/day (3 g/day in hot weather).
4. Over 5 years: 3 g/day (4 g/day in hot weather).

In infants, salt can be given as oral rehydration solutions (e.g. Glucolyte), or as pinches of salt added to the bottle. As children get older, they can switch to salt tablets with added drinks. The fluid component is important to reduce DIOS.

Other gastrointestinal problems

The spectrum of gastrointestinal involvement is as follows:

1. Pancreas: insufficiency (see above); pancreatitis (in patients with pancreatic sufficiency).
2. Liver: focal biliary cirrhosis, multilobular biliary cirrhosis (complications include portal hypertension, liver failure), intrahepatic stones and sludge.
3. Gallbladder: non-functioning, stones.
4. Common bile duct: stones, stricture, rarely carcinoma.
5. Oesophagus: gastro-oesophageal reflux, oesophagitis.
6. Duodenum: ulcer.
7. Small intestine: meconium ileus (with or without the associated complications of volvulus, atresia, perforation), meconium ileus equivalent (DIOS), intussusception.

8. Large intestine: rectal prolapse, constipation with acquired megacolon, meconium plug, fibrosing colonopathy.
9. Gastrointestinal malignancy: occurs more frequently in CF, although overall risk of cancer anywhere is no different to general population.

These complications are managed by standard therapy, but some deserve particular consideration.

Meconium ileus

Meconium ileus (MI) occurs in association with PI almost exclusively. Management may include careful monitoring of fluid status and conservative enema (e.g. Urograffin and Tween 80 isotonic mixture) if uncomplicated. In some patients with MI refractory to Urograffin enemas, T-tube ileostomy with installation of N-acetylcysteine or Gastrografin has been tried with success as an alternative to surgical decompression. Operative management is needed if complicated (includes meconium peritonitis from in utero perforation, gangrene, volvulus and atresia), or if more conservative means fail. Usually the Bishop-Koop procedure is used.

Meconium ileus equivalent (distal intestinal obstruction syndrome, DIOS)

DIOS is due to abnormally viscid mucofaeculent material in the terminal ileum and right colon, presenting with attacks of bowel obstruction with pain and vomiting, but with normal stool frequency and consistency initially. If obstruction becomes complete, management may include nasogastric decompression, intravenous hydration and enemas. In incomplete obstruction, paraffin oil, stool softeners, low-residue diet, enemas or a colonic electrolyte lavage formulation (Golytely) flush, by nasogastric tube, may be used. Once an episode has resolved, review PERT; consider high-fibre diet and laxatives. If problem persists, consider cisapride, stimulant laxatives, or even oral N-acetylcysteine or Gastrografin. It often presents as a mass in the right iliac fossa and may be asymptomatic. Acute episodes may be confused with appendicitis or appendix mass. Management needs CF team involvement and careful multidisciplinary assessment. Prevention needs to be focused on improving fluid and salt intake.

Rectal prolapse

This usually occurs in the first few years of life; spontaneous resolution by 5 years is usual. It is associated with inadequate control of steatorrhoea, and may resolve with adequate PERT. Conservative management is with manual reduction, stool softeners (mineral oil or lactulose) and improved nutrition. Not infrequently, patients learn to self-reduce the prolapse with pelvic floor muscles, and do not need manual pressure on the prolapsed rectum. If prolapse is persistent, it may require general anaesthesia and pararectal triple saline injection, but this is very rare.

Liver and biliary tract disease

The incidence of liver disease and cirrhosis in CF are 1% and 0.8% respectively. The average age of onset is 7 years, with the peak incidence at 16–20 years. Once cirrhosis has developed, the duration of survival is 4–5 years: hepatobiliary disease is the second most common cause of mortality in CF. In the liver, only intrahepatic biliary epithelial cells express CFTR chloride channels. CF-associated liver disease (CFLD) is more common with PI. Management of cholestasis may include giving ursodeoxycholic acid (URSO). Management of portal hypertension may include sclerotherapy, variceal bonding, endoscopic variceal ligation, portosystemic shunting or transjugular intra-hepatic portosystemic shunt placement. If progressive, irreversible hepatic insufficiency develops, liver transplantation (LTx) is the treatment of choice. Long-term survival after LTx in CF is comparable to LTx performed for other indications (see the section on LTx in Chapter 8, Gastroenterology). Distal common bile duct stricture, recurrent pain or biliary tree obstruction can be managed with surgical intervention: cholecystojejunostomy if the gall bladder is functioning, or choledochojejunostomy for nonvisualised gallbladder, or microgallbladder.

Fibrosing colonopathy

This is an iatrogenic complication of the treatment of CF. The risk is greatest in children under 12 or with a history of DIOS. Colonic strictures/stenoses, frequently long segment, occur from submucosal thickening by fibrous connective tissue, leading to intraluminal narrowing related to high-dose PERT. Patients may present with abdominal pain, diarrhoea and haematochezia, before strictures form. It seems likely that a methacrylic acid co-polymer in the enteric coatings of some PERT preparations is the putative agent. Since particular PERTs were withdrawn from the market, it is reported less. Management in the past has included colectomy.

Abdominal pain

This can be a diagnostic and management problem. The possibilities include intestinal causes (e.g. DIOS, gastro-oesophageal reflux, duodenal ulcer, oesophagitis), biliary causes (e.g. cholelithiasis, common bile duct stricture, cholecystitis), pancreatitis, renal stones, related to respiratory disease (e.g. muscle strain with coughing, lower lobe infection), functional (e.g. grief reaction with death of close friend with CF, or patient's own deteriorating health), or unrelated to CF.

Treatment of other complications

Cystic-fibrosis–related diabetes (CFRD)

CFRD is becoming more common, due to increased lifespan of CF patients: it occurs in 10–15% of patients and is increasing. It is linked to the common delta-F508 mutation. It is managed in the standard fashion, but particular difficulties can occur with concomitant corticosteroid usage and dietary requirements. Ketoacidosis is very rare in CFRD, but microvascular complications have been recorded. See the long and short cases on diabetes in Chapter 7, Endocrinology, for further discussion.

Musculoskeletal complications

These are increasingly recognised with longer life span.

- Hypertrophic pulmonary osteoarthropathy (HPOA) is the most common disorder (it occurs in 2-7% patients with CF). It is characterised by digital clubbing, long-bone and joint pain (especially wrists, knees and ankles), worsened by pulmonary exacerbations. The aetiology remains unclear. Bone scan can detect HPOA early. Management includes optimising pulmonary care and aggressive treatment of exacerbations. Non-steroidal anti-inflammatory drugs (NSAIDs) may relieve discomfort.
- Kyphosis with an angle over 40 degrees occurs in over 75% of adult female CF patients, and around one-third of adult male patients. Both HPOA and kyphosis are associated with deteriorating lung function and are seen as markers of poor prognosis.
- Low bone mass is common, despite supplementation with vitamin D, calcium and PERT. Osteoporosis and crush fractures can lead to significant back problems. Rib fractures are also reported. Severe bone loss occurs in transplant patients.

- CF episodic arthritis usually presents with recurrent (non-destructive) mono-articular involvement or a symmetrical polyarthritis. It can be managed by standard therapy (NSAIDs or aspirin). Glucocorticoids may be required, orally or intra-articularly. It has been observed that antibiotic therapy for lung disease can improve joint symptoms. Eruptions resembling erythema nodosum may occur in association with it.
- Rheumatoid arthritis has been reported, and treated successfully with hydroxy-chloroquine and gold.
- Ciprofloxacin-induced arthralgia is treated by stopping the drug.

Growth and recombinant human growth hormone (rhGH)
Poor linear growth and inadequate weight gain are very common, and adults with CF have lower than average final adult heights. Poor weight gain and worsening of clinical state are well known. It has been hypothesised that improved linear growth can allow greater lung mass, leading to improved lung function. Many studies of rhGH in children with CF have shown significant improvement in height velocity, weight velocity, bone accumulation, forced vital capacity and exercise tolerance.

Adolescence and fertility
Females with CF are mildly subfertile (related to suboptimal body weight, thick cervical mucus, low body fat and associated oestrogen deficiency). Many pregnancies are successful, although pregnancy can be associated with risk of cardiorespiratory failure and fetal loss; however, the only contraindication is cor pulmonale. Tolerance of pregnancy depends on the severity of lung disease, and is better tolerated in those with milder disease and in those with a certain ideal body weight before conception.

Implanon and 3-monthly Depo-Provera are frequently used for contraception. All oral contraceptives are avoided in adolescent females, because frequent use of different antibiotic therapies may affect drug levels and effectiveness, and patients may have liver disease. The only time oral contraceptives would be used is for medical/hormonal purposes like acne or painful menses.

With increased survival, many CF patients request genetic counselling and fertility assessment. Genetic screening of partners detects around 90% of carriers. Females with CF can overcome difficulties with conception by in-vitro fertilisation techniques.

Males with CF usually have congenital bilateral absence of the vas deferens (CBAVD) but the resultant infertility can be managed by having spermatazoa retrieved by direct aspiration from the head of the epididymis, then intracytoplasmic sperm injection (ICSI) into an oocyte obtained by egg harvesting.

Common management issues

What should the patient know about the illness?

Most patients are diagnosed through neonatal screening, so that the parents receive education about the condition. As children get older, simple explanations are required to explain why they require physiotherapy and medications. Fertility should be discussed around 13–17 years of age, explaining infertility to the boys and implications of pregnancy to the girls. With the advent of the Internet and acceleration in the ease of information retrieval, most children and parents will have 'surfed the Net' and will be asking challenging questions regarding these issues earlier than in the past.

How much should school/peers be told?

School should be told about the diagnosis, the need for exceptions to school rules (e.g. running late for class due to treatment at home, running to toilet, being exempt from sport) when necessary, and the need for free access to bronchodilator therapy. School friends can be supplied with information when they ask, keeping answers simple, but there is little point in trying to keep the diagnosis secret. It is important that the school is aware that if there is more than one patient with CF in the school the children should not be in the same class, to avoid prolonged contact and the risk of transmission of organisms from patient to patient. It is of key importance that children and parents have a positive attitude to prognosis and ensure adequate education. The majority of children born with CF today will live to adult life, will need to work and may have a family of their own.

When should the patient take responsibility for self-care?

Children can generally manage to swallow their pancreatic enzymes by 5 years. Adolescents often start to have some time alone with the doctor during consultations by around 14 years and achieve total self-care by the end of adolescence.

When should the patient transfer to adult care?

The appropriate time is more dependent on maturity and physical health than age. Some units feel the year after leaving school is the appropriate time, with prior introduction to the adult physician. A common problem with transfer is decreased compliance (factors include loyalty, rapport with new doctors, physiotherapists, change in treatment, clinic environment, drug costs, loss of parental supervision). Positive reasons for transfer include recognition of transition to adulthood, and patient preference (but a problem can be disease stability at the time). Negative reasons include crowding of paediatric outpatient clinics and disinclination of paediatricians to manage adult problems. Most young people are happy to transfer care when they finish school or if they take on adult responsibilities and behaviours earlier. Many units make the transition to adult care after completion of grade 12. Most patients are happy with this and, although most parents are worried, the doctors and therapists usually have no concerns.

Is modification of current medical treatments warranted?

Alternate daily oral steroids may impact negatively on growth and bone density, and increase the risk of diabetes, although previously reported positive effects have included increased growth and appetite, decreased infection and increased well-being in some patients. Home intravenous antibiotics using venous access ports had appeared promising, and seemed as effective as hospital antibiotics, but now many studies have shown that home IV treatment may require longer time on therapy, compared to hospital care, to achieve the same end points. Many units reserve this for patients who are very well motivated and have a lot of support. Home oxygen is useful for later stage 'restless' nights and morning headache with significant oxygen desaturation overnight: this needs assessment (e.g. overnight oxygen saturation monitoring, echocardiography to detect cor pulmonale).

Is lung transplantation an option for this patient?

This is an area to be evaluated in any terminal patient with CF. Bilateral sequential single lung transplantation is the sole option for long-term survival of such patients. See the discussion in the section on the treatment of lung disease.

If there is a second major organ failure, a second organ transplant may be appropriate (for coexistent liver failure, liver-lung transplantation; for coexistent heart failure, heart-lung transplantation). In the past, heart-lung transplant had been considered for cor pulmonale associated with pulmonary hypertension; however, it is now recognised that the right-sided heart dysfunction of cor pulmonale resolves after lung transplantation.

Are the family coping at present?

There may be a need for increased financial and social support. Depending on the state of the child's illness, there may be a need for grief counselling. This is useful at any of the more stressful times in the parents' lives, including the initial diagnosis, the next hospital admission, the death of someone else's child, crisis times (e.g. increased hospitalisation, start of school), antenatal diagnosis and termination of pregnancy, transfer to adult hospital. Grief reactions can include shock, denial, sadness (e.g. loss of expected healthy child/life span), anger (why me?) that may be directed at health workers, relief (symptoms have a name), guilt (they transmitted the disease), resentment, anxiety (fear for future), somatic problems (e.g. headaches).

Are the parents planning more children?

Discussion must include prenatal diagnosis and the ethical problem of what to do should the result be positive. The education of the parents in the genetic considerations should be explored to prevent misunderstanding (e.g. 'The next three will be all right because the risk is 1 in 4').

Prognosis

Life expectancy is increasing. Median survival is 36 years. Over 90% of mortality is due to lung disease; cirrhosis is a second life-threatening complication. Poor prognostic factors include:

- Female sex (teenage and young adult age period).
- Pancreatic insufficiency.
- Complications, including CFRD or CFLD, or ABPA.
- Abnormal chest X-ray 12 months after diagnosis.
- Age of acquisition of chronic pulmonary infection with *P. aeruginosa* and, in particular, mucoid *P. aeruginosa* under 6 years.
- Lung infection with *Burkholderia cepacia*.
- Fall off in growth curves.
- Recurrent haemoptysis.
- Pneumothorax.
- Onset of cor pulmonale.
- Cigarette smoke exposure.
- Poor socioeconomic status.
- Non-CF-clinic care.

Short cases

The respiratory system

This is a common case, expected to be performed well. On occasion, the patient may have a chronic rare condition such as hypoplastic lung, congenital lobar emphysema or Kartagener's syndrome (primary ciliary dyskinesia), but more common problems include CF and CLD. Specific approaches for the latter two cases are given in the long-case section. The approaches for 'stridor' and for a 'chest' examination are described after this section.

'Examine the respiratory system' implies something different from 'Examine the chest'. The former includes the hands (starting with the nails for clubbing), chest wall, praecordium, lungs, ears, nose, throat and regional lymph nodes. The latter includes chest wall (starting with this, not the hands), heart and lungs, as the primary focus of the examination, only then followed by more peripheral signs. The key is to do exactly what the examiners ask, not interpret their instructions inappropriately.

Commence the examination of the respiratory system by introducing yourself. Note the child's voice, which may be hoarse (e.g. in laryngotracheobronchitis). Stand back and give a general description of the child, in particular noting the growth parameters (e.g. failure to thrive with CF, BPD), nutritional status (e.g. poor fat stores in CF) and any dysmorphic features (e.g. Pierre Robin's facies, with micrognathia). At this point, the child's chest should be fully exposed, except in the case of an infant, where more subtle manoeuvring may be necessary to avoid upsetting the patient.

Note whether the child looks well or unwell, cyanosed or acyanotic, and describe any notable respiratory noises, such as stridor or wheeze, any cough and the nature of the cry in infants. Note the degree of respiratory distress (e.g. tracheal tug, intercostal, substernal and subcostal recession) and count the respiratory rate. Describe any IV lines (look at what is in the fluid being given: e.g. salbutamol, aminophylline, hydrocortisone, antibiotics), oxygen being administered (at what rate), nebuliser or spacer at the end of bed.

Note any monitoring devices present, such as pulse oximetry or transcutaneous monitoring devices, and their readings. Also note any useful signs on the cot or bed. Describe any chest deformity, asymmetry, any scars, venous access devices and ask the child to cough. Request inspection of sputum if there is a moist, productive cough in an older child, and no sputum cup to be seen in the vicinity of the bed.

Commence general systematic examination of the child with the hands. Then examine the head, followed by the chest, abdomen, ears, nose, palate, throat and regional lymph nodes, the lower limbs, and request the temperature chart.

Only ask the PEFR if it would be relevant (making sure you know the appropriate expected values for that patient). Depending on the prior findings, further examination of the fundi, skin and the neurological system may be required. The various findings sought are listed in Figure 15.1, and a comprehensive listing of possible signs on initial inspection is given in Table 15.3.

After inspection, ask the child to take a deep breath in and observe the chest expansion for asymmetry. This tends to be more useful than actually palpating during deep inspiration. Next, palpate for the apex beat, parasternal heave, palpable pulmonary valve closure and tracheal position, before percussion. Tactile fremitus can be omitted, as it is unlikely to be helpful in most children. Percussion must be performed well; have consultants check your technique while practising cases. Ensure that percussion is performed symmetrically. The apices are best percussed from behind. When percussing the axillae, it is easier with the child's hands on his or her head. Next, auscultate in the standard manner, again symmetrically. Vocal resonance can usually be omitted. If any rhonchi are noted, it is worth asking the examiners when the last nebuliser was given.

Consultants differ in their approach to examining the chest. Some prefer to examine the anterior chest wall completely, and then the posterior aspect of the chest completely. Others prefer percussion of front and back, then auscultation in a similar manner. There is no right or wrong way to do it: the important thing is sticking to one method with which you are comfortable; do not change it on exam day.

At the completion of the physical examination, the chest X-ray (CXR) can be requested; logical and succinct interpretation is expected (see the section on reading CXRs at the end of this chapter).

Figure 15.1 The respiratory system

1. Introduce self
Voice: hoarse (e.g. laryngitis)

2. General inspection
Position patient: standing, fully
  undressed; then sitting
Well or unwell
Parameters
- Height
- Weight
- Head circumference
Dysmorphic features
Nutritional status
Intervention (e.g. IV line, oxygen mask,
  nasogastric tube)
Monitoring devices
Colour
Respiratory rate
Respiratory noises
Respiratory distress
Chest deformity
Asymmetry
Scars
Venous access devices
Cough

3. Upper limbs
Nails
Palms
Joints
Pulse
Asterixis

4. Head
Face
- Dysmorphic
- 'Ex-premmie' (BPD)
- Cushingoid (treatment with
  corticosteroids)
Mouth
- Cyanosis
- Cleft lip
- Tongue: cyanosis

5. Chest
Reinspect (for anything missed on
  general inspection)
Palpate
- Apex beat (displacement)
- Parasternal area (RV heave)
- Pulmonary area (palpable
  pulmonary valve closure)
- Trachea (displacement)
Chest expansion (symmetry in older
  children; inspection better in
  younger children)

Percuss
Auscultate
- Lungs
- Praecordium, for evidence of
  pulmonary hypertension, cor
  pulmonale

6. Abdomen
Liver
- Ptosis (hyperinflated chest)
- Enlarged (right heart failure)
Spleen
- Enlarged (portal hypertension in
  CF)

7. ENT and lymph nodes
Ears: otitis media, acute or chronic
  serous
Nose: polyps (CF)
Mouth: cleft palate
Throat: tonsillitis
Lymph nodes
- Occipital, postauricular (from in
  front)

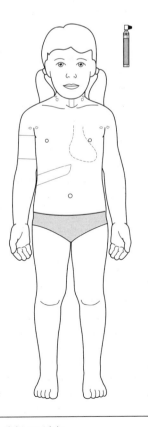

BPD = bronchopulmonary dysplasia; CF = cystic fibrosis; RV = right ventricle.

Table 15.3 Additional information: details of possible findings on respiratory examination

Inspection
Dysmorphic features
- Robin sequence
- Down syndrome
- Apert's syndrome
- Cleft lip sequence

Nutritional status
- Muscle bulk
- Subcutaneous fat

Intervention
- Intravenous line
- Oxygen mask or catheter
- Nebuliser at end of bed
- Mist tent
- Nasogastric tube

Monitoring devices
- Pulse oximeter
- Transcutaneous O_2 and CO_2 monitor
- Oxygen analyser in oxygen tent or head box
- Cardiorespiratory monitor

Colour
Respiratory rate
Respiratory noises: stridor, wheeze, cough, cry

Respiratory distress, degree of
- Tracheal tug
- Sternal recession
- Intercostal, subcostal, substernal or supraclavicular retraction

Chest deformity: barrel chest, Harrison's sulcus, pectus carinatum or excavatum, rib flaring, scoliosis, kyphosis

Asymmetry (e.g. hypoplastic lung, congenital lobar emphysema)

Scars (e.g. multiple intercostal drain tubes, lobectomy, associated congenital heart defects)

Venous access devices (e.g. for antibiotics, in CF patients)

Cough (ask patient to do this and request inspection of sputum)

Upper limbs
Nails: clubbing (suppurative lung disease, pulmonary fibrosis, coexistent cyanotic heart disease)

Fingertips: prickmarks (BSL testing in CF patients with diabetes)

Palms: crease pallor (anaemia)

Dorsum of hand: scars of previous multiple IVs (NICU graduate)

Joints: swollen (HPOA)

Pulse
- Tachycardia (hypoxia, fever, treatment with beta-2 agonists)
- Pulsus paradoxus (e.g. in severe asthma)

Asterixis: CO_2 retention

Other
Lower limbs
- Toenail clubbing
- Ankle oedema (right ventricular failure)

Temperature chart
Peak flow meter readings

Fundi: retinal venous dilatation (CO_2 retention)

Skin: eczema (e.g. with asthma)

Neurological system for predisposing causes of respiratory distress, e.g. bulbar palsy (aspiration), spinal muscular atrophy (diaphragmatic breathing)

BSL = blood sugar level; CF = cystic fibrosis; HFOA = hypertrophic pulmonary osteoarthropathy; NICU = neonatal intensive care unit.

The chest

With this introduction, the examiners want you to start with the chest, not the hands. After general inspection, looking for the various findings sought in a cardiac or respiratory short case, with the child's chest fully exposed, perform a thorough examination of the lungs (as in a respiratory case) and the heart (as thoroughly as in a cardiac short case), as well as the bony structures (sternum, ribs, clavicles, spine), for findings such as scoliosis. Only when every component of the chest per se has been assessed should the systematic examination move peripherally, the direction this takes depending on the findings noted.

Stridor

This is a variation of the respiratory examination. The patients seen are usually infants, often with congenital stridor. There is a wide differential diagnosis.

After introducing yourself, stand back and give a general description of the child. Note if he or she appears well or unwell, note the growth parameters, and look for any dysmorphic/syndromal features (e.g. Opitz's syndrome, with hypertelorism, cleft lips, protruding ears and laryngeal cleft), or the features of the 'ex-premmie' NICU graduate (prolonged intubation, resultant subglottic stenosis). Scan the child for any evidence of capillary haemangiomata, particularly in the 'beard' distribution of the face and neck (associated subglottic haemangioma).

Note the infant's colour, posture (e.g. hyperextended neck with supralaryngeal problems, hypertonic spastic posturing in infants with cerebral palsy and pseudobulbar palsy), activity (paucity of movement with some neurological causes), and the degree of respiratory distress. Note respiratory rate, tracheal tug, degree of chest recession (sternal, intercostal, substernal, subcostal or supraclavicular). Also note the following:

1. Whether the child is receiving any supports, such as nasogastric feeding (which implies at least one patent choanal opening), intravenous fluids, oxygen.
2. Whether the child has been receiving supports (which are temporarily unnecessary), such as nebulised therapy, an oropharyngeal airway on the bedside cupboard, or whether there is perinasal linear skin reddening, suggesting recent removal of tape securing a nasogastric tube.
3. Whether the child is being monitored, e.g. with pulse oximetry.

Observe if the child is a nose or mouth breather (mouth breathing inferring nasal obstruction: e.g. due to choanal atresia), if there is any drooling (suggesting supralaryngeal obstruction) or pooling of secretions (neurological causes).

Listen to the child's breathing to determine in which phase of respiration the noise occurs. Note that fixed obstructive lesions causing significant cross-sectional area reduction of the airway (anywhere) can cause inspiratory and expiratory (biphasic) stridor, irrespective of whether the lesion is extrathoracic (above the clavicles) or intrathoracic (below the clavicles). Purely inspiratory stridor suggests a non-fixed obstruction, usually above the clavicles/extrathoracic, such as a laryngeal or supralaryngeal obstruction. Inspiratory and expiratory (biphasic) stridor may infer a non-fixed lesion with tracheal involvement. Expiratory noises alone are more likely non-fixed and below the clavicles (tracheal). Laryngeal problems may change the character of the voice (e.g. a hoarse voice with unilateral vocal cord paralysis, or with laryngitis) or the cry (e.g. weak with vocal cord problems; note that bilateral vocal cord palsy is more often associated with a normal cry and normal voice). Crying itself worsens the stridor in laryngomalacia or subglottic haemangioma. Note the relative timing of inspiration and expiration: in laryngeal disorders, inspiration is prolonged, while in bronchial obstruction expiration is prolonged.

If the mother changes the infant's position when the child is distressed, note any change in the stridor with the crying and with the repositioning.

The child's head posturing must be noted, as it may give a clue to the level of the problem. Laryngeal or supralaryngeal narrowing tends to make a child hyperextend the neck (classic example: epiglottitis) to increase the upper airway diameter.

Inspect the nose, noting whether it permits passage of a nasogastric tube and whether there is any movement of mucus with respiration, inferring patent nostrils. Inspect the mouth for any scars from repaired cleft lip, glossoptosis or micrognathia (syndromal diagnoses) and, when the child opens the mouth, note any obvious cleft palate. Inspect the neck for any asymmetry (e.g. lymphatic malformation ['cystic hygroma'], neoplasm). Inspect the chest for scars (e.g. previous tracheostomy, previous multiple intercostal drain tubes in the NICU graduate), deformity (e.g. pectus excavatum, Harrison's sulci), increased anteroposterior diameter (e.g. in coexistent CLD in the NICU graduate), degree of chest recession.

Before the child is too distressed, if you suspect nasal obstruction, the 'metal condensation test' can be performed in a few seconds. Simply hold the metal arm of your stethoscope under the infant's nostrils, and as the metal is (usually) cold, any nasal breathing will result in moisture condensing on the metal, confirming nostril and choanal patency.

Some aspects of the examination of the mouth are unpleasant and are best deferred until the end of the examination, but must not be omitted (see below).

Palpate the neck for any masses (e.g. lymphatic malformation [cystic hygroma]). If any masses are present, examine these in the standard manner for any lump (i.e. size, shape, consistency, pulsatility, attachments, fluctuation, transillumination, auscultation, regional lymph nodes). At this stage, if there is a neck mass, turn the child's head to either side, then flex and extend the neck to assess if this worsens or alleviates the stridor.

Palpate the trachea to detect any deviation. Also palpate the apex beat (deviation), any parasternal heave or palpable pulmonary valve closure (pulmonary hypertension and cor pulmonale), and then percuss across the upper chest to detect any retrosternal mass compressing the airway. Auscultate the lungs (to confirm the timing of the stridor, and detect associated respiratory disease: e.g. CLD) and the heart, for loud second sound and any evidence of right-heart failure or coexistent heart disease (as in some syndromal diagnoses). Now, with auscultation completed, move the infant into a supine and then a prone position, to detect any change in the stridor: in laryngomalacia, the stridor diminishes when prone.

At this point, it may be worthwhile looking carefully at the skin for any 'strawberry' haemangiomata that may have passed unnoticed.

Now come the least pleasant aspects to the examination:

1. Inspect the oral cavity, using a spatula and torch, looking for cleft palate and any obvious swellings or tumours (e.g. retropharyngeal or tonsillar).
2. Test the gag reflex and the suck (for bulbar dysfunction in neurological causes).
3. Palpate the tongue all the way back, to detect any mucus retention, cyst or other obstructive lesion.
4. If the condensation test suggests complete obstruction, it is now the time to request a feeding tube, and pass this down each nostril. Only do this at the very end of the examination, as it always upsets the child.

If a syndrome seems likely, look for other dysmorphic features.

If there is a suggestion of a neurological aetiology, perform a gross motor assessment, followed by testing the long tracts, and then motor cranial nerves (starting from cranial nerve XII and progressing upward to III).

Always request the temperature chart at the completion of your examination (e.g. for retropharyngeal abscess).

Give a brief, logical differential diagnosis, and after this request a posteroanterior (P-A) chest X-ray (CXR) and a lateral airways film.

Chest X-rays

Accurate interpretation is expected. Note the date of the X-ray and the name, to check that it is the correct film. Then note which side is labelled 'right' to avoid missing dextrocardia (although it should have been noted clinically), particularly in the child with clubbing and purulent sputum, who has Kartagener's syndrome (immotile cilia/primary ciliary dyskinesia) and not CF. Note whether the film is well centred. This is the time to quickly scan the bony structures, as rotated films will show asymmetry of clavicles on the P-A view. Check chest symmetry and note any scoliosis or rib crowding. Check that the film is well penetrated, and has been taken during a full inspiration. Expiratory films are notoriously difficult to interpret and may be quite misleading. Note the centring of the trachea and the cardiac shadow, checking for any deviation. Assess the cardiac size: the cardiac diameter is normally 50% or less of the cardiothoracic diameter (except in neonates, where it can be 60%). The heart may be enlarged due to pathology related to the lungs, such as cor pulmonale. The cardiac contour is then inspected, looking for evidence of the following.

1. Loss of right-heart border definition, which indicates right middle-lobe involvement.
2. Loss of apex definition, which indicates lingula involvement.
3. Increased opacification behind the heart, usually in a 'sail' or triangular shape, indicating left lower-lobe involvement.
4. Prominent pulmonary artery shadow, which can indicate pulmonary hypertension (PHT).
5. Prominent right-atrial shadow, which can occur with PHT.
6. Prominent right ventricular region, which can occur with PHT.

Focus on the lung fields. Note any asymmetry in lucency of the lungs (e.g. in congenital lobar emphysema), any hyperinflation (as in asthma, with 'flattened' diaphragm shadows and increased lucency). Focus on the diaphragm shadows, looking for the following:

1. Loss of line of left hemidiaphragm suggests left lower-lobe involvement.
2. Loss of line of right hemidiaphragm suggests right lower-lobe involvement.
3. Loss of clear costophrenic angle suggests pleural effusion (remember to examine the apices for a pleural cap).
4. Right hemidiaphragm is normally higher than the left, due to the liver; if the lungs are hyperinflated, the hemidiaphragms may be at almost the same level.

Note any focal areas of increased opacification, generalised increase in opacification in perihilar or peripheral areas. If it is unclear on assessing the P-A film which region of the lung is involved (as is particularly the case in consolidation affecting the 'midzone' of the lung fields), request a lateral film.

In assessing the lateral film, first note the bony structures. Note the degree of opacification of the vertebrae: normally the upper vertebrae are quite opaque, due to the overlying shoulder region, and as one progresses down the spine, the vertebral bodies appear increasingly lucent, because of the lack of overlying soft tissues in that region. Thus, if there is increased opacification of the lower vertebral area, there may be consolidation, or other process, involving the posterior segments of the affected lobe. Also note any kyphosis (rare) or rib abnormalities. Check tracheal position followed by assessing the positions of the hemidiaphragms. Now inspect the lung fields; they are normally obscured in the postero-superior aspect (by the shoulders) and in the anteroinferior aspect (by the heart). Look for the interlobar fissures, which may delineate a collapsed or consolidated area.

Rheumatology

Long cases

Juvenile idiopathic arthritis

There have been major advances in the development of therapeutic agents available to treat juvenile idiopathic arthritis (JIA), and the acceptance of an internationally recognised unifying classification by the International League of Associations for Rheumatology (ILAR) and the World Health Organization (WHO) encompassing seven types of JIA. A shift in the approach to therapy has occurred, with continued use of non-steroidal anti-inflammatory drugs (NSAIDs), and much greater emphasis on earlier use of intra-articular steroids, use of methotrexate (MTX) as a first-line disease-modifying antirheumatic drug (DMARD), and establishment of newer biological agents effective in resistant disease. Children with JIA are often used as long-case subjects, as their care is multifaceted and often difficult. The candidate should be well versed in the range of drugs and newer biologic agents employed, their important adverse effects, the role of physical and other support therapies, the associated disorders, and the long-term outcomes.

Current classification of JIA

Oligoarthritis (four or fewer joints involved)

This is the most common form of JIA. Approximately 45% of all JIA, this form predominantly occurs in females aged between 12 months and 5 years (peak 3 years). This group is at risk (up to 35%) of eye involvement: this is a chronic uveitis, which is almost always asymptomatic, but can cause blindness due to band keratopathy, cataract and glaucoma. All children in this group require regular slit-lamp examination, every 3–4 months, by an ophthalmologist. ANA positivity (which occurs in about 50% of this group) increases this risk. Joints involved: often one or two large joints (e.g. knees, ankles [including subtalar joints], wrists and elbows); hip involvement is very rare. The arthritis is rarely erosive.

   Oligoarthritis is defined as arthritis affecting one to four joints during the first 6 months after onset of the disease. Specific exclusions are: (a) positive family history of psoriasis; (b) positive family history of spondyloarthropathy; or (c) positive rheumatoid factor. The prognosis in this group is good, with remission usually within 5 years. A functional result is dependent on appropriate management (e.g. physiotherapy and exercise, in addition to anti-inflammatory medication, can prevent complications of asymmetrical growth in the inflamed joint). Intra-articular steroids are often very useful here. The associated uveitis has better prognosis when discovered by screening than by symptomatic referral.

Extended oligoarthritis

Extended oligoarthritis is defined as arthritis affecting one to four joints during the first six months of the disease, and a cumulative total of five joints or more after the first six months of the disease. Specific exclusions are: (a) positive family history of psoriasis; (b) positive rheumatoid factor. This group has the best response to MTX. This type of JIA can be quite severe and can continue into adult life.

Polyarticular RF-negative (five joints or more involved)

This accounts for around 25% of JIA with female predominance, at any age. There is arthritis involving both large and small joints of upper and lower limbs, usually asymmetrical. Uveitis may occur in approximately 10% and requires surveillance. ANA is positive in over 25%. Joint destruction occurs in 10–15%. It can remit in late childhood. 'Polyarthritis RF-negative' is defined as arthritis affecting five or more joints during the first 6 months after onset of the disease. NSAIDs and MTX are effective. Some need higher doses of MTX; as absorption of oral MTX is finite, parenteral administration may be required. Subcutaneous MTX is as effective as intramuscular MTX, but better tolerated.

Polyarthritis RF-positive (five joints or more involved)

This accounts for around 5–10% of JIA with female predominance and late childhood/teenage onset. Resembles adult rheumatoid arthritis, with a *symmetrical* polyarthritis affecting upper (e.g. metacarpophalangeal joints most common) and lower limbs. Other features include subcutaneous nodules and early erosive changes radiologically. It often follows a progressive course, with eventual joint destruction. Unremitting severe disease and poor functional outcome occur in over 50%. Polyarthritis RF-positive is defined as arthritis affecting five or more joints during the first 6 months of the disease, associated with positive rheumatoid factor tests on at least two occasions 3 months apart. This group responds to the same drugs as adult rheumatoid arthritis.

Systemic onset juvenile idiopathic arthritis (SOJIA), previously known as Still's disease

1. Early onset (1–4 years; peak at 2), equal sex incidence, up to 10% of JIA.
2. Systemic symptoms: fever (typically double quotidian pattern with two high spikes daily); rash (evanescent, coming and going with fever spikes; discrete salmon pink macules 2–10 mm, usually around upper trunk and axillae; show Koebner phenomenon; rarely pruritic; not purpuric); polyarticular arthritis (can be late feature).
3. Other features: lymphadenopathy, hepatosplenomegaly, serositis, pericarditis (often asymptomatic), haematological changes (anaemia, leucocytosis).
4. An occasional feature is myocarditis.
5. Systemic features can precede arthritis by months. Natural evolution: systemic features followed by polyarthritis; this remains while systemic features regress.
6. Rheumatoid factor (RF) negative and usually antinuclear antibody (ANA) negative.
7. Approximately 50% remit in 2–3 years.
8. Joint destruction occurs in 20% of cases.

9. SOJIA is the only type of JIA without a specific age, gender or HLA association.
10. Most mortality from JIA is in this subgroup. Deaths can be due to infection secondary to immunosuppression, myocardial involvement or macrophage activation syndrome (MAS). MAS is a rare complication of SOJIA, involving increased activation of histiophagocytosis. Triggers include preceding viral illness and additional medications (particularly NSAIDs, sulfasalazine and etanercept). Clinical findings include lymphadenopathy, hepatosplenomegaly, purpura, mucosal bleeding, multiple organ failure. Investigations may show pancytopenia, prolonged prothrombin time and partial thromboplastin time, elevated fibrin degradation products, hyperferritinaemia, hypertriglyceridaemia, low ESR. Treatment involves pulse methylprednisolone and cyclosporine A, or dexamethasone and etoposide.
11. Uveitis is rare.

The ILAR classification lists three criteria that are *definite*: (a) documented quotidian fever for at least 2 weeks; (b) evanescent, non-fixed erythematous rash; (c) arthritis. There are also criteria for *probable* systemic disease, in the absence of arthritis, criteria (a) and (b) above together with any two of: generalised lymph node enlargement; hepatomegaly or splenomegaly; serositis.

Enthesitis-related arthritis (ERA)

Approximately 15% of all JIA, it predominantly occurs in males in pre-teenage years, with lower limb involvement, especially hips and sacroiliac joints. Many show features common to spondylo-arthropathies (e.g. enthesitis, decreased lumbar flexion). The difference is that the main clinical feature here is peripheral arthritis, not sacroiliitis. Involvement of the spine is uncommon in childhood. Rarely buttock pain occurs, reflecting sacroiliitis. Imaging the sacroiliac (SI) joints with CT, MRI or bone scans is useful, and may detect earlier involvement based on the shape of the SI joint, compared with SI changes on plain X-ray films, which are typically delayed. At risk (25%) of uveitis (acute symptomatic 'red eye'; this is quite different from the chronic asymptomatic uveitis that occurs in oligoarthritis or extended oligoarthritis). HLA-B27 positive in 80%; ANA- and RF-negative.

ERA is defined by (1) arthritis and enthesitis, or (2) arthritis with at least two of the following: sacroiliac joint tenderness, inflammatory spinal pain, HLA-B27 positive family history (first- or second-degree relatives: at least one of (a) anterior uveitis with pain, redness or photophobia, (b) spondylo-arthopathy confirmed by a rheumatologist, or (c) inflammatory bowel disease), or anterior uveitis with pain, redness or photophobia. Specific exclusions are positive rheumatoid factor or antinuclear antibody. The treatment of choice for the peripheral arthritis is sulphasalazine (SSZ) in addition to an NSAID (e.g. indomethacin); if unsuccessful or not tolerated, MTX is the next choice.

ERA includes patients with juvenile ankylosing spondylitis. There are two forms of arthritis associated with inflammatory bowel disease (IBD): an acute polyarticular form that tends to reflect the disease activity of the coexistent IBD, and the second more common form that runs independently of the IBD. Extra-articular manifestations of ERA, in addition to anterior uveitis, include aortitis, aortic incompetence, muscle weakness and fever (usually low grade).

Psoriatic arthritis (JPsA)

This shows a female predominance, tending to occur in mid-childhood. The arthritis frequently is *asymmetrical*, may start as oligoarticular but most progress to polyarticular. It can affect fingers and toes (sausage digits), one or more large joints (particularly the knee) and can involve flexor tendons. The distal interphalangeal joints may be involved. There is often a family history of psoriasis. Fingernail pitting and onycholysis may be seen. Half the patients have the rash of psoriasis before the arthritis, and half after (it may not occur until many years later). Only a few children develop both symptoms simultaneously. Uveitis can occur, and is seen in about 10% (chronic asymptomatic, as with extended oligoarthritis). ANA positivity is more common, and HLA-B27 is less common, than in the ERA group (where JPsA used to be listed). The arthritis can be quite erosive. MTX has been used, but definitive studies have yet to be done to confirm its efficacy here. Severity of joint involvement is independent of the rash.

Presentation of a long case with JIA

The child with JIA may have a very long and complicated history. Clarity of presentation to the examiners is essential. Long cases with JIA particularly lend themselves to pictorial display. This method can be used for recording the history and allows the examiners to appreciate clearly the progress of the illness. If the candidate wishes to try this technique, it should be practised on trial cases before the exam. Figure 16.1 demonstrates an example: a 15-year-old girl with difficult-to-control polyarthritis RF-positive JIA. The diagram shows progress over a 5-year period, with arthritis activity and drugs used. Investigation results can be shown on the same diagram.

History

The history given here includes questions regarding possible differential diagnoses, which would be relevant only in a newly presenting patient. Differentials are given after their symptoms, in parentheses. Ask about the following.

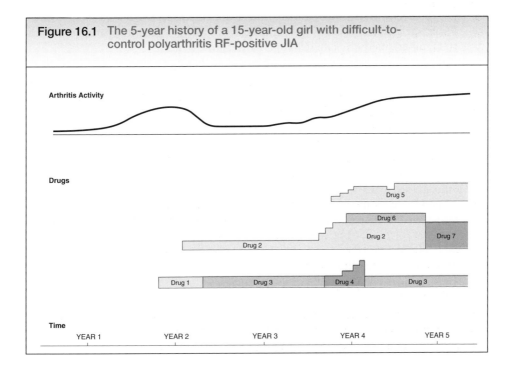

Figure 16.1 The 5-year history of a 15-year-old girl with difficult-to-control polyarthritis RF-positive JIA

Presenting complaint

Reason for current admission.

Current symptoms

1. General health: e.g. fever, pallor, weight loss, quality of sleep.
2. Joint symptoms: e.g. early morning stiffness, nocturnal discomfort, pain, tenderness, swelling, limitation of movement, problem joints (e.g. knees, hands), splints and orthoses used.
3. Level of functioning with activities of daily living (ADLs): e.g. eating (jaw opening reflecting temporo-mandibular joint (TMJ) involvement), dressing, writing, walking, aids required (e.g. dressing sticks, adaptive utensils, wheelchair, computer), home modifications required (e.g. ramps, bathroom fittings), ability to attend/manage school, limitations of sporting and social activities, depression.
4. Skin rashes: e.g. salmon rash of systemic JIA, malar flush (SLE), heliotrope of eyelids (dermatomyositis), psoriasis, rheumatoid nodules.
5. Chest symptoms: e.g. pain from pleuritis, pericarditis.
6. Bowel symptoms: e.g. diarrhoea with inflammatory bowel disease (IBD).
7. Eye problems: e.g. uveitis, cataract, glaucoma.
8. Neurological symptoms: e.g. seizures, drowsiness (JIA or SLE), personality change or headache with SLE.
9. Growth concerns: e.g. short stature, delayed puberty, requirement for growth hormone, self-image effects.
10. Nutritional issues: e.g. anorexia from drug side effects, cachexia from TNF alpha and IL-1, mechanical issues (TMJ involvement), bone mineral density (BMD) measurements (increased fracture risk with osteopenia [low bone mass for age, BMD −2.5 SD below the mean for age and sex] or osteoporosis [BMD more than 2.5 SD below the mean for age and sex]), whether taking calcium or vitamin D supplements, muscle mass measurements.
11. Jaw involvement: e.g. micrognathia, effect on self-image.
12. Drug/agent side effects: e.g. steroid effects (poor height gain, myopathy), NSAIDs (GIT upset), methotrexate (leukopenia, hepatotoxicity).

Past history

Initial diagnosis (when, where, presenting symptoms, initial investigations), apparent triggers (e.g. rubella), number of hospitalisations, sequence of joint involvement, development of complications and their management.

Management

Present treatment in hospital, usual treatment at home (including occupational and physiotherapy, exercises, sports, drugs), previous treatments used (including effects, and why stopped), side effects, monitoring of levels, compliance, use of identification bracelet, alternative therapies tried (e.g. naturopathy), elimination diets.

Social history

1. Disease impact on child: e.g. school absenteeism, limitation of ADLs, self-image.
2. Impact on parents: e.g. financial considerations such as cost of home modifications, splints, wheelchairs, transport, frequent hospitalisations, drugs.
3. Impact on siblings: e.g. sibling rivalry.
4. Benefits received: e.g. Child Disability Allowance.
5. Social supports: e.g. Arthritis Foundation of Australia.

Family history

Arthritis, inflammatory bowel disease, psoriasis, enthesitis, uveitis.

At the completion of presenting the history, the examiners should have a clear impression of the following:

1. The patient's current functioning (e.g. ADLs).
2. The patient's current (and past) treatment modalities, such as physiotherapy, drugs and alternative therapies (e.g. naturopathic) tried.
3. Social situation (e.g. child's expectations for the future, geographic situation relative to treating hospital).

Examination

See the short case on joints in this chapter. This gives an approach to the lead-in 'Please examine this child's joints', so that it covers not only signs found in JIA, but also signs indicating other diseases such as SLE. These latter features are not usually relevant in the JIA long case, unless a diagnostic dilemma exists.

Diagnosis

Although it is the most common chronic inflammatory arthropathy in children, JIA remains a clinical diagnosis of exclusion. Some of the diseases to be excluded are enumerated above. The diagnosis has been made categorically in patients used as long-case subjects. However, the candidate may be asked which investigations would have been appropriate when the child was initially seen. Thus, a differential diagnosis is worth considering, even in established cases, if only for possible discussion purposes.

Investigations

In terms of differential diagnoses, there are too many to allow a brief but worthwhile list to be given. The most appropriate investigations obviously depend on the clinical situation. Texts of paediatric rheumatology will give further information.

The following investigations may be helpful in JIA.

Blood tests

Serology

1. IgM rheumatoid factor (RF): 10% seropositive. High IgM RF titres carry a worse prognosis as regards permanent disability, and a greater likelihood of systemic features.
2. Antinuclear antibody (ANA): positive in 50%.

Haematology

1. Full blood examination may reveal normochromic normocytic anaemia, neutrophil leucocytosis or thrombocytosis.
2. ESR: often raised; sometimes normal. May be a useful monitor.

Immunology

1. Immunoglobulins: IgG may be raised; occasionally IgA may be low or absent (associated IgA deficiency).
2. Complement: C3 often elevated; a low C2 may occasionally be found (associated C2 complement deficiency); raised alpha-2-globulin.

HLA typing

1. B27: e.g. enthesitis-related arthritis in older males, psoriatic arthritis, arthritis associated with bowel disorders such as IBD.
2. DR4 (polyarthritis: RF-positive).

Imaging

Plain radiography

Plain radiographs are useful in excluding other differential diagnoses such as osteomyelitis, septic arthritis, trauma and malignancy. It is not necessary to X-ray the lumbosacral region in most children with JIA, as sacroiliac involvement appears fairly late in childhood, and the radiation dose is high. Common findings on plain X-rays include:

1. Soft-tissue swelling.
2. Joint-space narrowing.
3. Periarticular osteoporosis.

(The above three are the most common findings in RF-negative JIA.)

4. Joint erosions (development may lead to changed management).
5. Leg-length discrepancy (accelerated maturation due to hyperaemia around the joint and low grade inflammation).

Ultrasound

Ultrasound can be useful in:
1. Effusions (especially useful assessing hips, shoulders).
2. Synovitis/tenosynovitis (increased echogenicity with inflamed tissues).
3. Acute synovitis (assessing for increased vascularity on Doppler).
4. Guiding intra-articular therapy.

Magnetic resonance imaging (MRI)

MRI is useful in demonstrating anatomy, including cartilage, to assess:

1. Early joint damage.
2. Positive effects of treatment before they are clinically apparent.
3. Amount of inflamed synovium (when performed with gadolinium enhancement).
4. Long-term effects in difficult-to-monitor joints (cervical spine, TMJ, hips).

Management

The goals of JIA management are the following:

1. Provide analgesia.
2. Control inflammation.
3. Maintain joint function.
4. Prevent deformities.
5. Treat complications and extra-articular manifestations.
6. Ensure optimal nutrition.
7. Rehabilitation.
8. Ensure optimal psychosocial health.
9. Educate parents/patient regarding disease.

Provide analgesia

Pain

1. Assess severity, timing.
2. Analgesic (e.g. paracetamol).
3. Ice packs (e.g. pack of frozen peas wrapped in a moist towel) for acutely inflamed joints or hot packs (especially if there is associated stiffness) may be useful.

Morning stiffness

1. Warm bath or hot packs may be helpful.
2. Rest (but too little activity may cause muscle atrophy).
3. Nocturnal non-steroidal anti-inflammatory drugs (NSAIDs) (e.g. dispersible piroxicam, naproxen, indomethacin).

Control inflammation

Local corticosteroid injections

Long-acting steroid preparations (e.g. triamcinolone hexatonide) injected intra-articularly are safe, effective, and useful for particular joints with flexion deformities (contractures) not responding to physiotherapy, for epiphyseal overgrowth or for persistent synovitis in a few joints. Often they obviate the need for NSAID treatment. Joint injections can be performed as a day case, under conscious sedation for older children (over 10), or under general anaesthesia for those under 10 years or when multiple joints are being injected. Image intensification or ultrasound may be useful, particularly in the shoulders, hips and subtalar joints. Paediatric rheumatologists are using intra-articular therapy much earlier in the evolution of JIA than previously, often deciding on this course of treatment after their initial consultation with patients who have had a previous unsatisfactory response to NSAIDs or who have joint complications already. The positive effects of the steroid are noted usually within a few days, with effects lasting several months.

NSAIDs

NSAIDs do not modify the natural history of the condition, but do decrease pain and stiffness, as well as increase the range of movement. Analgesic response is rapid; anti-inflammatory effect takes longer. The average time to achieve a therapeutic response is around 1 month. Nearly all patients who are going to respond to a particular NSAID will do so within 3 months. The most common side effects are anorexia and abdominal pain, although some children may also have behavioural effects. Gastrointestinal ulceration is rarer in children than in adults; however, medications such as antacids or H_2 blockers may well be required. More significant side effects can include bruising from abnormal coagulation, and pseudoporphyria skin rashes on sun exposed areas. Probably all NSAIDs can cause pseudoporphyria rashes, although the highest relative risk and the early descriptions were with naproxen. Unfortunately NSAIDs are unpredictable, their effectiveness being largely idiosyncratic. Around 50% of JIA children respond to their first NSAID.

NSAIDs include naproxen, diclofenac (avoid if there is a history of aspirin allergy, as there is cross-sensitivity with aspirin), ibuprofen (can be used if intolerant to other drugs in this group), indomethacin (especially enthesitis arthritis or unresponsive systemic onset patients), piroxicam, aspirin, and tolmetin sodium (not available in Australia).

With the past adverse publicity relating to salicylate usage and Reye's syndrome, aspirin is used rarely and is not recommended. The toxicity to therapeutic efficacy ratio is low. The usual maximum dosage is 100 mg/kg/day. Starting dosage is 50 to 60 mg/kg/day. Use a buffered form. Monitor with salicylate levels, particularly if high doses are used (take at 2 hours post-dose, after 5 days of treatment). It is unwise to adjust the dose by any more than 10% at any time. Levels are lowered by systemic steroids (so be aware that when steroids are ceased, salicylate levels may rise acutely). Liver function tests (LFTs) should be performed before commencing treatment and regularly during treatment (for hepatic dysfunction, especially in the systemic onset group). If LFT results are abnormal initially, aspirin should be avoided.

COX-2 (cyclo-oxygenase isoenzyme 2) inhibitors

These have been used in adults extensively. They block the prostaglandins (PGs) responsible for inflammation, pain and fever, but not the PGs that protect the gastric antrum: hence, they have a lower incidence of upper GIT symptoms than the older NSAIDs. They have similar efficacy to NSAIDs. They are reserved for patients with gastrointestinal intolerance to conventional NSAIDs. Recent concern in post-licensing adult studies about an increased relative risk of cardiovascular events has led to the withdrawal of rofecoxib from the market, and caution with the use of other COX-2 inhibitors.

Disease-modifying antirheumatic drugs (DMARDs)

DMARDs that are known to be effective include methotrexate (MTX), leflunomide, sulphasalazine (SSZ) and etanercept (see under biological agents below). Previously used DMARDs including penicillamine and gold preparations have not shown efficacy in double-blind placebo-controlled trials. Hydroxychloroquine has been shown in a RCT in polyarticular-onset JIA to be effective in comparison with placebo. If the response to NSAIDs is unsatisfactory, then more potent agents may be required. In polyarticular JIA, if there is not an early NSAID response, NSAIDs and DMARDs are used together. About two-thirds of JIA patients require a DMARD.

Methotrexate (MTX)

MTX is effective in all forms of JIA, and represents the gold standard for DMARDs. Low-dose, once-a-week MTX is safe and reliable. Folate supplementation decreases side effects. MTX is given at a dose of 10–20 mg per square metre of surface area once a week, orally. Higher doses are more effective but may require intramuscular or subcutaneous injection (oral doses limited by finite absorption). Side effects include nausea and oral ulcers (lessened by treating with folate), gastrointestinal and bone marrow toxicities. Regular blood tests are performed to detect any liver impairment or marrow involvement. Long-term studies of MTX in JIA have yet to be published. Theoretical risks of carcinogenesis, infertility or interstitial lung disease have not transpired with several years of treatment. It has been shown to slow and even stop the progression of bone destruction in adults with rheumatoid arthritis. MTX has allowed remission to be achieved early in many patients.

Leflunomide

This is a pyrimidine synthesis inhibitor of dihydro-orotate dehydrogenase. It appears safe and effective, and compares favourably to MTX, both in efficacy and in having fewer side effects. It is currently being studied for use in JIA. Its side effects include diarrhoea, elevated liver enzyme levels, and mucocutaneous abnormalities. Leflunomide may have teratogenic effects and in patients of child-bearing age effective contraception is required during and for up to 2 years after use ('washout' regimens are available to shorten this interval if needed).

Sulphasalazine (SSZ)

Some rheumatologists use this before MTX, particularly in ERA. The effective moiety of the drug is 5-aminosalicylic acid. A trial of at least three months, and usually longer, is needed to judge efficacy. Side effects include hypersensitivity reactions, hepatotoxicity and bone marrow alterations. In adults with rheumatoid arthritis (RA), it is used in triple therapy with MTX and hydroxychloroquine (see below).

Corticosteroids

Systemic use

Generally, steroids are used in systemic disease (usually required for a substantial period). Steroids are indicated in any serious complications (such as cardiac involvement, hepatitis, encephalitis or uveitis (topical, or oral/systemic if uveitis is severe). They also have a place as an adjunct to other therapy (e.g. in polyarthritis not responding to other drugs). There tends to be a very individual response to steroids. Oral steroids should be taken on an alternate-day basis to decrease the incidence of Cushingoid side effects.

Pulse intravenous steroids are worth trying initially in severe systemic illness (e.g. pericarditis) or blinding iridocyclitis. IV methylprednisolone (30 mg/kg [up to one gram maximum dose] for 3 consecutive days; some units repeat this a week later) can be used as an inducing agent for systemic JIA. It is combined with cyclosporine to treat macrophage activation syndrome (haemophagocytic syndrome), which occurs in systemic arthritis and has a high mortality rate.

Biological agents

Etanercept (recombinant p75 soluble tumour necrosis factor receptor (sTNFR): Fc fusion protein)

The first anticytokine therapy used in JIA, it is recommended for patients with extended oligoarticular and polyarticular JIA, who have failed to respond to NSAIDs or MTX. At the time of writing (2006) it remains the only biological agent that has been proved to be effective in JIA. The dose in children/adolescents aged 4–17 is 0.4 mg/kg twice weekly by subcutaneous (SC) injection. Parents are trained in reconstituting the etanercept and administering the injection using an aseptic technique. Autoinjectors (as used for diabetics) can be useful. Injection site reactions are common. It is contraindicated in sepsis. It has been trialled in hundreds of adults with RA with good effect, causing significant reductions in disease activity within 2 weeks of starting it (in adults) with prolonged benefit for 6 months, in patients with disease refractory to other DMARDs. In polyarticular JIA it has been used in MTX-refractory disease with clinically significant improvement in up to 70% of patients: it controlled pain and swelling, improved laboratory parameters and slowed radiographic progression of disease. The drug is named to indicate that it intercepts TNF-alpha, a cytokine thought to be most crucial in the pathogenesis of RA. As well as binding and inhibiting TNF-alpha, it has similar effects on lymphotoxin-alpha (also called TNF-beta). It is made up of two components: the extracellular ligand-binding domain of the 75kD human receptor for TNF-alpha, and the constant portion of human immunoglobulin (IgG1): hence the term 'fusion protein'. Its initial success suggests it will become a major agent in JIA.

In Australia, Medicare requirements for the funded supply of etanercept are that application must be made for an authority for specialised drug use, and that the patient must be under the care of a recognised paediatric rheumatology service.

Other biological agents

- **Infliximab** is a chimeric monoclonal anti-TNF-alpha antibody. Preliminary studies suggest it is as efficacious as etanercept in treating SOJIA, polyarthritis and JPsA, but has more frequent and more severe side effects, including increased rates of new infections. It is given intravenously.

- **Adalimumab** also is a monoclonal anti–TNF-alpha antibody, but is completely humanised, and given by SC injection. Early studies suggest it may be useful in the treatment of polyarticular disease.
- **Anakinra** is a recombinant IL-1 receptor antagonist, which may be useful in recalcitrant SOJIA.
- **Humanised anti-interleukin-6 receptor antibody** also appears promising in the therapy of recalcitrant SOJIA.

Autologous haemopoietic stem cell transplantation (HSCT)

This is experimental. A small number of studies have shown it can be successful in the short term, but long-term effects are not known, and side effects can be substantial. At least four deaths as a complication of an HSCT for JIA have been recorded, related to MAS (see page 454) and many rheumatologists would not consider the procedure because of the inherent risks.

Monitoring disease activity

An essential component of controlling the inflammatory process is that of clinical and laboratory monitoring.

1. Clinical disease (e.g. fever, worsening joint count, worsening joint function).
2. Erythrocyte sedimentation rate.
3. MRI/X-ray showing disease progression.
4. Degree of anaemia.

Sequence of drugs/agents

The examiners may ask your approach to the use of the drugs noted above.

1. For life-threatening SOJIA, pulse corticosteroids are the agents of choice. If pulse steroids are ineffective, then MTX. If MTX is unsuccessful, then leflunomide. If the condition is not responding, consider biological agents.
2. For non–life-threatening and non-systemic disease, try the following sequentially:
   - In oligoarthritis, intra-articular corticosteroids with NSAIDs. If unsuccessful, add MTX (or SSZ for ERA). If not responding, consider biological agents ($\pm$ repeating intra-articular steroid injections).
   - In polyarthritis, MTX with NSAIDs, $\pm$ intra-articular corticosteroids. If unsuccessful, try systemic steroids. If unsuccessful, consider leflunomide. If not responding, consider biological agents.
   - In extended oligoarthritis, and JPsA patients who do not respond to first-line therapy, follow the sequence for polyarthritis.

The management algorithm for each type ends with biological agents, after steroids and/or MTX along the way.

Maintain joint function

1. Physiotherapy (including hydrotherapy) to maintain joint range of movement (ROM) (e.g. by gentle stretching), muscle strength (exercise) and gait education. Particularly useful types of exercise that help joint range and strength are cycling and swimming.
2. Attention to footwear (e.g. 'jogging' or 'tennis' shoes are comfortable and often appropriate), leg length (for development of epiphyseal overgrowth), deformities

(e.g. genu valgus, from epiphyseal overgrowth; measure intermalleolar distance to monitor this).

3. Even in acute flare-ups of disease, continue passive movement to maintain joint range of movement (e.g. in the hydrotherapy pool).

4. Occupational therapy assistance for those with upper limb involvement, particularly for wrist, metacarpophalangeal and interphalangeal joint involvement. This assists with fine motor movement, and ADLs such as dressing, feeding and toileting, and for writing and keyboard use.

Prevent deformities

1. Splinting
   a. Resting splint (to rest an acutely inflamed joint).
   b. Corrective splint (to increase joint ROM; by serial splinting, placing in maximal ROM or dynamic splinting).
   c. Functional splinting (to protect joint during ADLs: e.g. ankle–foot orthoses, wrist cock-up splint).
2. Insoles and medial arch support (for ankle valgus).
3. Prone lying (for hip contractures in particular).
4. Nocturnal traction (especially for hip pain).
5. Cervical collar (for torticollis, pain, occipito-atlanto dislocation, and before general anaesthesia requiring intubation).
6. Surgical intervention may be needed where conservative treatment has failed to prevent deformity. Possible interventions include soft-tissue releases (e.g. for fixed flexion deformities at hips, knees), stapling (e.g. of medial femoral and tibial epiphyses to correct valgus deformity), osteotomy, fusion. Synovectomy is occasionally needed for persistent pain and swelling (e.g. hips, knees). Occasionally, total joint replacement (e.g. hips, knees) is required.

Treat complications

Eye involvement

All sero-negative patients are at risk of uveitis.

1. Chronic uveitis: all patients need regular eye checks: if ANA-positive, every 3–4 months if under the age of 7 years at onset of disease; every 6 months if older than 7 years at onset of disease; then annually. For RF-positive or systemic onset disease, eye checks annually.
2. Active uveitis is treated with steroid eye drops and mydriatics.

Infection

Treat with appropriate antibiotics and general supportive measures.

Amyloidosis

Fortunately this is now extremely rare. It may present with hepatosplenomegaly, abdominal pain, diarrhoea or albuminuria, and is diagnosed by rectal or renal biopsy. Treatment is with chlorambucil. Children with severe SOJIA are more likely to have this complication: the overall incidence of amyloidosis in some studies in this group has been up to 9%, but it is now much less likely with early and appropriate treatment.

Ensure optimal nutrition

Nutritional status may be inadvertently overlooked. Drug-treatment side effects, active disease or TMJ involvement can lead to suboptimal intake, inadequate energy and muscle bulk, which can negatively impact on many aspects of treatment.

Rehabilitation

Occupational therapy

1. School: use of adaptive pencil holder, standing desks, ramps, decreasing inter-class distances, avoiding stairs, potential for use of laptops in place of writing.
2. Home: dressing sticks and hoops, large buttons, Velcro fasteners, adaptive utensils, hand-held shower, use of computers, tape recorders (if writing difficult).

Physiotherapy

Exercise: passive to improve joint ROM; active to prevent weakness; resistive to strengthen muscles. Also aim for better endurance.

Family support

Social worker, parent support groups, child disability allowances, disabled parking authorisation.

Ensure optimal psychosocial health

1. Promote as much independence as possible.
2. Encourage child to take responsibility for management, as appropriate for age.
3. Build self-esteem.
4. Help child deal with peer-group problems.
5. Family psychosocial support, including siblings.

Educate parents and patient regarding disease

1. Ensure adequate understanding by parents, patients and siblings of disease, treatment, drug side effects, importance of compliance and prognosis.
2. Dispel myths and false beliefs (e.g. held by other, older family members) regarding JIA, drugs used, alternative therapies (unproven therapies that are popular [despite no data in existence to support their use], including glucosamine and hyaluronic acid).
3. No significant familial incidence of JIA; no association with later onset in adult life of RF-positive disease.

Prognosis

One-third of patients with JIA will still have active disease as adults, which may well interfere with their ADLs and lifestyle. The prognosis depends on the type of JIA. RF-positive patients have the worst prognosis: these are usually females with onset as teenagers. Children with only a few joints involved do better than children with systemic disease or polyarthritis with regard to joint deformities and complications (e.g. osteoporosis, growth impairment [local and general] and psychosocial development). Children with oligoarthritis tend to have a good functional outcome with respect to joints. Serious ocular damage occurs in 10–20%. In SOJIA, 60–85% of patients will go into remission; up to one-third develop destructive polyarthritis; the average duration of disease activity is 6 years. In a follow up study of JIA patients with disease duration over 10 years, around one-third had depression, related directly to disability and ongoing disease activity. Death from complications is extremely rare (less than 0.3% in North America).

Idiopathic inflammatory myopathies (IIMs): juvenile dermatomyositis (JDM)

The IIMs of childhood are rare diseases, but not uncommon in examination settings.

Background

Since 1975, the criteria of Bohan and Peter have been used widely. The five diagnostic criteria include:

1. Characteristic rashes. Two are pathognomonic: (a) Gottron's papules—scaly red papular areas over the knuckles (MP) and IP joints [papules can also overlay elbows, knees and malleoli]; (b) heliotrope rash—a violaceous or purplish, somewhat oedematous discolouration around the eyes, particularly over the eyelids (capillary telangiectasia), which may cross the nasal bridge and include the nasolabial folds. Other rashes encountered include scaly red rash on the face, neck and upper chest (V-sign), the shawl area (shawl sign) and over the extensor tendons, particularly of the hands (linear extensor erythema).
    The other criteria, of which three out of four are required, are:
2. Symmetrical proximal muscle weakness.
3. Elevated muscle-derived enzymes (creatine kinase [CK], aldolase, lactate dehydrogenase [LDH] and transaminases [AST and ALT]).
4. Muscle histopathology confirming chronic inflammation.
5. Electromyography [EMG] changes of inflammatory myopathy [fasciculations at rest, bizarre high-frequency discharges]. EMG interpretation is dependent on appropriate placing of the electrode in areas of inflammation. Magnetic resonance imaging (MRI) is used to select the sample site (inflammatory muscle involvement causes non-uniform changes in muscle, abnormal increased signal on T2-weighted images and normal signal on T1).

JDM is an occlusive small-vessel vasculopathy, involving arterioles and capillaries. There can be very diffuse vasculitis (which may include nail-bed telangiectasia, digital ulceration, infarction of oral epithelium, gastrointestinal ulceration) and vasomotor instability. In 1997, Rider and Miller suggested a clinicopathological classification of the juvenile IIMs, listing 11 subsets in keeping with the myositis subsets recognised in adults.

The incidence of JDM is around 2–3 per million. Gender ratio varies around the world: in the UK and USA girls are affected more often (up to twice as often), but in India and Japan boys are affected more often. Mean age of onset varies also: it is around 7 years in the USA and in the UK, but in the UK it has bimodal incidence, with one peak at 2–6 and the other at 12–13. Susceptibility to developing JDM has been associated with several HLA alleles, including the class II major histocompatibility allele HLA-DQA1*0501, and the course of the disease and the development of complications are associated with polymorphisms at the tumour necrosis factor (TNF) alpha-308 locus.

At diagnosis, all children have weakness and rash, most have muscle pain and fever, and 20–50% have dysphagia, abdominal pain and/or arthritis. Soft-tissue calcification (calcinosis) is seen in 30–70%, in sites exposed to trauma (buttocks, knees, elbows) and seems to reflect the severity and duration of disease. Calcification can resolve spontaneously, and drain a white exudate, leaving pitted scars. They can persist in fibrotic muscle in sheath-like forms, impairing function. Both the skin and the muscle manifestations may be precipitated by sun exposure.

Gastrointestinal involvement, through muscle weakness and/or vasculitis, can lead to impaired speech from tongue involvement, decreased oesophageal motility with impaired swallowing, oesophageal reflux, aspiration pneumonia, ulceration, perforation, haemorrhage, pneumatosis intestinalis and malabsorption.

Cardiopulmonary involvement can cause asymptomatic conduction abnormalities and pulmonary fibrosis.

Other manifestations include:

1. Vasculitis involving the central nervous system (causing seizures, organic psychosis; even fatal brainstem infarction has been described).
2. Ophthalmologic complications include retinopathy (retinal exudates, 'cotton-wool' spots, optic atrophy, visual impairment), glaucoma (from steroids) and cataracts (from steroids).
3. Renal tract: renal failure secondary to myoglobinuria from muscle breakdown; ureteral (middle third) necrosis secondary to vasculopathy.
4. Reproductive system: active disease can delay menarche, interrupt menses or adversely affect pregnancy outcomes.
5. Raynaud's phenomenon.

There are recognised subgroups based on the course of the disease: monocyclic (full recovery without relapse), chronic polycyclic (prolonged relapsing course), chronic continuous (persistent disease despite daily steroids), and ulcerative.

In recent years, a number of groups have collaborated internationally and produced accurate, reliable and validated outcome measurement tools. The three commonly used are the Childhood Health Assessment Questionnaire (CHAQ; initially developed to measure physical function in children with arthritis), Manual Muscle Testing (MMT; a score that assesses muscle strength of seven proximal and five distal muscle groups, bilaterally; predicts disease activity) and the Childhood Myositis Assessment Scale (CMAS; a 14-activity assessment of physical function, strength and endurance). These standardised tools allow comparisons between groups throughout the world.

History

At the completion of presenting the history, the examiners should have a clear impression of the patient's current functioning (e.g. ADLs), current (and past) treatment modalities (such as physiotherapy, drugs and alternative therapies [e.g. naturopathic] tried), and social situation (e.g. transport issues, distance from home to treating hospital).

Ask about the following:

Presenting complaint

Reason for current admission.

Current symptoms

1. General health (e.g. fever, weight loss, nutritional status).
2. Musculoskeletal symptoms: e.g. muscle tenderness, cramps, weakness, joint symptoms (early morning stiffness, nocturnal discomfort, pain, tenderness, swelling, limitation of movement [calcinosis of tendon sheaths], problem joints), contractures, requirement for serial casting.

3. Skin rashes: e.g. heliotrope of eyelids, Gottron's papules (knuckles), photosensitive rashes, scarring, atrophy.
4. Calcinosis: e.g. problem areas (e.g. buttocks).
5. Level of functioning with activities of daily living (ADLs): e.g. speech (tongue involvement), eating (chewing difficulties from masseter involvement), swallowing (abnormal oesophageal motility), sitting (buttock soft-tissue calcification), walking, negotiating stairs, squatting, assistance devices (e.g. adaptive utensils, wheelchair, computer), home modifications required (e.g. ramps, bathroom fittings).
6. Gastrointestinal (GIT) symptoms: oral, upper GIT, lower GIT (e.g. ulceration, perforation, haemorrhage, malabsorption).
7. Genitourinary symptoms: e.g. episodes of myoglobinuria, renal impairment, ureteral involvement, interference with menstruation.
8. Eye problems: e.g. visual impairment, retinopathy, glaucoma.
9. Neurological symptoms: e.g. mood swings, depression.
10. Drug side effects: e.g. steroid effects (Cushing's syndrome, poor height gain, myopathy), cytotoxics (e.g. myelosuppression, opportunistic infection, hepatotoxicity [MTX], hypertension [CPA]), IVIG (infusion-related toxicities, other IVIG complications such as aseptic meningitis, thromboembolism).
11. Other systems review: e.g. cardiopulmonary symptoms, Raynaud's phenomenon.

Past history

Initial diagnosis (when, where, presenting symptoms, initial investigations), possible triggers (e.g. infectious agents [parvovirus, enteroviruses, hepatitis B], excessive sun exposure), pattern of illness (monocyclic, chronic polycyclic, continuous), hospitalisations, development of complications and their management.

Management

Current treatment in hospital, usual treatment at home (e.g. occupational therapy and physiotherapy, exercises, medications), previous treatments used (e.g. azathioprine, IVIG), responses to treatment, side effects, monitoring of effect, alternative therapies tried.

Social history

1. Disease impact on: (a) child (school absenteeism, limited ADLs, poor self-image); (b) parents (financial considerations: home modifications, wheelchairs, computers, transport, frequent hospitalisations, drugs); (c) siblings (rivalry).
2. Benefits received: e.g. Child Disability Allowance.
3. Social supports.

Family history

Any connective tissue diseases.

Examination

The approach given in Table 16.1 could be used for a short case or clinic follow-up.

The following is the sequence suggested for the joint examination (for detail see joints short case). Inspect distribution of joint involvement (symmetry); note swelling, loss of normal contours, angulation, deformity, redness, muscle wasting. Next, feel the joint and periarticular areas for tenderness, warmth, effusion, 'boggy' swelling

Table 16.1 Examination for juvenile dermatomyositis (JDM)

Initial impression
Well or unwell
Face
- Cushingoid (steroids)
- Heliotrope eyelid rash
- 'Chipmunk' facies (masseter atrophy)
Parameters
- Height (short from steroids)
- Weight (obese from steroids; thin from hypercatabolism or malabsorption)
Lipodystrophy (symmetrical loss of subcutaneous fatty tissue, mainly upper body; occasionally asymmetrical; usually in females; can be associated with acanthosis nigricans, hirsutism and clitoral hypertrophy)

Skin
Photosensitive rashes (distribution of sun exposure)
Vasculitic rash
Subcutaneous calcification (buttocks, elbows, knees), scars/pits of old calcinosis
Atrophy
Hypertrichosis (cyclosporine)

Upper limbs
Hands
- Raynaud's phenomenon
- Digital ulcers/scars
Nails: nail fold capillary bed telangiectasia
Palms
- Anaemia (drug side effects, e.g. cytotoxics)
Knuckles
- Gottron's papules
Blood pressure
- Elevated (e.g. steroids, nephropathy, cyclosporine); if elevated, make a point of requesting urinalysis now
Neuromuscular assessment
- Palpate muscles (tenderness)
- Range of movement of joints (active then passive)/tone (contractures from sheathing of tendons)
- Power
- Reflexes
Joint assessment
- All joints of upper limbs (as for joints short case)
Functional assessment
- Activities of daily living (e.g. writing,

brushing teeth, combing hair, turning taps on or off, feeding self, carrying household objects)

Head and neck
Eyes
- Conjunctival pallor
- Visual acuity
- Glaucoma (steroids)
- Cataract (steroids)
- Retinopathy (retinal 'cottonwool' spots; optic atrophy)
Mouth
- Inflamed mucous membrane
- Gum hyperplasia (CPA)
- Dysphonia

Cardiorespiratory
Auscultate
- Praecordium
- Lung fields

Abdomen
Tenderness (gastrointestinal haemorrhage/ulceration)
Buttock rash

Gait, lower limbs and back
Neuromuscular assessment
- Full gait examination
Squat
- Proximal weakness (JDM per se; steroids)
Test for truncal weakness: get child to do a sit up from lying position on the bed, or resisted head lift off the bed (truncal weakness can take quite some time to return to normal, often lagging behind limb strength improvements)
Lower limbs (neurologically)
- Palpate muscles (tenderness)
- Range of movement of joints (active then passive)/tone (contractures from sheathing of tendons)
- Power
- Reflexes
Back
- Palpate for tenderness (osteoporosis)
- Examine joints
Joint assessment
- All joints of lower limbs (as per joints short case)

Continued

Table 16.1 *(Continued)*	

Functional assessment
  • Activities of daily living (e.g. sitting,
    getting out of chair, climbing stairs)
Other
Temperature chart
  • Fever (intercurrent illness, from
    steroids/cytotoxics)
Urinalysis
  • Myoglobinuria
	• Proteinuria (nephropathy: JDM per
	  se, or cytotoxics)
	• Haematuria (nephropathy: JDM per
	  se, or cytotoxics)
	Stool analysis
	  • Blood

CPA = cyclophosphamide.

(thickened synovium and fluid), contractures. Range of movement (ROM) is then examined, active movement first. Only test passive movement if active movement does not produce the full range. The angle from neutral should be recorded using your own joints (hopefully normal) as reference. A suggested order for a systematic examination of all the joints is as follows: hands, wrists, elbows, shoulders, temporo-mandibular joints, cervical spine, lumbar spine, hips, knees, ankles, feet (i.e. hand to head, and head to toe). A good initial position is with the child sitting in a chair, or on the side of a bed, with the hands resting on the thighs.

The easiest places on the body to visualise capillaries are the nail folds and along the teeth–gum line. This is where the underlying pathological lesion, capillary vasculopathy, can best be assessed. The findings of capillary branching and dilation, areas of haemor-rhage, fewer capillaries per millimetre, can all be seen with nail-fold capillaroscopy. Paediatric rheumatologists may use a stereomicroscope with microscopic oil to cut down on skin reflection, or simply a magnifying glass with water-soluble gel. Counting capillaries at distal nail fold can predict disease activity, muscle strength and function, as well as skin activity.

Management

Goals of JDM management

1. Control inflammation.
2. Restore muscle strength.
3. Maintain functional abilities.
4. Prevent and treat complications.
5. Minimise treatment side effects.
6. Educate parent and patient regarding disease.

First-line treatment

There is a lack of randomised controlled trials in JDM. Corticosteroids (CS) remain the conventional first-line agents in conjunction with physiotherapy. CS have been used for over 40 years in JDM. Around 80% of patients improve on CS treatment. The previous pre-CS mortality of 40% has decreased to 3%, substantially due to daily oral CS therapy. It is likely that residual disability and extent of calcinosis have been diminished by CS as well (although CS themselves can cause muscle weakness, osteoporotic fractures and avascular necrosis, which can adversely affect residual disability). The oral prednisolone dosage is usually 1–3 mg/kg/day. The dose can be weaned, once normal (or near normal) muscle strength is established, slowly to lower-dose daily therapy.

The use of intravenous pulse methylprednisolone seems to lead to less relapsing disease, residual weakness or calcinosis, compared to daily oral prednisolone treatment. Pulse methylprednisolone also may be useful for treating serious complications such as myocarditis or dysphagia, as well as for treating the skin manifestations.

If remission is not induced by CS quickly, then use of immunomodulating agents is the next step. Many rheumatologists now would use combination methotrexate (MTX) and CS from day 1.

Other drugs previously used have included azathioprine (AZA), cyclosporine (CSA), and cyclophosphamide (CPA). Other immuno-modulating agents include intravenous immunoglobulin (IVIG), plasmapheresis and tacrolimus.

Second-line treatment

Methotrexate (MTX)

This inhibits dihydrofolate reductase, which is needed to make DNA and some amino acids. Lower doses are used in rheumatology than in oncology. MTX was originally a second-line agent used with steroids for refractory disease, but recently there has been a shift towards earlier use of MTX as a steroid-sparing agent. Benefit is apparent within 4–8 weeks after the dosage is optimised (though it can take up to 12 weeks before a positive effect is seen). Side effects include (mnemonic: MTX):

M **M**ucositis and **M**yelosuppression
T **T**ransaminase increase (i.e. hepatotoxicity)
X **X**-rays warranted (*chest* X-ray for pulmonary toxicity and/or pulmonary infection [e.g. varicella pneumonia, *Pneumocystis carinii* pneumonia]; *skeletal* X-ray for osteopathy or osteomyelitis) and **X**tra folate recommended.

Other opportunistic infections can occur: e.g. cutaneous herpes zoster, herpes simplex, *Listeria monocytogenes* meningitis, tuberculosis. In combination with CS, there is an increased risk of opportunistic infection. Unfortunately, not all patients will respond to the combination of steroids and MTX.

Cyclophosphamide (CPA)

Pulse IV-CPA has been used for skin and gut ulceration, and interstitial lung disease. Side effects are (mnemonic: CPA):

C **C**ystitis (haemorrhagic)
P **P**ancytopenia
A **A**ctivation of herpes zoster (i.e. opportunistic infection).

Intravenous immunoglobulin (IVIG)

This has, presumably, multiple mechanisms of action. A regimen of 2 days consecutive treatment monthly leads to peak effect after 3 months. Response is comparable to that of pulse methylprednisolone and cyclosporine. Side effects include infusion-related toxicities (e.g. hypotension, fever), aseptic meningitis, thromboembolic events caused by increased viscosity.

Azathioprine (AZA)

This is a purine analogue, metabolised to 6-mercaptopurine, inhibits purine ribo-nucleotide synthesis. It can lead to complete or partial remission in up to 70% of patients when used as the second-line immunosuppressive. It has fewer side effects than the other cytotoxics. Its onset peak effect is at 3–6 months after initiating treatment. It can cause gastrointestinal upset, and bone marrow suppression with leukopenia. In combination with CS, there is an increased risk of opportunistic infection.

Cyclosporine (CSA)

A prodrug derived from fungi, binds to an intracellular protein 'cyclophilin' which inhibits activity of a calcium-regulated enzyme, calcineurin, required for transmitting activating signals from T-cell receptors. There are several noteworthy side effects (mnemonic: CSA):

C   **C**ompromised kidneys (nephrotoxicity includes irreversible vasculopathy, interstitial fibrosis, tubular damage)

S   **S**econdary malignancy potential (especially lymphoproliferative)

A   **A**naemia and **A**ccelerated blood pressure (hypertension), hair growth (hypertrichosis) and gums (gingival hyperplasia), and **A**dditional myopathy (caused by CSA per se; this can contribute to osteoporosis).

There is little published evidence to support the use of CSA in JDM, though anecdotally some paediatric rheumatologists will quote it as effective.

Prognostic predictors

Some units use second-line agents in patients with factors known to portend a worse prognosis, including those with: (a) severe disease, particularly with complications of calcification, ulceration, interstitial lung disease or significant dysphagia; (b) particular myositis-specific autoantibodies (MSAs); (c) delayed treatment.

Life-threatening disease (e.g. myocarditis, severe dysphagia)

Treatments have included pulse methylprednisolone, oral CPA, pulse IV-CPA, plasmapheresis, or combination therapies (e,g. MTX + AZA; IVIG + CSA).

Extramuscular disease

1. Calcinosis

This is more common where there has been a delay in starting treatment, and in polycyclic disease, local trauma and treatment with low CS doses. All the following treatments are anecdotal and there is no evidence they are better than the natural history, as many cases with calcinosis resolve. These include aggressive therapy for underlying disease (as calcinosis reflects ongoing disease activity); colchicine; surgical removal (some cases); diltiazem (but can induce flares of myositis); aluminium hydroxide; oral, intralesional and intravenous magnesium sulphate and magnesium lactate; pamidronate (a bisphosphonate); lithotripsy.

2. Skin disease

Sun protection using sunscreens, sun avoidance and topical steroids are useful. Hydroxychloroquine is also useful. Antihistamines may be needed for associated pruritus. Other agents that can improve rashes include methylprednisolone, MTX, CSA, IVIG and dapsone.

3. Osteoporosis

Multifactorial: (a) steroid use; (b) decreased muscle bulk and mobility; (c) deposition of resorbed bone calcium in calcinosis; (d) decreased GIT calcium absorption; (e) production of cytokines that resorb bone (during active disease). With steroid therapy, if dietary intake is inadequate, supplementation with calcium and vitamin D can prevent osteoporosis occurring.

Prognosis

Mortality is 3%. Morbidity remains high, from delay of treatment, or medication side effects. Daily steroids are often needed for 2 years: toxicities include growth failure, hypertension, cataracts and Cushingoid features.

Systemic lupus erythematosus (SLE)

SLE is a multisystem disease traditionally labelled as autoimmune and usually affecting older children and adolescents. The main problem is persistent nonspecific polyclonal B-cell activation, which causes immune complexes to be deposited widely in various organs. Compared to adults with SLE, there is a change (increase) in frequency of several aspects of SLE in children (mnemonic: CHANGE):

C	**C**horea
H	**H**epatosplenomegaly
AN	**A**vascular **N**ecrosis
G	**G**lomerulonephritis
E	**E**xclusively paediatric problems: growth abnormalities, and neonatal lupus.

As paediatric SLE (pSLE) is a chronic illness, whose sufferers are generally fairly well, but in which there are still a wide range of management issues for discussion, affected children may be ideal long-case subjects. Over the last 5 years there have been improvements in outcomes in many aspects of pSLE, with earlier use of powerful immunosuppressive therapy, increased 5- and 10-year survival rates, and joint revision of a comprehensive renal biopsy classification in 2003 by the World Health Organization (WHO), the International Society of Nephrology and the Renal Pathological Society. Lupus nephritis is categorised from class I to class VI, with many subgroups in between. Treatment for lupus nephritis is based on the renal histology.

Background information

The incidence of SLE is 1 in 2500: it is ten times more common in females. It usually becomes apparent in the second or third decade. It is more common in African Americans, Asians and Arabs. There is a genetic component, with 30% concordance in monozygotic twins, an increased susceptibility to SLE with certain HLA haplotypes (HLA-DQ loci), and deficiency of complement components (homozygous deficiency of C1q, C1r, C1s, C4, C2). These deficiencies remain the strongest susceptibility factors to SLE yet identified.

It has been hypothesised that the cause of SLE could be failure to maintain self-tolerance, secondary to defective removal of apoptotic cells. A common feature of the autoantigens in SLE, particularly chromatin and phospholipids, is that they are components of the surface blebs of apoptotic cells. Apoptosis is programmed cell death. Condensation and fragmentation of the nucleus, plus internucleosomal cleavage of chromatin, lead to formation of apoptotic bodies and blebs. If there is disturbed removal of apoptotic cells, these could become antigenic targets for autoantibodies. Other non-genetic factors that increase the likelihood of developing SLE include oestrogens (androgens protect), UV light and certain medications. There is a range of medications definitely associated (e.g. procainamide, hydralazine), and several possibly associated (e.g. minocycline) with SLE.

History

Presenting complaint

Reason for current admission.

Symptoms

Essentially an extensive systems review. The three common organ systems involved in pSLE are the skin, musculoskeletal and renal systems. The most common clinical features include (in approximate descending order): rash (any type), arthritis, fever, nephritis (all of these are present in over 50% at presentation), lymphadenopathy, hepatosplenomegaly, malar rash (specifically, these present in about one-third at presentation), neuropsychiatric disease, gastrointestinal disease, pulmonary disease and cardiovascular disease (these last four are uncommon in pSLE). Constitutional symptoms such as fever, fatigue/malaise and weight loss are very common at presentation and with flares of disease.

1. General (anorexia, malaise, pallor, weight loss, fatigue).
2. Skin (malar rash [in 33%], purpura), mucous membrane (palate ulcers), hair loss.
3. Joints (morning stiffness, pain, swelling).
4. Cardiovascular (Raynaud's phenomenon, cardiac failure symptoms due to myocarditis, chest pain from serositis, or, less likely, myocardial ischaemia).
5. Respiratory (recurrent chest infections, pleuritic chest pain, dyspnoea).
6. Renal (hypertension, oedema).
7. Neurological (seizures, headache, chorea, personality change, depression).
8. Abdominal pain (e.g. serositis, pancreatitis).
9. Menstrual abnormalties (due to SLE per se or steroids).
10. Endocrine (diabetes).
11. Drug effects (e.g. steroid effects: Cushing syndrome, hypertension, poor height gain, myopathy).

Past history

Initial diagnosis (when, where, presenting symptoms, initial investigations), recognised aetiologies such as complement deficiencies, drug-induced disease (e.g. hydralazine, alpha-methyldopa, penicillamine, isoniazid, chlorpromazine), number of hospitalisations, sequence of complication developments and their management.

Management

Present treatment in hospital, usual treatment at home, previous treatments tried, side effects, compliance, use of identification bracelet.

Social history

Disease impact on child (e.g. amount of school missed, limitation of activities of daily living, impact of disease manifestations and side effects of treatment such as malar rash, hair loss from cyclophosphamide or weight gain from steroids). Impact on family (financial considerations such as cost of frequent hospitalisation, private health insurance), impact on siblings (e.g. sibling rivalry), benefits received (e.g. Child Disability Allowance), social supports (e.g. Lupus Association).

Understanding of disease

By child and by parents. Ask about the degree of previous education (e.g. in hospital, by local paediatrician), contingency plans (e.g. who to contact first when the child is unwell).

Examination

The procedure outlined here would also be suitable for a short-case approach.

General observation

1.   Well or unwell.
2.   Pallor (anaemia; various mechanisms).
3.   Cushingoid features (steroid treatment).
4.   Parameters: height (e.g. short due to steroids); weight (e.g. obese due to steroids).
5.   Skin rashes.
6.   Joint swelling.
7.   Peripheral oedema (renal disease).
8.   Posturing (e.g. hemiplegic).
9.   Involuntary movements (e.g. chorea).
10.   Respiratory distress (e.g. pneumonitis, pulmonary oedema).
11.   Impression of mental state (e.g. depressed, or difficulty concentrating, with neuropsychiatric involvement).

In a short-case setting, request the following.

1.   Temperature chart (fever, e.g. infection from leucopenia, steroids or cytotoxics).
2.   Blood pressure (hypertension, from renal disease or steroids).
3.   Urinalysis (blood, protein [renal disease]; glucose [steroids, or frank diabetes]).

After this, the systems involved are screened sequentially.

Skin, hair and mucous membrane

Thorough inspection of skin for rashes (including: malar rash over cheeks and nasal bridge sparing nasolabial folds, photosensitive rash, vasculitic rash, discoid lesions, Raynaud's phenomenon), digital ulcers; hair for alopecia, broken hairs; mucous membranes (oral and nasal) for ulcers or infection.

Joints and bones

Full joint screening examination (after enquiring if the child has pain anywhere; always get the patient to move her/his joints first [active range of movement] before passive [the candidate moving the joints]; if this order is forgotten, the patient could be hurt). Particularly note wrists, hands, knees and feet, as these tend to be more commonly affected. Get patient to walk normally (looking particularly for limp; avascular necrosis of the hips or knees can occur in around 10% of pSLE). Perform Trendelenberg's test to detect proximal weakness (with unilateral or bilateral hip disease, or proximal myopathy; both can occur due to steroids). Detailed examination of any involved joints is important (but be aware of time constraints).

Neurological and eyes

Screening examination for common complications.

Gait and lower limbs

Full gait examination, to detect limp (e.g. from avascular necrosis of femoral head or knee due to steroids), hemiplegia, other focal deficits, cerebellar ataxia, peripheral neuropathy, proximal myopathy (steroids, SLE per se).

Upper limbs and/or cerebellar involvement

Arms held straight out in front of body (screen for chorea, tremor, monoplegic posturing). Finger–nose test (screen for cerebellar ataxia with eyes open, and for sensory neuropathy with eyes closed).

Cranial nerves

Test extraocular movements (cranial neuropathy). If the child has focal deficits, also check visual fields (e.g. for hemianopia). Inspect for episcleritis. Ophthalmoscopy: cataracts (steroids); retinal cottonwool exudates, haemorrhages.

Cardiorespiratory

Before palpating the chest, take the pulse (e.g. tachycardia or arrhythmia with myocarditis) and count the respiratory rate. Check the blood pressure (if you have not already requested this, in short case) for narrow pulse pressure (myocarditis), or hypertension (renal involvement). Examine the praecordium (for cardiac manifestations: e.g. pericarditis, myocarditis). Examine the posterior aspect of the chest: percuss lung fields for pleural effusion; percuss over vertebrae for compression fractures (steroid side effect); auscultate lung fields (e.g. for pleuritis, pneumonitis). Examine lymph nodes (lymphadenopathy).

Abdomen

Inspect for scars (e.g. peritoneal dialysis, renal transplant, laparotomy for acute abdomen). Palpate for tenderness (serositis), hepatosplenomegaly (SLE per se), inguinal lymphadenopathy (SLE per se). Percuss for shifting dullness if there is any peripheral oedema or pleural effusion.

Diagnosis

The diagnosis of SLE is aided by the revised 1982 American College of Rheumatology (ACR) criteria. A child is said to have SLE if 4 or more of 11 selected criteria are present, either serially or simultaneously. Each criterion has a specific definition (refer to the standard texts). The 11 criteria are: malar rash, discoid rash, photosensitivity, oral ulcers, arthritis, serositis, renal disorder, neurologic disorder, haematologic disorder, immunologic disorder and antinuclear antibody.

Investigations

SLE is characterised by the production of autoantibodies directed against a wide range of proteins: histone, non-histone, RNA-binding, cytoplasmic and nuclear proteins. The following lists the antibodies and their approximate frequency in SLE (derived from adult data):

- Antinuclear antibodies (ANA): up to 100%.
- Anti-U1 RNP antibodies (an RNA-binding protein): 70–90%.
- Anti-DNA antibodies: 60–70%.
- Anti-cardiolipin (aCL) antibodies (antiphospholipid antibodies): 50%.
- Anti-Sm antibodies (another RNA-binding protein): 40–50%.
- Anti-Ro antibodies: 30–40%.
- Lupus anticoagulant (LAC) antibodies (antiphospholipid antibodies): 20%.
- Anti-La antibodies: 15–20%.
- Antiribosomal antibodies: 15%.

This list is given for completeness, and does not indicate clinical usefulness, which is covered below. The following investigations may be useful.

Simple screening tests

1. Haemoglobin (e.g. haemolytic anaemia; relative macrocytosis).
2. White cell count (e.g. leukopenia).
3. Platelet count (e.g. thrombocytopenia).
4. Antinuclear antibodies (ANA), directed against a number of autoantigens. This is one of the hallmarks of SLE. This is the best simple screening test. Be aware that persistently positive ANA in the absence of other objective evidence of rheumatic disease does not suggest a chronic rheumatic disease by itself. The vast majority of ANA positive children do not have SLE. At least 10% of the normal paediatric population are positive for ANA.
5. Inflammatory markers: ESR and CRP are useful if elevated; if normal, this does not exclude SLE.
6. Urea, creatinine, electrolytes (to assess renal function).
7. Urinalysis (for protein, blood).

More specific tests for pSLE

Blood

1. Double-stranded DNA antibodies (relatively specific to SLE; correlates with more severe systemic involvement, e.g. renal disease); DNA-Farr (radioimmunoassay); DNA-Crithidia titre (immunofluorescence). DNA binding is also useful. These are the best tests for SLE. They are also useful in monitoring progress.
2. Antibodies to extractable nuclear antigens (e.g. Ro [SSA], La [SSB], Sm, RNP). Antibodies to Ro and La are associated with neonatal lupus, and occur with increased frequency in children of SLE patients. Antibodies to Sm are very specific for patients with SLE: they are found in about two-thirds of SLE patients.
3. CH 50, C3, C4 (usually low values in active disease). C3 and C4 are useful in monitoring disease activity. Isolated deficiencies (e.g. C2) may be found.
4. Coomb's test (e.g. positive with immune-mediated anaemias).
5. Clotting profile (e.g. prolonged PTT with circulating lupus anticoagulant; paradoxically a tendency for thrombotic events).
6. Antiphospholipid antibodies (aPL): includes anticardiolipin antibody (aCL) and lupus anticoagulant (LAC). Associated with recurrent thrombo-embolic events.
7. Liver function tests (raised enzymes in salicylate hepatotoxicity or active SLE).
8. Creatine phosphokinase (myositis).

Cerebrospinal fluid

No consistent CSF abnormalities are found with neurological sequelae of SLE, although pleocytosis, elevated protein level and low glucose level may occur. CSF examination helps to exclude haemorrhage and infection, but is not part of a standard assessment of a patient with SLE.

Imaging

1. Chest X-ray (e.g. pneumonitis, myocarditis).
2. Bone X-rays (e.g. vertebral collapse).
3. Neuroimaging (all but MRI scan are research tests so far):
   a. Cranial MRI scan (e.g. localised areas of vasculitis).
   b. SPECT (single-photon-emission computerised tomography) imaging (e.g. areas of hypoperfusion; often in parietal and cerebellar lobes).

    c. NMR (nuclear magnetic resonance) spectroscopy (e.g. areas with decreased ATP [adenosine triphosphate] levels).

    d. PET (positron emission tomography) scanning (areas of hypometabolism; often in temporal and parietal lobes).

    e. Cerebral angiography is not usually performed. It is usually normal in patients with neurological or psychiatric manifestations of SLE (perhaps due to small size of vessels affected by lupus vasculopathy).

  4. Cardiac imaging: echocardiography—M-mode, two-dimensional, Doppler and/or transoesophageal (endocarditis vegetations, mural thrombi, other cardiac source for emboli).

Neurophysiological testing
  1. EEG (abnormalities may occur in children with neurologic sequelae of SLE, but are non-specific).
  2. ECG (e.g. pericarditis, arrhythmias).

Urine
A 24-hour urine collection for creatinine clearance and protein.

Other
  1. Renal biopsy is indicated if an abnormality is detected in the urinalysis. Many children with SLE will have a renal biopsy. The vast majority of children with SLE have some form of renal disease. Various forms of glomerulonephritis (GN) can occur: e.g. mesangial GN, focal and segmental proliferative GN, diffuse proliferative GN (DPGN), membranous GN, mixed patterns.
  2. Pulmonary function testing (e.g. interstitial lung disease).
  3. Neuropsychological assessment (for children with neurologic involvement; there is some evidence that this may be the best test for CNS lupus).

Management

The treatment goals are as follows:

  1. Control disease activity (prevent and suppress disease flaring) to restore health towards normal.
  2. Prevent scarring of organs (e.g. kidneys, brain).
  3. Minimise adverse drug side effects (e.g. Cushing's syndrome).

A management 'tree' for increasing severity of SLE is as follows:

  1. Non-steroidal anti-inflammatory drugs (NSAIDs).
  2. NSAIDs plus antimalarial (for joint symptoms).
  3. NSAIDs plus steroids (low dose daily).
  4. Steroids and immunosuppressives.

General measures

The role of the general paediatrician (the candidate) is as a coordinator of overall care, in conjunction with a paediatric rheumatologist and other health professionals. The candidate should ensure that the family is appropriately educated regarding SLE, its complications and treatment (and its side effects), that there are adequate contingency plans in case of intercurrent illnesses or flares in disease activity. An identification bracelet should be worn (indicating whether taking steroids), and general measures such as adequate exercise and a well-balanced diet should be encouraged.

The child should receive the normal immunisations, unless receiving cytotoxics or high-dose steroids, when live viral vaccines are avoided. Sulphonamide drugs are best avoided as children with SLE may have severe toxic reactions to them.

There may well be a number of social issues, including those specifically related to adolescence. A chronic disease conflicts with the desires for independence, peer acceptance and sexual activity, and SLE can have particularly obvious physical stigmata (e.g. malar rash). Problems to be addressed can thus include low self-esteem, poor self-image, lack of compliance and even suicidal ideation.

The issue of pregnancy is a further problem. Although the majority of patients can probably tolerate an oral contraceptive pill, this should only be prescribed with caution as the pill can induce SLE, cause hypertension, thrombosis and chronic active hepatitis. Barrier methods should be encouraged (condom or diaphragm with spermicidal foam). The risks of pregnancy (which can be particularly hazardous if renal disease is present) must be discussed with the adolescent girl. She should be aware of the following.

1. The occurrence of the 'postpartum backlash'.
2. SLE association with increased miscarriage, and neonatal lupus with congenital heart block (see later).
3. Pregnancy must be carefully planned, i.e. with blood pressure, renal disease and haematological indices under control, and is best timed when in remission, or stable for over 12 months.

Steroid usage can cause amenorrhoea, without interfering with ovulation, giving the patient a false sense of security. This may lead to unprotected intercourse and an unplanned pregnancy. Male adolescents receiving cytotoxics should be informed about the availability of sperm banks.

A key to managing an adolescent is allowing the patient to look after their own disease as much as is practicable.

Specific measures

There is some variation between different centres regarding optimal treatment, including whether to treat only clinical disease flares, or to treat serological flares (e.g. rising anti-double-stranded DNA antibodies, falling complement: decreases in C4 preceding, and decreases in C3 coinciding with, disease flares), or a balance between these options. Treatment is individualised for each patient; in selected patients, serological measurements may be useful guides to timing of treatment courses. A staging system has been developed, mirroring the example of the oncologists, by the Hospital for Special Surgery in the USA. There are 10 stages of increasing severity.

Main agents used

Corticosteroids

Most children with SLE will need steroids at some stage of their management, as most children have systemic disease. Severe systemic disease (e.g. renal involvement, haematological complications, pleuritis, pericarditis) requires steroids. Steroids will rapidly bring more minor problems (e.g. fever, arthritis and myositis) under control. For severe active disease that does not respond to high-dose steroids, high-dose intravenous pulse doses can be tried (based on anecdotal evidence, not controlled trials; also be aware that side effects have included hypertensive crises and fatal cardiac arrhythmias).

Use of short-term, high doses of steroids is more effective and causes fewer adverse effects than long-term lower doses. The side effects of steroids are well known: children generally develop Cushingoid features if they take over 20 mg prednisolone per day for over a month. A radioreceptor assay can measure steroid activity (plasma prednisolone equivalents). Catch-up growth after cessation of treatment may not be complete. Children who have had more steroids are more likely to develop more significant sepsis.

Non-steroidal anti-inflammatory drugs (NSAIDs)

If only skin or joints are affected, aspirin or other NSAIDs may control the symptoms by themselves (or in combination with hydroxychloroquine), without resorting to steroids. Problems with aspirin include the risk of salicylate hepatotoxicity (if liver enzyme levels are increased twofold or threefold and persist, aspirin should be ceased), concern regarding Reye's syndrome, and possible alteration of glomerular filtration rate (GFR). Aspirin is also contraindicated in thrombocytopenia. All NSAIDs can adversely affect the GFR, so caution or avoidance in renal disease is recommended.

Hydroxychloroquine

This may be useful for skin and joint involvement. Side effects include renal and retinal toxicities (maculopathy) and gastrointestinal symptoms. Rarely cardiomyopathy and neuromyotoxicity have been reported. Eye checks every 4–6 months are mandatory.

Cytotoxics

Methotrexate (MTX) is effective as a steroid-sparing agent in musculoskeletal disease. Low dose, once-a-week MTX is safe; folate supplementation decreases side effects. It is given orally. Side effects include oral ulcers, gastrointestinal and bone marrow toxicities. Regular blood tests are performed to detect any liver impairment or marrow involvement. Long-term studies of MTX in SLE have yet to be published.

Other cytotoxics can be useful in children with uncontrolled progressive disease, or severe steroid side effects (e.g. significant growth failure), again based largely on anecdotal evidence. Agents used include oral azathioprine (AZA) or cyclophosphamide (CPA), intravenous cyclophosphamide (IV-CPA) pulses.

Short-term effects of IV-CPA pulses include bone marrow suppression and significant hyperemesis (which can be minimised, either by giving frusemide 8–12 hours after the CPA dose, or by using ondansetron, the 5-HT$_3$ receptor antagonist). Long-term effects of IV-CPA such as risks of infertility [around 17%] and neoplasia also need consideration. More recently mycophenolate mofetil (MMF) has been used in class III and IV nephritis, and is as effective as CPA, but has fewer side effects. Cyclosporine A (CSA) can used for class V nephritis, as an alternative to AZA or MMF. A paediatric rheumatologist should decide if, when, and which cytotoxics should be used, after careful discussion of the risk/benefit profile with the family.

A major use for these agents is severe renal pSLE. These children may need prolonged treatment. The role of cytotoxics treating extra-renal disease is less clear than it is for renal disease.

Approach to treatment of specific system involvement

Life-threatening systemic disease

Pulse intravenous steroids, IV-CPA and plasmapheresis.

Kidneys

Renal involvement in SLE is as follows (simplified schema of WHO classification):

WHO class I	Normal light microscopy
WHO class II	Mesangial lupus nephritis (around 20% of cases)

WHO class III	Focal proliferative glomerulonephritis (GN) (around 20% of cases)
WHO class IV	Diffuse proliferative GN (just under 50% of cases)
WHO class V	Membranous GN (around 10% of cases)
WHO class VI	Sclerosed glomeruli

Treatment is based on renal histology. Severe renal involvement requires intensive and prolonged treatment. Steroids (high-dose oral prednisone, or pulse intravenous doses of methylprednisolone, if required) and cytotoxics as above are often needed:

- WHO class II: low-dose steroids: short course, slow taper, excellent outcome.
- WHO class III and IV: high-dose steroids, slow taper, add second agent after biopsy to confirm histology. Second agent: MMF, AZA or CPA. MMF and AZA are safer. Class IV usually responds to steroids. For active SLE complicated by class IV, intravenous (IV-) CPA may be indicated. One effective regimen used monthly IV-CPA for 7 months, then IV-CPA every 3 months for the next 30 months. Any flare-up resulted in monthly IV-CPA for another 3 months. With this treatment, many children exhibited marked improvement in their overall well-being, including a decrease in infection, cerebritis, arthritis and emergency hospitalisation. If nephrotic syndrome occurs, AZA may be useful.
- WHO class V may well respond to low-dose steroids. Some patients require prolonged steroids, then CSA, AZA or MMF. Angiotensin-converting enzyme (ACE) inhibitors are used as well to decrease proteinuria. Anticoagulation may be required, due to the risk of renal vein thrombosis, and possible pulmonary embolism.

Some children have histology that demonstrates more than one pathology type: e.g. WHO classes II, III, IV and V. Treatment is directed against the most serious (proliferative) component.

Children with significant renal disease usually manifest haematuria and proteinuria within 6 months of initial diagnosis of their SLE. Progression to chronic renal failure (CRF) is associated with class IV, persistent hypertension lasting over 4 months, abnormal urinalysis, elevated creatinine, and anaemia. If CRF and then end-stage renal disease (ESRD) supervene, dialysis may be needed while awaiting renal transplantation (RTx). Lupus can recur in transplants, but only rarely. Children who receive RTx have a better prognosis than those on dialysis (see section on RTx in Chapter 13, Nephrology). Those children with poor prognostic factors are treated aggressively, and those with ESRD have transplants as soon as possible.

Hypertension

Thiazide diuretics and beta-blockers are the first line. If there is renal disease, especially with proteinuria, an ACE inhibitor, such as captopril, is first line. Avoid drugs that can cause SLE (e.g. hydralazine, methyldopa). Second-line agents include calcium channel blockers and minoxidil. If hypertension is uncontrolled, it can aggravate vasculitis and renal disease. Hypertension will be aggravated by steroid treatment.

Cardiovascular

The most common manifestation is pericarditis with pericardial effusion. Other forms of involvement include endocarditis and myocarditis, which can be treated with steroids. Pericarditis can respond to NSAIDs alone. Valvular heart disease can occur, in association with aPL antibodies or with non-infective endocarditis. Libman-Sacks verrucous endocarditis can occur in acutely ill children with pSLE. The most commonly affected valves in order (left two, then right two): mitral, aortic, pulmonary, tricuspid. There is an inflammatory infiltrate first, then formation of nodules of fibrinoid necrosis of the supporting connective tissue of the valve. Treatment may involve high-dose steroids, plasmapheresis, cytotoxics or surgery. The main cardiovascular morbidity, however, is premature atherosclerosis. The main risk factor for this is ongoing chronic inflammation of pSLE itself. Steroids could theoretically make atherosclerosis worse. Antimalarials like hydroxychloroquine have an advantage of lipid-lowering among their many effects. Input from dieticians and physiotherapists will help avoid high blood lipid levels and obesity, and will help optimise physical exercise. In North America, the Childhood Arthritis and Rheumatology Research Alliance (CARRA) has launched the Atherosclerosis Prevention in Pediatric Lupus Erythematosis (APPLE) prospective study, assessing the role of statins in the prevention of atherosclerosis—the largest prospective study ever undertaken in pSLE.

Pulmonary
Steroids, plus antibiotics if infection is suspected. If severe pulmonary haemorrhage occurs, use pulse steroids or cytotoxics. In severely ill patients, multiple antibiotics, high-dose steroids and positive pressure ventilation may be required. Children with pSLE should have opportunistic infections excluded (such as herpes, *Pneumocystis carinii*, legionella or fungal infections) before introducing cytotoxic agents.

Neuropsychiatric SLE (NP-SLE)
In 1999, the American College of Rheumatology divided NP-SLE into 19 separate conditions. Some of the more common ones are headache, psychosis, mood disorder/depression, cognitive dysfunction, cerebrovascular disease, seizures, and movement disorders. An infrequent manifestation of NP-SLE is neuropathy (cranial [more common] and peripheral). As the area is complex, treatment decisions should involve a team including psychiatrists, psychologists, neurologists and rheumatologists. In general, high-dose steroids and cytotoxics (AZA or CPA) are used. Psychotropic drugs, antidepressants and anticonvulsants may be needed as well. Analgesia can be ineffective in lupus headache. The underlying cause for the headache must be sought and that cause treated (e.g. cerebral vein thrombosis [CVT], raised intracranial pressure from CNS infection or pseudotumour cerebri, or active CNS vasculitis). A difficulty is determining whether behavioural problems are secondary to having a chronic illness or secondary to NP-SLE. Patients can die of NP-SLE. If questioning the diagnosis, it is better to give a short increased dose of prednisolone (oral or pulse IV). If symptoms improve, this indicates NP-SLE. If symptoms worsen, question if it could be steroid psychosis or if psychiatric therapy is needed.

Joints
Sequentially: NSAIDs, hydroxychloroquine or MTX, low-dose steroids; plus physiotherapy.

Skin
Avoid sun exposure wherever possible. Appropriate clothing and use of sunscreen (with sun protection factor over 15), topical steroids for discoid lesions; oral agents (sequentially: NSAIDs, hydroxychloroquine, low-dose steroids). Raynaud's phenomenon is less common in paediatric than in adult SLE: management is by avoidance of cold exposure, appropriate clothing (e.g. insulated mittens [rather than gloves], multiple layers of clothing, hats, hand and feet warmers) to keep extremities warm, low-dose aspirin (if there is no thrombocytopenia), and, if these are inadequate, oral nifedipine or low-dose steroids, or topical nitroglycerine paste.

Neonatal lupus

Adolescent girls with pSLE contemplating having children need to be fully aware that babies of mothers with SLE can develop features of SLE. Transient features are entirely due to transplacental passage of maternal antibodies, as they resolve with clearance of the antibodies. Examples include thrombocytopenia, leukopenia, hepatosplenomegaly, myocarditis, pericarditis and the photosensitive discoid skin rash. The other group of features are permanent, their aetiology only partially explained by transplacental antibody passage. Examples include congenital complete heart block (CCHB; associated with antibodies to SSA/Ro [particularly to the 52 kD Ro polypeptide rather than the 60kD Ro] and SSB/La), endomyocardial fibroelastosis and other forms of structural heart disease. Fetuses with congestive cardiac failure, CCHB and pericardial effusions have been treated with some success by giving the mother dexamethasone.

Prognosis

Overall survival in pSLE approximates 95–100% at 5 years, and 75–85% at 10 years. Mortality rates are connected to socioeconomic status and disease activity. The most common cause of death remains infection, usually associated with the use of steroids and cytotoxic agents. Other more common causes of mortality are cerebritis, pancreatitis, pulmonary haemorrhage, renal failure and myocardial infarction. The poorest prognosis is with class VI nephritis and severe CNS involvement. After the first 2 years of disease, new organs are much less likely to become involved, with the exception of the CNS.

Short case

Joints

This is not an infrequent case. The approach given here has three basic components:

1. Thorough general inspection.
2. Systematic examination of all joints.
3. Examination for extra-articular manifestations of JCA and other diseases affecting joints, plus detection of drug side effects.

Figure 16.2 outlines the findings sought on inspection, plus those sought on assessing for extra-articular manifestations and drug side effects. A suggested order for this is: skin, hands, blood pressure, hair, eyes, mouth, neck, chest, abdomen and lower limbs neurologically, plus temperature chart, urine and stool analysis.

Examination

The examination for each joint comprises inspection, palpation, movement (active first, as passive movements may cause distress and immediate loss of rapport with patient and examiners), measurement, and finally assessment of functional ability.

A useful initial screen, on being introduced to the patient, is to ask him or her to walk a short distance (for antalgic gait), take off a jumper or shirt (for upper limb function) and then write her or his name for you (hand function).

Although, ideally, the child should be undressed down to underwear, there are many children who can become embarrassed, particularly those approaching adolescence. Showing sensitivity to the child's modesty will be well received by examiners and parents alike. If the child is younger and does not get embarrassed, then watching the

Figure 16.2 Joint disease: extra-articular manifestations and drug side effects

1. Introduce self

2. General inspection
Well or unwell
Age and sex (e.g. JIA under 5 years usually female; JAS usually older male)
Cushingoid (steroids)
Obvious skin rash (e.g. SLE, psoriasis, HSP—see below)
Parameters
- Height (short from steroids)
- Weight (obese from steroids; thin from hypercatabolism)

3. Skin
Butterfly malar erythema (SLE)
Heliotrope eyelids (dermatomyositis)
Purpura (HSP, PAN)
Psoriasis
Vasculitic rash (e.g. SLE dermatomyositis, MCTD)
Maculopapular rash (systemic JIA)
Subcutaneous calcification (dermatomyositis)
Nodules (JIA, JRA)
Tight skin (scleroderma, MCTD)
Pigmentation and depigmentation (sclerodermal)

4. Upper limbs
Hands
- Raynaud's phenomenon (SLE, MCTD, scleroderma, PAN)
Nails
- Subungual haemorrhage (SLE)
- Pitting (psoriasis)
- Nail bed telangiectasia (dermatomyositis)
Palms
- Anaemia (systemic JIA, SLE, drug side effects)
- Flexor tendon nodules (scleroderma)
- Flexor tenosynovitis (JIA)
Elbow region
- Epitrochlear nodes (systemic JIA, SLE, MCTD)
- Nodules over elbows (scleroderma)
- Rheumatoid nodules (JRA)
Blood pressure
- Elevated (e.g. HSP, steroids, PAN, SLE with nephropathy); if elevated, make a point of requesting urinalysis now
Axillae
- Lymphadenopathy (e.g. systemic JIA, SLE, Kawasaki's, MCTD)

5. Head and neck
Hair: alopecia (SLE)
Eyes: signs of seronegative JIA
- Iridocyclitis (usually need slit lamp to see)
- Band keratopathy
- Posterior synechiae (pupil shape change)
- Glaucoma
Eyes: signs of seropositive JIA
- Dry eyes (Sjögren's)
- Scleritis, episcleritis
- Scleromalacia perforans
Eyes: less specific signs
- Conjunctival pallor
- Cataract (JIA, steroids or chloroquine)

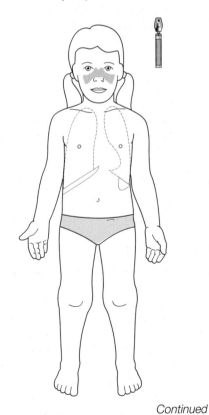

Continued

Figure 16.2 *(Continued)*

- Retinopathy (chloroquine)

Parotid: swelling (Sjögren's, MCTD)

Mouth
  - Inflamed mucous membrane (e.g. SLE, dermatomyositis)
  - Petechiae, purpura (e.g. SLE)
  - Ulcers (e.g. SLE, gold penicillamine)

Dysphonia (dermatomyositis)

Hoarseness (cricoarytenoid arthritis, laryngeal nodules with JRA)

Neck: lymphadenopathy (e.g. SLE, Kawasaki's, systemic JIA, MCTD)

6. Chest

Auscultate praecordium
  - Cardiomegaly (myocarditis with SLE or systemic JIA)
  - Pericarditis (SLE, systemic JIA)
  - Murmurs (SLE, SBE, rheumatic fever)

Auscultate lung fields

Pleuritis (systemic JIA, SLE)

Pleural effusion (SLE)

7. Abdomen

Tenderness (e.g. serositis with SLE, enteritis with IBD)

Hepatosplenomegaly (systemic JIA, SLE, MCTD)

Perianal disease (IBD)

Buttock rash (HSP)

8. Gait and lower limbs

Gait examination: screen for neurological signs (atlanto-axial subluxation with JIA; very uncommon)

Squat: proximal weakness (steroids, dermatomyositis, JA)

Lower limbs (neurologically)
  - Power (myopathy)
  - Reflexes (atlanto-axial subluxation)

9. Other

Temperature chart
  - Quotidian fever (systemic JIA)

Urinalysis
  - Proteinuria (penicillamine, amyloid, SLE, HSP, PAN, scleroderma)
  - Haematuria (SLE, HSP, PAN, naproxen)

Stool analysis
  - Blood (HSP, IBD, dermatomyositis)

HSP = Henoch-Schönlein purpura; IBD = inflammatory bowel disease; JAS = juvenile ankylosing spondylitis; JIA = juvenile idiopathic arthritis; JRA = juvenile rheumatoid arthritis (seropositive for IgM rheumatoid factor); MCTD = mixed connective tissue disease; PAN = polyarteritis nodosa; SBE = subacute bacterial endocarditis; SLE = systemic lupus erythematosus.

child undress may yield valuable clues regarding involved joints. A good position for the examination is confrontation (i.e. positioning yourself immediately opposite the child), so that you can demonstrate clearly what movements are required of the child, while using your own joints as reminders regarding normal range of movement.

The following is the sequence suggested for whichever joints are being examined. Inspect distribution of joint involvement (symmetry), note swelling, loss of normal contours, angulation, deformity, redness, muscle wasting. Next, feel the joint and peri-articular areas for tenderness, warmth, effusion, 'boggy' swelling (thickened synovium and fluid), enthesitis, contractures. Range of movement (ROM) is then examined, active movement first. Only test passive movement if active movement does not produce the full range, remembering to watch the child's face to detect any discomfort. The angle from neutral should be described (as mentioned, use your own joints as reference). Finally, function (which correlates with strength) should be tested.

A suggested order for a systematic examination of all the joints is as follows: hands, wrists, elbows, shoulders, temporomandibular joints, cervical spine, lumbar spine, hips, knees, ankles, feet (i.e. hand to head, and head to toe). A good initial position is with the child sitting in a chair, or on the side of a bed, with the hands resting on the thighs.

Specific joints

Note that the normal range of movement (ROM) at each joint is given in degrees, in parentheses.

Upper limbs
Hands and wrists

Look at the dorsum first: note any skin rash or muscle wasting. Methodically inspect the wrist, followed by the metacarpophalangeal (MCP) joints, proximal and distal inter-phalangeal (PIP and DIP) joints, and the nails. Then have the child turn the hands over and look at the palmar aspect in the same systematic fashion. Next, palpate each joint for tenderness and effusion. Flex and extend the child's fingers while palpating over the flexor tendon sheaths (for synovitis). Check ROM (active, then passive). Normal ROM values (in degrees) are as follows:

1. Wrist: flexion (80°), extension (70°), radial deviation (20°), ulnar deviation (30°).
2. MCP joints: flexion (90°), extension (30°).
3. PIP joints: flexion (100°).
4. DIP joints: flexion (90°), extension (10°).

Note that the thumb can flex to contact the tips of the other digits, and abduct from the index finger (50°).

Now, test the hands with respect to function. Simple tests include: grip strength; write with pencil; use knife, fork, spoon, cup; hold toothbrush; undo and do up buttons; turn key.

Elbows

Inspection and palpation are followed by checking ROM.

1. Flexion (135°).
2. Extension (0–10°).
3. Supination (90°).
4. Pronation (90°).

Note that supination and pronation should be tested with the elbow flexed (if possible) at 90°; a pencil held in the closed hand (making a fist) can simplify assessment of the position.

Functionally, check if the child can turn an (imaginary) doorknob, comb hair, hang out the washing, answer a telephone.

Shoulders

After inspection and palpation, test ROM. It is usually easier to test younger children with play-like activities that produce the required movements that are to be tested. For example, you can tell the child:

1. 'Put your hands above your head' (demonstrate to the child): tests flexion (90°) and abduction (180°).
2. 'Give yourself a hug' (demonstrate): tests adduction (45°).
3. 'Scratch your back' (demonstrate): tests external rotation (45°).
4. 'Hide your hands behind your back' (demonstrate): tests internal rotation (55°) and extension (45°).

Functionally, several of the tests overlap with those for the elbows: comb hair, take off clothing, hang out washing, scratch near bottom (toileting function), use a telephone.

Jaw and neck

Look at the jaw (especially for acquired micrognathia) and feel for crepitus over the temporomandibular joints (TMJs), with the child opening and closing the mouth. Note the interdental distance and show to the examiners (if relevant) that you are aware of the importance of measuring this to follow progress of TMJ disease.

Next examine the cervical spine: inspect, palpate and check ROM.

1. Flexion: chin touches chest (45°).
2. Extension: head touches back (50°).
3. Rotation: turning chin to be in line with shoulder (80°).
4. Lateral flexion: ear to shoulder (40°).

Thoracolumbar spine

Inspect with the child standing, and then bending forward (for scoliosis or kyphosis). Palpate for tenderness. Check ROM.

1. Flexion: should be able to touch toes.
2. Extension: arching back (30° at lumbar area).
3. Lateral bending (50° to each side).
4. Lateral rotation: most easily checked with child sitting (30° to each side).

To assess function, the child can be asked to pick an object up from the floor and to put on socks and shoes.

Schöber's test measuring lumbar spine flexion can be performed; in older children, more than 4 cm of movement should be measured.

Sacroiliac joints

Palpate for tenderness over the joint, plus press the pelvis from each side towards the midline to assess for pain (pelvic work test).

Lower limbs

Examination can commence with watching the child walk (for antalgic gait), stand on each leg (for Trendelenburg's sign) and squat (for proximal weakness or instability).

Hips

Inspect the resting position (e.g. external rotation with active synovitis) and muscle bulk. Palpate for tenderness. Measure the true leg length (anterior superior iliac spine [ASIS] to medial malleolus of ankle). With the child lying on the back, check ROM. Flexion (120°) can be checked first with active movement. Then perform Thomas' test for fixed flexion deformity. Then test:

1. Internal rotation (35°).
2. External rotation (45°).
   (Both of these are tested with hips at 90° flexion.)
3. Abduction (50°).
4. Adduction (30°).

Note that the pelvis should be stabilised (by one hand fixing the ASIS) when checking all these movements. Then, have the child turn over onto the abdomen and test extension (30°). Gait examination serves as a functional assessment.

Knees

Inspect, noting quadriceps bulk. Feel for temperature and tenderness, and palpate entheses (at 10, 2 and 6 o'clock positions on the patella) and any synovial thickening or effusion. Test for the 'bulge sign' by 'milking' any joint fluid down the lateral aspect of the joint (look for bulge medially) and then stroking upwards on the medial aspect, moving any fluid present into the suprapatellar bursa. Next, test for a patella tap. It may be appropriate to measure the muscle bulk of the thighs and calves if there appears to be a difference between the two sides: measure the circumference at a fixed distance (e.g. 5–10 cm) above the superior aspect of the patella, and at 10 cm below the tibial tuberosity. Also, if not already done, measure leg length.

Next, check the ROM: flexion (135°); extension (up to 10°).

Finally, check for knee stability. This should not be done if the knee is acutely inflamed, as the test will be painful and unnecessary. Test for anteroposterior movement with the knee joint flexed, with position fixed by sitting on the child's foot. Check for the 'drawer sign' signifying damage to the cruciate ligaments (anterior cruciate is ruptured if there is movement when the leg is pulled forwards; posterior cruciate is ruptured if movement when the leg is pushed backwards). Also check for lateral mobility with the knee fully extended, for lesions of the medial or lateral ligament; normally there is no lateral movement.

Ankles and feet

Inspect for swelling, and loss of definition of the Achilles tendon (synovial thickening at the ankle joint). Palpate the ankle joint, entheses (Achilles insertion into calcaneus, metatarsal heads, plantar fascia insertion to calcaneus). Check the ROM.

1. Ankle: plantar flexion (50°); extension (dorsiflexion) (20°).
2. Subtalar joint: inversion (5°); eversion (5°).
3. Midtarsal (talonavicular and calcaneocuboid) joints: abduction (10°); adduction (20°). The midtarsal joint is tested by stabilising the calcaneus with one hand and moving the forefoot with the other.
4. First metatarsophalangeal joint: plantar flexion (45°); extension (dorsiflexion)(70°). Note any crepitus or pain on moving the first metatarsal joint (may be selectively involved in spondyloarthropathies).

At the completion of the examination, summarise the positive findings, noting the number of joints involved, symmetry (symmetrical like juvenile rheumatoid arthritis, or asymmetrical like psoriatic arthritis), activity of disease (active with pain, redness), the functional severity (most important) and the differential diagnosis.

Suggested reading

The preparation for any examination, particularly the Fellowship Examination, requires the candidate to read widely. Reading allows the candidate to strengthen weaker areas and consolidate stronger ones.

The following list is incomplete, but contains textbooks that the author and his colleagues have found useful in preparing for the Fellowship Examination. It is not expected that the prospective candidate will read all these tomes, but reference to at least some of them will be necessary.

The edition or year of publication of the medical texts is not listed, as the candidate should seek the latest edition.

Medical books

Ansell BM. Rheumatic disorders in childhood. London: Butterworths. *Very good short textbook covering paediatric rheumatology.*

Behrman KE, Vaughan III VC (eds). Nelson textbook of pediatrics. Philadelphia: Saunders. *Standard text.*

Campbell I, Munro J. MacLeod's clinical examination. Edinburgh: Churchill Livingstone. *Standard text.*

Dale M, Moore P, Rang H, Ritter J. Pharmacology. Edinburgh: Churchill Livingstone. *Good coverage of pharmacology.*

Ekert H (ed). Clinical paediatric haematology and oncology. Oxford: Blackwell. *Very good short textbook on haematology and oncology in children.*

Fink BW. Congenital heart disease. Chicago: Year Book Medical Publishers. *Excellent little tome on the diagnosis of congenital heart disease, especially the 'pearls' at the end of each chapter. However, management of conditions is not addressed.*

Forfar JO, Arneil GC (eds). Textbook of paediatrics. Edinburgh: Churchill Livingstone. *Good text for clinical paediatrics, but coverage of basic sciences is insufficient for the written component of the Fellowship Examination.*

Ganong WF. Review of medical physiology. Connecticut: Appleton & Lange. *Good coverage of medical physiology.*

Guyton A, Hall J. Textbook of medical physiology. Philadelphia: Saunders. *Comprehensive coverage of medical physiology.*

Habel A. Aids to paediatrics. Edinburgh: Churchill Livingstone. *A little book with useful lists.*

Hardman J, Limbard L. Goodman and Gilman's the pharmacological basis of therapeutics. New York: McGraw-Hill. *Standard tome.*

Illingworth RS. The development of the infant and young child. Edinburgh: Churchill Livingstone. *Unless you have children of your own, this book should be read to learn about normal development and its assessment.*

Jordan SC, Scott O. Heart disease in paediatrics. London: Butterworths. *Probably the best short textbook on paediatric cardiology.*

Katzung B. Basic and clinical pharmacology. New York: McGraw-Hill. *Concise coverage of pharmacology.*

Kempe CH, Silver HK, O'Brien D, Fulginiti VA (eds). Current pediatric diagnosis and treatment. Connecticut: Appleton & Lange. *Concise text, but by itself is insufficient for the Fellowship Examination.*

Macleod J, Munro J. Clinical examination. Edinburgh: Churchill Livingstone. *Though intended for undergraduates, this book is valuable for postgraduate students revising their clinical examination methods (i.e. elicitation and interpretation of signs and symptoms).*

Menkes JH. Textbook of child neurology. Philadelphia: Lea & Febiger. *Excellent textbook on paediatric neurology.*

Oski F et al. Principles and practice of pediatrics. Philadelphia: JB Lippincott Company. *Standard text in the class of Nelson and Rudolph.*

Phelan PD, Landau LI, Olinsky A. Respiratory illness in children. Oxford: Blackwell. *Written by eminent Australian authors and **the** best short textbook on paediatric respiratory medicine.*

Robinson MJ (ed). Practical paediatrics. Edinburgh: Churchill Livingstone. *Australian text aimed at undergraduates. However, many of the contributors are examiners for the Fellowship Examinations, and it does contain some highly relevant material for the postgraduate student.*

Rudolph C, Rudolph A, Hostetter M, Lister G, Siegel N. Rudolph's pediatrics. New York: McGraw-Hill. *Standard text.*

Talley NJ, O'Connor S. Clinical examination. Sydney: Elsevier. *Comprehensive text on how to examine a patient.*

Walker-Smith JA, Hamilton JR, Walker WA. Practical paediatric gastroenterology. London: Butterworths. *Very good short textbook on paediatric gastroenterology.*

Weiner HL, Bresnan MJ, Levitt LP. Pediatric neurology for the house officer. Baltimore: Williams & Wilkins. *If you haven't already got a copy, then acquire one. It is inexpensive and packed with information on paediatric neurology.*

Wilson JD, Petersdorf RG, Adams RD et al (eds). Harrison's principles of internal medicine. New York: McGraw-Hill. *Yes, Harrison's! Excellent for preparation for Paper A (Principles of Medicine and Basic Sciences Applicable to Paediatrics).*

Medical journals

Paediatric journals

Since candidates are expected to know of the advances in physiology, biochemistry and pharmacology applicable to paediatrics, studying the review articles, leading articles, annotations and editorial comments in appropriate medical journals is essential in the candidate's preparation for the Fellowship Examination. The following journals are recommended:

Pediatrics
Journal of Pediatrics
Archives of Disease in Childhood
Journal of Paediatrics and Child Health
The Pediatric Clinics of North America

Internal medicine journals

Internal medicine journals that are recommended are:

Australian and New Zealand Journal of Medicine
The Lancet
The British Medical Journal
The New England Journal of Medicine
The American Journal of Medicine
Annals of Internal Medicine
Medicine International

Other paediatric journals

Other paediatric journals well worth looking at, especially in preparation for the clinical examination, are:

Pediatrics in Review
Current Problems in Pediatrics
Pediatric Annals

Audiotapes

If you learn and retain facts better by listening, then the Audio–Digest Pediatrics, and Audio–Digest Internal Medicine series (produced by the AudioDigest Foundation, a subsidiary of the California Medical Association) are certainly worth considering. These tapes also come with a summary sheet with questions, and a list of journal references. The Royal Australasian College of Physicians also produces audiotapes and CDs from recent meetings that are very useful. The author listened to audiotapes driving to and from work, and found this an efficient way of using what would otherwise be wasted time.

Medical examinations

Sewell Ivor A. Passing the FRCS. London: Butterworths, 1989. *A book that provided inspiration for some parts of this book. Although it deals with passing the FRCS, many of the ideas can be adapted for passing the FRACP.*

Pappworth MH. Passing medical examinations. London: Butterworths, 1975. *Well-known book, which gives practical advice regarding written and oral examinations and is worth looking at.*

Motivation and achievement

Finally, if you are interested in reading more about motivation and the psychology of achievement, then the following books are recommended.

Andreas S, Faulkner C. NLP, the new technology of achievement. London: Nicholas Brealey Publishing Limited, 1996.

Buzan T, Keene R. Buzan's book of genius. London: Stanley Paul, 1994.

De Bono E. Tactics. London: Collins, 1986.

Dibley J. Let's get motivated. Sydney: Corporate Publishing, 1986.

Feist E. The winning edge. Sydney: Golden Spurs Publications, 1989.

Garfield C. Peak performers. London: Hutchinson Business, 1986.

Gelb MJ. How to think like Leonardo Da Vinci: seven steps to genius every day. London: Dell, 2000.

Hopkins T. The official guide to success. New York: Champion Press, 1982.

Kriegel R, Kriegel MH. The C zone. New York: Doubleday, 1984.

Loehr JE. Toughness training for life. New York: Plume/Penguin Books, 1993.

Loehr JE. Stress for success. New York: Time Books, 1998.

Maltz M. Psycho-cybernetics. New York: Pocket Books, 1960.

Orlick T. In pursuit of excellence: how to win in sport and life through mental training, 3rd edn. Windsor, Ontario: Human Kinetics, 2000.

Orlick T. Embracing Your Potential. Windsor, Ontario: Human Kinetics, 1998.

Pease A. Body language. Sydney: Camel Publishing Company, 1981.

Robbins A. Unlimited power. New York: Simon & Schuster, 1986.

Robbins A. Awaken the giant within. New York: Simon & Schuster, 1991.

Rohn EJ. The five major pieces to the life puzzle. Prima, 1992.

Siegel PC. Supercharged! Dallas: Taylor Publishing Company, 1991.

Waitley D. The psychology of winning. New York: Berkley, 1979.

Waitley D. Seeds of greatness. New York: Simon & Schuster, 1983.

Waitley D. The new dynamics of winning. London: Nicholas Brealey Publishing Limited, 1994.

Webster R. Winning ways. Sydney: Fontana, 1984.

Ziglar Z. Over the top. Thomas Nelson, 1997

Ziglar Z. Success for dummies. IDG Books, 1998.

Index